Antenna and Sensor Technologies in Modern Medical Applications

Antenna and Sensor Technologies in Modern Medical Applications

Edited by
Yahya Rahmat-Samii
University of California
Los Angeles, CA 90095, USA

Erdem Topsakal
Virginia Commonwealth University
Richmond, VA 23224, USA

IEEE PRESS
WILEY

This edition first published 2021

Registered Office
John Wiley & Sons, Inc., 111 River Street, Hoboken, NJ 07030, USA

Editorial Office
111 River Street, Hoboken, NJ 07030, USA

For details of our global editorial offices, customer services, and more information about Wiley products visit us at www.wiley.com.

Wiley also publishes its books in a variety of electronic formats and by print-on-demand. Some content that appears in standard print versions of this book may not be available in other formats.

Library of Congress Cataloging-in-Publication Data

Names: Rahmat-Samii, Yahya, editor. | Topsakal, Erdem, editor.
Title: Antenna and sensor technologies in modern medical applications / edited by Yahya Rahmat-Samii, University of California, Los Angeles, CA, USA, Erdem Topsakal, Virginia Commonwealth University, Richmond, VA, US.
Description: Hoboken, NJ, USA : Wiley-IEEE, 2021. | Includes bibliographical references and index.
Identifiers: LCCN 2020026616 (print) | LCCN 2020026617 (ebook) | ISBN 9781119683308 (cloth) | ISBN 9781119683278 (adobe pdf) | ISBN 9781119683292 (epub)
Subjects: LCSH: Biosensors. | Wearable technology–Antennas. | Medical electronics. | Body area networks (Electronics) | Patient monitoring–Equipment and supplies.
Classification: LCC R857.B54 A58 2021 (print) | LCC R857.B54 (ebook) | DDC 610.285–dc23
LC record available at https://lccn.loc.gov/2020026616
LC ebook record available at https://lccn.loc.gov/2020026617

Cover Design: Wiley
Cover Images: Human anatomy © SciePro/Shutterstock, Abstractpurple and pink polygonal vector background © Tuomas Lehtinen/Getty Images, Connected World © Adyna/Getty Images

Set in 10/12pt Warnock by SPi Global, Chennai, India

MIX
Paper from responsible sources
FSC
www.fsc.org
FSC® C013604

COVID-19 has forever changed the face of humanity. We dedicate this book to all medical personnel, scientists, and frontline helpers who have tirelessly attempted to save humanity. It is our hope that this book constructs a stronger bridge between engineering and medicine.

Contents

List of Contributors

AJIBAYO O. ADEYEYE,
School of Electrical and Computer Engineering, Georgia Institute of Technology, Atlanta, GA, USA

GEORGE ALEXOPOULOS,
Department of Electrical Engineering, Stanford University, Stanford, CA, USA

NADER BEHDAD,
Department of Electrical and Computer Engineering, University of Wisconsin, Madison, WI, USA

SHUBHENDU BHARDWAJ,
Department of Electrical and Computer Engineering, Florida International University, Miami, FL, USA

TONI BJÖRNINEN,
Faculty of Medicine and Health Technology, Tampere University, Tampere, Finland

YEPU CUI,
School of Electrical and Computer Engineering, Georgia Institute of Technology, Atlanta, GA, USA

ALINE EID,
School of Electrical and Computer Engineering, Georgia Institute of Technology, Atlanta, GA, USA

SAM EMAMINEJAD,
Interconnected and Integrated Bioelectronics Lab (I^2BL), Department of Electrical and Computer Engineering, University of California, Los Angeles, CA, USA

ALEXEY ERMAKOV,
I.M. Sechenov First Moscow State Medical University, Moscow, Russia

RYAN B. GREEN,
Department of Electrical and Computer Engineering, Mississippi State University, Mississippi State, MS, USA

YONGXIN GUO,
Department of Electrical and Computer Engineering, National University of Singapore, Singapore

SUSAN C. HAGNESS,
Department of Electrical and Computer Engineering, University of Wisconsin, Madison, WI, USA

YANG HAO,
School of Electronic Engineering and Computer Science, Queen Mary University of London, London, UK

JIMMY G.D. HESTER,
School of Electrical and Computer Engineering, Georgia Institute of Technology, Atlanta, GA, USA

KOICHI ITO,
Center for Frontier Medical Engineering, Chiba University, Chiba, Japan

SIAVASH KANANIAN,
Department of Electrical Engineering, Stanford University, Stanford, CA, USA

AHSAN NOOR KHAN,
School of Electronic Engineering and Computer Science, Queen Mary University of London, London, UK

ASIMINA KIOURTI,
ElectroScience Laboratory, Department of Electrical and Computer Engineering, The Ohio State University, Columbus, OH, USA

GIANLUCA LAZZI,
Department of Electrical and Computer Engineering, University of Southern California, Los Angeles, CA, USA

PONGPHAN LEELATIEN,
Department of Electrical and Computer Engineering, Faculty of Engineering, Thammasat University, Pathumthani, Thailand

SHUYU LIN,
Interconnected and Integrated Bioelectronics Lab (I^2BL), Department of Electrical and Computer Engineering, University of California, Los Angeles, CA, USA

TONG-HONG LIN,
School of Electrical and Computer Engineering, Georgia Institute of Technology, Atlanta, GA, USA

HUNG LUYEN,
Department of Electrical and Computer Engineering, University of Wisconsin, Madison, WI, USA

SHUBIN MA,
Faculty of Medicine and Health Technology, Tampere University, Tampere, Finland

MANJUNATH MACHNOOR,
Department of Electrical and Computer Engineering, University of Southern California, Los Angeles, CA, USA

VIGYANSHU MISHRA,
ElectroScience Laboratory, Department of Electrical and Computer Engineering, The Ohio State University, Columbus, OH, USA

YAHYA MOHTASHAMI,
Department of Electrical and Computer Engineering, University of California, Santa Barbara, CA, USA

SYED A. NAUROZE,
School of Electrical and Computer Engineering, Georgia Institute of Technology, Atlanta, GA, USA

ADA POON,
Department of Electrical Engineering, Stanford University, Stanford, CA, USA

RAJ PULUGURTHA,
Department of Electrical and Computer Engineering, Florida International University, Miami, FL, USA

YAHYA RAHMAT-SAMII,
Department of Electrical and Computer Engineering, University of California at Los Angeles, Los Angeles, CA, USA

KAZUYUKI SAITO,
Center for Frontier Medical Engineering, Chiba University, Chiba, Japan

JAMES F. SAWICKI,
Direct Imaging Center of Excellence, Boston Scientific Corporation, Marlborough, MA, USA

GUOLIANG SHAO,
Department of Electrical and Computer Engineering, National University of Singapore, Singapore

RYAN SHIH,
Interconnected and Integrated Bioelectronics Lab (I^2BL), Department of Electrical and Computer Engineering, University of California, Los Angeles, CA, USA

MARY V. SMITH,
VERO Biotech, LLC, Atlanta, GA

LINGNAN SONG,
Department of Electrical and Computer Engineering, University of California, Los Angeles, CA, USA

GLEB SUKHORUKOV,
School of Engineering and Material Science, Queen Mary University of London, London, UK

LAURI SYDÄNHEIMO,
Faculty of Medicine and Health Technology, Tampere University, Tampere, Finland

BIJAN K. TEHRANI,
School of Electrical and Computer Engineering, Georgia Institute of Technology, Atlanta, GA, USA

MANOS M. TENTZERIS,
School of Electrical and Computer Engineering, Georgia Institute of Technology, Atlanta, GA, USA

ERDEM TOPSAKAL,
Department of Electrical and Computer Engineering, Virginia Commonwealth University, Richmond, VA, USA

LEENA UKKONEN,
Faculty of Medicine and Health Technology, Tampere University, Tampere, Finland

JOHN L. VOLAKIS,
Department of Electrical and Computer Engineering, Florida International University, Miami, FL, USA

BO WANG,
Interconnected and Integrated Bioelectronics Lab (I^2BL), Department of Electrical and Computer Engineering, University of California, Los Angeles, CA, USA

DAISONG ZHANG,
Department of Electrical and Computer Engineering, University of California at Los Angeles, Los Angeles, CA, USA

1

Introduction

We strongly believe that when history is looked back a century from now, the twenty-first century will be considered the dawn of convergence of engineering technology and its infusion into modern medical practice. Among various important engineering disciplines, customized antennas and sensors are going to be evaluated as paramount components. This book is the first of its kind in paving the way for helping engineering researchers, medical practitioners, educators, and students to appreciate the importance of the fundamentals and the state-of-the-art developments in antennas and sensors in medical applications. Every chapter of this book is written by well-known researchers in the field, and we, as the editors, thank them for their timely contributions and high-quality production.

This book consists of 14 chapters and an Appendix. We would like to encourage the readers who are not familiar with the topics of this book to first review the appendix, providing a representative literature review of antennas and sensors for medical applications, and then learn about the details of diversified subjects in various chapters of the book. Figure 1.1 shows a pictorial demonstration of chapters and their body-related significance. As can be seen from this figure, the book covers many applications that are relevant to multiple regions of the body varying from implantable to wearable devices.

In Chapter 2, the authors initially introduce some key features of magnetic resonance imaging (MRI). MRI has evolved into one of the most powerful imaging methods since its inception in the 1970s. Clinically, it is regarded as the ultimate imaging method for a wide variety of diseases. MRI has the most distinct feature of effectively differentiating between soft tissues both qualitatively and quantitatively, compared with other imaging methods. The powerful capability of MRI fundamentally depends on the image quality which is characterized by image signal-to-noise ratio (SNR). The ultraflexible 3 Tesla (3T) MRI radio-frequency (RF) coil array presented in Chapter 2 manages to increase the MRI image SNR by a noticeable amount in targeted regions. It utilizes high conductivity and flexible electrotextile designs to closely wrap around the regions of interest. The ultraflexible RF coil array for the neck region

Antenna and Sensor Technologies in Modern Medical Applications,
First Edition. Edited by Yahya Rahmat-Samii and Erdem Topsakal.

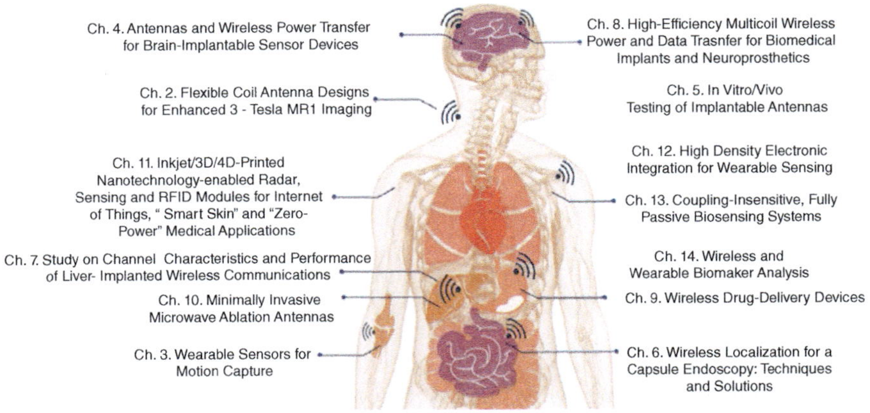

Figure 1.1 A pictorial demonstration of various chapters and their body-related significance.

is designed to significantly enhance the image quality of carotid artery, which is a key area for stroke being a leading cause of death in the United States. The chapter focuses on the challenges, requirements, and strategies for the design of ultraflexible electrotextile MRI RF coils. This is done by the characterization of several flexible materials and the development of roadmap to guide the design procedure. As a representative example, the neck RF coil array system is designed, prototyped, measured, and integrated into the MRI platform to perform phantom scanning and system-level characterizations. In order to confirm the effectiveness of the ultraflexible RF coil array, cadaver measurements are also conducted to demonstrate the enhanced MRI image quality. The flexible RF coil can be applied to other body areas such as wrist and knee and could potentially be extended to applications such as MRI-guided surgeries.

Chapter 3 will focus on human motion capture. Capturing motion as an intricate part of human existence can lead to tremendous improvements in our quality of life. Example applications range from health care to sports, gaming, training, and beyond. But what technologies are currently available for motion capture, and what are the associated benefits and limitations? What are the current research trends in the area? And what lies in the future? This chapter is dedicated to answering all these questions. Focus is primarily on wearable sensors for motion capture as attributed to their seamless nature and future potential. Examples include inertial measurement units, bending/deformation sensors, time-of-flight sensors, and received signal strength-based sensors. Nevertheless, several technologies that are relevant to motion capture are also discussed in this chapter (motion capture labs, electromagnetic-based sensors, magnetic motion capture, imaging methods, and more), indicating where wearable sensors find their place. Knowledge of the various available technologies, along with their advantages and limitations, provides guidelines to choose one or combination thereof per application requirements. Although the discussion in this chapter is geared toward human motion, nothing stops the reported technologies from capturing motion of any other moving beings (i.e. animals) and beyond (such as structures).

In Chapter 4, the authors outline the approaches to the electromagnetic optimization of antennas and wireless links for battery-free brain implantable devices where the wireless powering and data transmission are based on inductive coupling, far-field radiation, and platforms integrating both approaches. Progress in brain research has brought compelling approaches to managing neurological illnesses. In neurorehabilitation, bidirectional neural interfaces enabling mind control of prosthetics and assistive devices as well as versatile research platform. Deep brain stimulators have become available for the management of movement disorders, such as tremors in Parkinson's disease. In the experimental neuroscience, optogenetic methods are providing a powerful new research tool, and advances have been made toward optoelectronics methods for potential local cerebral tissue oxygenation monitoring. Apart from neurophysiological applications, new methods for the long-term monitoring of intracranial pressure (ICP) hold the potential for home monitoring for improving the safety of people predisposed to the elevation of ICP and becoming a research tool for cerebrospinal fluid research. In terms of medical technology, the enabling parts for all systems involving long-term brain implantable devices are antennas that must be small and flexible enough to be fully cranially concealed and function based on energy transmitted from an external source rather than relying on batteries. This technology will empower novel means to research in in vivo animal models and long-term implantable medical devices for humans alike. To demonstrate the research, the authors present three different wireless systems developed in our research group that rely on each of the three electromagnetic modalities.

Chapter 5 discusses tools and techniques for in vitro and in vivo testing of implantable antennas as well as the common materials used for fabricating them. Various factors go into the design of an implantable antenna, including the materials for the substrate and radiating element. Historically used materials for antennas (e.g. copper) can pose health effects with prolonged exposure, requiring either biocompatible encapsulation or biocompatible conductors. After the antenna is designed to operate within the body, bench testing is required to validate performance. One method is to test the antenna using ex vivo tissues; however, this method requires immediate testing of the antenna due to the decay of the tissues after extraction. As a result, this chapter presents the mixture and characterization of in vitro tissue-mimicking gels (for the dielectric properties of human skin, adipose, and muscle) to validate antenna performance. Tissue-mimicking gels have shelf, if refrigerated, life greater than three weeks. While in vitro testing provides a necessary step in the development of implantable antennas, it still remains lacking in some aspects. For example, tissue-mimicking gels only replicate the dielectric properties of human tissues, not the thermal or biological properties. In vivo, Latin for "in the living," testing is the next step after in vitro. A major difference between the two testing methodologies is the presence of an immune system, which seeks to encapsulate and expel foreign objects. Due to this, in vivo measurements are necessary for long-term studies for antenna performance and biological effects. Additionally, in vivo models are dynamic systems where dielectric properties can change with temperature and time. This chapter explores how the dielectric properties of three animal models change with temperature and age, and how implanted antennas are tested in vivo.

In Chapter 6, the focus is ingestible devices. The localization of ingestible (swallowable) biomedical devices is crucial for accurate diagnosis. Over the past decades, a variety of approaches have been proposed to increase the localization accuracy. However, localizing ingestible devices is very challenging by considering the complexity of the in-body environment. Focusing on wireless capsule endoscopy, various solutions for localizing ingestible devices are analyzed in this chapter. Firstly, the chapter starts from introducing various localization approaches, and performance comparisons are made in terms of positioning accuracy, system complexity, power consumption, and device size. Secondly, considering the unique requirements of wireless capsule endoscopy, the magnetic localization method is focused and analyzed. The research progress of the magnetic localization for wireless capsule endoscopy is introduced and analyzed. Two types of magnetic localization, static magnetic localization and inductive magnetic localization, are introduced in detail from the basic theory to the possible solutions for realization challenges. Thirdly, the performance comparison of each solution with different system configurations and position retrieval algorithms are discussed. An innovative method of combining the wireless charging and wireless positioning within the same hardware system is also introduced. The chapter concludes at the end that the selection of different solutions depends on different application scenarios.

Chapter 7 addresses the UWB channel characteristics for an application of transplanted liver monitoring after an operation using liver-implanted wireless devices in an example case scenario. The chapter presents quantitative information such as path loss models under various circumstances for two typical in-body communication scenarios, i.e. in-body to on-body and in-body to off-body, as well as assesses the system performance. Initially, simplified human equivalent multilayer semisolid phantoms were used in measurement and simulation studies. To gain the first approximation on liver-implanted channel characteristics and to confirm the feasibility of the wireless communications from the liver to the skin surface, channel characteristics in the frequency domain are discussed and analyzed. Thereafter, numerical studies on the characteristics of liver-implanted channel were done by means of simulations using digital human models. Accordingly, path loss data and path loss models are presented and discussed. Consequently, the evaluations of system performance are carried out by the approach of link budget analysis. The chapter also deals with the possibility of UWB communications for the liver-implanted channel considering the safety standard based on the FCC regulations of UWB transmission power and ICNIRP guidelines. These results demonstrated that it is feasible to achieve a reliable wireless communication link using UWB technology for the liver-implanted scenarios. The results can be used as guidelines for the analysis of in-body applications using wireless implant devices such as medical telemetry for not only the liver area but also other implant locations.

In Chapter 8, the authors describe an in-depth operation of inductive power transfer for the biomedical applications. The inductive wireless power transfer technique has been successfully applied to transmit power to commercial prosthetic systems, such as the artificial retina. The chapter describes the existing conventional techniques and focuses mainly on the multicoil approach to the system design. The chapter covers the design procedure of the traditional two- and three-coil systems and the advantages offered by the proposed circuit techniques. The reflected impedance concepts explain the operation and simplify the system design parameters such as efficiency, power delivery, and power factor of a wireless power and data transmission system. The proposed coil design technique enhances efficiency and operational tolerance and simplifies the coil design and data transmission capabilities.

Chapter 9 is devoted to precision wireless drug delivery. Precision medicine technology is an emerging facet of therapeutic regimen that is conducive for treating chronic ailments due to its ability to concentrate high drug potency at the targeted tumors as compared to traditional systemic administration. The recent developments in microchip and micromachined technology have leveraged the fabrication of miniaturized transdermal and implantable devices for delivering drugs in the human body. Profuse research is still in progress to devise an optimum drug delivery device that can be wirelessly triggered for releasing encapsulated drug compounds according to prescribed dosing schedule. Apart from drug release actuation, wireless systems of a drug delivery device are useful for wireless power transfer and data telemetry with an external interrogator. In addition, an embedded wireless system of a device provides patients and physicians the control on release mechanism for personalized drug delivery. This chapter recapitulates the state-of-the-art multifaceted drug delivery devices and discusses about imperative requirements for manifesting wireless power transfer, data telemetry, and user control on the release mechanism. The main emphasis is on wirelessly controlled devices that exhibit release mechanisms that can triggered wirelessly, enabling drug spouting from the device toward the targeted organ location in the human body. We have also delineated a wide ensemble of integrated components for drug delivery applications, such as microchips, microvalves, micropumps, and microrobots. Apart from integrated components, a wide assortment of nanomaterials-mediated drug delivery and the fabrication of RF-sensitive microcontainers have also been discussed in this chapter.

In Chapter 10, the authors discuss the recent advances in minimally invasive microwave ablation antenna designs. The emphasis is placed on a growing trend in miniaturization of interstitial antennas to reduce the invasiveness and increase the flexibility of the treatment. The effort toward length reduction for interstitial antennas is highlighted by a number of studies investigating the use of higher frequency microwaves for tissue ablation. Additionally, various novel microwave ablation antenna designs with reduced-diameter topologies, compared to conventional coax-fed, balun-equipped antennas, are presented. These innovative designs are classified into two general groups: one group represents solutions that target less-invasive implementations of coaxial baluns, and the other involves novel balun-free antenna designs that provide localized heating patterns. Moreover, this chapter also presents the authors' own effort in developing flexible antennas as well as directional-heating antennas, which are aimed at increasing the flexibility and customization of microwave ablation treatment.

Chapter 11 is devoted to additive manufacturing and 3D printing technologies for the state-of-the-art health wearables. The use of additive manufacturing technologies, such as the commonly encountered inkjet-printing technology or the popular forms of 3D printing approaches, enable, through their versatility, a surprising wealth of solutions to the limitations of the state-of-the-art health wearables. The innovations presented in this chapter, centered on the peculiar needs of wearable health devices, tackle their requirements from a variety of perspectives. New strategies enabling the powering of printed wearable systems using both legacy RF wireless networks and upcoming 5G mm-wave implementations are presented. Next are reported innovations required for the additive integration of the mature state-of-the-art RF and mm-wave chips into both partially printed flexible boards and compact fully 3D-printed mm-wave multilayer modules. Wearable systems also require—due to their need for energy autonomy and ultralow power consumption in an on-body setting—the development of new communications and shape-shifting electromagnetic shielding schemes. Finally, ultra-low-cost printed architectures are reported, which are capable of sensitizing printed devices to a near-infinite variety of gaseous and dissolved or dispersed (through microfluidic means) chemical analytes. The projects and results succinctly presented in this chapter set the foundation for the emergence of a greatly anticipated and socially transformative offering of smart wearable health devices that will be able to monitor (among others) their users' very movements, heart beats, physical and mental activities, and chemical and physical exposure and stress levels.

In Chapter 12, the authors present electronic textile technologies. Integration of computing, sensing, and communication electronics into clothing is an imminent trend. The need for such systems is supported by the desire toward ubiquitous electronic connectedness, medical and commercial sensing, hand-free communications, and for supporting 5G and future 6G campaigns. A cost-effective method to integrate RF circuits and sensors into clothing is that of embroidery conductive threads onto clothing. In this paper, we discuss developments of the past decade in using conductive embroidery (e-fiber) technology with a focus on RF and sensing applications. Several examples of antenna interfaces, RF power harvesting, and sensor integration using electronic textiles (e-textiles) are discussed. Challenges related to integration of hard components and conductivity limitations are discussed, and solutions are presented. The chapter also discusses techniques for high-density integration of RF-communication chains, antennas on flexible substrate, and interconnects for laminates and flex substrates. Pertinent packaging techniques are also presented for e-textile electronics, and conclusions are drawn.

Chapter 13 provides an overview of the existing readout techniques for fully passive sensors, discussing various aspects of such sensing systems for practical uses. The goal is to introduce the requirements of a complete and practical sensing system. The focus of the chapter is, therefore, on the near-field (NF) interrogation techniques that allow for a low power consumption and low complexity reader solution compared to far-field techniques. The main challenge in NF techniques has traditionally been reader complexity and dependence of the measurement on the coupling strength (or the readout distance). The chapter starts with the introduction of two general reader excitation techniques, forced and self-oscillating, where the first relies on either bulky and expensive lab equipment, such as a vector network analyzer (VNA), or complex and power-hungry custom circuitry. The latter, however, provides more simplified and easier sensor measurement. Next, two general approaches based on either a nonresonant or a resonant reader are introduced, analyzed, and compared. In each case, relevant works are listed, and the advantages and disadvantages of each technique are discussed; it will be shown that some of these techniques possess the tremendous advantage of coupling-independent operation. The chapter concludes that resonant, self-oscillating reader systems with multiple resonators provide a higher measurement sensitivity, enabling interrogation of smaller sensors, at the cost of higher mismatch sensitivity and implementation complexity.

In Chapter 14, the authors focus on wireless wearable biomarkers. Recent advances in wearable sensors have created unprecedented opportunities for addressing grand societal health-care challenges by enabling physiological monitoring at the point of person. Toward providing a complete view of individuals' health status, the measurement of chemical signals (e.g. endogenous biomarker molecules and xenobiotics) is necessary, which in turn requires the development of wearable chemical sensing technologies to analyze noninvasively retrievable biofluids (e.g. sweat and saliva) and to seamlessly process and relay the harvested information. The establishment of such technologies allows for reducing the chemical signal sampling interval from months and years (e.g. those obtained in the annual checkup) to minutes and hours. The subsequent enhancement—by several orders of magnitude—in the chemical signal acquisition frequency will create new dimensions (e.g. diurnal and longitudinal tracking of biomarker profiles) for personal health monitoring, presenting a high potential to transform the current practices in health care and to catalyze the transition from traditional reactive medicine to preventive and personalized medicine.

Appendix A presents a representative literature review on the development of antenna and sensor technologies for modern medical applications. Advanced wireless diagnosis and treatment technologies have recently and rapidly moved from largely a vision of science fiction to a widely spreading consumer and clinical products. Large numbers of valuable research and literature are published in different journals and conferences each year on the development of antennas and sensors targeting various health-care applications. The antenna-related topics are broken into three subsections according to their specific applications and operating mechanisms: medical imaging antennas and coils, miniature telemetry antennas for implantable and ingestible devices, and microwave ablation antennas for localized tumor treatments. The discussion on sensor technologies consists of mechanical, electrical, and chemical sensing devices, with emphasis on the advanced wearable and noninvasive sensing technologies that have been developed in the past decade. In each of the subtopics, the authors present the basic system-level principles, followed by the state-of-the-art developments with representative literature in each field. This review serves not only as an introductory platform for new researchers to the fields but also benefits experienced engineers and researchers by broadening their views about various related topics.

The editors would like to sincerely thank the chapter contributors for their timely preparation of their chapters and for graciously supporting us throughout the development of this book. We also like to acknowledge the support of many colleagues who have collaborated with us throughout the years on the research and developments of many topics discussed in this book. Wiley staff were most collaborative in helping us to publish an outstanding and unique book that we strongly believe will serve the scientific, engineering, medical, and educational communities for many years to come. Particularly, Sarah Lemore, Grace Paulin, Muralidharan Mourthy, Brett Kurzman, and Victoria Bradsha from Wiley are acknowledged for their constructive interactions with us to complete the book.

Yahya Rahmat-Samii
Erdem Topsakal
December, 2020

2

Ultraflexible Electrotextile Magnetic Resonance Imaging (MRI) Radio-Frequency Coils

Daisong Zhang and Yahya Rahmat-Samii

Department of Electrical and Computer Engineering, University of California at Los Angeles, Los Angeles, CA, USA

2.1 Introduction to MRI and the Basic Antenna Considerations

The primary purpose of this section is to provide a brief overview and background of MRI for the interested readers. For a more complete description, the reader is referred to [1, 2]. An overview of electromagnetics in MRI is given in [3], and it is discussed in more detail in [4]. The MRI introduction and basics for antenna design is also summarized in [5].

Magnetic resonance imaging(MRI) was developed in the 1970s, and the widespread clinical use of MRI started in the 1980s. In 2000, more than 20,000 MRI scanners were available worldwide, and more than 70 million magnetic resonance (MR) scans were performed every year [1]. Today, the number of MRI scanners has increased to 50,000 [6]. It is one of the most powerful and favorable imaging modalities for a few reasons. First, MR provides excellent differentiation between soft tissues and is quantitative. These unique features distinguish MRI from other imaging methods and leave much room for researchers and doctors to explore its potential. Active research areas such as perfusion, diffusion, and functional MRI are based on MRI's capability of giving access to biophysical and biochemical tissue properties. Second, MR is versatile: it is capable of imaging any arbitrary scan plane or 3D volume. This feature makes it applicable to large range of anatomical structures throughout the body. Last, MRI is noninvasive, and it does not use ionizing radiation. This is critical in the clinical applications and has a rising awareness as MRI progresses toward a more frequent imaging modality. This is also the reason that the ergonomic ultraflexible MRI radio-frequency (RF) coils become more essential candidates for next-generation MRI scanners.

Antenna and Sensor Technologies in Modern Medical Applications,
First Edition. Edited by Yahya Rahmat-Samii and Erdem Topsakal.

Modern MRI has been maturing rapidly over the years and has become a very powerful and comprehensive capability. Some cases are listed here as examples to show its capabilities in different applications. Carotid artery is one of the leading causes of stroke and thus plays a vital role in stroke prevention and treatment. Specific types of high-risk types of carotid artery plaques can be identified using multiple quantitative parameters overlaid with 3D images, with the help of specifically designed algorithm (sequence used to control the magnetic field variations) [7]. The most recent studies are focused on preventing the use of contrast agent for this application. For carotid artery area where signal-to-noise ratio (SNR) requirement is high, ultraflexible RF coil could efficiently reduce the imaging time and improve the image quality. Another example is the use of MRI to help place needle during motion using hydrostatic actuators [8]. MRI is not limited to disease diagnosis and treatment but is also used in surgeries. For these applications, ultraflexible RF coil can also greatly enhance image quality in combination with other techniques, given limited physical space.

MRI stems from the application of nuclear magnetic resonance (NMR) to radiological imaging. The adjective magnetic refers to the use of an assortment of magnetic fields, and resonance refers to the need to match the (radio) frequency of an oscillating magnetic field to the precessional frequency of the spin of a certain nucleus (hence the nuclear) of interest [1]. The NMR rises from the phenomenon called Zeeman splitting. Certain atomic nuclei assume one of two states when placed in a magnetic field, one is high energy state, and the other low energy state. When the outside field increases, the energy split between the two different states increases accordingly. The number of nuclei with higher energy state is slightly ($\sim 1/10^6$ for ^{1}H) less than that with the lower energy state (such as ^{1}H, ^{13}C, and ^{31}P nucleus), making it possible for the MRI. The detection of the magnetic signal stems from the lower energy state absorbing externally exerted photon and releasing photon after leaving the thermal equilibrium state [3].

A rigorous and accurate description of the basic MR physics requires quantum mechanics; however, in most cases, a classical treatment amply describes the macroscopic behavior. Atoms with an odd number of protons or neutrons possess a nuclear spin angular momentum and therefore exhibit the NMR phenomenon. Qualitatively, these nuclei can be visualized as spinning charged spheres that give rise to a small magnetic moment. We often refer to these MR-relevant nuclei as simply spins. Hydrogen with a single proton is the most abundant (the body consists largely of H_2O), the most sensitive, and by far the most studied in biomedical MRI. The angular frequency of the electromagnetic fields ω_r is given by the Larmor Equation (2.1)

$$\omega_r = \gamma B_0 \tag{2.1}$$

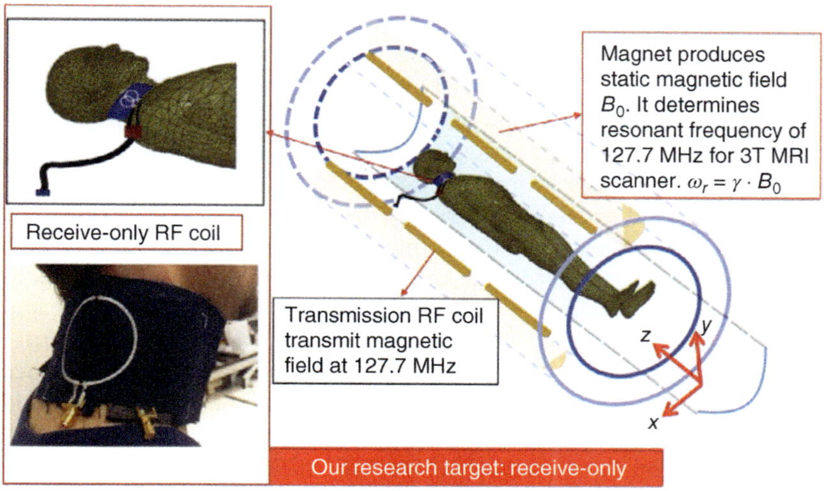

Figure 2.1 3T MRI scanner. After patients lie on top of the MRI bench, the technician puts RF coils around the patient's neck. Uncomfortable RF coils use heavy and rigid material around the neck. Patients move due to low comfort level. This may lead to low image quality and increase clinic time. Ultraflexible RF coil solves that problem. The MRI scanner cutaway exhibits (1) the main magnet that produces and receives the B_0 field in the *z*-direction, (2) the radio-frequency coil that produces the B_1 field in the *xy*-plane typically, and (3) the gradient coils to encode the spatial information [5]. (*Source*: Zhang, D. and Rahmat-Samii, Y., 2019. © IEEE.)

where B_0 denotes the strength of the static magnetic field, and γ is known as the gyromagnetic ratio. For protons, $\gamma/2\pi = 42.58$ MHz per Tesla. The nature of MR is based on the interaction of the spins with three types of magnetic fields: (i) main field B_0, (ii) RF field B_1, and (iii) linear gradient fields G. An MRI scanner is shown in Figure 2.1. The MRI scanner cutaway exhibits (i) the main magnet that produces B_0 field in z-direction, (ii) the RF coil that produces B_1 field in xy-plane typically, and (iii) the gradient coils that add incremental difference in the strength of the B_0 along the z-direction, with linear dependence on the x, y, or z directions, to encode the spatial information into the signal received.

When the B_0 is applied to the human body, the hydrogen nucleus begins to precess along the z-direction in the lab frame. In other words, the magnetization vector (M) points toward the z-direction. After the B_1 field is applied, the magnetization vector is rotated from the z-direction to the xy-plane in the rotating frame (the frame of reference that rotates with Larmor frequency). However, after the application of the B_1 field, the M is gradually relaxed to its equilibrium position along the z-direction. During this process, magnetic flux changes caused by the precessing spins induce voltage changes in receiver coils. The receiver RF coils at this point are used to detect the RF magnetic signals. These magnetic signals are subsequently transformed into anatomic images. The gradient coils are critical in making this transformation step possible by encoding the spatial information into the data acquisition process. Detailed encoding process requires an understanding of the MR pulse sequence design, where the application time point, duration, and waveform of the transmitted B_1 field, gradient field, and received B_1 field are carefully designed. The basic steps involve the use of B_1 and gradient fields to excite a specific imaging plane, then read out by the receiver coils, and repeat the process to get the data in different locations in the k-space (2-D Fourier transform spatial frequency domain). The image in the spatial domain is obtained using Fourier transform from the data in the k-space. More details on the pulse sequence design and MR imaging from the signal processing perspective can be found in [1, 2].

RF coils excite and receive magnetic signals in MRI scanners. The transmission RF coils require uniform magnetic field distribution in the area of interest and are usually embedded in the MRI scanners. In this chapter, we discuss receive-only RF coils, more specifically, the surface coils used to receive signals. Modern MRI scanners extensively use the surface coils for areas throughout the body to improve image quality. Surface coils are localized coils that are coupled to a limited region of the body at a time. Although they may operate as transmit/receive coils, they are often used in receive mode only, owing to their highly nonuniform B_1 distribution. They are appropriate for imaging superficial anatomical structures such as eyes, spine, extremities, and carotid arteries. Compared to using a head coil or body coil (in many cases birdcage coil is used) as the receiver coil, surface coils achieve a better SNR in superficial regions because of a higher image-volume to noise-volume ratio. However, simple single-element surface coils are less suitable for imaging deep-lying structures because of the falloff of sensitivity with depth. For a circular surface coil with radius a, situated at $x = 0$, the B_1 sensitivity at $x = a$ along the main axis falls off by a factor of 0.35 relative to its sensitivity at $x = 0$ as observed in Equation (2.2) [2].

$$B_1(x, a) \propto \frac{a^2}{(a^2 + x^2)^{\frac{3}{2}}} \tag{2.2}$$

A detailed discussion on the surface coil technology is given by Bendall [9]. While a single surface coil provides higher SNR in a localized region, surface coil arrays are commonly used because they extend the available field of view (FOV) while retaining the high SNR advantages [10]. Coil arrays are also useful for scan acceleration. Simplistically, imaging with each coil in the array requires fewer phase encodes because of the smaller FOV seen by the coil. The full-FOV image can be pieced together through appropriate processing of the outputs from the individual coils in the array.

It is discussed above that the SNR advantage of the surface coil array makes it the dominant type of RF-receiving coil. It is therefore important to characterize how the RF coils affect the SNR of an image. The performance of a coil can be predicted using Equation (2.3), where SNR_0 is the total available (or intrinsic) SNR described in [11]. Q_{loaded} and $Q_{unloaded}$ will be discussed in more detail in Section 2.4.1.

$$SNR = SNR_0 \sqrt{1 - \frac{Q_{loaded}}{Q_{unloaded}}} \tag{2.3}$$

The noise of the RF coil arrays come from two sources: the human body and the imperfect conductivity of the material used. The respective losses from these two sources vary with different coil diameters and frequencies as shown in [12]. The parameter of interest is the ratio of the unloaded over the loaded quality factor. A quick rule of thumb for an estimate is whether the Q ratio is over 5. When the quality factors ratio is 5, the $SNR = 0.9\ SNR_0$. In practice, it is usually time consuming and inaccurate to measure the loaded quality factor. In [12], a practical method is introduced to quickly measure the loaded and unloaded quality factors ratio without directly measuring the loaded quality factor.

2.2 Motivations, Challenges, and Strategies for MRI RF Coil Design

The previous section provided a brief overview of MRI in general, and in this section MRI RF coil design motivations, challenges, and strategies will be discussed.

2.2.1 Design Motivations and Challenges for MRI RF Coils

RF coil is a key component of the MRI, serving as the signal generation and reception device in MRI scanners. As mentioned previously, this chapter discusses solely receive-only RF coils. The SNR of the image is the key to any image modality including MRI. This is a hybrid of both hardware and algorithm improvement. Hardware upgrades lay the foundation and provide the platform for sequence optimizations. The current state-of-art hardware incorporates many technological breakthroughs in the past few years, including the better imaging analysis and processing capability, higher intensity, and homogeneity magnet and RF coils for specific areas. These breakthroughs render advanced imaging methods, such as 3D fast imaging and parallel imaging sequence techniques. As a result, the diagnosis and treatment capabilities toward cardiovascular diseases and strokes are improved. The receive-only RF coils fall into two categories: surface coil and birdcage coil. Birdcage coil has the advantage of higher homogeneity through the image space and is a good candidate for head coils [13]. It is widely used in research and clinical settings. Surface coils are more widely used in areas where surface SNR is of paramount importance, which generally cover all the body anatomies from neck to toe.

Here, we provide a design example of receive-only RF coil for stroke prevention using ultraflexible material to improve the image quality. The design requirements and principles can readily be applied to other receive-only RF surface coils and will be pointed out wherever necessary.

In the United States, stroke occurs around every 40 s, and there are deaths due to stroke every 4 min. Stroke is the no. 4 cause of death in the United States, killing nearly 130,000 people a year (128,978), that is, one in every 20 deaths based on the data in 2009 [14]. Among these stroke cases, one out of four is related to carotid artery diseases [15]. Carotid arteries are two major arteries near neck, as shown in Figure 2.2a. Pieces of plaque can break free, travel to the brain, and block blood vessels in the brain, neck, and face as shown in Figure 2.2a. Patients with substantial carotid narrowing are at large risk for a major stroke; however, the degree of stenosis alone is a relatively poor prediction of neurological events [16]. The clinical standard for measuring disease severity is the overall luminal stenosis, which is not enough for accurate prediction. The carotid artery provides an excellent location for imaging arterial plaques and the study of disease progression [16] involving more detailed artery information including plaque composition and microstructure. MRI of the carotid arteries are not only critical clinically but also important for the research of the “vulnerable plaque” mechanisms. As a result, a reliable in vivo image method monitoring the components of the plaques is needed. The RF coil is the fundamental limiting factor for a high-performance image that provides both high SNR high resolution and additional information about the plaque [17].

RF coils are integral part of the MRI scanners for transmission and reception of RF magnetic signals. When the imaging area is not the entire human body, surface RF coils are preferably used due to its advantageous SNR. They spatially reject noise from parts of the human body that are not imaged and as a result inherently have higher SNR than whole body coils. Current RF coils, however, have the disadvantage of not being comfortable to wear. Due to the comparatively long imaging time needed for MRI than other imaging modalities, this disadvantage may consequently lead to other problems such as repetitive imaging trials and MRI image motion artifact. Additionally, the high curvature of the neck area makes it hard to place the RF coils near it. Clinically used coils are either low in SNR (made with rigid material) or very uncomfortable to wear

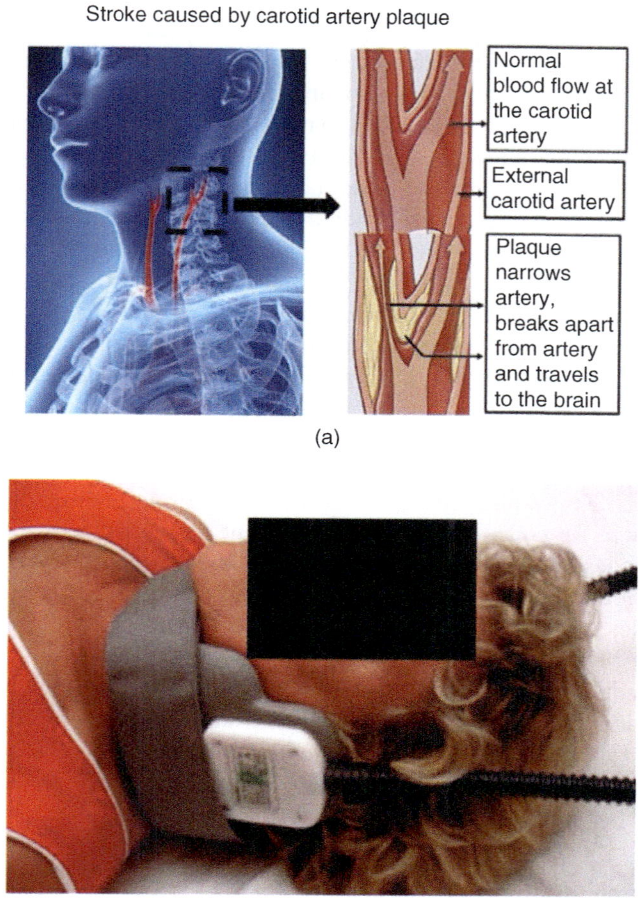

Figure 2.2 (a) Carotid arteries are two major arteries near the neck. Pieces of plaque narrow the artery, reduce the blood flow, break free, travel to the brain, and block blood vessels that supply blood to the brain. (b) Regular neck RF coils giving the patient uncomfortable experience while being scanned [5]. (*Source*: Zhang, D. and Rahmat-Samii, Y., 2019. © IEEE.)

with small SNR benefit, as shown in Figure 2.2b. As a result, flexible MRI RF coils are desired.

Flexible RF coils not only are more ergonomic but also bring another chance to increase SNR, which is a fundamental limiting factor of MRI image quality. The SNR of surface RF coils is very sensitive to the placement of the coil relative to the tissue for imaging. When the coil is placed near the tissue, an increase in signal sensitivity is expected. The noises in MRI come from two different sources: human tissue and coils along with its relevant circuitry. For most clinical applications of RF surface coils, noises from human tissue are much larger or at least comparable to those from coils and circuitry. This observation brings an opportunity to the various materials to be used in flexible MRI RF coils. A slight increase in losses by coils and circuitry is offset by the advantage of ergonomic consideration and potentially higher SNR of flexible RF surface coils. Flexible MRI RF coils were studied using screen printing in [18], ink-jet printing in [19], and copper braid in [20]. The substrate of the first two methods has limited flexibility compared with normal clothes. Additionally, the second method is limited by the layer thickness of the conductor it can print. As a result, its conductivity is limited at interested frequencies. The third method uses meandered copper braid and as a result may be worn out over the time. In this chapter, electrotextiles are explored and used as an alternative method to build flexible MRI RF coils. Electrotextiles have the advantages of being highly conductive, as flexible as normal cloth, and also enduring over the time.

Several challenges need to be overcome in designing high-quality electrotextile flexible RF coils. First of all, the current literature lacks a systematic approach to design MRI RF electrotextile RF coils. Secondly, the combined subtleness of the electrotextiles and the high accuracy requirement for the resonant tuning makes it difficult to get high SNR in the specified 127.7 MHz near human body for 3T MRI scanners. Thirdly, the trade-off between the coverage area and the single-coil SNR performance requires the use of RF coil array. Some specific difficulties are involved in the design of RF coil array system. They include the minimization of the mutual coupling between different coil elements, the integration of the coil elements into the multilayer coil array, and the system integration between the RF coils and the MRI scanner.

2.2.2 Design Strategies and Roadmap of MRI RF Coils

The design strategies for RF coil in general and the proposed systematic design roadmap are introduced in this section. In order to design MRI RF coils, the design goal needs to be specified. More specifically, the targeted anatomy and the type of scanner used need to be specified. The targeted anatomy determines the image depth and coverage, and the scanner type determines the resonant frequency. As discussed in Section 2.1, the magnetic field decreases as depth (the distance between coil center and the point of interest) increases. In general, coils with larger diameter are more suitable for deeper anatomies. Smaller coils, however, are more sensitive near the surface. In order to cover more area, larger number of coils are needed for smaller coils. As a result, the trade-offs between using larger or smaller coils include signal sensitivity in different depth, signal homogeneity between surface and deep tissues, coverage area, design complexity, and associated cost. After the goal is specified, the single-coil size, the number of coils elements, and the resonant frequency are determined. It is of paramount importance that each of the coil elements is designed at the specified frequency, given the size. Their relative positions need to be optimized for minimal mutual coupling. In general, $S_{21} < -15\,\text{dB}$ is regarded acceptable. Here, S_{21} denotes the transmission coefficient from port 1 to port 2 when all other ports are terminated in matched loads for an N port network. A detailed explanation can be found in [21]. The RF coil design needs to be verified in the MRI system by evaluating the SNR of the final image after it is integrated with preamplifiers and MRI scanner. According to the design goal, cadaver or human trials are essential to deliver a system-level solution.

In our work, systematic steps are proposed to explore the potential of electrotextiles for MRI RF coils. We start with (i) the design and analysis of RF coils using rigid materials, proceed to (ii) the single-coil element with electrotextiles, and finally come to (iii) the multilayer RF coil array using electrotextiles and resonant at exactly 127.7 MHz near the human neck. The overview and illustrative figure of the RF coil array by electrotextiles is shown in Figure 2.3. The highly flexible RF coils gently wrap around the patient's neck. It is noted that the RF coil elements are overlapped without touching each other with the multilayer structure. Two elements of the RF coils are needed to cover a large imaging area around the neck. The two elements are optimally overlapped to minimize the mutual coupling between the two elements. As mentioned previously, the roadmap of the RF coil array system design is divided into three steps as shown in Figure 2.3: in step 1, the coil elements using normal lithography etching methods are designed and serve as a reference for later prototypes; in step 2,

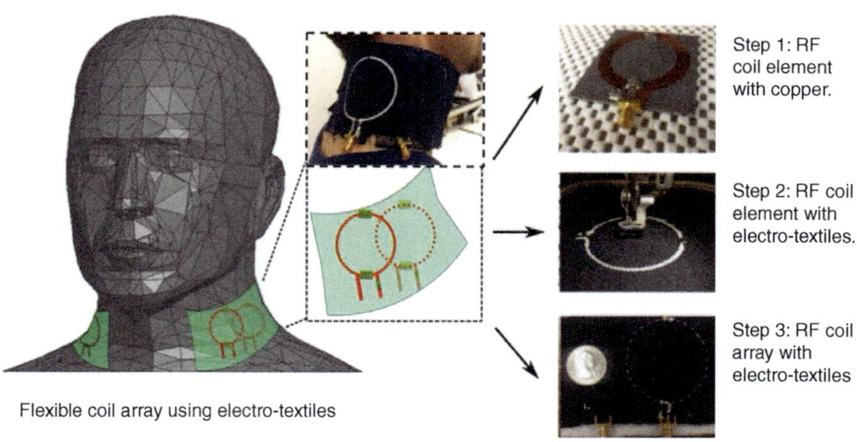

Figure 2.3 An illustrative figure of the RF coil array by electrotextiles that gently wraps around the patient's neck. The RF coil elements are overlapped without touching each other. Two coil elements are positioned in the front and back of the supporting layer. The roadmap to design RF coil array system using electrotextiles is shown on the right starting from the coil element using copper, textile element using electrotextiles, and finally coil array using electrotextiles [5]. (*Source*: Zhang, D. and Rahmat-Samii, Y., 2019. © IEEE.)

the electrotextiles are used to design the RF coil element; and in step 3, the coil array with the electrotextiles is designed, prototyped, and measured. It should be pointed out that the RF coils in the figure use conductive threads. Our research is not limited to using conductive threads but also conductive cloth, and it turns out that the cloth has a distinctive advantage of easier for integration.

2.3 Selection, Fabrication, and Characterization of Electrotextiles for RF Coils

This section discusses electrotextile candidates for high-performance MRI RF coils to pave the way for the next section of RF coil design. The use of appropriate electrotextile and integrating it into the RF coil design is the key and major challenge to achieve its high performance and to realize ergonomic benefit.

2.3.1 Selection and Fabrication of Flexible Material Candidate

The major criteria for an appropriate electrotextile for RF coil design are high electrical conductivity, nonmagnetic, and high flexibility. Besides that, other benefits such as robustness, easy to be fabricated, lightweight, and low cost are also essential. Considering all the above factors, electrotextile threads and electrotextile cloth made of silver and copper are the potential candidates for the ultraflexible RF coil.

Electrotextile threads used for the MRI RF coil arrays are the metal-coated textiles to achieve a balance between conductivity, tensile strength (improved robustness and easy to fabricate), and flexibility. All the conductive materials to be discussed in this section are either silver or copper to achieve nonmagnetic characteristic. An illustrative micro- and macroscale images of electrotextile from [22] are shown in Figure 2.4a. Two kinds of electrotextiles tested include Shieldex 110f34 dtex 2-ply HC found in and Liberator 40. Shieldex thread is created from two strands of raw yarn initially used in [23] for UHF RFID. Two of its major advantages are the appropriate diameter and flexibility. It has the diameter of 0.2 mm, which is very similar to the standard cotton-based threads used for embroidery machines. Because of the fact that the core of the thread is Nylon, the flexibility of the thread is close to standard nylon-based threads, making it suitable for embroidery machine integration. Despite the diameter and the flexibility advantage, the major disadvantage is the conductivity. The high and varied DC linear resistivity of $500\,\Omega\,m^{-1} \pm 100\ \ \Omega\,m^{-1}$ leads to difficulty in impedance matching and resonant tuning, as well as the quality factor performances. Low DC conductivity implies inferior performance in RF frequencies around 127 MHz for 3 Tesla (3T) scanners. The high variation of the DC conductivity makes it difficult to streamline the design process and involves lengthy trial-and-error process. The MRI scanner RF signal

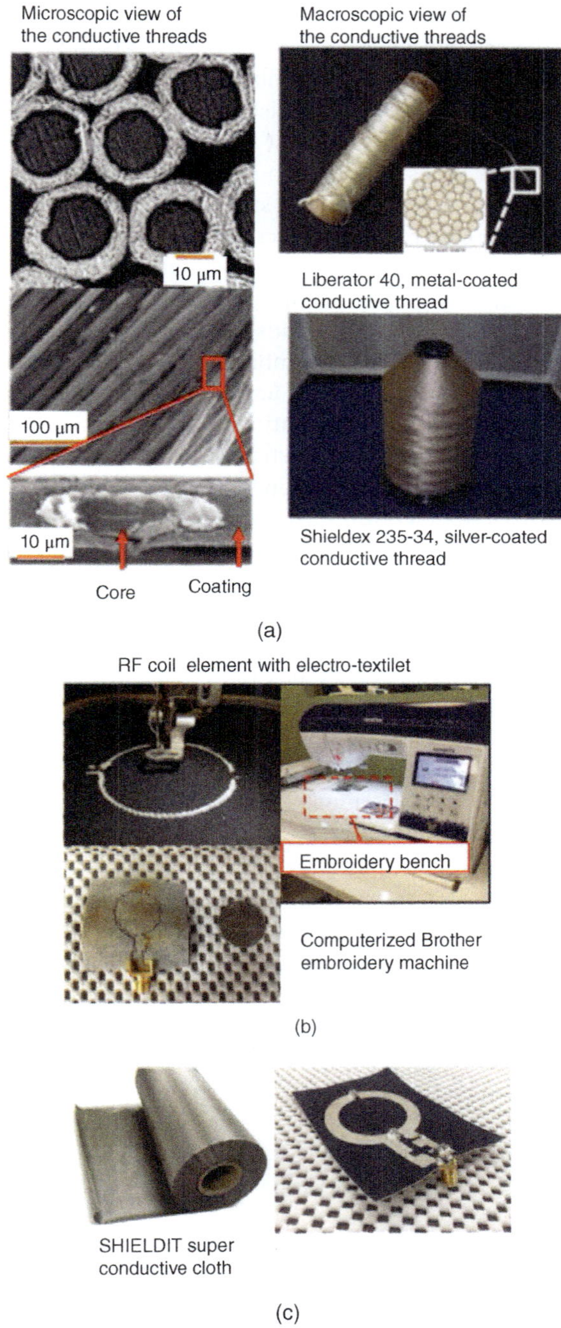

Figure 2.4 (a) Illustrative micro- and macroscale images of electrotextile from [20]. Liberator 40 and Shieldex are both electrotextiles. Liberator 40 is used to construct single-element coils due to its excellent performance in conductivity and tensile strength. (b) Front and back sides of the fabricated RF coil using electrotextiles and the embroidery machine Brother NQ1400. (c) Electrotextile cloth SHIELDIT Super (on the left) and the fabricated RF coil element (on the right) with this material [5]. (*Source*: Zhang, D. and Rahmat-Samii, Y., 2019. © IEEE.)

bandwidth is on the order of tens of kHz. A small change in conductivity leads to huge change in impedance matching.

The second type of electrotextile used is the Liberator 40, made of 40 filaments of Kururay Vectran fiber coated with 3 μm silver or copper layers used in [23, 24]. Its DC linear resistivity is $3\,\Omega\,\text{m}^{-1}$ with diameter of around 0.5 mm. The polymer-based Vectran fiber has a large tensile strength of 3 GPa, more than four times the strength of Nylon. Although its flexibility is not as high as the Shieldex, its high tensile strength makes it less vulnerable to be broken than the other electrotextiles. Vectran fiber has the necessary characteristics of high conductivity, flexibility, and being nonmagnetic, while having a decent balance in other factors. The major disadvantage is its diameter is a bit larger than the normal Nylon-based threads, and the flexibility is a bit different from other threads. As a result, the embroidery machine Brother NQ1400 in Figure 2.4b needs detailed calibration for smooth stitching. If the failure rate is not well controlled, both the fabrication time and cost surge. It should be noted that the coil element made with electrotextile threads to be discussed in the next section is shown in Figure 2.4b along with the embroidery machine used to fabricate the pattern on cotton substrate. The C_r and C_{m} in the figure are the capacitors used for tuning and matching.

The electrotextile cloth SHIELDIT Super shown in Figure 2.4c satisfies all the necessary requirements. Additionally, it is acceptable in all other factors mentioned at the beginning of the section. Compared with the electrotextile threads, cloth category has the major advantage of easier to be fabricated. Unlike the thread category, no embroidery machine is needed. As a result, the process is not very sensitive to the factors such as the thread diameter, flexibility, and tensile strength. A computerized cutting machine is used to cut and form the pattern on conductive cloth. It is less sensitive to the conductive material variations compared with embroidery machine. The accurate cutting technologies such as laser cutting can be used to form precise electrotextile patterns. The preparation of the electrotextile cloth pattern, however, needs modifications from the original trace due to the fact that the spacing between separated elements needs to be managed. More specifically, redundant traces connecting the separated RF coil elements in coil array need to be prepared before the fabrication and to be removed after the fabrication. The resistivity of the material as an appropriate candidate is less than $1\,\Omega/sq$. The variation of a specific type of electrotextile cloth is much below that of electrotextile threads. It is noted that the electrotextile cloth coil to be discussed in the next section is shown in Figure 2.4c along with how it looks like before fabrication.

2.3.2 Characterization of Electrotextiles

Characterization of the electrotextile is the major challenge and of great importance for the electrotextile antennas in general. The surfaces of the electrotextile patterns are not as smooth as the normal metal, making its electrical conductivity more complicated as discussed in [25–27].

In this design example, two scenarios are studied. In the first scenario, a single electrotextile thread is used for RF coil design. As a result, the linear conductivity is used as a starting point for coil tuning and matching. Since the linear resistance is usually given for the electrotextile threads, we can use this value to design in Keysight advanced design system (ADS) software and further optimize the design using full-wave electromagnetic solvers such as Ansys high-frequency simulation system (HFSS). In the second scenario, laser cut electrotextile cloth is used for both coil element and coil array design. A systematic characterization method applicable to MRI RF coils at other frequencies or electrotextile antennas in general will be discussed. In [25, 26], this characterization method is used for the design of microstrip patch antennas. The following discussion focuses on the second scenario of using electrotextile cloth.

Several researchers have made efforts in characterizing electrotextile patterns or threads using effective conductivities and surface resistance. In [24], a microstrip line-based method to get effective conductivity at 0–6 GHz was proposed, where the surface roughness is taken into consideration. Although this method includes the frequency from very low to 6 GHz, the major applications are focused on lower GHz range. The surface roughness factor was taken under the assumption that the surface roughness is much larger than the skin depth, which needs verification for low-frequency applications such as MRI around 127 MHz (3T). Another disadvantage is that the loss in theory is small at lower frequencies than the higher frequencies and introduces more error using this method. In [28], the authors combined the strip line and Method of Moments (MOM) to get the effective conductivities for different stitch types and embroidery methods. However, this method was limited to the single thread property characterization in RF frequencies. In our application, the parameter is usually provided by the vendor and serves as a good starting point for designs using single thread. Additionally, it had the difficulty to model dimensionally small conductor undulation for MOM simulation. In [23], a systematic method to characterize the electrical properties of electrotextiles at high frequency is applied using both the waveguide cavity method and the microstrip resonator method. This method is effective in high-frequency applications but not as convenient for the low-frequency application such as MRI because the size of the cavity and resonator may be really big, around 127 MHz. In [29], an experimental method was proposed to get the complex sheet impedance that has both resistive and reactive parts. This method is effective for the radio-frequency identification (RFID) development. However, its biggest disadvantage was that it took several iterations to get the accurate values of sheet impedance and was time consuming. Since these electrical properties depend on the stitch strategies, stitch densities, type of pattern, and type of electrotextiles, it is critical that we have a rapid characterization method. Although the above characterization methods are effective in some applications, there is a missing part in characterizing the electrical properties of both the single thread and the electrotextile pattern. As a summary, the current methods in the literature adopted a trial-and-error method that is not systematic, time consuming, or not generally applicable to various applications.

Here, we applied a modified method to get the effective conductivity of the electrotextile antenna pattern based on the method proposed in [24]. The major steps and equations are included in Figure 2.5. In step 1, microstrip lines with different length fabricated with the copper and the electrotextiles are constructed. In step 2, the total attenuation constants of these microstrip lines are calculated based on the measured S_{21}. It is noted that the S_{21} information is de-embedded from the loss and perturbation of the connectors using S-matrix or ABCD matrix de-embedding methods in [24, 30]. In step 3, the conductivity attenuation constants of the electrotextile patterns are separated from the dielectric and the radiation losses. In step 4, the effective conductivity is extracted considering the surface roughness. The effective conductive loss that accounts for the loss due to surface roughness is used. The surface roughness constant K is used in Equations (2.4) and (2.5) from [31, 32] to relate the effective attenuation constant and the ordinary attenuation constant derived based on "smooth" metallic surface.

$$\alpha_{\text{cond}-\text{eff}} = \alpha_{\text{cond}} \times K \tag{2.4}$$

where $\alpha_{\text{cond-eff}}$ is the effective conductivity, and α_{cond} is the ordinary conductivity. The surface roughness constant K is calculated in Equation (2.5):

$$K = 1 + \frac{2}{\pi}\tan^{-1}\left(1.4\frac{\Delta}{\delta}\right) \tag{2.5}$$

where Δ is the height of the rough surface triangle from the bottom to the top, when the 2D rough surface is modeled as triangles are laid back to back [24]. δ is the skin depth of the electrotextile. Although the height of the rough surface and the skin depth of the electrotextile are unknown, it is observed that when the Δ is greater than 6, K begins to plateau. In [24], the surface roughness constant $K = 2$ is used considering the large surface roughness compared with the skin depth. In our application, this assumption may no longer hold because of the skin depth increase at lower frequencies. At the frequency of 127 MHz, the skin depth of the copper is around 6 μm. In order for the K factor to reach 2, the surface roughness needs to be greater than 36 μm, which is not always the case for the electrotextile pattern, especially when the stitch density is high or the electrotextile cloth surface is relatively smooth. We used $K = 2$ in our design case and achieved accurate impedance matching.

As a summary, the electrotextile cloth is the most ideal material for our application. The well-selected electrotextile thread is also a good candidate although the fabrication process is more complicated. The characterization of electrotextile pattern requires a systematic four-step measurement process to obtain

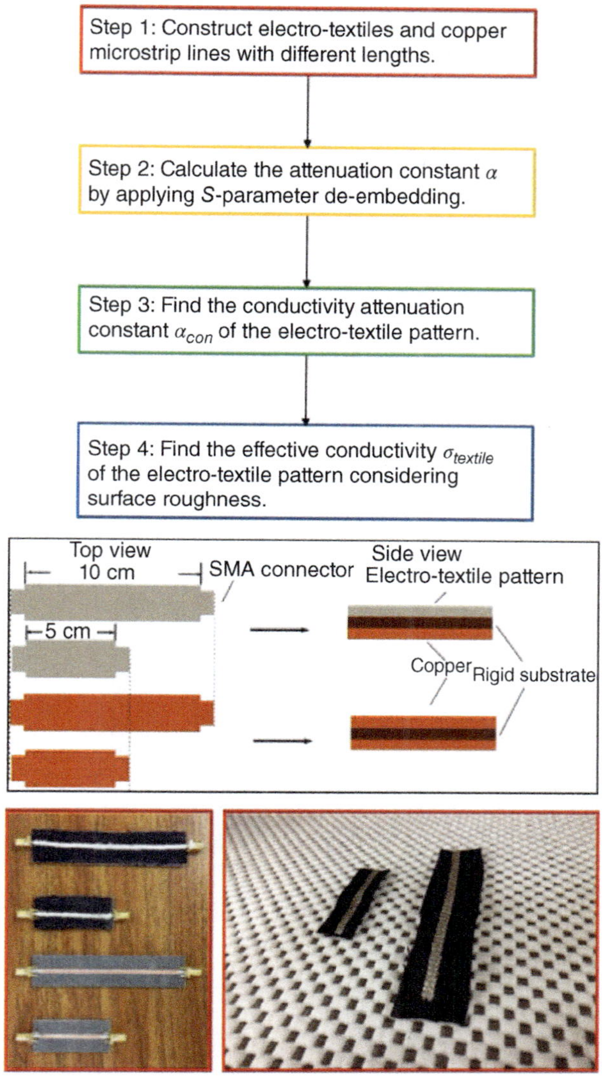

Figure 2.5 The steps to obtain the effective conductivities of the electrotextile patterns using microstrip line method. In step 1, build four lines with electrotextile and metal. In step 2, calculate the total attenuation constant with S-parameter method to de-embed the connector factor. In step 3, obtain the electrotextile conductivity attenuation constant. In step 4, obtain the effective conductivity using surface roughness estimate for certain frequencies [5]. (*Source*: Zhang, D. and Rahmat-Samii, Y., 2019. © IEEE.)

the effective conductivity of the material. The obtained value for electrotextile pattern effective conductivity can be used for full-wave electromagnetic simulation to facilitate accurate RF coil design.

2.4 Design of Single-Element Flexible RF Coil

The design of single-element flexible RF coil starts with the design of RF coil using regular metal and substrates following the strategy and roadmap discussed in Section 2.2. The design details will be introduced. The performances of the coil element using rigid material and electrotextiles are characterized. The key figure of merits including S_{11}, S_{21}, and H field are studied and compared.

2.4.1 RF Coil Element Design with a Rigid Material

The coil element design is shown in Figure 2.6. The proposed coil can be used in transmit/receive coil systems. The total size of the coil and substrate is 30 mm × 35 mm. The diameter of the circle is 20 mm. It can evolve in subsequent steps as a receiving-only coil and a coil array by adding transmission decoupling

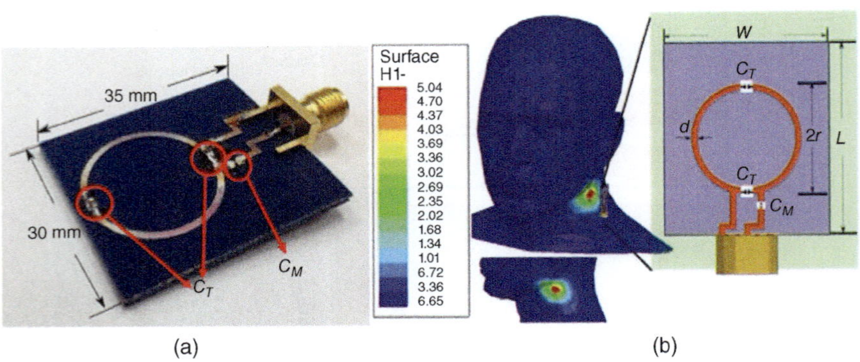

(c)

Parameter	Substrate width, W	Substrate length, L	Loop radius, r
Value	30 mm	35 mm	10 mm
Parameter	Loop width, d	C_T	C_M
Value	1 mm	83.5 pF	7 pF

Figure 2.6 (a) Fabricated neck RF coil with a resonant frequency at 127.7 MHz. RF coil position relative to the human neck and its structure including tuning capacitors [5]. (*Source*: Zhang, D. and Rahmat-Samii, Y., 2019. © IEEE.) (b) H_1-field distribution on the surface of the human neck with an input power of 1 W. It is noted that the examination of the coil magnetic field is necessary for parallel imaging acceleration in later development. (c) Parameter values of the RF coil structure are listed.

mechanism. The structure of the proposed RF coil and its performance near human neck are shown in Figure 2.6a,b. H_1-field is the left-hand circular polarized (LHCP) RF magnetic field at 127 MHz with the z-axis shown in Figure 2.1. It should be noted that only the LHCP signal is emanated from the human body. The most popular coil shape is a linearly polarized circular shape element due to its structural simplicity. As a result, the SNR can be further improved by adopting a LHCP coil element. The H_1-field distribution on the surface of the human neck with an input power of 1 W is shown in Figure 2.6b. It is noted that the examination of the coil magnetic field is necessary for parallel imaging acceleration but not necessary for other MRI image sequences. Modern MRI scanners usually perform this step of evaluating the coil sensitivity distribution every time it runs parallel imaging automatically. The detailed dimensions and capacitor values of the RF coil can be found in Figure 2.6c. The RF coil is placed 10 mm away from the human neck. The coil is connected to edge mount 50 Ω SMA connector. The proposed coil shown in Figure 2.6a is fabricated with photolithography on FR4 substrate with $\varepsilon_r = 4.4$, $\tan\sigma = 0.02$, and thickness of 0.4 mm. It should be noted that no balun is included in the design. The full-wave simulation shows that the current on the outer side of the coaxial cable is negligible. As a result, no balun is needed. The experiment also shows that the simulated and measured S-parameter results agree well. The interested readers may refer to [33–35] for more details.

Here, the rigid RF coil design is used in simulation as an example to study the bending effect. The S_{11} performance, however, does not have significant change when conformal to cylinders of different diameters. This is because the resonant frequency is mainly determined by the inductance of the coil and the capacitance of the frequency tuning capacitors, which do not have significant change when conformal to cylinders with reasonable diameters. On the contrary, it brings the advantage of potential higher SNR compared with the flat case. The human head model provided by HFSS with the minimum voxel length of 4 mm is used. The H_1-distribution of 30×35 mm cut 10 mm away from coil center is shown in Figure 2.7a. The cut is highlighted with pink color. The input power at the feeding point is 1 W as a reference. Without having the transmission decoupling mechanism incorporated in the RF coil elements, they can also be used as transmission/reception coils when the specific absorption rate (SAR) is important to consider. Although the major focus of this paper is on the receive-only surface coils, the SAR performance is also provided in Figure 2.7b with the reference input power of 1 W, which is at the same order of magnitude as real MRI scanner systems. The SAR maximum averaged over 1 g is $0.32\ \mathrm{W\,kg^{-1}}$. This is much below the SAR requirement of $1.6\ \mathrm{W\,kg^{-1}}$ by the Federal Communication Commission (FCC), which is the lowest SAR maximum average over 1 g. More detailed SAR requirements can be found in International Electrotechnical Commission (IEC) 60601-2-33 including the imaging time and peak SAR. Homogeneous mass (human tissue using the data based

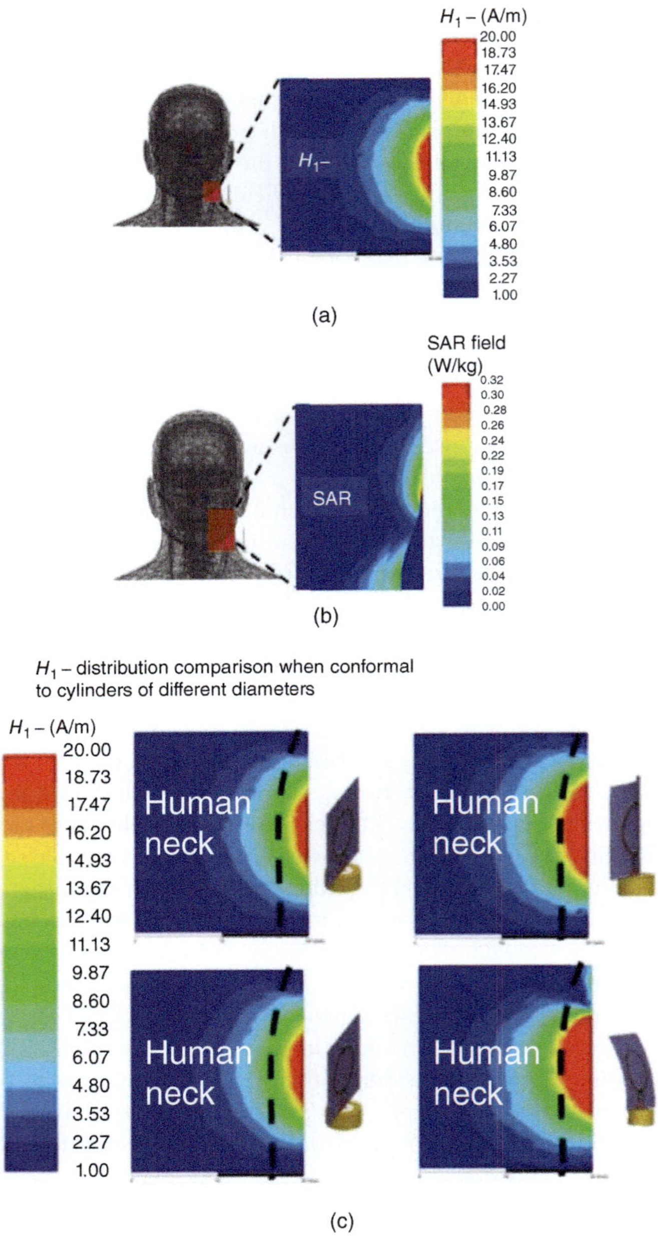

Figure 2.7 (a) H_1 distribution of 30 ×35 mm cut 10 mm away from the coil center; the cut is highlighted with pink color. (b) SAR distribution of 50 × 70 mm cut 10 mm away from the coil center; the cut is highlighted with pink color. (c) H_1-distribution comparison when conformal to cylinders of different sizes. A 30 × 35 mm cut 10 mm away from the coil center is shown. The input power of 1 W is used as a reference power level.

on Aarkid, East Lothian, Scotland [36]) distribution is used in the simulation. The database of the biological tissues can be found in [37]. The H_1-distribution when the coil is conformal to cylinders with 60 mm cross-sectional diameter is shown in Figure 2.7c. The penetration depth is increased when the coil is conformal to the cylinder according to the magnetic field distribution. The increase of SNR is also confirmed through the comparison of the MRI images after system integration. The SNR of conformal electrotextile coil is higher than the nonconformal RF coil with the rigid material at the same distance from the phantom in the same depth of 1 cm.

A commonly used preliminary method to predict the effect of RF coil on the SNR performance is to measure the quality factor ratio with Equation (2.6). Q_{loaded} and $Q_{unloaded}$ denote the quality factor of the RF coil with and without human loading, respectively. They are also introduced in Section 2.1. The Q-factor ratio quantifies how dominant the loss from the human loading is among the total loss. Meanwhile, it should be noted that the contribution to the loss from the two sources varies with different coil diameters and frequencies as shown in [12]. As a result, a fair comparison of the Q ratio requires a fixed coil size, frequency, and measurement setup. It is measured that the designed RF coil in copper and electrotextile with a diameter of 5 cm has Q ratio of 2.1 and 1.5 at 127.7 MHz, respectively, using the measurement setup in Figure 2.8. It indicates that the copper coil is less lossy compared with the electrotextile coils as expected. The SNR of the final MRI image is one order of magnitude higher at the depth of 0.5 cm even with the more lossy coil. This Q ratio value

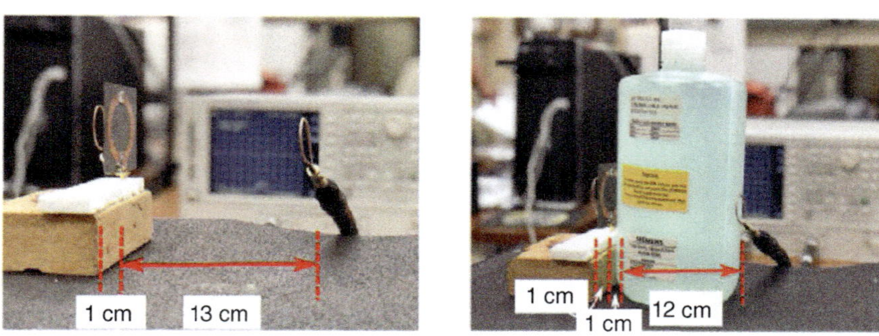

(a) (b)

Figure 2.8 The quality factor measurement setup. (a) $Q_{unloaded}$ measurement setup [5]. (*Source*: Zhang, D. and Rahmat-Samii, Y., 2019. © IEEE.) The two broadband RF probes are separated by 14 cm to guarantee that they are weakly coupled. (b) Q_{loaded} measurement setup. The RF coil under test is placed 1 cm away from the outer perimeter of the phantom. The phantom is filled with 1900 ml solution (per 1000 g H_2O dist.: 3.75 g $NiSO_4 \times 6\,H_2O + 5$ g NaCl). The conductivity is 1.109 S m^{-1}, and the relative permittivity is 72.84 at 127 MHz. (*Source*: Zhang, D. and Rahmat-Samii, Y., 2019. © IEEE.)

can be used as a reference for a quick check for later electrotextile designs.

$$Q_{\text{ratio}} = Q_{\text{unloaded}}/Q_{\text{loaded}} \tag{2.6}$$

In order to directly link the loss of RF coil material to SNR of the coil, the relationship between the total available SNR and Q ratio is shown in Equation(2.7) (the same as Equation(2.3)), where SNR_0 is the total available (or intrinsic) SNR described in [38]. Additionally, it can also be derived that the SNR is linearly proportional to $\sqrt{Q_{\text{loaded}}}$ under the condition that the same phantom loading is used. As a result, $\sqrt{Q_{\text{unloaded}}}$ indicates how much RF coil noise impacts the total available SNR. In order to compare the performance of RF coil made with electrotextile and copper, relative SNR can be defined in Equation (2.8)[39]. Here, $Q_{\text{loaded-test}}$ is the loaded quality factor of the coil under test, in our case the electrotextile RF coil, and the $Q_{\text{loaded-control}}$ is the loaded quality factor of the coil under control, in our case the rigid RF coil. Figure 2.8a shows the Q_{unloaded} measurement setup. The two broadband RF probes are separated by 14 cm to guarantee that they are weakly coupled. Figure 2.8b shows the Q_{loaded} measurement setup. The RF coil under test is placed 1 cm away from the outer perimeter of the phantom. The phantom is filled with 1900 ml solution (per 1000 g H_2O dist.: 3.75 g $NiSO_4 \times 6\,H_2O$+5 g NaCl). The conductivity is 1.109 S m^{-1}, and the relative permittivity is 72.84 at 127 MHz. Utilizing the Q_{loaded} measured using the setup in Figure 2.8, we find that the relative SNR of the electrotextile coil is 80% of that using copper and dielectric substrate. Due to the complexity involved in measuring Q_{loaded}, the author in [39] also proposed a method of using a controlled quality factor to find relative SNR by only measuring unloaded quality factor of test coils.

$$\text{SNR} = \text{SNR}_0\sqrt{1 - \frac{Q_{\text{loaded}}}{Q_{\text{unloaded}}}} \tag{2.7}$$

(same as Equation(2.3))

$$\text{SNR}_{\text{relative}} = \sqrt{Q_{\text{loaded-test}}}/\sqrt{Q_{\text{loaded-control}}} \tag{2.8}$$

2.4.2 RF Coil Element Design with Electrotextile Cloth

Electrotextile single thread can also make decent performance RF coil. The interested readers may refer to [33–35]. The electrotextile cloth RF coil in Figure 2.9 is designed to have a width of $W = 7$ mm, wider than the copper coil shown previously to reduce the coil loss, because most of the current flow directions are along the circular shape of the coil. Additionally, the diameter D_1 of the coil is 36 mm to have enough coverage for the targeted carotid artery region near the neck. The S-parameter at 127 MHz is below −20 dB and will be shown in Section 2.5. The bending study observations discussed in Section 2.4.1 also apply to the electrotextile cloth RF coil. In Figure 2.9a, the

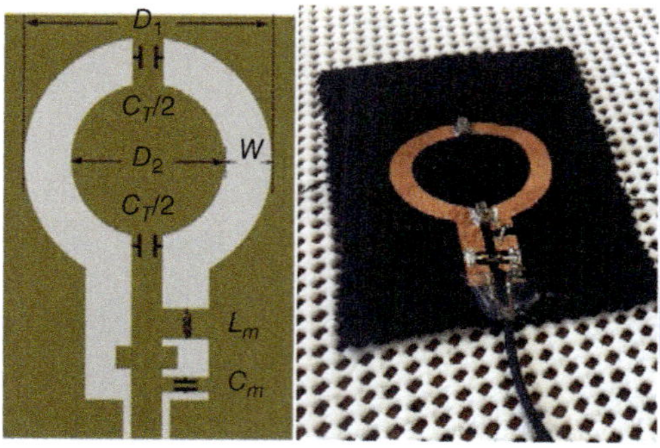

(a)

D_1	D_2	W
36 mm	50 mm	7 mm
C_T	C_m	L_m
88.4 pF	8.4 pF	35.2 nH

(b)

Figure 2.9 Electrotextile cloth RF coil. (a) the illustrative figure and the fabricated ultraflexible RF coil and (b) parameter values of the RF coil structure.

electrotextile cloth RF coil illustrative figure and the fabricated ultraflexible RF coil are shown. In Figure 2.9b, the parameter values of the RF coil structure are also presented.

2.4.3 RF Coil Element Design with Tunable Circuitry

One of the key difficulties of the coil element design using electrotextiles at 3T is to accurately tune the resonant frequency exactly at 127.7 MHz, given the narrow bandwidth of the coil and the RF transmission signal, as discussed in [35]. It is shown in the previous two sections that appropriate designs without tunable circuitry are achievable. Alternatively, in order to expedite the development process, we proposed a tunable circuitry with varactors and variable capacitors shown in Figure 2.10a to accurately tune the resonant frequency exactly at the designated frequency, saving the time-consuming process of the changing components. PELCO propanol-graphite-based paint is used for DC bias line. The measured S_{11} of the fabricated tunable RF coil element is −24.5 dB at exactly 127.7 MHz shown in Figure 2.10b. It can be seen that the simulated result agrees well with the measured result. It should also be noted that the series resistance associated with the varactors needs to be considered in full-wave simulation for accurate modeling.

2.5 Design of Flexible RF Coil Array and System Integration with MRI Scanner

This section discusses RF coil array using electrotextiles and its integration with MRI scanners. The major design goal is to maintain low mutual coupling so as to keep every element independent of other channels. The RF coil array

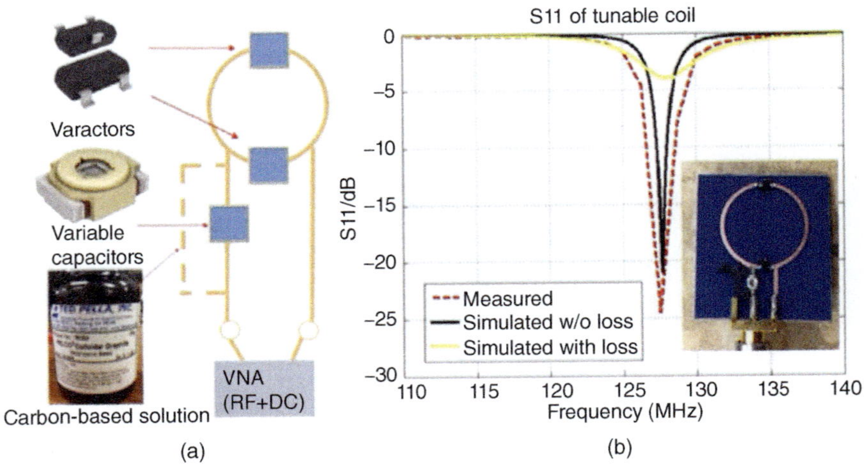

Figure 2.10 Tunable circuitry. (a) Components and the design of the coil element with the accurate resonant frequency. (b) Measured S_{11} of the fabricated tunable RF coil element is −24.5 dB at exactly 127.7 MHz. Fabricated coil element with tuning circuitry is also shown. It can be seen that the simulation result agrees well with the measured result. In addition, the series resistance associated with the varactors needs to be considered in full-wave simulation for accurate modeling [5]. (*Source*: Zhang, D. and Rahmat-Samii, Y., 2019. © IEEE.)

characterizations include the S_{11} and S_{21} measurements. The integration with the MRI scanner requires the use of preamplifier and the capability of being identified. PIN diodes were used to detune the coil during the RF transmission phase. The preamplifier was noise matched to achieve 0.5 dB noise figure (NF) and 28.5 dB gain [40].

2.5.1 RF Coil Array Design and Characterization

In our design, two overlapped (zeroing the mutual magnetic flux) circular coil elements are designed to consider low mutual coupling; 12 mm (approximately 0.48× radius) overlap is used to obtain the lowest coupling [41]. The radius of the coil element in the coil array is 25 mm, as shown in Figure 2.11a, to achieve large covering area. A four-layer structure is proposed for the coil array with one coil element in the front and the other in the back in Figure 2.11b. A cotton interlayer is used to avoid the direct touch of the two elements. In order to reduce the influence of human body, the direct touch of human body and the coil is avoided by adding the cotton cushion at the bottom as shown in Figure 2.11b.

The RF coils with electrotextiles are simulated and measured based on the effective conductivity method in Section 2.3. As shown in Figure 2.11c, the S_{11} performance is tuned to exactly 127.7 MHz with the minimum of −18 dB, which

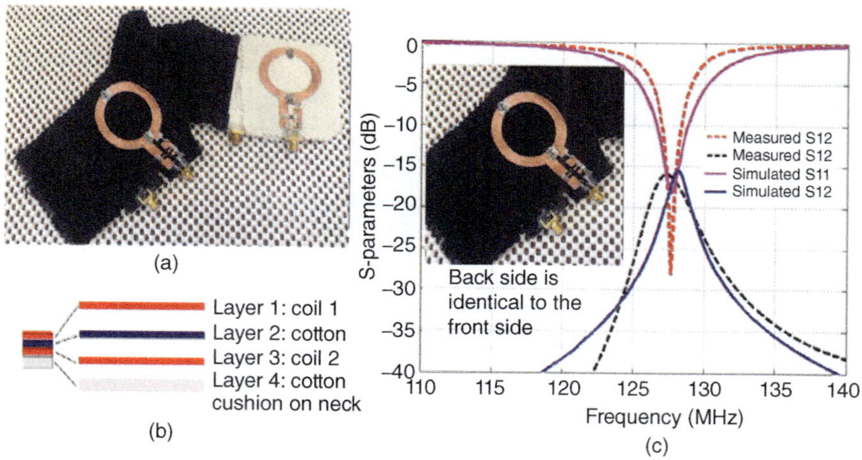

Figure 2.11 Coil array structure. (a) Front view of the fabricated coil array with electrotextiles. One coil element is in the front, and the other coil element is in the back. (b) Side view of the four-layer coil array structure with electrotextiles. The overall thickness is 1.88 mm. Note that the location of the front and back coils is shown in red. (c) Simulated and measured S_{11} and S_{12} of the fabricated coil array. Note that one coil is in the front and another coil is in the back [5]. (*Source*: Zhang, D. and Rahmat-Samii, Y., 2019. © IEEE.)

agrees well with the simulated value. In addition, the measured S_{12} has a maximum of around −16 dB, which is within the acceptable range. It is also found that S_{11} and S_{12} would change noticeably if the overlap distance is smaller than 12 mm or larger than 14 mm.

2.5.2 RF Coil Array System Integration with MRI Scanner

The close-up look of the RF coil array system configuration is shown in Figure 2.12, including the RF coil array, the transmission decoupling circuitry, and RF coil interface with the MRI scanner. The RF coil array and transmission decoupling circuitry are connected with coaxial cables. The transmission decoupling circuitry is further connected with the RF coil interface using coaxial cables. The major component of the interface is a preamplifier. One of the most critical modules is the transmission decoupling circuitry. The transmission decoupling circuitry is used to show high impedance when the MRI scanner is working in the transmission mode. During the transmission phase, the transmission coils usually embedded in the MRI scanners are turned on, and the hydrogen nucleus is flipped to the *xy*-plane (coordinate shown in Figure 2.1). To keep the homogeneity of the static magnetic field and the desired effect by the gradient coils, receive-only coils should not affect the transmission process at this time and enter a transmission decoupling mode.

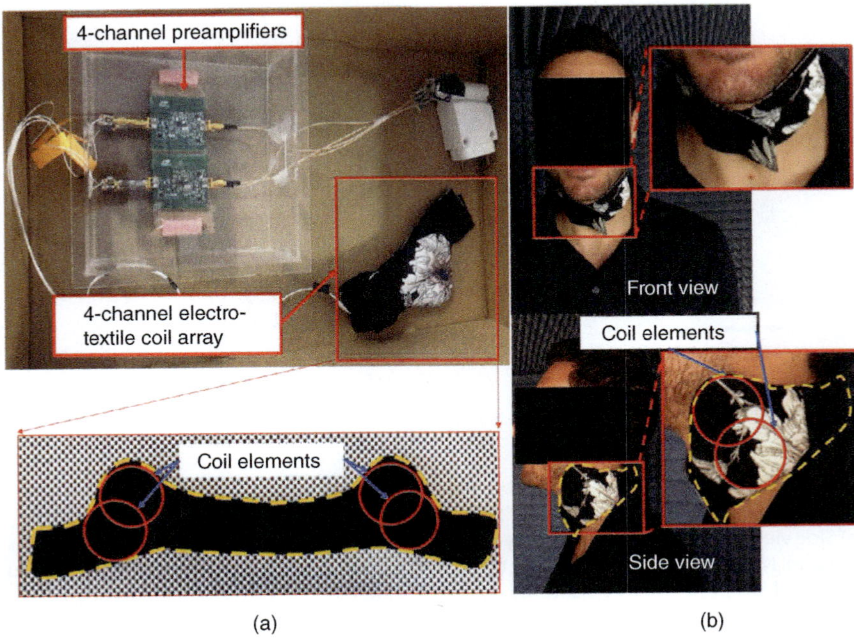

Figure 2.12 Ultraflexible electrotextile RF coil array. (a) The four-channel e-textile coil array includes four elements and preamplifiers. In the close-up figure, the coil array contains two elements on each side. (b) The model wears the e-textile coil around the neck. It is noted that this is only for the purpose of demonstration and not testing.

In our design shown in Figure 2.12, an ultraflexible four-channel electrotextile RF coil array is connected with four-channel preamplifiers, which is connected with the plug-in of the MRI scanner. Each channel in the coil array is connected with a specific preamplifier channel. The total imaging coverage includes the two sides around the neck Figure 2.12b targeting carotid arteries. The ultraflexible RF coil array covered in cotton case gently wraps around the model's neck. It is noted that this is only for the purpose of demonstration and not testing.

2.6 Characterization of RF Coil Array

In order to verify the effectiveness of the ultraflexible MRI RF coil platform, the ultraflexible coil array is connected with the MRI scanner and shows its improvement in the final images compared with the standard RF coil. The characterization results using both phantom and human cadaver are presented and discussed.

2.6.1 Characterization of RF Coil Array System with Phantom

The system-level performance of the UCLA ultraflexible RF coil array is measured with the setup shown in Figure 2.13. The UCLA electrotextile RF coil array is taped to the phantom with a 1-cm-thick foam in between. The image is obtained at UCLA School of Medicine using 3T MRI scanner. The authors acknowledge the support they received from UCLA medical center.

The ultraflexible electrotextile coil and a four-channel standard surface coil (small flex coil, Siemens) were used to scan a water phantom (Figure 2.14f) and the neck of an unembalmed cadaver at room temperature at 3T (Prisma, Siemens) (Figure 2.15). Biosafety approval was obtained for human cadaver research [42]. The coil locations are indicated by the yellow ellipses. A T_1-weighted spin-echo sequence was used for both the phantom and cadaver, with $1 \times 1\,\text{mm}^2$ in-plane resolution, 0.8 mm slice thickness, and $\text{FOV} = 320 \times 320\,\text{mm}^2$. For phantom scans: TR = 573 ms, TE = 20 ms. For cadaver scans: TR = 309 ms, TE = 11 ms.

The signal strength of electrotextile coil near the surface is noticeably stronger than a standard surface coil (Figure 2.14a,b). The SNRs calculated using the difference method in [43] at the depths of 0.5 and 3 cm were 4.2 and 3.4 times (Table 2.1) higher than the standard coil, respectively, at the indicated Region of Interest (ROI) (Figure 2.14c,d). The noise correlation matrix (NCM) quantifies the noise from each individual element and provides information about the correlations between channels which degrade the final image SNR [44]. The NCM of the image with ultraflexible coil shows that the minimum on-diagonal value is 77.6% of the maximum. The off-diagonal maximum is

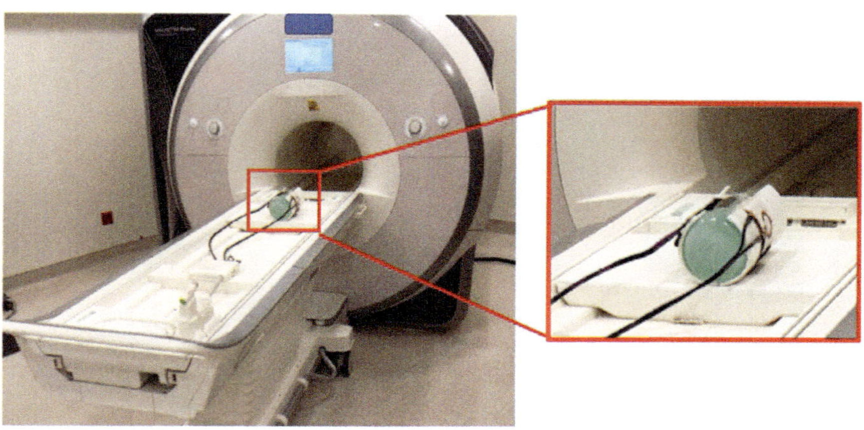

Figure 2.13 The UCLA electrotextile RF coil array is taped to the phantom with a 1-cm-thick foam in between. The image is obtained at UCLA School of Medicine using 3T MRI scanner. *Source*: UCLA School of Medicine.

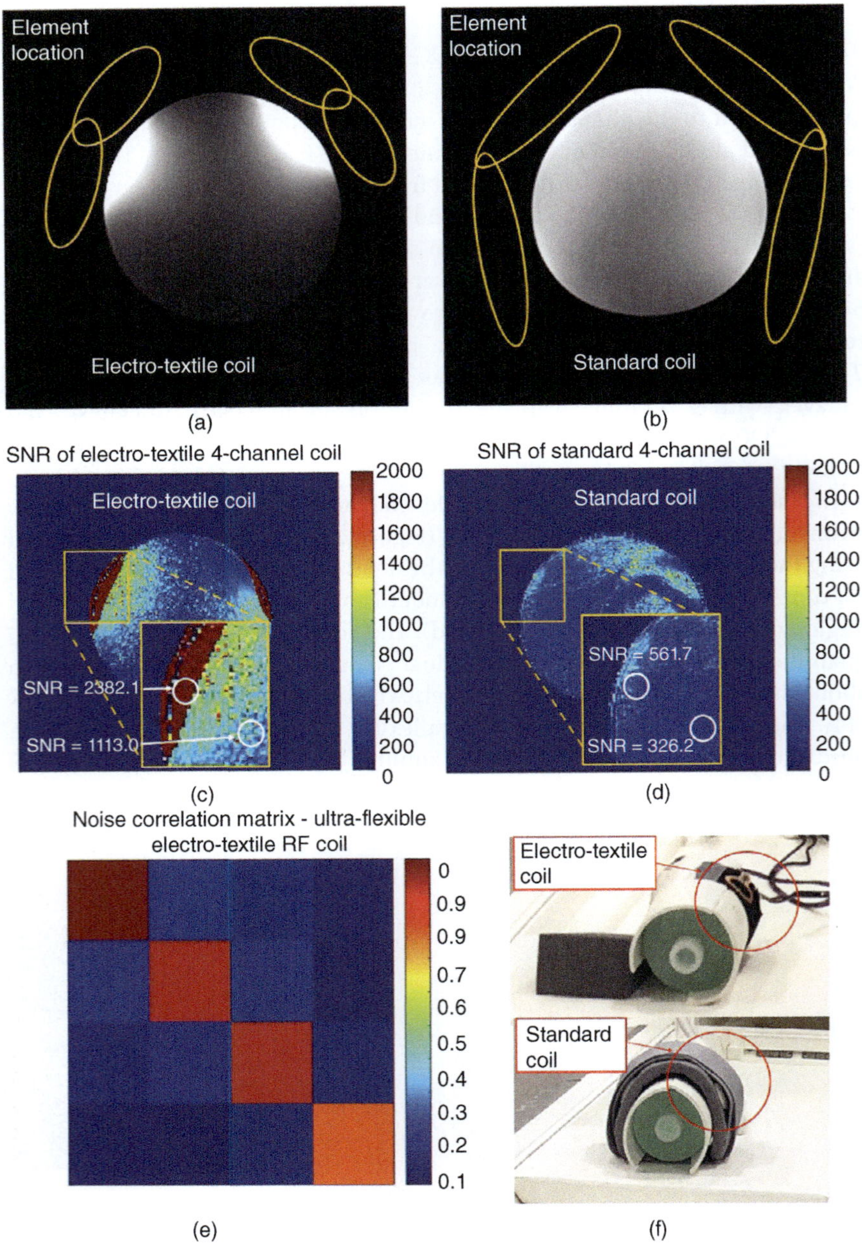

Figure 2.14 The electrotextile RF coil performance on a water phantom. (a) Image acquired using the four-channel electrotextile coil array. (b) Image acquired using a four-channel standard coil array. (c) The SNR map of the phantom image for the ultraflexible electrotextile coil. (d) The SNR map of the phantom image for the standard coil. (e) The noise correlation matrix (NCM) of the electrotextile coil wrapped around the phantom. (f) The scanning setup of the ultraflexible electrotextile coil array and standard coil array. These images were generated with the help of H. Wu, L. Zhang and S. Mikaiel of UCLA School of Medicine.

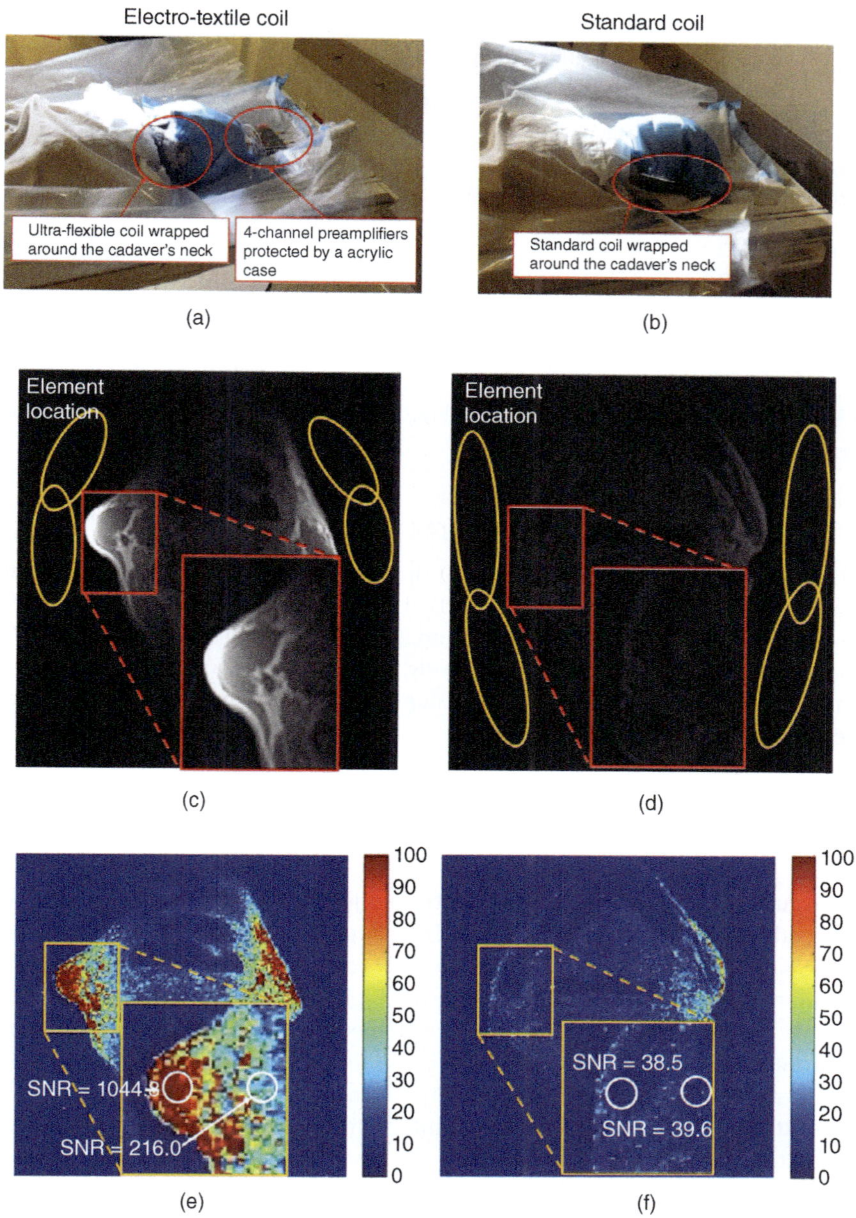

Figure 2.15 The electrotextile coil performance for cadaver neck MRI in comparison with a standard surface coil. (a) The scanning setup of the electrotextile coil array. (b) The scanning setup of the standard coil array. (c) An image of the neck using electrotextile coil. (d) An image of the neck using standard coil. (e) The SNR map of the neck using the electrotextile coil. (f) The SNR map of the neck using a standard coil. These images were generated with the help of H. Wu, L. Zhang and S. Mikaiel of UCLA School of Medicine.

Table 2.1 Signal-to-noise ratio (SNR) comparison between the ultraflexible e-textile and standard coils when imaging phantom and cadaver at the depths of 0.5 and 3 cm from the surface of the imaging area.

	Water phantom			Cadaver		
Depth (cm)	Ultraflexible coil SNR	Standard coil SNR	$SNR_{flexible}$/ $SNR_{standard}$	Ultraflexible coil SNR	Standard coil SNR	$SNR_{flexible}$/ $SNR_{standard}$
0.5	2382.1	561.7	4.2	1044.8	38.5	27
3	1113.0	326.2	3.4	216.0	39.6	5.5

The e-textile coil achieved multifold improvement in SNR compared to a standard coil.

13.4% of the on-diagonal maximum (Figure 2.14e), indicating satisfactory coil array performance [44].

2.6.2 Characterization of RF Coil Array System with Cadaver

The signal strength near the surface of the cadaver is noticeably stronger than a standard surface coil (Figure 2.15c,d). The SNRs calculated using the difference method [43] at the depths of 0.5 and 3 cm were 27 and 5.5 times (Table 2.1) higher than the standard coil, respectively, at the indicated ROI (Figure 2.15e,f). An expert radiologist reported good depiction of vertebral artery and sternocleidomastoid muscle in the images.

2.7 Conclusion

In summary, the new ultraflexible electrotextile RF array coil shows substantial SNR advantage over a standard coil. In cadaver images at a depth of 0.5 cm, the SNR of the ultraflexible electrotextile coil was 27 times higher than a standard coil. The cadaver images showed high-quality anatomical features in the neck. As the size and number of coil elements can be modified for different anatomies of interest, this technology is not limited to neck MRI. The electrotextile material can be readily applied to more areas including pediatric, joint, and extremity MRI and MRI-guided interventions. Future works include the evaluation of new coils on the human body for different diagnostic applications.

References

1 Liang, Z.P. and Lauterbur, P.C. (2000). *Principles of Magnetic Resonance Imaging: A Signal Processing Perspective*. New York: Wiley-IEEE Press.

2 Nishimura, D.G. (2010). *Principles of magnetic resonance imaging*, 1.1e. California: Electrical Engineering Department, Stanford University.
3 Jin, J.M. (1998). Electromagnetics in magnetic resonance imaging. *IEEE Antennas and Propagation Magazine* 40 (6): 7–22.
4 Jin, J.M. (1998). *Electromagnetic Analysis and Design in Magnetic Resonance Imaging. Department of Electrical and Computer Engineering, University of Illinois at Urbana-Champaign Urbana*. Illinois: CRC Press.
5 Zhang, D. and Rahmat-Samii, Y. (2019). A novel flexible electro-textile 3T MRI RF coil array for stroke prevention: design, characterization and prototyping. *IEEE Transaction on Antennas and Propagation*, Special issue Wireless Healthcare Biotechnology 67: 5115–5125.
6 Magnetic Resonance Facts and Figures.https://www.magnetic-resonance.org/ch/21-01.html
7 Wang, N., Christodoulou, A., Christodoulou, G. et al. (2019). Quantitative 3D dynamic contrast-enhanced (DCE) MR imaging of carotid vessel wall by fast T1 mapping using multitasking. *Magnetic Resonance in Medicine* 81: 2302–2314.
8 Mikaiel, S., Simonelli, J., Li, X. et al. (2019). MRI-guided targeted needle placement during motion using hydrostatic actuators. *The International Journal of Medical Robotics and Computer Assisted Surgery* 16: e2041.
9 Bendall, M.R. (1988). *Magnetic Resonance Imaging* (eds. C.L. Partain, R.R. Price, J.A. Patton, et al.). Philadelphia: Saunders.
10 Roemer, P.B., Edelstein, W.A., Hayes, C.E. et al. (1990). The NMR phased array. *Magnetic Resonance in Medicine* 16: 192–225.
11 Edelstein, W.A., Glover, G.H., Hardy, C.J., and Redington, R.W. (1986). The intrinsic signal-to-noise ratio in NMR imaging. *Magnetic Resonance in Medicine* 3: 604–618.
12 Corea, J.R., Flynn, A.M., Lechene, B. et al. (2016). Screen-printed flexible MRI receive coils. *Nature Communications* 7: 10839.
13 Thomas Vaughan, J. and Griffth, J.R. *RF Coils for MRI*. Hoboken, NJ: Wiley ISBN-13: 9780470770764, ISBN-10: 470770767.
14 American Heart Association. https://www.heart.org/idc/groups/heart-public/@wcm/@adv/documents/downloadable/ucm_305054.pdf
15 Mayo Clinics, Carotid Artery Disease. https://dovemed.com/diseases-conditions/carotid-artery-disease/
16 Yuan, C., Oikawa, M., Miller, Z., and Hatsukami, T. (2008). MRI of carotid atherosclerosis. *Journal of Nuclear Cardiology* 15: 266–275.
17 Zhang, D. and Rahmat-Samii, Y. (2016). An ergonomic design for 3Tesla MRI neck coil.IEEE International Symposium on Antennas and Propagation & USNC/URSI National Radio Science Meeting, IEEE, 463–464.
18 Corea, J.R. et al. (2016). Screen-printed flexible MRI receive coils. *Nature Communications* 7: 10839-1–10839-11.

19 Mager, D. et al. (2010). An MRI receiver coil produced by inkjet printing directly on to a flexible substrate. *IEEE Transactions on Medical Imaging* 29 (2): 482–487.

20 Nordmeyer-Massner, J.A., De Zanche, N., and Pruessmann, K.P. (2012). Stretchable coil arrays: Application to knee imaging under varying flexion angles. *Magnetic Resonance in Medicine* 67 (3): 872–879.

21 Pozar, D.M. (2005). *Microwave Engineering*, 3e. New Jersey: Wiley, ISBN: 978-0-471-44878-5.

22 Lobodzinski, S.S. and Laks, M. (2009). New material for implantable cardiac leads. *Journal of Electrocardiology* 42 (6): 566–573.

23 S. A. Materials (2017). Liberator 40, Syscom Advanced Material.

24 Wang, Z. (2014). Electronic textile antennas and radio frequency circuits for body-worn applications. Ph.D. Thesis.

25 Song, L., Zhang, D., and Rahmat-Samii, Y. (2018).Towards embroidered textile antenna systematic design and accurate modeling: rectangular patch antenna case studies. IEEE International Symposium on Antennas and Propagation & USNC/URSI National Radio Science Meeting.

26 Song, L., Zhang, D., and Rahmat-Samii, Y. (2018). Towards embroidered textile antenna systematic design and accurate modeling: rectangular patch antenna case studies. IEEE Antenna and Propagation Society International Symposium.

27 Zhang, D. and Rahmat-Samii, Y. (2018). Integration of electro-textile RF coil array with magnetic resonance imaging (MRI) system: design strategies and characterization methods. International Workshop on Antenna Technology (iWAT)(5 March 2018).

28 Shawl, R.K., Longj, B.R., and Werner, D.H. (2007). The characterization of conductive textile materials intended for radio frequency applications. *IEEE Antennas and Propagation Magazine* 49 (3): 28–40.

29 Koski, K. and Sydänheimo, L. (2014). Fundamental characteristics of electro-textiles in wearable UHF RFID patch antennas for body-centric sensing systems. *IEEE Transactions on Antennas and Propagation* 62 (12): 6454–6462.

30 Collin, R.E. (2007). *Foundations for Microwave Engineering*. New Delhi: Wiley.

31 Morgan, S.P. Jr., (1949). Effect of surface roughness on eddy current losses at microwave frequencies. *Journal of Applied Physics* 20: 352–362.

32 Lukic, M.V. and Filipovic, D.S. (2007). Modeling of 3-D surface roughness effects with application to u-coaxial lines. *IEEE Transactions on Microwave Theory and Techniques* 55 (3): 518–525.

33 Zhang, D. and Rahmat-Samii, Y. (2017). Electro-textiles as potential candidate of flexible MRI RF coil for stroke prevention. Proceedings of the United States National Committee of URSI National Radio Science Meeting

(USNC-URSI NRSM)(4 January 2017), 1–2(Student paper competition 2nd prize).

34 Zhang, D. and Rahmat-Samii, Y. (2017). Flexible RF coil array system utilizing electro-textiles for 3T MRI carotid artery imaging. IEEE Antenna and Propagation Society International Symposium(12 July 2017, Student paper competition finalist).

35 Zhang, D. and Rahmat-Samii, Y. (2016). An ergonomic design for 3Tesla MRI neckcoil. Proceedings of the IEEE Antenna and Propagation Society International Symposium(28June 2016), 463–464.

36 Homann, H., Börnert, P., Eggers, H. et al. (2011). Toward individualized SAR models and in vivo validation. *Magnetic Resonance in Medicine* 66: 1767–1776. https://doi.org/10.1002/mrm.22948.

37 Lobodzinski, S.S. and Laks, M. (2009). New material for implantable cardiac 731 leads. *Journal of Electrocardiology* 42 (6): 566–573.

38 Edelstein, W.A., Glover, G.H., Hardy, C.J., and Redington, R.W. (1986). The intrinsic signal-to-noise ratio in NMR imaging. *Magnetic Resonance in Medicine* 3: 604–618.

39 Corea, J.R., Lechene, P.B., Lustig, M., and Arias, A.C. (2016). Materials and methods for higher performance screen-printed flexible MRI receive coils. *Magnetic Resonance in Medicine* 16: 1–9.

40 Roemer, P. et al. (1990). The NMR phased array. *MRM* 16 (2): 192–225.

41 Angelidis, P., Vassiliadis, K., and Sergiadis, G.D. (1991). Lowest mutual coupling between closely spaced loop antennas. *IEEE Transaction on Antenna and Propagation* 39 (7): 949–953.

42 Zhang, D., Zhang, L., Prosper, A., Wu, H.H., and Rahmat-Samii, Y. (2019). Ultra-flexible electro-textile 4-channel MRI RF coil array for neck MRI, ISMRM.

43 Dietrich, O., Raya, J.G., Reeder, S.B. et al. (2007). Measurement of signal-to-noise ratios in MR images: influence of multichannel coils, parallel imaging, and reconstruction filters. *Journal of Magnetic Resonance Imaging* 26: 375–385.

44 Tunnicliffe, E.M. et al. (2011). Use of the noise covariance matrix in array coil quality assurance. *ISMRM* 19: 4548–4548.

45 Ouyang, Y. and Chappell, W.J. (2008). High frequency properties of electro-textiles for wearable antenna applications. *IEEE Transactions on Antennas and Propagation* 56 (2): 381–389.

3

Wearable Sensors for Motion Capture

Vigyanshu Mishra and Asimina Kiourti

ElectroScience Laboratory, Department of Electrical and Computer Engineering, The Ohio State University, Columbus, OH, USA

3.1 Introduction

Human motion is ubiquitous. Running, walking, jumping, cooking, driving, playing, throwing, climbing, swimming, and several other activities can be listed as examples of human motion. Interestingly enough, human motion is highly complex. Indeed, from an anatomical perspective, human movements can be classified into numerous types (Figure 3.1), including, but not limited to, flexion (decreases the angle between the bones or bending of joint, e.g. decrease of angle between the forearm and upper arm in the case of elbow joint), extension (opposite of flexion—increases the angle and straightens the joint), abduction (moving the body part away from the midline of body, e.g. lifting of arms away from the body using the shoulder joint), adduction (opposite of abduction—bringing it closer to midline), and rotation (rotation of a body part, e.g. pronation and supination of arms and medial (internal) and lateral (external) rotation of legs) [1]. Simple activities, such as lifting a lightweight object by hand, may involve combination of a few different types of such movements, while more sophisticated tasks, such as running or swimming, may involve combinations of multiple of these tasks. A small example of this is a movement called circumduction (also shown in Figure 3.1), which involves sequential combination of flexion, adduction, extension, and abduction at a joint [1]. The above help us appreciate how complex certain tasks that we perform on a daily basis can be.

Capturing motion as an intricate part of human existence can lead to tremendous improvements in our quality of life. Example applications that may benefit from such motion capture technologies range from healthcare to sports, gaming, training, and beyond. But what technologies are currently available for motion capture, and what are the associated benefits and limitations? What

Antenna and Sensor Technologies in Modern Medical Applications,
First Edition. Edited by Yahya Rahmat-Samii and Erdem Topsakal.

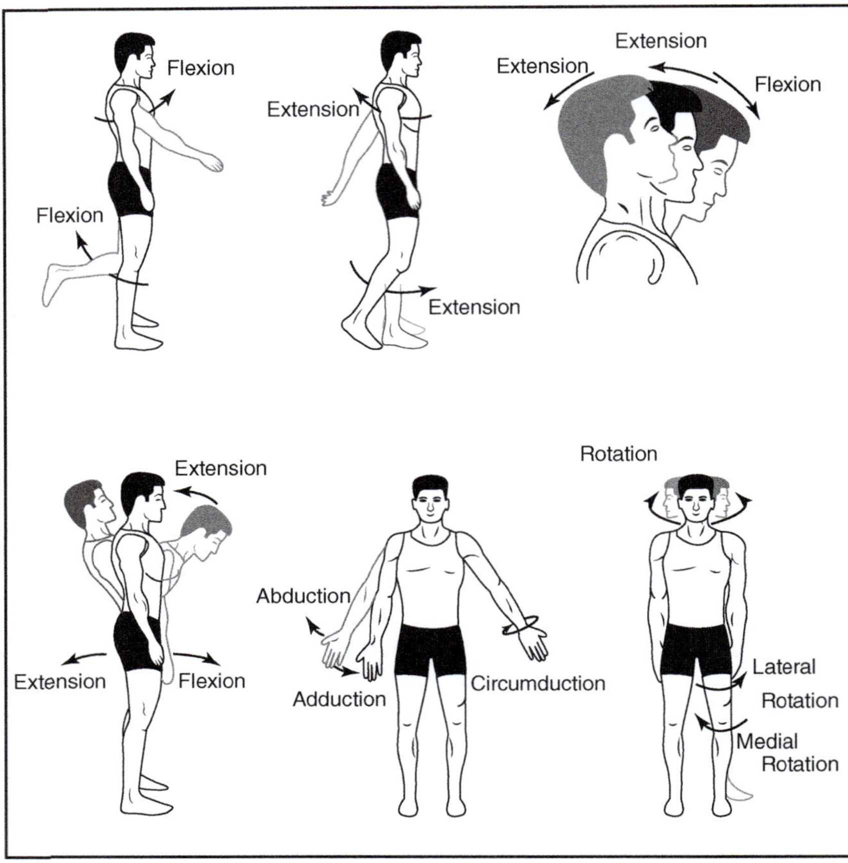

Figure 3.1 Examples of anatomical classification of different types of human movements [1]. *Source*: Types of Body Movements, in "Joints," in Anatomy and Physiology, OpenStax. License under CC 4.0.

are the current research trends in the area? And what lies in the future? This chapter is dedicated to answering all these questions. Expectedly, the impact of motion capture technology is not limited to the discussion in this chapter, as creative ways of leveraging motion capture are unfolding at unprecedented paces. However, this chapter intends to provide a comprehensive overview of the state of the art in the field, build a complete picture that surrounds this technology, and trigger the reader's interest toward further explorations in the field. To this end, the chapter focuses primarily on wearable sensors for motion capture as attributed to their seamless nature and future potential and also covers a wide variety of technologies that are relevant to motion capture, indicating where wearable sensors find their place. Notably, although the discussion in this chapter is geared toward human motion, nothing stops the reported technologies from capturing motion of any other moving beings (i.e. animals) and beyond (such as structures).

The rest of the chapter is organized as follows. First, we discuss various application sectors where motion capture technology can be employed and highlight the merits of employing wearable motion capture in each of these sectors. In doing so, it will become evident how motion capture technology can improve our quality of life and why the ultimate aim is often about making such technology wearable. Second, we explore various methods and sensors that can be used to capture human motion in confined or contrived settings, including motion capture labs, electromagnetic-based sensors, magnetic motion capture, imaging methods, and more. Third, we discuss wearable approaches to motion capture, including inertial measurement units, bending/deformation sensors, time-of-flight sensors, and received signal strength (RSS)-based sensors. Finally, we conclude the chapter with a summary of the reported technologies, a lookout into the future, and a comparative table summarizing the advantages and limitations of the technologies described throughout the chapter.

3.2 The Promise of Motion Capture

Referring to Figure 3.2, motion capture opens doors for widespread applications. Example sectors where such technology has already been employed or is envisioned to be employed are discussed next.

3.2.1 Healthcare

Health is indispensable for human life, and hence, employing motion capture in this sector can directly impact the individuals' quality of life. In brief, motion capture technology for healthcare can be subdivided into two main classes of applications.

(a) *Rehabilitation*: Considering health conditions that may cause motor disability, such as athletic injuries, Parkinson's, traumatic brain injury (TBI), concussion, falls (e.g. in the case of elderly), or accidents; motion capture technology can play a crucial role in personalizing rehabilitation. Indeed, motion capture performed within contrived environments (either manually by a physical therapist or via cameras) has long been used to adjust the patients' rehabilitation program for applications as diverse as anterior cruciate ligament reconstruction (ACLR) [2], stroke [3], etc. The above implies a known medical condition and the individual being located in a dedicated setting to have his/her motion monitored. However, rehabilitation monitoring should not ultimately be restricted to specific

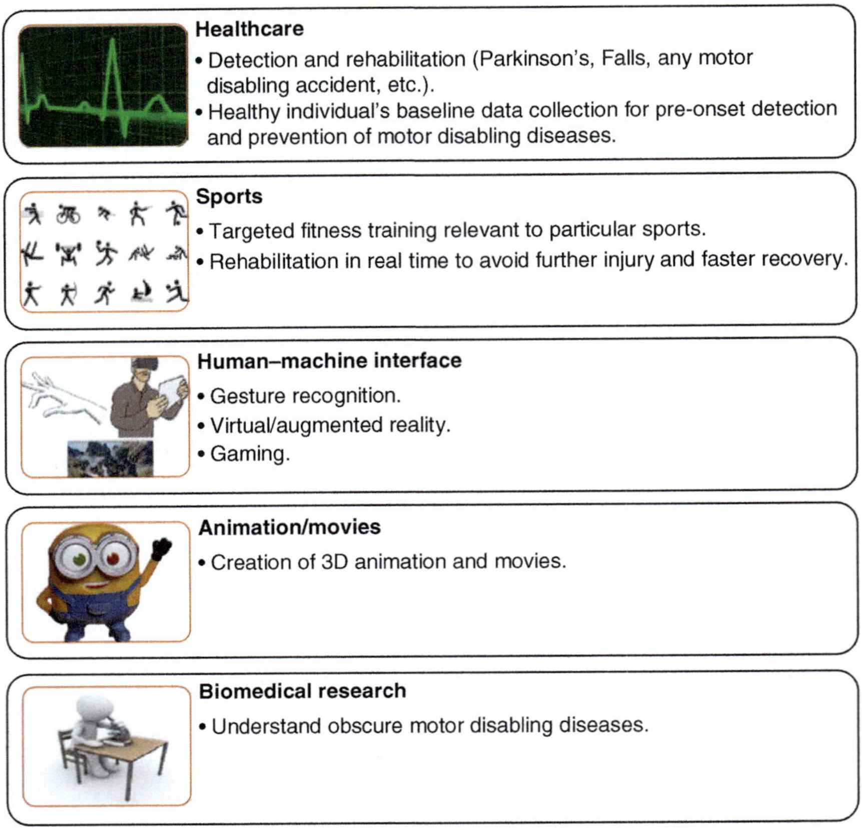

Figure 3.2 The promise of motion capture technology.

hours and intervals spent at the hospital/clinic. Using wearables, kinematics data can eventually be recorded in the individual's natural environment, enabling round-the-clock monitoring and real-time feedback on the rehabilitation program and patient performance. As another example, there are times when a patient may complain about pain or discomfort during certain hours of the day or while carrying out a specific activity. With wearable motion capture, it is possible to track such issues much easily, get to the root of the problem, and solve it more efficiently and faster. The importance of such data is immense for the future of personalized rehabilitation.

(b) *Preonset detection and prevention*: While the former class of applications encompasses patients suffering from motor disabling conditions, this second category accounts for healthy individuals who may be at risk of developing such conditions. This category is practically possible only through wearable motion capture technologies that can record continuous, real-time data related to one's motion. Such data captured over a period of time can form the baseline for a certain individual, while any deviation from the baseline will raise an alarm. By identifying the signature of any such deviation, it is possible to narrow down the possibility of a specific disease or condition that might have started to onset. Notably, such diagnostics may be feasible at a very early stage when they would otherwise go unnoticed. With preonset detection enabled by wearables, it becomes much easier to prevent and/or manage a disabling condition much more effectively.

Whether it is taking care of the diseased/injured or notifying healthy individuals of a possible upcoming motor disability, wearable motion capture technology has immense potential to transform human life as reflected in the healthcare arena.

3.2.2 Sports

Sports applications entail the fitness and training of players/athletes, as well as their rehabilitation when injured. As per today's "gold standard," it is possible to rehabilitate athletes with motion capture technology that is contrived to laboratory environments [4, 5]. However, completely wearable counterparts open up new opportunities in this sector. For example, with wearable motion capture technology, it is possible to monitor the motion of players in real time. In turn, it now becomes possible to develop quantifiable measures that assess fitness and performance pertinent to a particular sport. This may prevent injuries caused during training (e.g. due to the choice of wrong techniques with respect to the physical/health status of the player/athlete) and may help athletes optimize their performance. In case of injury, such wearable technology may readily provide a mechanism for personalized rehabilitation that uses real-time feedback and enables faster and more efficient recovery.

3.2.3 Human–Machine Interfaces

Interfaces that enable communication between humans and machines are all around us. Examples include computers (where interaction is made possible through keyboards, mouse, or touchscreen), mobile phones (where interaction is mostly through touch screens in modern devices and keypads in older ones), industrial equipment with interactive panels (interaction based on touch or haptic feedback or keypads), and measurement equipment found in laboratories (for example, oscilloscopes with the interaction mechanism relying on touch or keypads). However, human–machine interaction can be implemented via diverse other means, including noncontact methods. Gesture recognition is one such method where gestures made by humans are captured by machines as an input to generate a certain output. As would be expected, gesture recognition is linked to motion capture, and hence, wearable motion capture technology provides a big impetus for gesture recognition. Another exciting development is happening at the forefront of virtual and augmented reality [6–8] may that be for education, training, or rehabilitation purposes, among others. It is highly desirable to make such environments interactive, which can again be made possible by capturing human motion and providing it as input to the system. In doing so, wearable motion capture technology can enable much more seamless virtual and augmented reality systems than ever before. Finally, gaming is yet another area where virtual reality and gesture recognition hold prime importance [9] and, hence, necessitate the deployment of wearable motion capture technology.

3.2.4 Animation/Movies

Numerous animations/movies rely strongly on motion capture technology. Various scenes of movies such as the King Kong and the Lord of the Rings, for instance, have been filmed using optical camera-based technology (to be discussed in detail in the next section) in contrived settings [10]. It is none other than the motion capture technology that enables such exciting and entertaining marvels possible.

3.2.5 Biomedical Research

Motion capture technology, and especially its wearable versions, can prove highly useful in biomedical research to ultimately unravel the causes of diverse obscure motor disabling diseases and conditions. For instance, there are certain neural injuries that may cause changes in gait patterns, such as TBI [11]. Researchers have found some correlation between the two, as attributed to possible effects of the injury on parts of the brain that control motor functions [11]. However, ongoing research in the biomedical area is still trying to understand this complex problem [12], alongside several other conditions of similar nature that involve changes in motor patterns and/or motor disability.

In order to study and understand such phenomena, a typical methodology being used by clinicians is to form experimental and control groups of individuals; test their gait patterns based on diverse (application-specific) conditions and during regular intervals; and compare the results between the two groups [11, 12]. Limitations of such studies are obvious and relate to challenges in recruiting participants who are willing to visit a dedicated lab environment during the aforementioned regular intervals, as well as the restriction of these studies to contrived settings, which unavoidably restricts their duration. However, all these drawbacks can be eliminated if wearable motion capture technology were to be used. In the latter case, kinematics data can be captured in real time,

24 × 7, in the individuals' natural setting. Further to overcome the limitations above, wearable technology also provides large amounts of data to be eventually used for more thorough analysis and deeper understanding. Leveraging these big data and tools, such as machine learning, it will eventually be much easier to track down the exact cause of diverse types of motor disabling conditions.

3.3 Motion Capture in Contrived Settings

This section begins by discussing one of the most popular technologies used for motion capture in contrived settings, namely camera-based motion capture. The discussion is followed by a thorough overview of electromagnetics-based sensors for motion capture which may be radar-, Wi-Fi-, or radio-frequency identification (RFID) based. Next, medical imaging techniques, such as dual fluoroscopy and magnetic resonance imaging (MRI), are discussed within the framework of motion capture. At the end, some additional sensors/tools are reported which are typically limited in terms of kinematics monitoring capabilities and are most often used in conjunction with the aforementioned motion capture technologies.

3.3.1 Camera-Based Motion Capture Laboratory

Motion capture laboratories, also known as MoCap labs, employ cameras to capture motion. This technology operates at the intersection of three main areas, i.e. biomechanics, computer graphics, and computer vision [13]. Specifically, biomechanics serve to understand and interpret the kinematics, while computer graphics and computer vision serve to capture the motion and further process it to derive meaningful results. This technology may be of two types.

(a) *Marker based*: Marker-based systems are currently one of the most widespread and reliable means of capturing human motion. Typical resources required for such systems include a capture room, body suit(s) with markers (as is clear from the name), camera equipment, and an acquisition system [14]. A typical motion capture lab schematic, along with a subject in a motion capture suit inside motion capture lab and animation created from it, is shown in Figure 3.3. The capture room can neither be too small as it restricts the motion nor can it be too large as it is difficult to capture the markers for a fixed number of cameras [16]. Proper lighting is important for high-quality capture [14]. Markers are generally placed at locations where the skin is close to the bone, e.g. at joint locations [14], as a means of avoiding skin sliding. Along these lines, body suits are generally made of spandex [16] with markers attached to them. In turn, these markers can be of two types: (i) passive and (ii) active.

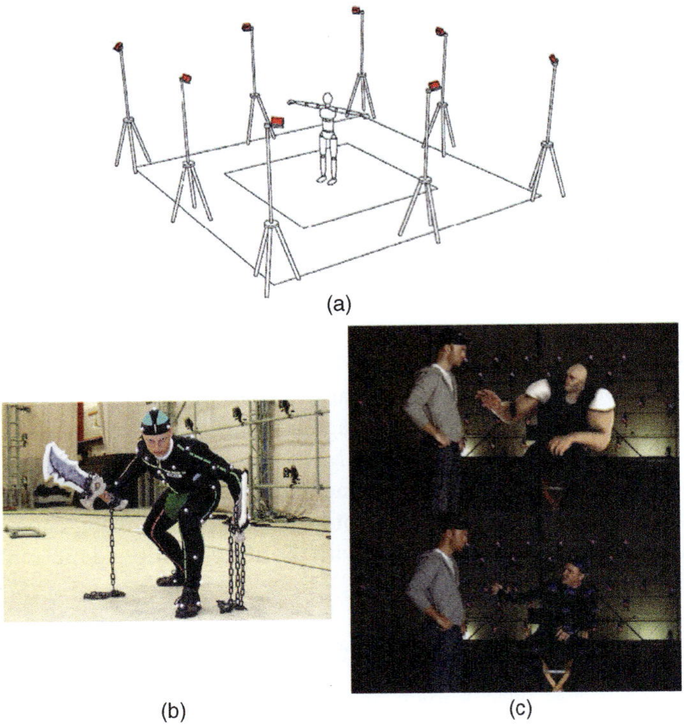

Figure 3.3 (a) Motion capture lab with cameras installed around and subject within capture area [15]. (b) Subject posing for the animation with motion capture suit (with markers) and cameras installed around. (c) Subject with motion capture suit (bottom) and animation produced by the technology (top).

Passive markers reflect off the light impinged by strobe lights fitted on the cameras (mainly infrared), hence enabling the tracking [16]. By contrast, active markers use LEDs (light emitting diodes) to shine light on the cameras. It is, thus, possible to change the frequency of active markers so that it becomes easier to track them [16]. However, this technology comes with a disadvantage: active markers have wires coming out, which, in turn, hinder with the individual's natural motion [16]. As for optical cameras, they typically operate in the infrared regime so as to reduce noise, given the minimal ambient interference in this spectrum [16].

Such cameras are placed all around within the capture room as shown in Figure 3.3. The operating principle is that motion is monitored from across different angles as a means of capturing an entire three-dimensional (3-D) view, sometimes also referred to as stereophotogrammetry [17]. Depending on the type of motion to be captured, the number of cameras may change. For instance, one or two cameras are generally enough to capture the human head motion, but a much larger number of cameras would be required to capture the complete motion of an individual running. Hence, in gist, multiple cameras located across the capture room record the real-time position of different markers placed across the human body, thereby generating the complete motion picture as a function of time. These details are acquired by the acquisition system and can be accessed using software on a computer.

Marker-based systems have been heavily used in the creation of movies and animations (e.g. the Avatar movie was made using this technology [16]). They have also found widespread application in the healthcare sector for applications ranging from rehabilitation to research on understanding various motor disabling conditions. The main advantages of marker-based MoCap labs lie in their accuracy and reliability because of which they are considered as the "gold standard" in the area. However, marker-based systems do suffer from several disadvantages, including operation in constrained environments, high cost, high susceptibility to line-of-sight problems (any obstacle between the camera and the person can completely obstruct the motion capture), and errors caused due to markers sliding on the skin. Some of the most popular commercially available systems are offered by Vicon [18], Qualisys [19], and OptiTrack [20].

(b) *Markerless*: As the name suggests, markerless camera-based motion capture does not rely on markers and hence is relatively easier to use as compared to its marker-based counterpart. This system utilizes infrared cameras along with depth-sensitive sensors [21] (can be viewed as compensation for markers) to capture human motion. Its evolution is mainly attributed to the gaming industry. This is because recent gaming platforms often necessitate motion capture and gesture recognition to integrate virtual reality capabilities and/or enable 3-D gaming experiences. As an example, a markerless system with subjects and corresponding output is depicted in Figure 3.4. However, even beyond gaming, the aforementioned markerless systems have frequently been translated to motion capture in diverse other applications, including the healthcare sector. For example, markerless camera-based motion capture has long been integrated with virtual reality to enhance the impact of rehabilitation [21].

The major advantage of markerless MoCap labs lies in their simplicity as compared to marker-based systems. There are versions that can be built just with a laptop, a webcam, and a software to capture motion. Since they do not require markers, such systems have the added advantage of not restricting natural motion and further adding to the convenience. Further, these systems cost much less than their marker-based counterparts. However, the above come at the expense of reduced accuracy and reliability as compared to

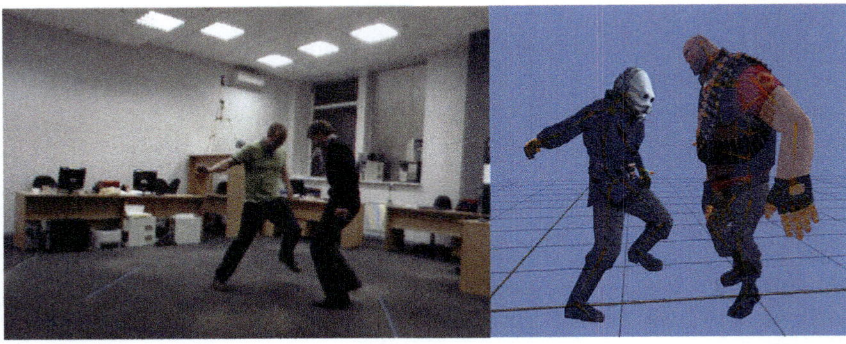

Figure 3.4 Markerless motion capture with subjects and its corresponding output.

marker-based systems. Also, similar to marker-based systems, markerless versions are also restrained to operation in confined spaces and are susceptible to line-of-sight problems. One of the most commonly used options is the Microsoft Kinect, which is derived from the Microsoft Xbox 360 gaming console [22]. There are other gaming consoles, such as the Sony PlayStation Move and the Nintendo Wii; however, the Microsoft Kinect is most often reported as a preferable choice [22]. Similar products include the Xtion Pro Live, Intel-Creative camera, and LeapMotion controller, but they have not been used as extensively as Kinect [22].

3.3.2 Electromagnetics-Based Sensors

Electromagnetics-based sensors rely on electromagnetic waves to capture human movement. Most of these technologies are still in the research phase, with only a few being close to commercialization (e.g. the Google Soli project discussed in the subsequent section). Sensors utilizing electromagnetic waves to capture human motion can be broadly categorized into three types: (i) RADAR-, (ii) Wi-Fi-, and (ii) RFID based.

3.3.2.1 RADAR Based

RADAR stands for RAdio Detection And Ranging. It is a well-known technique that utilizes transmitted and received electromagnetic waves to detect distance, angle, position, and other such information about an intended target. RADARs are most commonly used in defense, space, and weather applications (e.g. for aircraft, missile, or spacecraft detection). Depending on the application, RADAR operation can be modulated or unmodulated, and the frequency, bandwidth, and postprocessing approaches may differ.

When applied in the biomedical area, RADAR systems are sometimes also termed as bioradars. The latter have been reported for diverse application scenarios, including the monitoring of physiological signals (such as respiration and heart rate) and the detection of human motion (such as for gait analysis and activity classification [23]). The latter is more pertinent to our discussion in this chapter.

Doppler-based radars are shown to perform quite well for the detection of human movement [24] and gesture recognition [23]. As is clear from the name, human movement is captured in the received signal due to the Doppler effect (i.e. modulation in frequency as the target moves closer or away from the source). The system works using time–frequency analysis and capturing the micro-Doppler effects (i.e. additional frequency modulation with respect to time due to small changes such as different gestures or human movement) [23] (Figure 3.5g depicts one such example). In [24], the roots of this method are traced to the detection of human movement by Geisheimer et al. [26]. This work is followed by several studies, including the estimation of parameters related to human gait using FMCW (frequency-modulated continuous wave) radar [27]; the distinguishing between animals, humans, and vehicles [28–32]; and the classification of different activities such as walking, running, and crawling [24]. As we move to higher frequencies, higher resolution is possible, implying that radars can capture even fine motions, such as finger movement patterns. For instance, gesture recognition using FMCW radar has been demonstrated (i) at 60 GHz under the Google Soli project [25, 33] for human–machine interfaces (Figure 3.5a–f) and (ii) at 25 GHz at NVIDIA Research [34] for intelligent driver assistance systems. In order to recognize or distinguish between different activities or gestures, generally, a machine-learning technique is used. The latter models are trained using the data obtained from the RADARs.

The main advantage of RADAR-based motion capture is that it does not require any markers or sensors attached to the human body. This allows for unhindered natural motion similar to markerless camera-based systems. An added advantage is that RADARs can detect movement through nonmetallic obstacles (clothes, brick walls, or ruins), whereas this is not the case with markerless camera systems [35]. Notably, with the advancement in semiconductor technology and embedded systems, the size of RADARs has reduced considerably, making them portable [23]. Further, and as also stated earlier, operation at high frequencies improves resolution and allows monitoring of very fine movements. Despite these advantages, however, RADAR-based technology does suffer from certain limitations. Although it is possible to detect movement through walls, this is generally challenging because of the presence of environmental noise which may decrease the accuracy and resolution. Further, electromagnetic wave propagation is not possible through metallic obstacles. Finally, until RADARs can be miniaturized enough to be carried around easily (which has

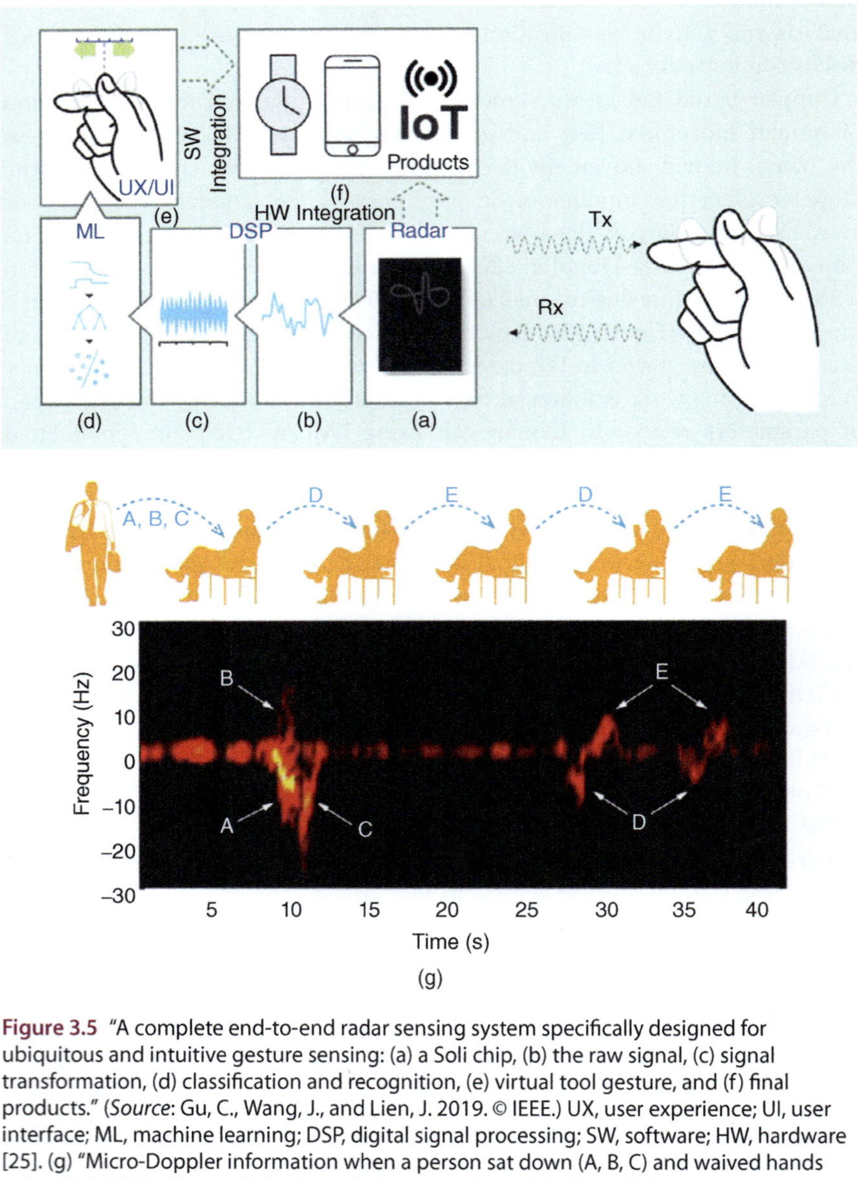

Figure 3.5 "A complete end-to-end radar sensing system specifically designed for ubiquitous and intuitive gesture sensing: (a) a Soli chip, (b) the raw signal, (c) signal transformation, (d) classification and recognition, (e) virtual tool gesture, and (f) final products." (*Source*: Gu, C., Wang, J., and Lien, J. 2019. © IEEE.) UX, user experience; UI, user interface; ML, machine learning; DSP, digital signal processing; SW, software; HW, hardware [25]. (g) "Micro-Doppler information when a person sat down (A, B, C) and waived hands twice (D, E)" [23]. (*Source*: Li, C., Peng, Z., Huang, T.-Y., et al., 2017. © IEEE.)

become possible now with the Google Soli project), this technique is restricted to fixed locations where the entire system is physically located.

3.3.2.2 Wi-Fi Based

Wi-Fi-based electromagnetic motion capture works in wireless environments, more specifically in environments with Wi-Fi signals. In [36], the roots of these systems are traced back to [37] where the concept of device-free passive localization was first introduced in wireless environments. Due to the presence of any entity (such as human) and his/her movement, RF signals (here Wi-Fi signals) will be affected. By tracking parameters such as signal strength and time of flight, entities can be localized and tracked [37]. Thus, Wi-Fi-based systems utilize the existing Wi-Fi infrastructure, and no sensor needs to be attached to the human body, hence the name device-free passive localization. There are other works by [38–40] based on RSSI (received signal strength indicator); however, these are limited to detection and localization only and, hence, are more geared toward surveillance. There are several other works along these lines which utilize the channel state information (CSI) combined with the RSS to obtain more information and achieve better detection [36]. A simplified schematic depicting the idea of detecting human movement using Wi-Fi is shown in Figure 3.6a. Also, once information of human movement captured in CSI (for instance) is received, it can be used in two different ways to retrieve information of movement from this data. Either pattern- or model-based method can be used to retrieve the required information (as explained in Figure 3.6b).

Over the years, such methods have been gradually applied to human activity recognition (such as walking and running) [42, 43] as well as gesture recognition. For instance, Pu et al. [44] demonstrated a system termed as WiSee which utilizes Wi-Fi signals for gesture recognition and relies on the Doppler shift as reported in RADAR-based methods. This system was demonstrated in home and office environments and was presented as an alternative to camera-based systems as it can monitor gestures and activity even through walls. This implies NLOS (non-line-of-sight) environments, such that movements can be tracked in private places (e.g. restrooms or bedrooms) where camera-based systems cannot be installed. Another system, namely AllSee, was demonstrated by Kellogg et al. [45] for gesture recognition, promising to utilize minimal power consumption in detecting gestures. This is achieved by utilizing the amplitude of environmental RF signals (such as TV or RFID) rather than the Doppler-based method. In another case, Wang et al. [46] demonstrated real-time fall detection for the elderly that utilized amplitude and phase (more important than amplitude here) information of the Wi-Fi CSI and an associated power profile. Features were extracted both in time and frequency domain. SVM (support vector machine), a machine-learning technique, was used to distinguish actual fall and fall-like activities in this work. In general, CSI-based and related methods have been utilized for different types of (behavioral) studies and have been nicely

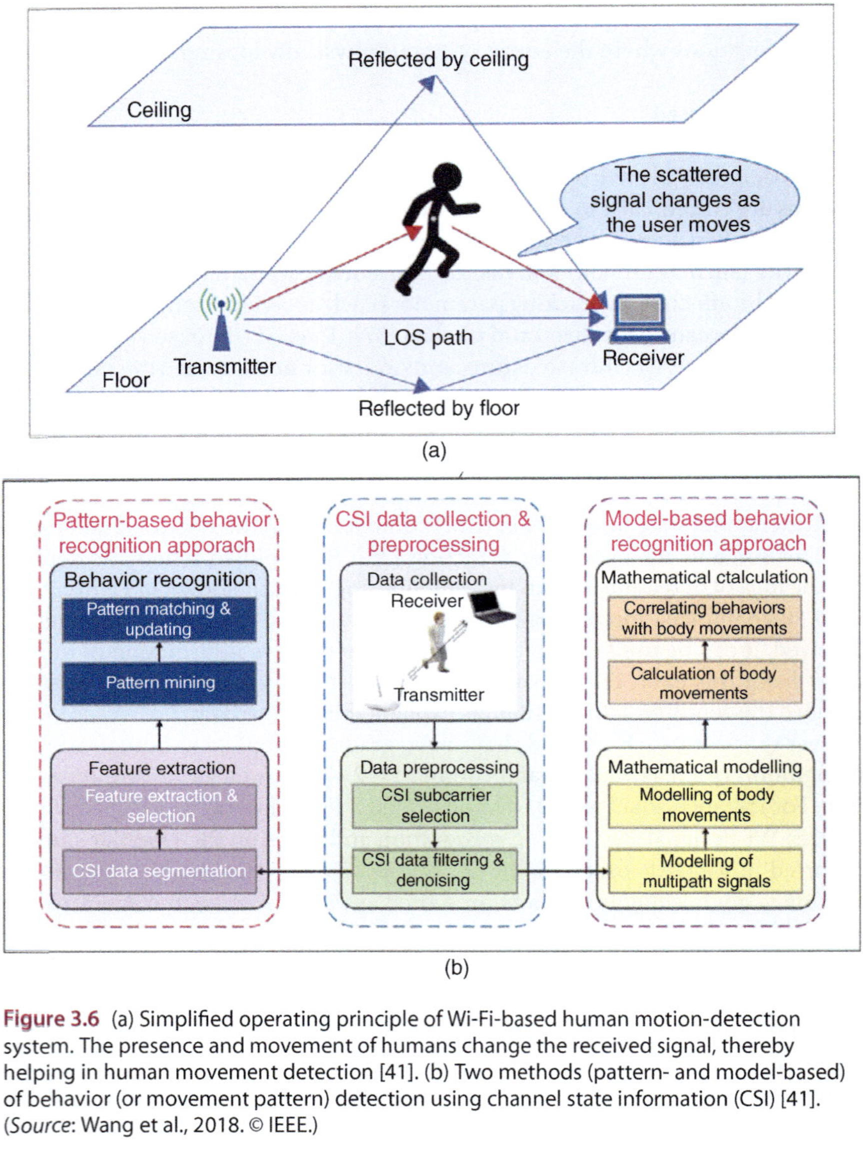

Figure 3.6 (a) Simplified operating principle of Wi-Fi-based human motion-detection system. The presence and movement of humans change the received signal, thereby helping in human movement detection [41]. (b) Two methods (pattern- and model-based) of behavior (or movement pattern) detection using channel state information (CSI) [41]. (*Source*: Wang et al., 2018. © IEEE.)

tabulated by Wang et al. [41]. In fact, both subtle behaviors such as breathing, respiration rate, and heart rate and pronounced movement (behaviors) such as hand motion, finger movement, lip reading (e.g. human talk), gait patterns, and human identity have been captured using this technology. There are several other works in this area, among which some of the recent ones are summarized in the guest editorials [47, 48].

The main advantage of Wi-Fi-based systems is that they allow for human motion capture without any sensor placed on the body. By contrast, these systems rely solely on the existing Wi-Fi (or similar) infrastructure. Nevertheless, this implies that such systems operate in contrived and wireless environments only. There are inherent challenges associated with the technology as well, such as (i) lack of fundamental theories that correlate CSI information and motion patterns, in turn limiting potential guidance toward robust system designs, (ii) difficulty in tackling noise, (iii) difficulty in capturing motion of multiple users and complex movements (due to different activities having similar profiles and leading to underdetermined systems of equations or ill-posed problems), and (iv) limited flexibility, meaning that the system is highly sensitive to changes in the environment (e.g. addition of any extra antenna or Wi-Fi access point or even a change in the arrangement of the room such as furniture) [41]. The above have restricted the technology from moving toward commercialization [41]. Nevertheless, Wi-Fi-based systems clearly have huge potential, and open challenges are currently being tackled in order to bring them to the service of the general public.

3.3.2.3 RFID Based

RFID-based systems are yet another way of capturing human motion by utilizing electromagnetic waves. Some preliminary proof-of-concept studies in the literature support this idea. For instance, one approach utilizes the amplitude information [49], while another approach utilizes the polarization information of RFID tags placed on the body [50] as a means of capturing motion. More specifically, Amendola et al. [49] placed passive RFID tags on different parts of the body. An external reader antenna was used to send electromagnetic waves which were subsequently backscattered by the body-worn RFID tags. These backscattered signals were shown to contain information related to motion (amplitude modulated by movement) which was collected and classified into different types of activities via machine-learning algorithms (Figure 3.7a, b). In the case of [50], the angle formed between the thigh and shank was measured using the polarization information captured by an external reader communicating with RFID tags placed on the thigh and shank. The results were further compared vs. camera-based motion capture and were shown to be in good agreement (Figure 3.7c,d).

As would be expected, RFID-based motion capture is restricted to contrived environments as a reader is always needed in the vicinity of the subject. Placement of RFID tags on the body segments and the need for a reader in close proximity make the requirements of this system very similar to those of marker-based MoCap labs. However, RFID-based motion capture does exhibit advantages over MoCap labs, as it enables (i) lower cost and (ii) uniquely identifiable tags which can, in turn, uniquely identify different body parts

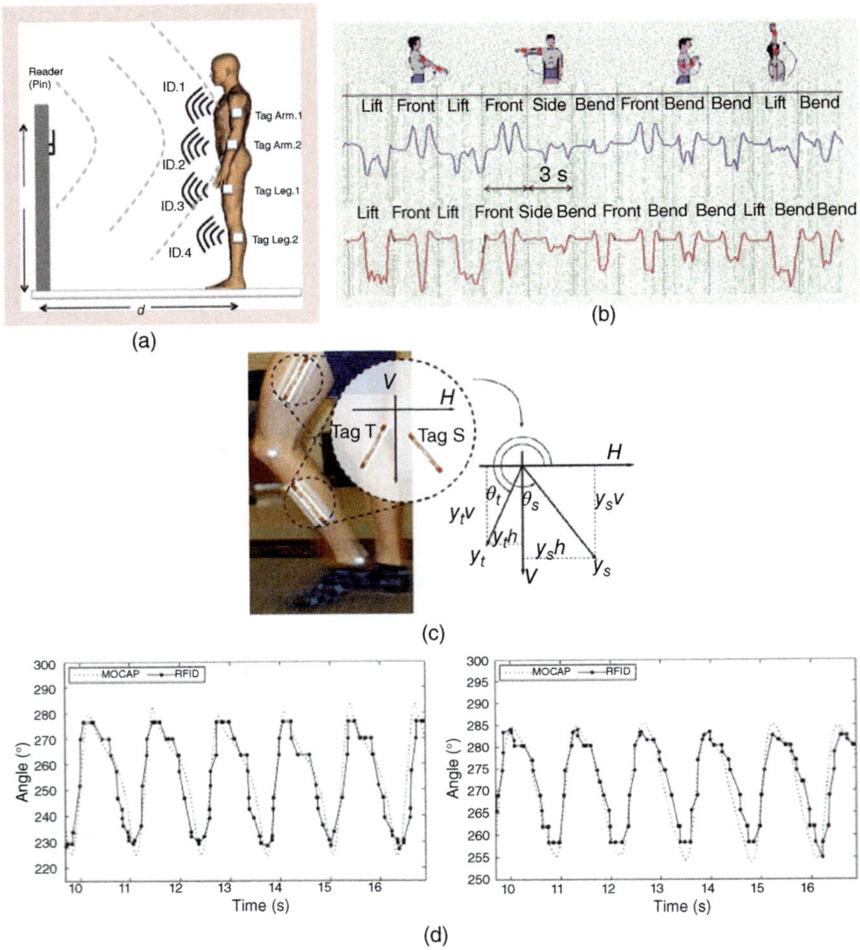

Figure 3.7 RFID-based human movement detection: (a) setup using amplitude information, (b) classification of different activities using this information [49]. (*Source*: Amendola, S., Bianchi, L., and Marrocco, G., 2015. © IEEE.) (c) Setup using polarization information, and (d) shank (left) and thigh (right) angles captured [50]. (*Source*: Krigslund, R., Dosen, S., Popovski, P., et al., 2013. © IEEE.)

(this is, however, also possible via active markers in the case of MoCap labs). Here, it is worth noting that results reported to date for RFID-based motion capture are proof of concept and have yet to be verified in practical settings. As such, reliability and accuracy of these systems still need to go through further research and testing.

3.3.3 Magnetic Motion Capture System

Magnetic motion capture systems generally consist of a transmitter and various receivers placed upon different parts of the body [51]: the transmitter generates a magnetic field, which is subsequently intercepted by the receivers. Given that receivers are body worn, movement of the human body in the presence of the external magnetic field (as generated by the transmitter) also changes the position of the receivers. Given the spatial variation of the receivers with respect to the transmitter, movement can be detected.

More specifically, both the transmitter and the receiver(s) of magnetic motion capture systems contain three orthogonal coils. Movement leads to change in the relative flux linkage, which, in turn, can be captured and postprocessed to monitor movement [52]. The presence of three orthogonal coils allows for both translation and orientation in 3-D, leading to information for all six degrees of freedom [51]. The received signals are filtered and amplified in the control unit and are then sent to a central computer where software is used to figure out the coordinates of movement [51]. These systems can work in two variants, i.e. under (i) DC (direct current) magnetic field and (ii) low-frequency AC (alternating current) magnetic field [51]. Here, it is interesting to note that apart from monitoring movement, magnetic motion capture systems also find application in real-time minimal invasive surgeries, for example to guide small biopsy needles to lesions [53].

As any other system, magnetic motion capture systems are associated with their own advantages and disadvantages. For instance, they are cheaper than optical camera-based systems and provide similar performance and with relatively less markers on the body [52], without suffering from line-of-sight issues (no occlusions). A disadvantage, however, is brought up in the case where receivers are tethered to a control unit. In doing so, subject mobility is restricted. Nevertheless, wireless versions of these systems are also available [54]. Another main drawback is the sensitivity of magnetic motion capture to the presence of metals in the building or the surrounding environment. This is attributed to the generation of eddy currents (in the presence of external magnetic fields) and the fields produced by them. Though algorithms exist to compensate for these effects, any related calibration would be only valid for a predefined scenario (for instance, specific metal structure used in the building) [51]. Hence, it is better to avoid proximity to metals while using these systems. Indeed, the brochure of the G4 by Polhemus, which relies on the aforementioned operating principle, clearly states that "Large metallic objects, such as desks or cabinets, located near the source or sensor, may adversely affect the performance of the system."[55] Examples of some of the commercially available systems include the Polhemus [56], TRACKLAB by FREEDSPACE [57], and, Ascension Technology Corporation [58] (acquired

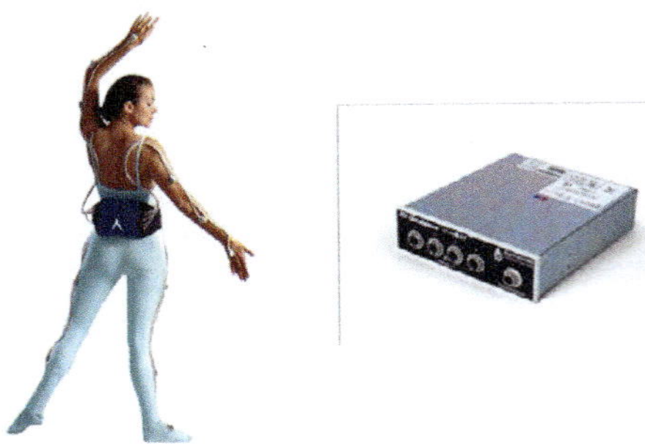

(a) (b)

Figure 3.8 Two different versions of the magnetic motion capture technology produced by Ascension Technology corporation (a) MotionStar™ Wireless and (b) driveBAY™. Images courtesy of Northern Digital Inc. (NDI)

by Roper Industries Inc.), becoming an affiliate company of NDI (Northern Digital Inc.) in 2012. These companies have different variants to choose from based on the need and application, i.e. ranging from subtle to swift movements. Figure 3.8 shows the evolution of two different versions of the system over the years, as reported by the Ascension Technology Corporation.

3.3.4 Imaging Methods

Conventional medical imaging methods such as CT (computed tomography) scans and MRI have been shown to capture human motion [59]. For instance, Li et al. [60] demonstrated measurement of in vivo knee joint kinematics using a dual fluoroscopic imaging system (which uses X-rays) (shown in Figure 3.9a), while [61] demonstrated 3-D lumbar spine posture measurements using MRI reconstruction (shown in Figure 3.9b). Advantages of such systems lie mainly in the accuracy with which different kinematics can be captured and for specific tasks where movement of bones/joints needs observation. However, these imaging methods are restricted to contrived environments and rely on machines that are typically quite heavy and expensive. In addition to the above, several of these methods (such as CT) use ionizing radiation, implying potential health risks and hence may not be applicable for day to day use of an individual.

3.3.5 Additional Sensors/Tools

This section discusses sensors/tools that are commonly used in the motion capture world. These are included separately as they either cannot capture all types of movement or are used as additional tools to the aforementioned motion capture technologies to provide complementary information.

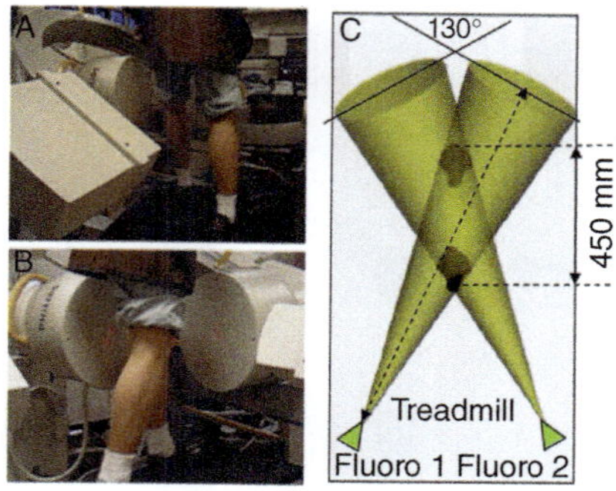

(a)

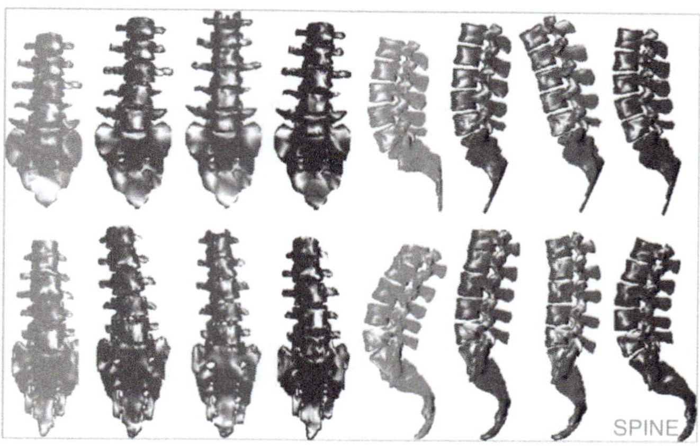

(b)

Figure 3.9 (a) Setup of the dual fluoroscopy imaging method used to capture gait patterns [60]. (*Source*: Li, G., Van de Velde, S. K., and Bingham, J. T., 2008. © Elsevier.) (b) Image showing how MRI images capture differences of lumbar spine during different postures (along row) for two different subjects (top and bottom) [61].

3.3.5.1 Goniometers

Goniometers are quite commonly used in clinical practice as a means of measuring the angles or range of motion (i.e. extreme angles to which a joint can bend and extend) of joints such as the knee and the elbow. For operation, the center of the goniometer is placed on the center of the joint of interest, while the arms of the goniometer are aligned with the body parts connected by the joint. One body part is then moved relative to the other along with the goniometer. During the process, the center of the goniometer and the joint should remain

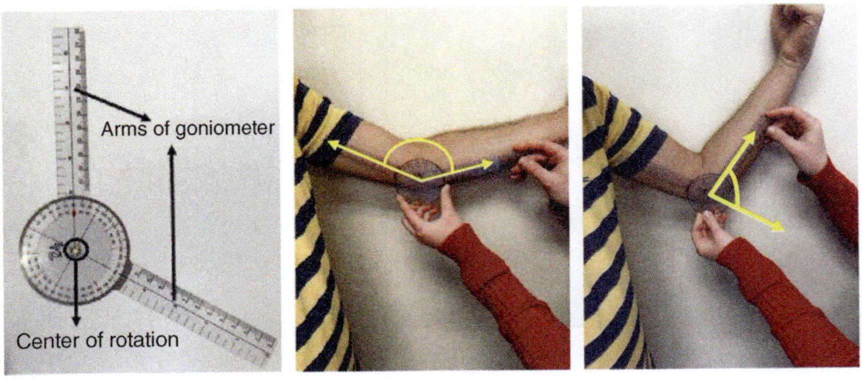

(a) (b) (c)

Figure 3.10 (a) A simple manual goniometer. (b) and (c) Measurements of elbow joint using goniometer at two different flexion angles and using two different conventions.

aligned. Concurrently, the arms of the goniometer should remain aligned with the body parts. In doing so, the angle recorded by the goniometer provides a measurement of the corresponding angle formed between the two body parts under consideration. For instance, to measure flexion (bend) angle of the elbow joint, the center of the goniometer should be aligned with the center of the elbow joint, and the two arms of the goniometer should be aligned with the forearm and upper arm, respectively. The flexion (bend) angle can be measured by keeping the goniometer aligned at the center and moving its two arms along with the two limbs as the elbow flexes (or arms bend about elbow) or extends. As an example, a simple manual goniometer and a setup of a goniometer measuring elbow flexion for two different flexion angles are shown in Figure 3.10.

Goniometers are available in different variants and sizes and can be made of plastic or metal. They are quite cheap and serve the purpose of day-to-day use. Electronic variants are also commercially available. Though quite costly, the latter can be used to monitor more specific tasks that require higher accuracy and precision. To name a few, commercial electronic goniometers are currently available by Biometrics Ltd., JTECH Medical, and ADINSTRUMENTS, among others [62–64].

3.3.5.2 Force Plates

Force plates rely on transducers to measure triaxial forces [65] and are typically placed on treadmills or on the ground so that the individual can stand/walk on them. To serve as transducers, strain gauges, piezoelectric/piezoresistive sensors, and capacitive gauges can be used [66]. Two or multiple force plates (sometimes also referred to as load cells) are typically placed side by side and serve to capture the reaction forces as the person walks or runs on them. Using

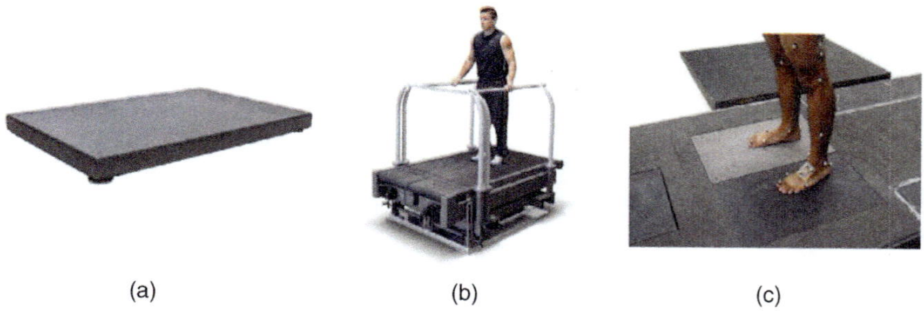

Figure 3.11 (a) Force plate. (b) Force plate integrated in treadmill to aid in gait analysis, both (a) and (b) produced by BERTEC. (c) Force plates used along with MoCap system (markers can be seen in the figure) to aid in measurements.

such force data, different parameters related to gait can be measured [67]. However, force plates cannot provide the complete picture of motion and, hence, are generally used in conjunction with other systems, such as camera-based motion capture (Figure 3.11).

3.4 Wearable Motion Capture (Noncontrived Settings)

This section is dedicated to wearable motion capture, the advantages of which have become obvious from the discussion in Section 3.2. Similar to contrived motion capture technology outlined in Section 3.3, there are several wearable or noncontrived motion capture technologies reported to date. We begin with one of the most popular technologies, namely inertial measurement units (IMUs), followed by discussion on bending/deformation-based, time-of-flight, and RSS-based sensors.

3.4.1 Inertial Measurement Units (IMUs)

IMUs are most often composed of an accelerometer and a gyroscope. The former serves to measure the sum of gravitational and inertial linear acceleration, while the latter measures angular velocity [68]. IMUs are also termed as inertial sensors as they utilize the principle of inertia [68]. Sometimes, they are further combined with a magnetometer which provides information about the local magnetic field vector components. In such cases, IMUs are often termed as MIMUs (or magnetic inertial measurement units) [68]. Single-, dual-, and triaxial sensors exist for the above. In the triaxial case, the three sensing axes are mutually orthogonal [68], serving to provide three degrees of freedom for the accelerometer, gyroscope, and magnetometer [69].

To capture motion, IMUs are first calibrated and then placed on different parts of the human body. The goal is to detect the orientation of diverse

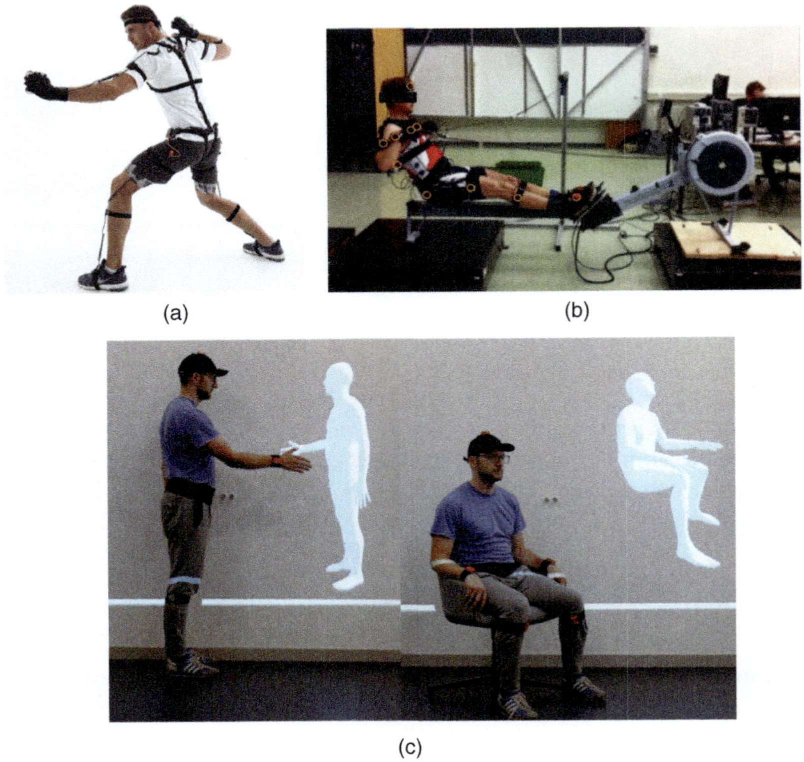

Figure 3.12 (a) IMUs produced by Noitom. (b) XSENS IMUs used to measure rower's center of mass horizontal acceleration (orange circles denote the visible IMUs on body of the subject) [72]. (*Source*: Lintmeijer, L. L., Faber, G. S., Kruk, H. R. et al., 2018. Taylor & Francis Group). (c) Reconstruction of human pose using IMUs [73]. (*Source*: Huang, Y., Kaufmann, M., Aksan, E. et al., 2018).

body segments and, eventually, monitor motion. This is mentioned in a very simple way here; however, the process of deriving motion from IMUs is highly complex, and there are several methods of doing so [68, 70, 71] (for visualization, Figure 3.12 [72, 73] depicts IMUs on the human body and their use in two different example applications). More specifically, IMUs rely strongly on the accelerometer data which can be integrated once and twice to obtain velocity and position, respectively. Similarly, the gyroscope provides angular velocity, which can be integrated and differentiated to obtain angular position and angular acceleration, respectively. Expectedly, the aim is to determine the orientation of the rigid body on which the sensor is placed. This can be achieved solely by the accelerometer itself; however, combination of the information obtained by the accelerometer and gyroscope can help in determining the body's orientation more accurately and precisely. Nevertheless, the aforementioned process of integration introduces errors, which further cause the sensors to drift. This is one of the biggest disadvantages of IMUs, with drift issues increasing linearly (integrated once) or quadratically (integrated twice) with time [68]. For mitigation, hardware and/or algorithmic solutions may be pursued [70]. Notably, the magnetometer becomes handy here as a hardware solution which provides an additional reference (i.e. using the local earth's magnetic field). But, unfortunately, magnetometers are susceptible to magnetic interference from the environment and the presence of ferromagnetic materials. As an alternative, algorithmic-based or combined hardware and algorithmic solutions may be used. Another source of error inherent to IMUs relates to the movement of sensor with respect to the skin which introduces soft body artifacts [68] (note that, while obtaining the data, rigid body assumptions are made that do not take skin movements into account). In addition to the above, IMUs are reported as not injury safe [74].

Though IMUs are commonly encountered in navigation systems (airplanes, missiles, spacecrafts, etc.) and smartphones (the reason why smartphones can detect and respond to changes in the phone's orientation and any acceleration), our focus in this section is primarily on human motion capture. Literature describes IMUs as wearable and cost-effective alternatives to Mocap labs (discussed in Section 3.1), while certain works [71] are referring to IMUs as a contemporary of optical camera-based systems. Being a wearable technology, IMUs allow for real-time motion capture in noncontrived settings and, hence, find application in healthcare, sports, gesture recognition, and more. With the advent of MEMS-based IMUs, they are expected to ultimately become increasingly popular for diverse motion capture applications [71]. Commercially available IMUs are currently provided by XSENS [75], APDM wearable technologies [76], TDK InvenSense [77], TRIVISIO [78], NOITM [79], and many more.

3.4.2 Bending/Deformation Sensors

Bending/deformation sensors are typically worn over the joint to be monitored. During motion of the joint, the sensor gets bent/deformed, and this mechanical deformation is further sensed as a means of quantifying movement. Depending on their operating principle, bending/deformation sensors can be subdivided into two types, i.e. strain based (further subdivided as resistance- and permeability based) and fiber-optic based.

3.4.2.1 Strain Based

Strain-sensing sensors, when placed on joints or body parts, experience variable strain with different movements. This strain gets reflected as either change in resistance (piezoresistive) or change in inductance (permeability) (Villari effect) and can serve to monitor human motion, as detailed below.

(a) *Resistance based:* In 2004, Gibbs and Asada [80] demonstrated the feasibility of integrating conductive fibers into stretchable fabrics. These fabrics can be worn such that the integrated conductive fibers cover the joint (for instance, upon knee or hip, as shown by Gibbs and Asada [80]) and stretch or contract along with the joint. In doing so, stretching of the conductive fabric changes its resistance. In turn, these resistance changes are further monitored for conversion into the corresponding movement (for instance, knee joint flexion/extension angles or hip joint flexion/extension and abduction/adduction movements). Related sensor designs can be of either single axis (measuring movement along one direction) or multiaxis (measuring movement along multiple directions). As would be expected, resistance-based sensors are not limited to conductive fiber-based solutions, and their performance ultimately depends on how well they can be manufactured by material scientists. Indeed, with recent advances in technology, numerous sensitive sensors have been reported that operate on the resistance-based principle. For example, Carbon nanotubes (CNTs) have been shown to measure stretch (or strain) from 410% [81] to 900% [82] at high sensitivity. In doing so, a wide range of kinematics activities can be monitored. For example, Li et al. [81] demonstrated hand (finger) motion capture with CNT-based sensors and its use to control mechanical hand movement (shown in Figure 3.13a), while [82] demonstrated both finger and arm motion capture. It was demonstrated in [82] that CNT-based sensors can be used biaxially to monitor movement in two different directions as their strain is almost independent in those two directions. Another example of resistance-based sensors entails the use of graphene-based fibers. It was shown in [84] that such sensors can have very high sensitivity, detecting deformations as small as 0.2% (and up to 30%), which can be used to monitor subtle motions such as breathing, phonation, expression changes, and pulse. In another case, Cheng et al. [83] reported graphene-based sensors which are capable of monitoring from 0.2% to 100% strain and, hence, were shown to capture not just subtle movements (e.g. pulse monitoring and speech recognition) but also vigorous movements (e.g. walking, jogging and jumping), shown in Figure 3.13b–d.
Resistance-based sensors have several advantages in terms of being conformal, having no line-of-sight issues, exhibiting high sensitivity, and demonstrating strong potential for easy integration into fabrics toward seamless kinematics monitoring. However, they suffer from certain disadvantages. For instance, there is an appreciable finite response time associated with the sensors' mechanical strain response (100 ms [83] to

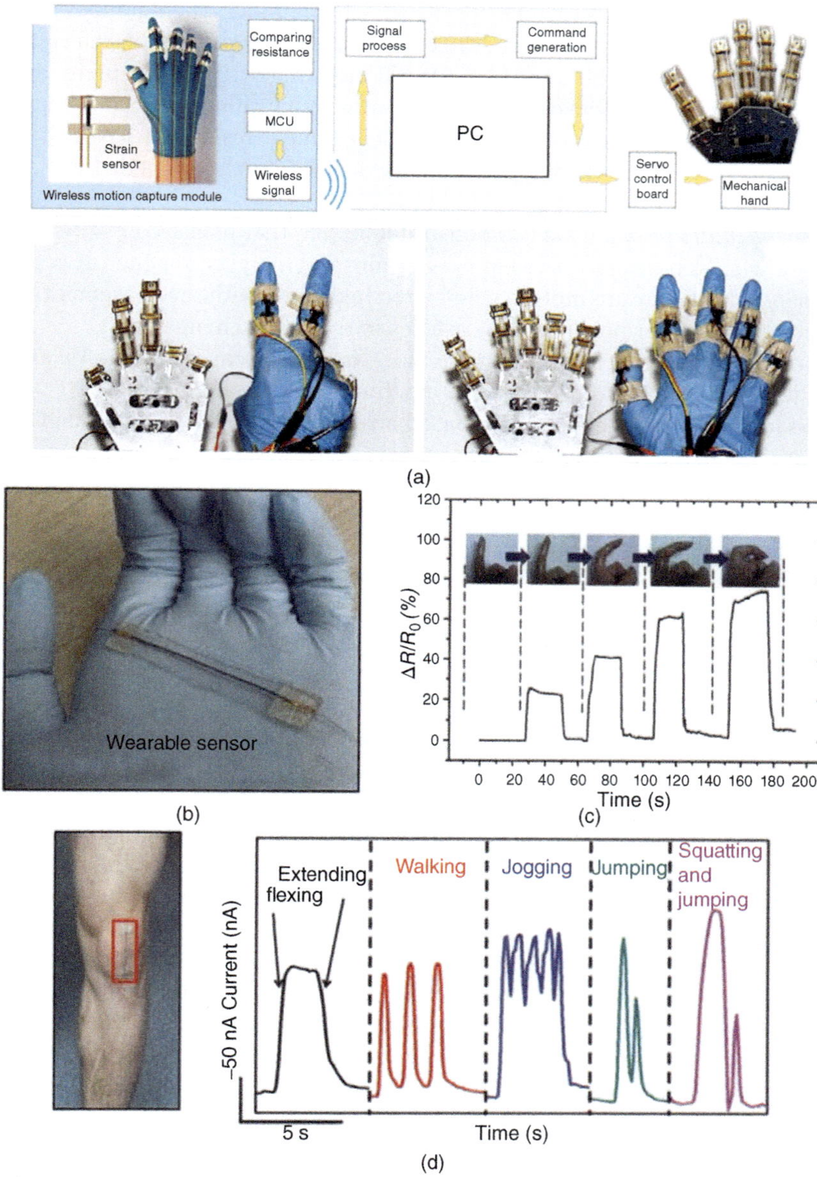

Figure 3.13 (a) Human hand motion capture using CNT-based strain sensor and its use to control movement of a mechanical hand (top) and demonstration of controlling mechanical hand gesture using human hand (bottom) [81]. (*Source*: Li C., Cui, Y.-L., Tian, L. et al., 2015.) (b) Graphene-based wearable sensor and its use to capture movements ranging from (c) finger movement to (d) knee movement (captures different activities such as walking, jogging, jumping, and squatting and jumping) [83]. (*Source*: Cheng, Y., Wang, R., Sun, J., et al., 2015.)

0.5 s [81] even for advanced techniques), which hinders their ability to capture fast movements. Also, since strain-based sensors are placed right on the joint, they tend to restrict natural motion. Further, the repetitive stretching of these sensors restricts the maximum number of cycles they can withstand (typically to ~10,000 cycles). Finally, resistance-based sensors often suffer from hysteresis effects which further impede their widespread deployment.

(b) *Permeability based*: It was demonstrated in [85] that planar coil sandwiched between flexible polyester film and metglass magnetostrictive material can capture motion when stretched along with the movement. The operating principle in this case lies in recording changes in permeability (reflected in the inductance values), as caused by the Villari effect. Permeability-based sensors exhibit similar advantages and disadvantages as the resistance-based ones. However, they are at much earlier stages of development as compared to resistance-based sensors.

3.4.2.2 Fiber Optics Based

There are different variants of fiber optics-based sensors used for motion capture. One variant relies on the optical fiber's place on the body part to be monitored and across the joint and measures the change in optical intensity as the fiber deforms. For instance, Nishiyama and Watanabe [86] employed hetero-core fiber optic sensors that utilized single-mode transmission fibers integrated into gloves to monitor joint flexion. Single-mode fibers were selected as opposed to multimode ones, given the limitations involved in conventional cases, such as Fiber Bragg Gratings being temperature dependent and cost-inefficient, and plastic optical fibers exhibiting limited stability. Nevertheless, Donno et al. [87] point out that utilizing the change in attenuation of the transmitted light as the fiber bends along with the joint presents several challenges because of variable losses caused by factors other than joint motion. To this effect, Donno et al. [87] demonstrated an alternative technique that uses intensity modulation of a laser beam in a single-mode fiber due to change in polarization (Figure 3.14a and its test setup in Figure 3.14b). This is caused by controlled birefringence induced by joint motion. As another example, Guo et al. [88] developed dye-doped polydimethylsiloxane optical fibers which can detect the strain caused due to joint motion by changes in the absorption of light passing through it. In this case, the sensor can be characterized like a strain-based sensor per Section 3.4.2.1, except that here optical loss is used instead of change in resistance or permeability (Figure 3.14c).

This technology does not face line-of-sight issues. It also has advantages in terms of performance but is still in exploratory phase. One of its disadvantages is that, when implemented on cloth, the performance is highly susceptible to any wrinkles present or created on the fabric [86]. In general, this technology seems promising but is still restricted in terms of practical implementation as

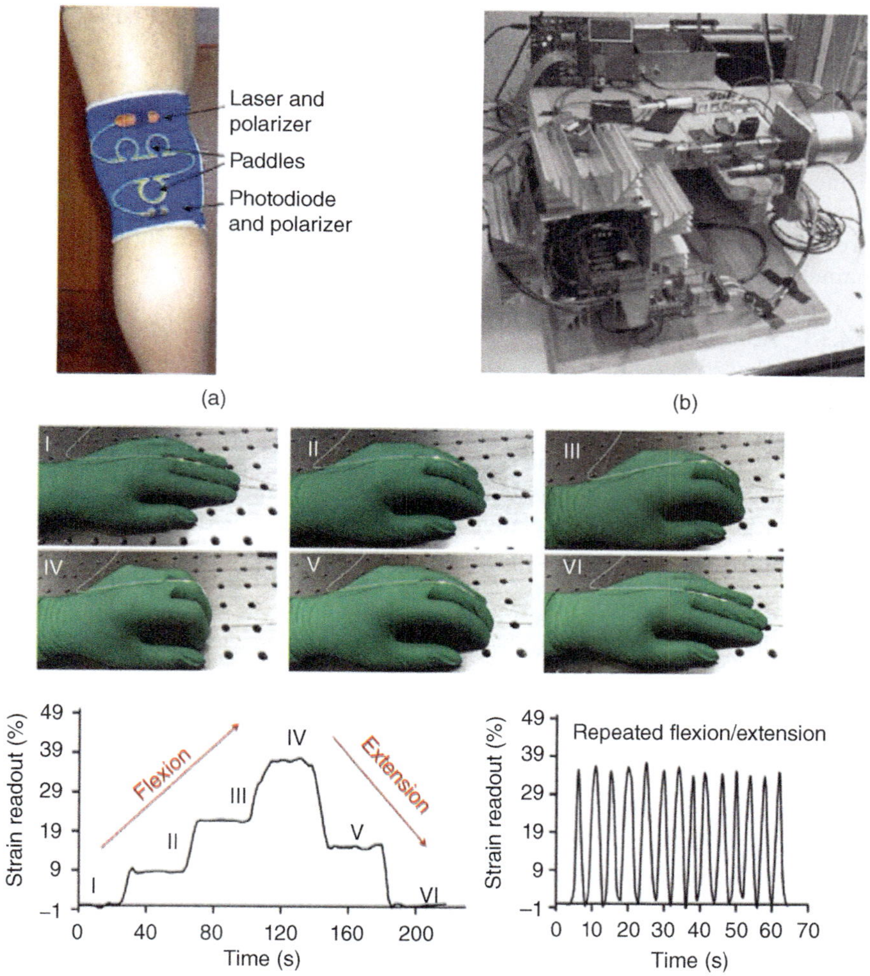

Figure 3.14 (a) Polarization-based fiber optic wearable joint sensor [87]. (*Source*: Donno, M., Palange, E., Di Nicola, F., et al., 2008.) (b) Setup used to perform measurements. (c) Fiber optics-based strain sensor shown to record finger movements (flexion (I–IV) and extension (V and VI)) (top) and corresponding result (bottom left) and for repeated flexion and extension (bottom right) [88]. (*Source*: Guo, J., Niu, M., and Yang, C., 2017.)

optical measurement devices are generally bulky (see Figure 3.14b) and costly and require very precise and controlled environments. However, the technology can become more pragmatic to apply in future when optical-based measurements are far less cheap and lightweight.

3.4.3 Time-of-Flight (TOF) Sensors

Time-of-flight sensors work on the principle of measuring distance using the time of flight of the signal given that speed of the signal is already known. There are mainly two different variants of these systems available in the literature, namely, acoustic and radio based.

3.4.3.1 Acoustic Based

Acoustic-based systems rely on the process of lateration, viz. estimation of the position by measuring the distance using multiple reference points. For instance, the global positioning system (GPS) uses this same process to track our position on earth, in which case the reference points are satellites. To better understand this concept, one can consider an example of tracking a target's position in a 2-D plane. To accurately predict the position, each transmitter will create a circle around the target (transmitter's coverage area). On a plane, if we can have three circles (using three transmitters), then these three circles will intersect at a unique point, the location of the target. So, for 2-D localization we need three references, for 3-D we need four references, and so on.

Utilizing a similar principle, acoustic transmitters and receivers can be used to track the position of different parts of the body, thereby enabling motion capture. For instance, contrived systems have been reported that entail either a fixed transmitter and a mobile receiver [89] (for target movement tracking) or a fixed receiver and a mobile transmitter [90] (for 3-D foot displacement) (Figure 3.15a–d). A wearable counterpart of such systems has been demonstrated by [91]. In this work, both the transmitter and receiver were located on the body, and their distance was calculated based on the time of flight which, when combined with lateration (example of lateration here is depicted in Figure 3.15e), provided the position of the body parts.

When used with a fixed frame of reference, acoustic-based systems can produce good results, much like the case of GPS. However, usage of these systems is most often limited to contrived settings. When translated into wearable versions, errors creep in as the reference points are no longer fixed [91]. Further to the above, acoustic-based systems are also sensitive to line-of-sight issues and are relatively big in size to be completely used as wearables (Figure 3.15c, d).

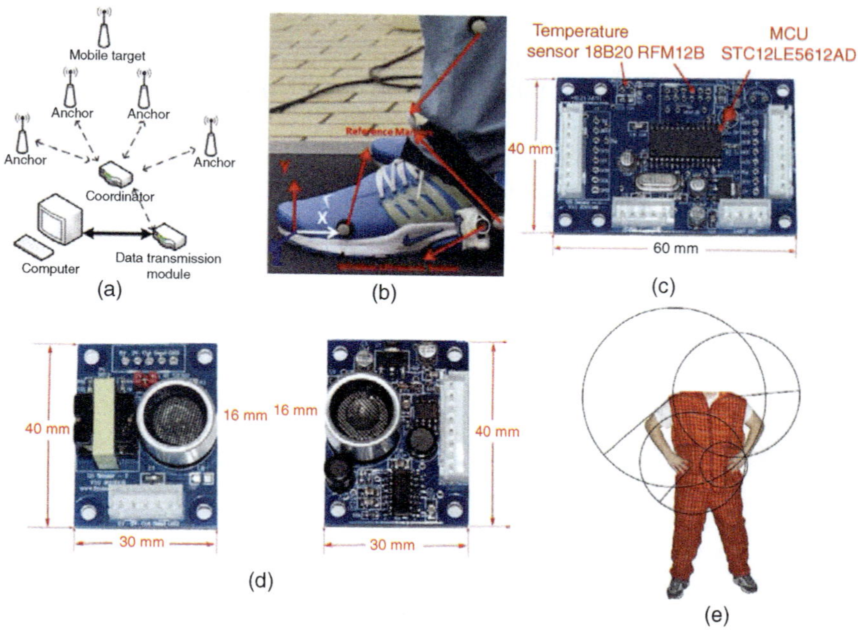

Figure 3.15 (a) Architecture of acoustic-based time-of-flight sensor with both fixed (hence not completely wearable) and mobile anchors. (b) Mobile anchor (with ultrasonic transmitter, controller, and reflective markers (for reference measurements using MoCaps) placed on shoes). (c) Ultrasonic controller. (d) Ultrasonic transmitter and receiver [90]. (*Source*: Qi, Y., Soh, C.B., Gunawan, E., et al., 2015. © IEEE.) (e) Complete wearable version of acoustic-based method depicting how four spheres intersect at a point to determine the target's position (lateration) [91]. (*Source*: Einsmann, C., Quirk, M., Muzal, B., et al., 2015. © IEEE.)

3.4.3.2 Radio Based

Radio-based systems again utilize the time-of-arrival technique to assess distance, but their operating principle is different than that discussed for acoustic-based systems. In [91], the authors mention that UWB radios can be used to implement wearable systems for motion capture using the lateration technique. However, this approach has yet to be demonstrated in practice. A feasibility study of UWB radios used for human motion capture has been reported by Di Renzo et al. [92]. This work studied the interaction of UWB electromagnetic pulses and the human body, the associated modeling, and the performance of different algorithms in the presence of pulse distortion and receiver noise. In another work, Hamie et al. [93] demonstrated the use of impulse radio-ultra wideband (IR-UWB) and narrowband technology (at 2.4 GHz) as a means of acquiring the time-of-arrival information when also combined with RSSI. The goal was to demonstrate large-scale individual motion capture functionality using two different algorithms. In this case, nodes were located both on body and off body, and hence, the system could not be considered as a truly wearable one. By contrast, Qi et al. [94] did demonstrate a wearable system, where two UWB radios were shown to monitor joint angles (knee or elbow). In this case, the transmitter and receiver were placed on the two sides of the joint, and the time-of-arrival principle was used to estimate the distance between the two. The latter was then used to predict the angle formed between the body parts using the trigonometry law of cosines (Figure 3.16).

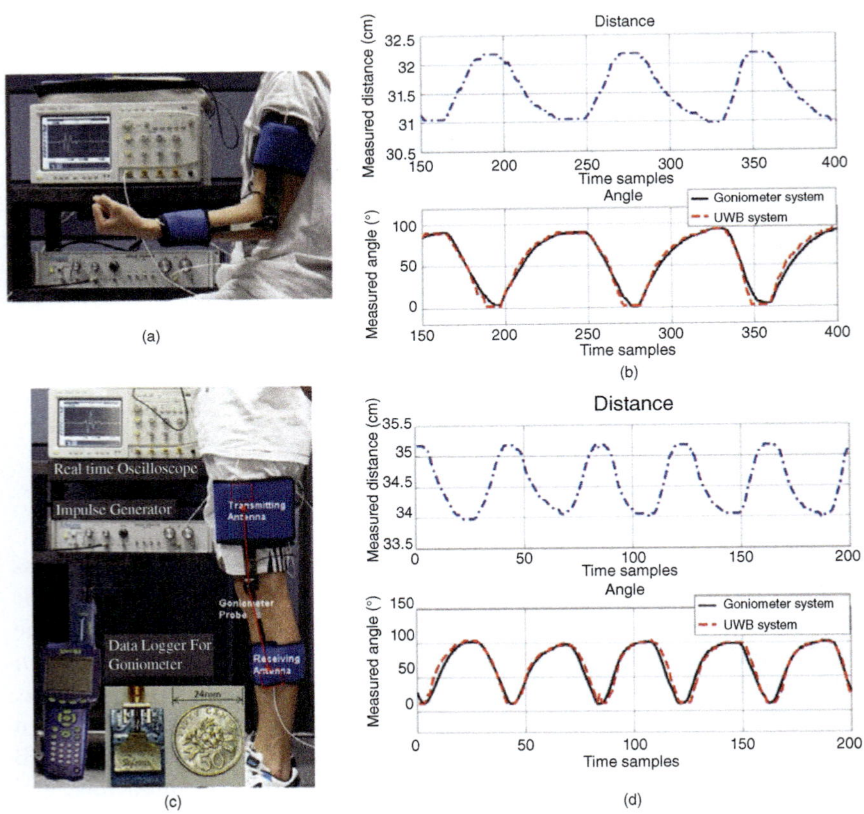

Figure 3.16 (a) Experimental setup to capture elbow flexion/extension and (b) the corresponding result compared against goniometer system. (c) Experimental setup for knee flexion/extension and (d) the corresponding result compared against goniometer system. Impulse generator is used to send impulse using UWB radio, and the received signal is captured on oscilloscope to perform further calculations [94]. (*Source*: Qi, Y., Soh, C.B., Gunawan, E., et al., 2014. © IEEE.)

Much like the acoustic-based systems, radio-based systems can be implemented via wearable versions and employed in noncontrived settings. However, radio-based systems suffer from line-of-sight issues, are of relatively large size, and also susceptible to channel variation (both because of the environment and human tissue property changes) and are still at a nascent stage of research.

3.4.4 Received Signal Strength-based Sensors

In RSS-based sensors, transmitting and receiving nodes are placed upon different parts of the human body. When the body is moving, the RSS across the nodes changes, in turn serving to quantify the corresponding motion. These sensors can be categorized into two types, namely antenna- and magnetoinductive sensors/electrically small loop antenna based.

3.4.4.1 Antenna Based

A 2.4-GHz antenna-based wearable system was reported in [95] wherein the transmitter was placed on the front side of the waist, and receivers were placed on the forearm, upper arm, thigh, and shank (Figure 3.17a). The RSS was monitored, and machine-learning classification techniques (support vector machine (SVM) and K-nearest neighbor [K-NN]) were used to classify different activities, such as different types of arm and leg movements (Figure 3.17b). In another case, Mishra and Kiourti [96] showed that two loop antennas working at 927 MHz can be wrapped around the human limbs (legs or arms) and across the joint, with one serving as a transmitter and the other as a receiver. With flexion/extension, the RSS or transmission coefficient ($|S_{21}|$) changes and can be used to monitor the corresponding movement. Such designs are advantageous as they can readily be implemented via conductive e-threads and, hence, seamlessly integrated into garments, thereby considerably reducing the size, weight, and cost and significantly improving the mobility of the subject. Notably, studies indicate that antennas based on e-threads around these frequencies exhibit similar electromagnetic performance to their copper equivalents [97].

Antenna-based technology is a clear example of capturing human motion in noncontrived settings. However, it does suffer from certain disadvantages. Antennas can be of relatively large size and hence difficult to integrate as complete wearables (especially at low frequencies of operation). This can be resolved using e-threads to fabricate wearable antennas as demonstrated in [96]. Still, antennas use electromagnetic waves (i.e. the radiative region of operation), which is susceptible to line-of-sight issues, and suffer significant loss during transmission through tissues. Also, their performance varies with changes in human tissue properties, which are known to occur from one individual to another and from time to time for the same individual. A solution for this would be to move to the inductive region of operation, as discussed

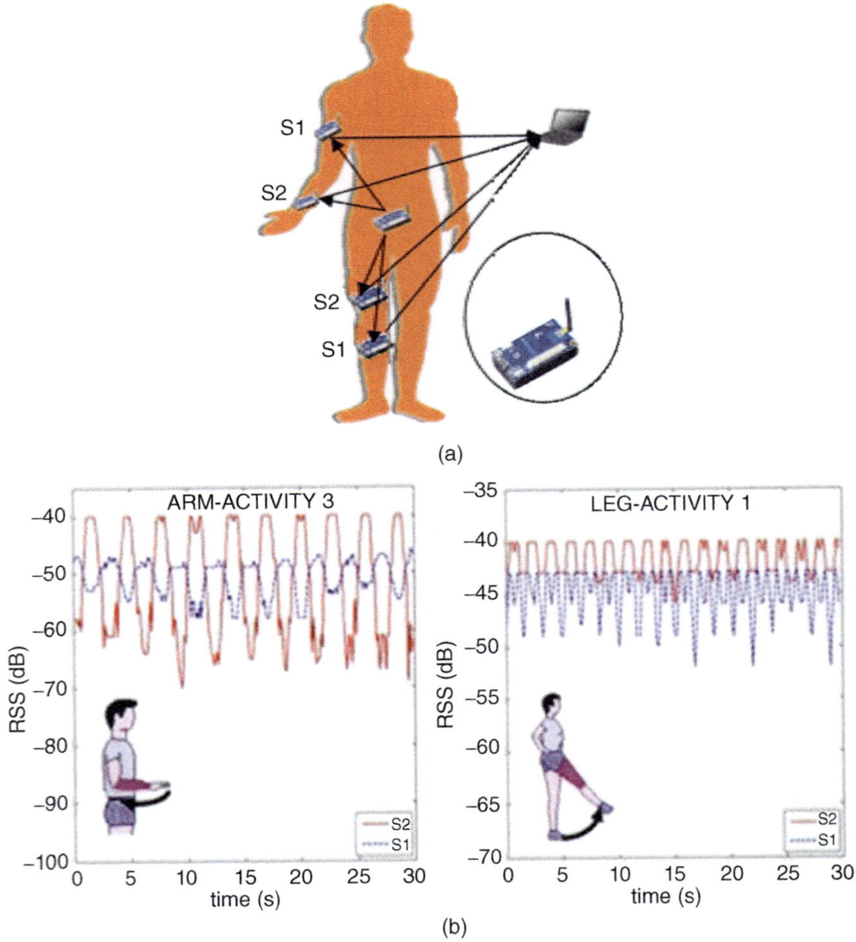

Figure 3.17 (a) Setup used to classify different activities involving arm and leg wherein transmitter (Tx) is placed on the front waist, while two receivers are placed both across elbow and knee joints [95]. (b) Results for received signal strength (RSS) vs. time for two different activities performed using arm and leg obtained via the setup shown in (a). [95]. (*Source*: Guraliuc, A. R., Barsocchi, P., Potortì, F., et al., 2011. © IEEE.)

in the following subsection. Also, operation of antenna-based motion capture in an already overloaded frequency spectrum can lead to interference and, in fact, can saturate the receiver and severely degrade the performance.

3.4.4.2 Magnetoinductive Sensors/Electrically Small Loop Antennas

Wearable magnetoinductive sensors have been introduced quite recently and, as clear from the name, are based on the principle of Faraday's law of magnetic

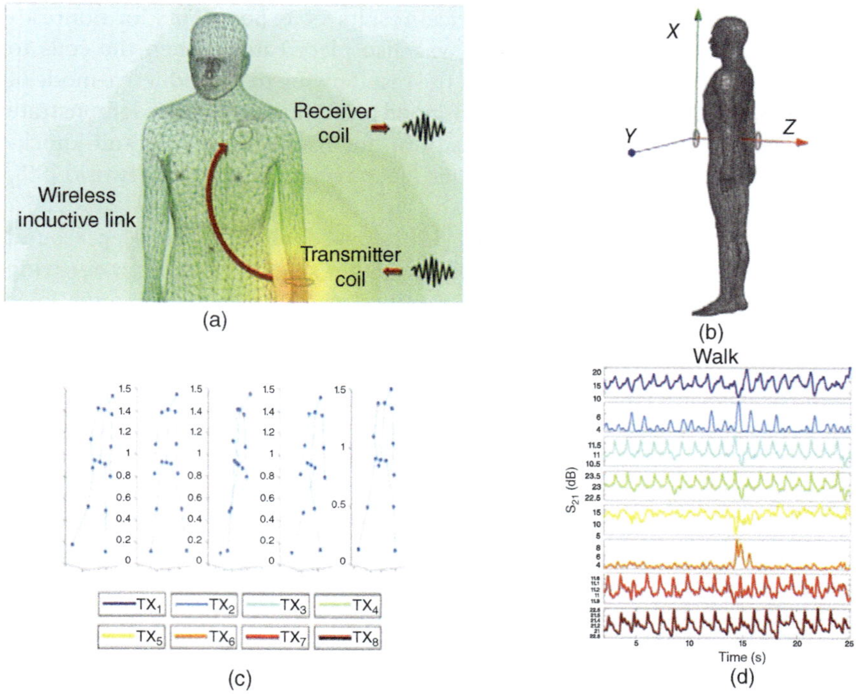

Figure 3.18 (a) Generic configuration of a magnetoinductive system [98]. (b) Simulation setup of magnetic induction coils with human body for testing against theoretical model and experiments [98]. (*Source*: Golestani, N., & Moghaddam, M., et al., 2018. © IEEE.) (c) Setup to capture and classify different activities of humans using this approach combined with machine learning and (d) results obtained from this setup showing walking activity [99]. (*Source*: Golestani, N., & Moghaddam, M., et al., 2019. © IEEE.)

induction. The general idea is that mutually coupled coils are placed on different parts of the body (Figure 3.18a); when these body parts move relative to each other, they cause changes in flux linkage; the latter is eventually detected as the change in induced voltage or transmission coefficient (RSS), thereby serving to capture the corresponding movement. In only a short span of time, this technology has been demonstrated for motion capture ranging from human activity recognition (via machine-learning techniques) to intricate measurements, such as measuring flexion/extension and rotation angles of different joints precisely and accurately.

In [98], the authors recently reported theoretical modeling of mutually coupled coils, wherein an analytical expression for the mutual inductance between two circular coils oriented randomly in free space was derived. This result was then used to derive the transmission coefficient between two coils ($|S_{21}|$) and further leveraged to compare numerical results vs. experiments for nonresonant coils. A human body medium was also placed in between the coils to confirm that its presence did not alter the result owing to the inductive mode of operation, Figure 3.18b. The aforementioned principle was used to demonstrate human activity recognition (classification), for instance walking and knocking, using machine-learning techniques (deep recurrent neural network) [99], Figure 3.18c, d.

In another case, Mishra and Kiourti [100] showed that resonant wrap-around coils on the limbs placed symmetrically on either side of the joint (one serving as the transmitter and the other as receiver) can be used to monitor joint flexion and extension (for instance, elbow flexion and extension when the coils are wrapped around the upper arm and forearm or knee flexion and extension when the coils are wrapped around the shank and thigh) (Figure 3.19a, b). A key advantage to this joint flexion monitoring approach is that it is robust to rotation (e.g. pronation and supination in the case of the elbow joint). The study indicated that operation deep in the inductive mode and around ~34 MHz was preferable. Experiments were also conducted using coils made of e-threads which were shown to be in agreement with numerical results and experiments conducted with copper coils, thereby demonstrating the possibility of seamless integration of these coils into garments (Figure 3.19c). Several design considerations such as gap between the coils and radius of the coils (to take into account changes with respect to individual's limb size) were shown to influence the levels of received power as well as the range of motion that can be captured. Safety considerations were also taken into account by calculating the specific absorption rate (SAR), showing that the technology is safe for human use. In fact, it was quantitatively demonstrated that this method exhibits equivalent or superior performance to state-of-the-art IMUs for flexion angles greater than 20°.

More recently, Mishra and Kiourti [101] reported an alternate setup in which the aforementioned resonant coils (or electrically small loop antennas (ESLAs)) can be placed longitudinally upon the body instead of wrapped around the limb (Figure 3.19d, e). In this longitudinal setup, the plane of the coil is parallel to the axis of the limb. This configuration allows to break the symmetry and hence enables monitoring of both joint flexion and rotation (Figure 3.19f). Using numerical and experimental results, this work demonstrated that much higher resolution is now possible as compared to the wraparound configuration. However, since the parameter used for monitoring both flexion and rotation is the transmission coefficient (i.e. $|S_{21}|$), there are ambiguities in detecting the state of motion. In other words, there can be multiple states of motion for a single value. To tackle this, a single-transmitter and multiple-receiver configuration was demonstrated which utilizes the asymmetry among receivers to resolve the ambiguities and achieve resolution as high as 2°. It was also shown that, by utilizing parameters such as coil

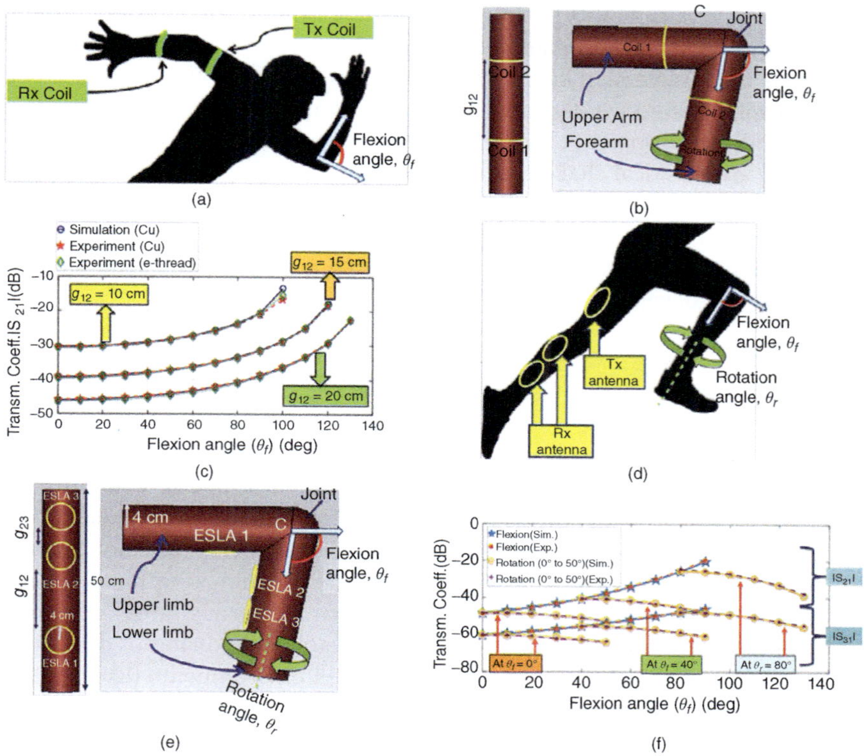

Figure 3.19 (a) Transmit (Tx) and receive (Rx) coils wrapped around (or in transverse configuration) limbs to capture joint (elbow) flexion/extension, (b) the corresponding simulation setup with cylindrical approximation of limbs and 2/3 muscle as material property, and (c) the corresponding result of $|S_{21}|$ vs. θ_f for three different gaps comparing simulation and experimental results (both for copper and e-thread) [100]. (*Source*: Mishra, V. and Kiourti, A., 2019.) (d) Transmit (Tx) and two receive (Rx) electrically small loop antennas (ESLAs) placed longitudinally on the thigh and shank respectively, (e) the corresponding simulation setup with cylindrical limb and 2/3 muscle material property approximation, and (f) the result (simulation and experiment) capturing flexion/extension and rotation at different flexion angles using both receivers [101]. (*Source*: Mishra, V. and Kiourti, A., 2020. © IEEE.)

gap and radius, this resolution limit can be further improved, yet with some trade-offs.

Magnetoinductive sensors have several advantages. Specifically, their ability to be implemented on e-threads allows for their seamless integration into garments, making the technology inconspicuous and lightweight, unlike other wearable technologies (most of which are relatively bulky and hence not quite convenient). This is one of the major advantages of this technology which brings forward a new perspective for fully wearable motion capture. Further, placement of these sensors above and below the joint (but not right atop) does not impede natural movement in any way. Also, it does not suffer from line-of-sight issues despite being a wireless technology. This is attributed to the fact that the human body is transparent to magnetic fields. However, like any other technology, there are practical challenges to be addressed. Examples include slipping of the coils with clothes or operation in the presence of external magnetic fields or in vicinity of magnetic materials and conductors. However, this technology is still in its nascent phase, and hence, research is ongoing to surmount the challenges and develop it to its true potential.

3.5 Conclusion

Capturing one of the most basic and essential parts of human life, i.e. human movement, opens doors for a plethora of new applications as well as solutions to several existing problems. Indeed, this chapter illuminated how motion capture can revolutionize various sectors including, but not limited to, healthcare, sports, human–machine interfaces, animation/movies, and biomedical research. It was also highlighted that numerous motion capture technologies are currently available or being researched upon in this direction. Some of these technologies operate in contrived environments (like Mocap labs, electromagnetic-based technologies, magnetic motion capture, and imaging methods), while others are intended to be wearable (like IMUs, deformation/bending sensors, time-of-flight sensors and RSS-based sensors). It became evident that wearable technology has several advantages over technologies working in contrived environments.

Scanning through the different technologies described in the chapter, it becomes obvious that there are different operating principles based on which motion can be sensed. These can be broadly categorized into three types. (i) Some technologies detect position of each body part, which is then used to derive any intended specific type of movement (e.g. flexion angle). Example technologies in this category entail MoCap labs, time-of-flight acoustic method, and magnetic motion capture systems. Notably, this is the most generic way of capturing movement as it includes knowledge of the exact position of each body part which can be further postprocessed to derive any intended motion. (ii) Other technologies focus on detecting specific movements and, hence, are designed for monitoring specific tasks. Alternatively, these can be designed so as to combine different movements as a means of eventually assessing full body movement. Example technologies in this category entail strain sensors, fiber optic sensors, and magnetoinductive/electrically small loop antennas. (iii) In other cases, technologies rely on identifying movement signatures and employing machine-learning

Table 3.1 Summary of motion capture technologies: advantages and limitations.

Technologies		Advantages	Limitations
MotionCapture (MoCap) Labs	Marker based	1. Highly accurate and reliable with precision of few millimeters 2. Gold standard	1. Restricted to contrived settings 2. Highly sensitive to line of sight 3. Soft tissue artifacts (markers sliding on skin) 4. High cost
	Markerless	1. No markers, so relatively simple and convenient to use with unhindered natural movement 2. Relatively low cost	1. Restricted to contrived settings 2. Relatively less reliable and accurate 3. Highly sensitive to line of sight
Electromagnetics based	Radar based	1. No sensor or marker on body (convenient to use) 2. Can detect movement through wall 3. Improved resolution at high frequencies (possible to capture fine movements)	1. Sensitivity to line-of-sight issues (especially at high frequencies). 2. Environmental noise (especially through wall) can degrade accuracy and resolution) 3. Generally restricted to fixed location
	Wi-Fi based	1. No sensor or marker on body (convenient to use)	1. Restricted to contrived and wireless environment only. 2. Highly susceptible to changes in environment 3. Difficult to capture complex movements
	RFID based	1. Uniquely identifiable tags for each body part 2. Lower cost	1. Restricted to contrived settings 2. Reliability and accuracy need further research and testing
Magnetic motion capture		1. Relatively less markers and cheaper than marker-based MoCap system 2. Reliable and accurate 3. No line-of-sight issue	1. Restricted to contrived setting 2. Subject mobility restricted in the case of tethered units 3. Sensitivity to metals located in close proximity to the system

(Continued)

Table 3.1 (Continued)

Technologies		Advantages	Limitations
Imaging methods		1. Provides relatively good accuracy	1. Restricted to contrived settings 2. Machines are typically quite heavy and expensive 3. Potential health risks (especially with ionizing radiation)
Inertial measurement units (IMUs)		1. Not restricted to contrived settings 2. No line-of-sight issues	1. Suffer from drift issues 2. Errors due to soft-body artifacts 3. Not injury safe 4. Relatively large size
Deformation/ bending sensors	Resistance Strain based (Resistance)	1. Not restricted to contrived settings 2. Conformal 3. Can have high sensitivity 4. No line-of-sight issue	1. Finite response time can hinder in recording fast movements 2. Restrict natural movement (worn on joint) 3. Restricted by number of cycle of use
	Strain-based (Permeability)	1. Not restricted to contrived setting 2. No line-of-sight issue	1. New idea and needs extensive further exploration
	Fiber optic based	1. Promising in terms of performance 2. No line-of-sight issue	1. Performance susceptible to wrinkles (e.g. on gloves) 2. Equipment used for demonstration are quite bulky and costly to be realized as wearables
Time of flight	Acoustic based	1. Good results with fixed reference	1. Errors introduced when implemented on wearables (nonfixed reference) 2. Sensitive to line of sight 3. Relatively large in size

(Continued)

Table 3.1 (Continued)

Technologies		Advantages	Limitations
	Radio based	1. Shows good performance in lab setting	1. Suffers from line-of-sight issue 2. Susceptible to change in channel (environment) and human tissue property variation 3. Relatively large in size 4. More research required to implement in practical scenario
Received signal strength based	Antennas	1. Shows the feasibility of capturing human motion	1. Suffers from line-of-sight issues 2. Susceptible to change in tissue property
	Magnetoinductive sensors	1. Seamless integration of e-threads with clothes makes the technology inconspicuous and extremely light weight (an initiative toward true wearables) 2. Conformal 3. No line-of-sight issue 4. Allows natural movement	1. Slipping of coils on loose clothes 2. More research needed to implement in practical scenario 3. Operation close to conductive or magnetic material is not yet tested and may need further research if any challenge is observed

techniques to eventually classify activities (e.g. running and walking). Example technologies in this category entail radar-, magnetoinductive-, RFID-, and antenna-based technologies. Of course, it is important to note that the first two categories of sensors can also be used for activity classification, as they are much more generic and can utilize their raw data to this end. For example, once the position of different body parts is known (first category discussed above), their relative movement can easily depict the type of movement. Similarly, sensors detecting specific movements in the second category discussed above, let us say flexion/extension of the knee, can also distinguish between different activities involving the knee (such as running, walking, and jumping).

In the present time, the most widely percolated technologies are (i) camera-based motion capture labs for operation in contrived environments and (ii) IMUs for operation in noncontrived environments. However, other technologies are catching up fast and have immense potential to revolutionize the area of motion capture. In fact, it was seen that each technology brings forward its own advantages and limitations and may ultimately be used for given applications. A comparative table for all technologies discussed in this chapter along with their corresponding advantages and limitations is provided in Table 3.1. A careful observation shows that most of these advantages and limitations are complementary for different technologies. Hence, in future, it is possible to use any one of the technologies described in the chapter, depending on the specifications (advantages) required for a given application. Alternatively, it is also possible to use combinations of two or more than two complementary technologies to achieve the requirements of a given application. Hence, attention to all the technologies is important so that they grow to their full potential and can contribute to the future of human motion capture and beyond.

References

1 J. Gordon Betts, Kelly A. Young, James A. Wise, et al. Types of Body Movements, in Joints, *Anatomy and Physiology*, OpenStax. CC by License. https://openstax.org/books/anatomy-and-physiology/pages/9-5-types-of-body-movements (accessed 7 July 2020).

2 Kiefer, A.W., Kushner, A.M., Groene, J. et al. (2015). A commentary on real-time biofeedback to augment neuromuscular training for ACL injury prevention in adolescent athletes. *Journal of Sports Science & Medicine* 14 (1): 1–8.

3 Saini, S., Rambli, D.R.A., Sulaiman, S. et al. (2012). A low-cost game framework for a home-based stroke rehabilitation system. 2012 International Conference on Computer Information Science (ICCIS), vol. 1, 55–60. doi: https://doi.org/10.1109/ICCISci.2012.6297212.

4 Pueo, B. and Jimenez-Olmedo, J.M. (2017). Application of motion capture technology for sport performance analysis," *El uso de la tecnología de captura de movimiento para el análisis del rendimiento deportivo. Retos: nuevas tendencias en educación física, deporte y recreación* 32: 241–247.

5 Vicon|Award Winning Motion Capture Systems, *Vicon*. [Online]. https://www.vicon.com/ (accessed 21 December 2019).

6 Alaraj, A., Charbel, F.T., Birk, D. et al. (2013). Role of cranial and spinal virtual and augmented reality simulation using immersive touch modules in neurosurgical training. *Neurosurgery* 72 (suppl. 1): A115–A123. https://doi.org/10.1227/NEU.0b013e3182753093.

7 Freina, L. and Ott, M. (2015). A literature review on immersive virtual reality in education: state of the art and perspectives. *The International Scientific Conference Elearning and Software for Education* 1: 133–141. https://doi.org/10.12753/2066-026X-15-020.

8 Rose, F.D., Brooks, B.M., and Rizzo, A.A. (2005). Virtual reality in brain damage rehabilitation: review. *Cyberpsychology & Behavior* 8 (3): 241–262. https://doi.org/10.1089/cpb.2005.8.241.

9 Virtual reality in gaming. *Thinkmobiles*. [Online]. https://thinkmobiles.com/blog/virtual-reality-gaming/ (accessed 21 December 2019).

10 Nogueira, P. (2012). Motion capture fundamentals: a critical and comparative analysis on real world applications. Proceedings of the 7th Doctoral Symposium in Informatics Engineering 2012, 303–314.

11 Niechwiej-Szwedo, E., Inness, E.L., Howe, J.A. et al. (2007). Changes in gait variability during different challenges to mobility in patients with traumatic brain injury. *Gait Posture* 25 (1): 70–77. https://doi.org/10.1016/j.gaitpost.2006.01.002.

12 Klima, D., Morgan, L., Baylor, M. et al. (2019). Physical performance and fall risk in persons with traumatic brain injury. *Perceptual and Motor Skills* 126 (1): 50–69. https://doi.org/10.1177/0031512518809203.

13 Klette, R. and Tee, G. (2008). Understanding human motion: a historic review. *Human Motion Understanding, Modelling, Capture and Animation* 36: 1–22.

14 Guerra-filho, G.B. (2005). Optical motion capture: theory and implementation. *Journal of Theoretical and Applied Information* 12: 61–89.

15 Takeuchi, A., Hasegawa, D. and Sakuta, H. (2015). Web-based avatar represented lecture viewer toward interactive e-Lecture performed by 3D avatar. 2015 IEEE Global Engineering Education Conference (EDUCON), Tallinn, 283–286. doi: 10.1109/EDUCON.2015.7095984.

16 Optical motion capture guide. [Online]. http://physbam.stanford.edu/cs448x/old/Optical_Motion_Capture_Guide.html (accessed 20 December 2019).

17 Cappozzo, A., Della Croce, U., Leardini, A., and Chiari, L. (2005). Human movement analysis using stereophotogrammetry: part 1: theoretical background. *Gait Posture* 21 (2): 186–196. https://doi.org/10.1016/j.gaitpost.2004.01.010.

18 Vicon|Award winning motion capture systems. *Vicon*. [Online]. https://www.vicon.com/ (accessed 21 December 2019).

19 Qualisys|motion capture systems. [Online]. https://www.qualisys.com/ (accessed 21 December 2019).

20 Motion capture systems. *OptiTrack*. [Online]. http://optitrack.com/index.html (accessed 21 December 2019).

21 Knippenberg, E., Verbrugghe, J., Lamers, I. et al. (2017). Markerless motion capture systems as training device in neurological rehabilitation: a systematic review of their use, application, target population and efficacy. *Journal of NeuroEngineering and Rehabilitation* 14 (1): 61. https://doi.org/10.1186/s12984-017-0270x.

22 Mousavi Hondori, H. and Khademi, M. (2014). A review on technical and clinical impact of microsoft kinect on physical therapy and rehabilitation. *Journal of Medical Engineering*. https://www.hindawi.com/journals/jme/2014/846514/abs/ (accessed 21 December 2019).

23 Li, C., Peng, Z., Huang, T.-Y. et al. (2017). A review on recent progress of portable short-range noncontact microwave radar systems. *IEEE Transactions on Microwave Theory and Techniques* 65 (5): 1692–1706. https://doi.org/10.1109/TMTT.2017.2650911.

24 Kim, Y. and Ling, H. (2009). Human activity classification based on micro-Doppler signatures using a support vector machine. *IEEE Transactions on Geoscience and Remote Sensing* 47 (5): 1328–1337. https://doi.org/10.1109/TGRS.2009.2012849.

25 Gu, C., Wang, J., and Lien, J. (2019). Motion sensing using radar: gesture interaction and beyond. *IEEE Microwave Magazine* 20 (8): 44–57. https://doi.org/10.1109/MMM.2019.2915490.

26 Geisheimer, J.L., Iii, E.F.G., and Marshall, W.S. (2002). High-resolution Doppler model of the human gait. *Radar Sensor Technology and Data Visualization* 4744: 8–18. https://doi.org/10.1117/12.488286.

27 van Dorp, P. and Groen, F.C.A. (2003). Human walking estimation with radar. *IEE Proceedings Radar, Sonar and Navigation* 150 (5): 356–365.

28 Stove, A.G. and Sykes, S.R. (2002). A Doppler-based automatic target classifier for a battlefield surveillance radar. *Proceedings of the 2004 IEEE Radar Conference*: 419–423. https://doi.org/10.1049/cp:20020320.

29 Bilik, I., Tabrikian, J., and Cohen, A. (2006). GMM-based target classification for ground surveillance Doppler radar. *IEEE Transactions on Aerospace and Electronic Systems* 42 (1): 267–278. https://doi.org/10.1109/TAES.2006.1603422.

30 Smith, G.E., Woodbridge, K., and Baker, C.J. (2006). Template based micro-Doppler signature classification. *2006 European Radar Conference*: 158–161. https://doi.org/10.1109/EURAD.2006.280298.

31 Anderson, M.G. and Rogers, R.L. (2007). Micro-Doppler analysis of multiple frequency continuous wave radar signatures. *Radar Sensor Technology XI* 6547: 65470A. https://doi.org/10.1117/12.719800.

32 Smith, G.E., Woodbridge, K., and Baker, C.J. (2008). Naïve Bayesian radar micro-Doppler recognition. 2008 International Conference on Radar, 111–116. doi: https://doi.org/10.1109/RADAR.2008.4653901.

33 Lien, J., Gillian, N., Karagozler, M.E. et al. (2016). Soli: ubiquitous gesture sensing with millimeter wave radar. *ACM Transactions on Graphics* 35 (4): 142:1–142:19. https://doi.org/10.1145/2897824.2925953.

34 Molchanov, P., Gupta, S., Kim, K., and Pulli, K. (2015). Short-range FMCW monopulse radar for hand-gesture sensing. 2015 IEEE Radar Conference (RadarCon), 1491–1496. doi: https://doi.org/10.1109/RADAR.2015.7131232.

35 Qi, F., Liang, F., Liu, M. et al. (2019). Position-information-indexed classifier for improved through-wall detection and classification of human activities using UWB bio-radar. *IEEE Antennas and Wireless Propagation Letters* 18 (3): 437–441. https://doi.org/10.1109/LAWP.2019.2893358.

36 Liu, J., Wang, L., Fang, J. et al. (2018). Multi-target intense human motion analysis and detection using channel state information. *Sensors* 18 (10) https://doi.org/10.3390/s18103379.

37 Youssef, M., Mah, M., and Agrawala, A. (2007). Challenges: device-free passive localization for wireless environments. Proceedings of the 13th Annual ACM International Conference on Mobile Computing and Networking, New York, NY, USA, 222–229. doi: https://doi.org/10.1145/1287853.1287880.

38 Yang, J., Ge, Y., Xiong, H. et al. (2010). Performing joint learning for passive intrusion detection in pervasive wireless environments. 2010 Proceedings IEEE INFOCOM, 1–9. doi: https://doi.org/10.1109/INFCOM.2010.5462148.

39 Zheng, X., Yang, J., Chen, Y., and Xiong, H. (2015). An adaptive framework coping with dynamic target speed for device-free passive localization. *IEEE Transactions on Mobile Computing* 14 (6): 1138–1150. https://doi.org/10.1109/TMC.2014.2347303.

40 Kaltiokallio, O.and Bocca, M. (2011). Real-time intrusion detection and tracking in indoor environment through distributed RSSI processing. 2011 IEEE 17th International Conference on Embedded and Real-Time Computing Systems and Applications, vol. 1, 61–70. doi: https://doi.org/10.1109/RTCSA.2011.38.

41 Wang, Z., Guo, B., Yu, Z., and Zhou, X. (2018). Wi-Fi CSI-based behavior recognition: from signals and actions to activities. *IEEE Communications Magazine* 56 (5): 109–115. https://doi.org/10.1109/MCOM.2018.1700144.

42 Adib, F. and Katabi, D. (2013). See through walls with WiFi! Proceedings of the ACM SIGCOMM 2013 Conference on SIGCOMM, New York, NY, USA, 75–86. doi: https://doi.org/10.1145/2486001.2486039.

43 Chetty, K., Smith, G.E., and Woodbridge, K. (2012). Through-the-wall sensing of personnel using passive bistatic WiFi radar at standoff distances. *IEEE Transactions on Geoscience and Remote Sensing* 50 (4): 1218–1226. https://doi.org/10.1109/TGRS.2011.2164411.

44 Pu, Q., Gupta, S., Gollakota, S., and Patel, S. (2013). Whole-home gesture recognition using wireless signals. Proceedings of the 19th Annual International Conference on MobileComputing & Networking, New York, NY, USA, 27–38. doi:https://doi.org/10.1145/2500423.2500436.

45 Kellogg, B., Talla, V. and Gollakota, S. (2014). Bringing gesture recognition to all devices. Presented at the 11th {USENIX} Symposium on Networked Systems Design and Implementation ({NSDI} 14), 303–316.

46 Wang, H., Zhang, D., Wang, Y. et al. (2017). RT-fall: areal-time and contactless fall detection system with commodity WiFi devices. *IEEE Transactions on Mobile Computing* 16 (2): 511–526. https://doi.org/10.1109/TMC.2016.2557795.

47 Guo, B., Chen, Y.J., Lane, N. et al. (2017). Behavior recognition based on Wi-Fi CSI: part 1. *IEEE Communications Magazine* 55 (10): 90–90. https://doi.org/10.1109/MCOM.2017.8067691.

48 Guo, B., Chen, Y.J., Lane, N. et al. (2018). Behavior recognition based on Wi-Fi CSI: part 2. *IEEE Communications Magazine* 56 (5): 108–108. https://doi.org/10.1109/MCOM.2018.8360859.

49 Amendola, S., Bianchi, L., and Marrocco, G. (2015). Movement detection of human body segments: passive radio-frequency identification and machine-learning technologies. *IEEE Antennas and Propagation Magazine* 57 (3): 23–37. https://doi.org/10.1109/MAP.2015.2437274.

50 Krigslund, R., Dosen, S., Popovski, P. et al. (2013). A novel technology for motion capture using passive UHF RFID tags. *IEEE Transactions on Biomedical Engineering* 60 (5): 1453–1457. https://doi.org/10.1109/TBME.2012.2209649.

51 Menache, A. (2011). 1 - Motion Capture Primer. In: *Understanding Motion Capture for Computer Animation*, 2e (ed. A. Menache), 1–46. Boston: Morgan Kaufmann.

52 Magnetic motion capture systems. *Tracklab*. [Online]. https://tracklab.com.au/magnetic-motion-capture-systems/ (accessed 20 December 2019).

53 Ascension trakSTAR 2.*Tracklab*16August2016. [Online]. https://tracklab.com.au/products/hardware/ascension-trakstar-2/ (accessed 21December2019).

54 Polhemus wireless motion trackers. [Online]. https://polhemus.com/motiontracking/wireless-trackers/ (accessed 21 December 2019).

55 Polhemus G4. [Online]. https://polhemus.com/motion-tracking/all-trackers/g4 (accessed 21 December 2019).

56 Polhemus is the premier precision motion tracking company. [Online]. https://polhemus.com/ (accessed 21 December 2019).

57 Tracklab –motion capture systems Australia.*Tracklab*. [Online]. https://tracklab.com.au/ (accessed 21 December 2019).

58 Ascension Technology Corp. [Online]. https://www.ascension-tech.com/ (accessed 21 December 2019).

59 do Rosário, J.L.P. (2014). Biomechanical assessment of human posture: A literature review. *Journal of Bodywork and Movement Therapies* 18 (3): 368–373. https://doi.org/10.1016/j.jbmt.2013.11.018.

60 Li, G., Van de Velde, S.K., and Bingham, J.T. (2008). Validation of a non-invasive fluoroscopic imaging technique for the measurement of dynamic knee joint motion. *Journal of Biomechanics* 41 (7): 1616–1622. https://doi.org/10.1016/j.jbiomech.2008.01.034.

61 Cargill, S.C., Pearcy, M., and Barry, M.D. (2007). Three-dimensional lumbar spine postures measured by magnetic resonance imaging reconstruction. *Spine* 32 (11): 1242–1248. https://doi.org/10.1097/01.brs.0000263404.66369.a5.

62 Unique equipment for data acquisition research and clinical applications. [Online]. http://www.biometricsltd.com/ (accessed 21December2019).

63 Functional status assessment tools|JTECH medical. [Online]. https://www.jtechmedical.com/ (accessed 21 December 2019).

64 ADInstruments.*ADInstruments*. [Online]. Available: https://www.adinstruments.com/ (accessed 21 December 2019).

65 Bonde-Petersen, F. (1975). A simple force platform. *European Journal of Applied Physiology* 34 (1): 51–54. https://doi.org/10.1007/BF00999915.

66 Griffiths, I.W. *Principles of Biomechanics & Motion Analysis*. Lippincott Williams &Wilkins. [Online]. https://textbookday.com/principles-of-biomechanics-motionanalysis/ (accessed 21 December 2019).

67 O'Connor, C.M., Thorpe, S.K., O'Malley, M.J., and Vaughan, C.L. (2007). Automatic detection of gait events using kinematic data. *Gait Posture* 25 (3): 469–474. https://doi.org/10.1016/j.gaitpost.2006.05.016.

68 Camomilla, V., Bergamini, E., Fantozzi, S., and Vannozzi, G. (2018). Trends supporting the in-field use of wearable inertial sensors for sport performance evaluation: a systematic review. *Sensors* 18 (3): 873. https://doi.org/10.3390/s18030873.

69 Ahmad, N., Ghazilla, R.A.R., Khairi, N.M., and Kasi, V. (2013). Reviews on various inertial measurement unit (IMU) sensor applications. *International Journal of Signal Processing* 1 (2): 256–262. https://doi.org/10.12720/ijsps.1.2.256-262.

70 Filippeschi, A., Schmitz, N., Miezal, M. et al. (2017). Survey of motion tracking methods based on inertial sensors: a focus on upper limb human motion. *Sensors* 17 (6) https://doi.org/10.3390/s17061257.

71 Picerno, P. (2017). 25 years of lower limb joint kinematics by using inertial and magnetic sensors: a review of methodological approaches. *Gait Posture* 51: 239–246. https://doi.org/10.1016/j.gaitpost.2016.11.008.

72 Lintmeijer, L.L., Faber, G.S., Kruk, H.R. et al. (2018). An accurate estimation of the horizontal acceleration of a rower's centre of mass using inertial sensors: a validation. *European Journal of Sport Science* 18 (7): 940–946. https://doi.org/10.1080/17461391.2018.1465126.

73 Huang, Y., Kaufmann, M., Aksan, E. et al. (2018). Deep inertial poser: learning to reconstruct human pose from sparse inertial measurements in real time. *ACM Transactions on Graphics* 37 (6): 185:1–185:15. https://doi.org/10.1145/3272127.3275108.

74 Mukhopadhyay, S.C. (2015). Wearable sensors for human activity monitoring: a review. *IEEE Sensors Journal* 15 (3): 1321–1330. https://doi.org/10.1109/JSEN.2014.2370945.

75 Xsens.Home –Xsens 3D motion tracking. [Online]. https://www.xsens.com (accessed 21 December 2019).

76 APDM wearable technologies.*APDM*. [Online]. https://www.apdm.com/ (accessed 21 December 2019).

77 TDK|Attracting tomorrow. [Online]. Available: https://www.invensense.com/ (accessed 21 December 2019).

78 TRIVISIO –Home.*trivisio*. [Online]. https://www.trivisio.com (accessed 21 December 2019).

79 NOITOM. [Online]. https://www.noitom.com/ (accessed 2 November 2020).

80 Gibbs, P. and Asada, H.H. (2004). Wearable conductive fiber sensor arrays for measuring multiaxis joint motion. The 26th Annual International Conference of the IEEE Engineering in Medicine and Biology Society, vol. 2, 4755–4758. doi: https://doi.org/10.1109/IEMBS.2004.1404316.

81 Li, C., Cui, Y.-L., Tian, G.-L. et al. (2015). Flexible CNT-array double helices strain sensor with high stretchability for motion capture. *Scientific Reports* 5 (1): 1–8. https://doi.org/10.1038/srep15554.

82 Ryu, S., Lee, P., Chou, J.B. et al. (2015). Extremely elastic wearable carbon nanotube fiber strain sensor for monitoring of human motion. *ACS Nano* 9 (6): 5929–5936. https://doi.org/10.1021/acsnano.5b00599.

83 Cheng, Y., Wang, R., Sun, J., and Gao, L. (2015). A stretchable and highly sensitive graphenebased fiber for sensing tensile strain, bending, and torsion. *Advanced Materials* 27 (45): 7365–7371. https://doi.org/10.1002/adma.201503558.

84 Wang, Y., Wang, L., Yang, T. et al. (2014). Wearable and highly sensitive graphene strain sensors for human motion monitoring. *Advanced Functional Materials* 24 (29): 4666–4670. https://doi.org/10.1002/adfm.201400379.

85 Moreton, G., Meydan, T., and Williams, P. (2017). Investigation and characterization of a planar figure-of-eight coil as a curvature sensor. 2017 IEEE SENSORS, 1–3. doi: https://doi.org/10.1109/ICSENS.2017.8234138.

86 Nishiyama, M. and Watanabe, K. (2009). Wearable sensing glove with embedded hetero-core fiber-optic nerves for unconstrained hand motion capture. *IEEE Transactions on Instrumentation and Measurement* 58 (12): 3995–4000. https://doi.org/10.1109/TIM.2009.2021640.

87 Donno, M., Palange, E., Di Nicola, F. et al. (2008). A new flexible optical fiber goniometer for dynamic angular measurements: application to human joint movement monitoring. *IEEE Transactions on Instrumentation and Measurement* 57 (8): 1614–1620. https://doi.org/10.1109/TIM.2008.925336.

88 Guo, J., Niu, M., and Yang, C. (2017). Highly flexible and stretchable optical strain sensing for human motion detection. *Optica* 4 (10): 1285–1288. https://doi.org/10.1364/OPTICA.4.001285.

89 Laurijssen, D., Truijen, S., Saeys, W., and Steckel, J. (2015). Three sources, three receivers, six degrees of freedom: an ultrasonic sensor for pose estimation motion capture. 2015 IEEE SENSORS, 1–4. doi: https://doi.org/10.1109/ICSENS.2015.7370689.

90 Qi, Y., Soh, C.B., Gunawan, E., and Low, K.-S. (2015). Ambulatory measurement of threedimensional foot displacement during treadmill walking using wearable wireless ultrasonic sensor network. *IEEE Journal of Biomedical and Health Informatics* 19 (2): 446–452. https://doi.org/10.1109/JBHI.2014.2316998.

91 Einsmann, C., Quirk, M., Muzal, B. et al. (2005) Modeling a wearable full-body motion capture system. Ninth IEEE International Symposium on Wearable Computers (ISWC'05), 144–151. doi: https://doi.org/10.1109/ISWC.2005.34.

92 Di Renzo, M., Buehrer, R.M. and Torres, J. (2017). Pulse shape distortion and ranging accuracy in UWB-based body area networks for full-body motion capture and gait analysis. IEEE GLOBECOM 2007 – IEEE Global Telecommunications Conference, 3775–3780. doi: https://doi.org/10.1109/GLOCOM.2007.717.

93 Hamie, J., Denis, B., and Richard, C. (2013). Joint motion capture and navigation in heterogeneous Body Area Networks with distance estimation over neighborhood graph. 2013 10th Workshop on Positioning, Navigation and Communication (WPNC), 1–6. doi: https://doi.org/10.1109/WPNC.2013.6533282.

94 Qi, Y., Soh, C.B., Gunawan, E. et al. (2014). A novel approach to joint flexion/extension angles measurement based on wearable UWB radios. *IEEE Journal of Biomedical and Health Informatics* 18 (1): 300–308. https://doi.org/10.1109/JBHI.2013.2253487.

95 Guraliuc, A.R., Barsocchi, P., Potortì, F., and Nepa, P. (2011). Limb movements classification using wearable wireless transceivers. *IEEE Transactions on Information Technology in Biomedicine* 15 (3): 474–480. https://doi.org/10.1109/TITB.2011.2118763.

96 Mishra, V. and Kiourti, A. (2019). Breaking the boundaries: monitoring joint flexion using radiofrequency coils. 2019 United States National Committee of URSI National Radio Science Meeting (USNC-URSI NRSM), 1–2. doi: https://doi.org/10.23919/USNC-URSINRSM.2019.8712863.

97 Mishra, V. and Kiourti, A. (2019). Electromagnetic components realized on conductive wires: a copper vs. E-thread comparison. 2019 IEEE International Symposium on Antennas and Propagation and USNC-URSI Radio Science Meeting, 359–360. doi: https://doi.org/10.1109/APUSNCURSINRSM.2019.8889214.

98 Golestani, N. and Moghaddam, M. (2018). Theoretical modeling and analysis of magnetic induction communication in wireless body area networks (WBANs). *IEEE Journal of Electromagnetics, RF and Microwaves in Medicine and Biology* 2 (1): 48–55. https://doi.org/10.1109/JERM.2018.2810603.

99 Golestani, N. and Moghaddam, M. (2019).Magnetic induction-based human activity recognition (MI-HAR). 2019 IEEE International Symposium on Antennas and Propagation and USNC-URSI Radio Science Meeting, 17–18. doi: https://doi.org/10.1109/APUSNCURSINRSM.2019.8888468.

100 Mishra, V. and Kiourti, A. (2019). Wrap-around wearable coils for seamless monitoring of joint flexion. *IEEE Transactions on Biomedical Engineering* 66 (10): 2753–2760. https://doi.org/10.1109/TBME.2019.2895293.

101 Mishra, V. and Kiourti, A. (2020). Wearable electrically small loop antennas for monitoring joint flexion and rotation. *IEEE Transactions on Antennas and Propagation* 68 (1): 134–141. https://doi.org/10.1109/TAP.2019.2935147.

4

Antennas and Wireless Power Transfer for Brain-Implantable Sensors

Leena Ukkonen, Lauri Sydänheimo, Toni Björninen and Shubin Ma

Faculty of Medicine and Health Technology, Tampere University, Tampere, Finland

4.1 Introduction

The first human brain implant can be traced back as early as 1874 when Roberts Bartholow implanted a pair of electrolytic needles into the meninges of his patient Mary Rafferty [1]. At that time, this experiment aroused a storm of ethical controversy and criticism, even though the experimental results revealed the fact that the sensorimotor function of brain is excitable with electric current. Later, in the twentieth century, the understanding of the brain and the nervous system became progressively precise, and effective treatments for neurophysiological diseases were put forward in succession. For instance, in the year 1924, Hans Berger recorded the first human brain electroencephalogram. His discovery of the brain electrical activity directly led to the concept of brain machine interface that helps to establish the bidirectional neural pathway between the brain and the external devices for the paralyzed in the late 1970s [2, 3]. Nearly concurrently, a neuroprosthetic device was invented to substitute or augment the damaged sensory with an implant electrode array simulating the neural electrical signals, such as the cochlear implant for the patients with sensorineural hearing loss [4]. Meanwhile, a deep brain implant with neurostimulator for direct alternation of brain activity to manage the movement disorders has been approved for clinical implementation around 2000. These deep brain implants treat essential tremor and have significantly improved the life quality of patients with Parkinson's disease, obsessive–compulsive disorder, or epilepsy [5]. Typically, the brain implant in treatments for neurological illnesses needs a chronical implantation under the skull for high-resolution neural signal recording [6–8], intracranial physiologically parameters monitoring [9–11], or deep brain stimulation [12–14]. Currently, implants are often connected with an off-body signal processor via percutaneous cables through a bone-anchored socket. This bulky

Antenna and Sensor Technologies in Modern Medical Applications,
First Edition. Edited by Yahya Rahmat-Samii and Erdem Topsakal.

and fragile structure is unlikely a favorable solution for the sake of patients' mobility and safety in a long-term implementation. For this reason, wireless solutions are presently sought for substituting the cable-based data and power transfer between the implants and the off-body devices for achieving safe and cranially concealed solutions that last for a lifetime.

4.2 Implantable Antennas for Wireless Biomedical Devices

The major challenge in developing a wireless brain implant is to establish a stable and efficient trans-cranial wireless link with an integrated implantable antenna. From the perspective of electromagnetics (EM) and wireless communications, a human head is a complex dielectric environment comprising biological materials that are dispersive and characterized with relative permittivity and conductivity tens of times higher than materials present in regular electronic devices and wireless signal ambience. In addition, different tissue types are dissimilar in terms of their dielectric properties. Thus, models comprising multiple tissue types are required in EM modeling of implanted wireless devices. The brain implant typically needs a deep implant depth under the skull, usually up to 15 mm for neural signal recording and even several centimeters for deep brain stimulation. This deep implant depth with the highly lossy intracranial tissues surrounding the implantable antenna will notably limit the antenna's radiation efficiency and overall worsen the efficiency of the wireless link of the implant. To achieve a long-term implementation of the implant and minimize the biological intrusiveness causing scar tissue aggregating on the implant that potentially affects the implant performance, the implant should meet extreme structural requirements in terms of device miniaturization, thinness, and flexibility. These physical constraints pose even strict requirements on antenna development in terms of antenna form factors and miniaturization.

Near-field communication with inductive links has long been utilized for wireless implants [15]. These wireless implants utilize the inductively coupled antenna pairs for communication: usually one to be implanted and the other one attached on the skin. These antenna pairs are co-optimized for maximizing the inductive coupling strength between them. Since the magnetic field is more resistive to the deterioration caused by the high lossy tissue materials, the wireless link can be efficient and cause less heating in the surrounding tissues. Due to the high efficiency of the inductive link, a near-field communication system is usually combined with wireless power transfer (WPT), which will be further discussed in the following section. In near-field communication systems, the amplitude of the magnetic field falls off with the third power of the distance from the antenna. Therefore, the operating distance of a near-field antenna is normally limited to several centimeters. As a rule of thumb, the near-field radius of an electrical small antenna is about one wavelength of its operation frequency; to prolong the operation distance of the antenna, a near-field antenna generally works in the low-frequency band, for example 5–60 MHz for the commercial cochlear implant systems [16]. Due to the relative long wavelength of the operation frequency, the near-field antennas are generally bulky and coil based. Moreover, since the magnetic field only dominates in proximity to the antenna, the near-field link is also sensitive to the misalignment between the antenna pairs. To alleviate the deterioration by this misalignment, the off-body antenna is usually made with even larger size to expand the effective coverage of the magnetic field. The lower frequency band also restricts the bandwidth of the antenna and limits the attainable data rates to a range of only 106–424 kbit s^{-1} [17].

On the other hand, far-field antennas with potentially higher data rates, smaller antenna dimension, and longer operation distance have been increasingly adopted in wireless implant development. Currently, a frequency band from 402 to 405 MHz (U.S. FCC) is specifically allocated for Medical Implant Communications Systems (MICS), and the Industrial, Scientific, and Medical (ISM) bands (e.g. 433.05–434.79 MHz in Region 1, 902–928 MHz in Region 2, and 2400–2500 MHz in Region 3) are recommended for implantable medical devices. Moreover, the radio-frequency identification (RFID) systems based on backscattering radio communication enable ultra-low-power radios that are also a compelling approach for medical implant communications and the RFID frequency bands centered at 866 and 915 MHz. These frequency bands provide wider bandwidth and more flexibility in implantable antenna development.

In the past decade, various techniques to develop the far-field miniature implantable antennas have been proposed and analyzed. Table 4.1 lists some of the implantable antennas with prior arts. Among them, the multilayer patch antenna and the planar inverted-F antenna (PIFA) are the most extensively studied antenna types. The main reason for their prevalence is their outstanding flexibility in design and well-understood miniaturization principles. Generally, the patch antenna consists of two conductor planes (a radiation plane and a ground plane) and high permittivity dielectric superstrate and substrate. The high permittivity of the superstrates and substrate shortens the effective wavelength and helps to decrease the antenna size. The radiation plane, as its name implies, is responsible for EM wave radiation, with careful and ingenious arrangement of the slots and the traces on the radiation plane, a patch antenna can offer advanced EM features, such as the multiband [18], wideband [19], or circular polarized (CP) [20–23] operations. The ground plane of the patch antenna ensures a good directivity and detuning resistance in the lossy tissue environment. A short pin between the two conductor planes is also commonly used to further decrease the antenna size. For example, in [20], the size of the proposed antenna is successfully decreased to 3% of the

Table 4.1 Comparison of different implantable antennas.

Refs	Year	Type	Frequency (MHz)	Dimension	Implant depth	Dielectric material	Gain	Stacking layer	Short pin	Features
[23]	2014	Patch	2450	$10 \times 10 \times 1.27\ mm^3$	4 mm in skin	Rogers 3010	−19.2 dBi	2	Yes	CP
[88]	2017	Patch	1900	$10.2 \times 4.2 \times 0.4\ mm^3$	5 mm in head	Rogers 3010	−14.5 dBi	2	Yes	
[21]	2017	Patch	2450	$8.5 \times 8.5 \times 1.27\ mm^3$	2 mm in skin	Rogers 3210	−17 dBi	2	No	CP
[20]	2018	Patch	915	$\pi \times (4.7)^2 \times 1.27\ mm^3$	4 mm in skin	Rogers 3010	−32.8 dBi	2	Yes	CP
[19]	2018	Patch	2450	$10 \times 10 \times 0.4\ mm^3$	4 mm in skin	Rogers 6010	−9 dBi	2	No	Wideband
[18]	2018	Patch	915, 2450	$8 \times 6 \times 0.5\ mm^3$	4 mm in skin	Rogers 6010	−28.5 dBi	2	No	Dual-band
[89]	2019	Patch	2450	$10 \times 10 \times 1\ mm^3$	12 mm in CSF	Taconic RF-35	−25 dBi	3	No	Broadside radiation
[24]	2005	PIFA	403	$24 \times 20 \times 2.4\ mm^3$	3.8 mm in skin	Rogers 3010	N/A	2	No	
[90]	2008	PIFA	403, 2450	$22.5 \times 22.5 \times 2.5\ mm^3$	3 mm in skin	Rogers 3210	−24 dBi (403 MHz) −7.5 (2480 MHz)	2	Yes	Dual-band
[91]	2014	PIFA	403, 2450	$13.4 \times 16 \times 0.835\ mm^3$	3 mm in skin	Rogers 3010	−30.5 dBi (403 MHz) −22.2 dBi (2480 MHz)	1	Yes	Dual-band
[25]	2014	PIFA	2450	$8 \times 4 \times 1.27\ mm^3$	4 mm in skin	Rogers 3010	−10.7 dBi	2	Yes	
[92]	2015	PIFA	403	$12.5 \times 12.5 \times 1.27\ mm^3$	18 mm in muscle	Rogers 3010	−32.49 dBi	2	Yes	
[93]	2019	PIFA	673	$10 \times 10 \times 3.2\ mm^3$	50 mm in muscle	FR 4	−29.4 dBi	2	Yes	
[24]	2014	Dipole	403, 2450	$10 \times 10 \times 0.67\ mm^3$	3 mm in skin	Rogers 3010	−30.5 dBi (403 MHz) −19.2 dBi (2480 MHz)	2	Yes	Dual-band
[22]	2015	Loop	915	$13 \times 13 \times 1.27\ mm^3$	3 mm in skin	Rogers 3010	−32 dBi	2	Yes	CP
[29]	2017	Loop	915	$\pi \times (12.5)^2 \times 3\ mm^3$	11 mm in brain	Rogers 4003	N/A	No	No	
[28]	2019	Loop	403	$16 \times 16 \times 1\ mm^3$	14 mm in CSF	FR 4	N/A	No	No	
[30]	2019	Loop	307–3500	$18 \times 18 \times 3\ mm^3$	50 mm in stomach	Rogers 3010	~ −30 dBi	No	No	Wideband

wavelength at the operation frequency. Likewise, the PIFA is composed of a ground plane and a parallel planar radiation element that is shorted to the ground by a pin or plate conductor. The PIFA is widely adopted in implantable devices for its small size and good specific absorption rate (SAR) properties. In [24], the authors elaborately outline the procedure of developing the PIFA for implantable applications. Different miniaturization approaches are compared and evaluated. In [25], the authors report a PIFA based on a spiral radiation element and a folded ground. With such configuration, the antenna with a size less than 1 cm was obtained. Besides the patch antenna and the PIFA, a loop antenna, for its good conformability and small electric field in the vicinity of the surrounding tissues [26, 27], is another good option for wireless implants. In [28, 29], two miniature loop antennas were proposed and evaluated with the implant placed as deep as 11 mm in the brain tissue. In [30], a split ring-loaded loop antenna was presented for capsule endoscopy with the implant placed 50 mm deep in the abdominal cavity.

4.3 Wireless Power Transfer Techniques for Implantable Devices

The supply of stable and continuous power is essential to ensure a proper operation of the implant devices. Conventionally, bioimplantable devices use battery as their power source. Even though the recent advances in battery technology have improved the battery's power density with optimized form factors, the lifetime of the battery is still limited, and the periodical surgery to replace the battery will increase the hospitalization time and risk the patients' safety. Therefore, powering the implant wirelessly from the external source outside the human body and meanwhile getting rid of the battery have significance in prolonging the implant's service life, decreasing the implant's overall size, and most importantly improving the patient's comfort and safety. To establish the wireless power link between the off-body device and the implant, various approaches have been proposed and evaluated, such as the inductive power transfer, ultrasonic power transfer, near-field capacitive power transfer, and far-field EM radiation-based power transfer.

4.3.1 Inductive Power Transfer

Inductive power transfer is the most extensively studied approach to establish the wireless power link between the off-body devices and the implants. Multiple research involving the inductive power transfer system can be found in the literature, including the analyses of the inductive link over biotissue [31–33], power link optimization [34], and coil designs [35–38]. The block diagram in Figure 4.1 shows a typical structure of the inductive power transfer system that

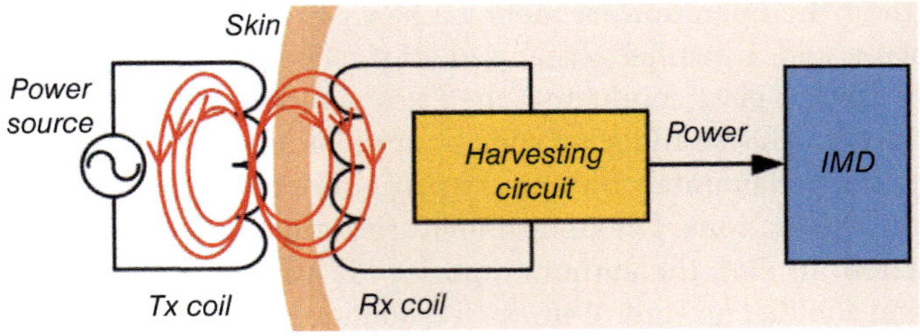

Figure 4.1 Structure of an inductive power transfer system.

consists of two coils, namely the transmit (TX) coil placed externally near the skin and the receive (RX) coil to be implanted into the tissue environment. The basic mechanism of inductive power transfer is the EM induction, which is as follows: an applied alternating current to the TX coil generates a time-varying magnetic field, and the alternating magnetic flux passing through the RX coil will induct an electromotive force (EMF) across the RX coil. Then, the inducted current on the RX coil can be rectified to power the implant. Table 4.2 lists several recent inductive power transfer systems for implantable applications.

As the magnetic field barely interacts with biotissues, the attainable efficiency of inductive power transfer can be higher than that of the ultrasonic-based ones. In [44], the proposed inductive power link reaches an efficiency of 66% with an operation distance of 15 mm in the skin tissue environment. However, since the intensity of the magnetic field decays as $1/d^3$ away from the TX coil, the operation distance is usually limited to 1–2 cm as the RX coil needs to be in

Table 4.2 Comparison of different inductive power transfer systems.

Refs	Year	Efficiency (%)	Frequency (MHz)	Received power	Diameter of implant coil	Operation range	Medium type
[39]	2014	0.0006	1600	200 μW	2 mm	50 mm	Brain
[40]	2015	17	4	20 mW	22 mm	15 mm	Rat brain
[41]	2016	13	1.5	15.9 mW	4 mm	110 mm	Rat and air
[42]	2016	2.2	20	1.4 mW	1 mm	10 mm	Skin
[43]	2016	0.56	200	224 μW	1 mm	12 mm	Gray mater
[44]	2017	66	13.56	100 mW	16 mm	15 mm	Skin
[45]	2017	2.4	60	N/A	1 mm	16 mm	Dura
[46]	2017	0.1	100	N/A	5 mm	50–100 mm	Body average
[47]	2018	0.1	400	N/A	1 mm	15 mm	CSF
[48]	2018	1.7	4	N/A	40 mm	30 mm	Muscle
[49]	2019	40	5	N/A	35 mm	50 mm	Fat
[50]	2019	12.82	100	N/A	2 mm	1.8 mm	Skull

the near field of the TX coil for a strong mutual coupling. This implant depth is generally sufficient for subcutaneous implants, however not quite enough for deep implant devices, e.g. the neural implants. To boost the operation range and enable the power transfer to the deep implants, the authors in [45, 46, 49] developed passive repeaters in between the TX and RX coils to strengthen the mutual coupling between the coils. With such configuration, the attainable operation distance improves to a maximum of 100 mm. Since the tissue loss increases with the frequency, most of the inductive power transfer systems operate in the low-frequency band (≤20 MHz); the necessary multiturn coil [50] makes the implant bulky and adds difficulties to implant miniaturization. In [51], the author proved that when the two coils are weakly coupled, for instance, the deep implant with a millimeter-sized receiving antenna, the power transfer efficiency can be improved by increasing the operation frequency to gigahertz range when the transmitting antenna is much smaller than the wavelength and subgigahertz range when comparable to the wavelength. Based on this finding, several midfield inductive power transfer systems with millimeter-sized receiving antennas were proposed. In [47], a 0.9-mm^3 3D bowtie antenna with a codesigned off-body loop antenna is developed for intracranial power transfer system at 400 MHz. When the bowtie antenna is placed in the cerebrospinal fluid (CSF) layer with an implant depth of 15 mm, a −30.12-dB wireless power link is obtained. In [39], a 2-mm receiving coil with a patterned metal plate antenna is developed for adaptive power transfer to the deep implants at 1.6 GHz. With a 50-mm implant depth in the brain, a −54-dB (0.0006%) power link is established.

4.3.2 Ultrasonic Power Transfer

The ultrasonic power transfer system is generally composed of an off-body transducer, converting the electrical power to the ultrasonic wave, and an implanted receiver, which is usually a microelectromechanical system (MEMS)-based piezoelectric energy harvester. In such a system, the ultrasonic wave transmitted by the off-body transducer (usually an ultrasonic gun) first generates the ultrasonic pressure on the implanted piezoelectric energy harvester. Due to the piezoelectric effect, this mechanical force will then cause the generation of the internal electric charges and potentials inside the piezoelectric material. The operating frequency of ultrasonic power transfer is usually in the range of 35 kHz to 30 MHz, and the attainable maximum operation range can be up to dozens of centimeters with an efficiency up to around 40% [52]. At the same operation frequency, acoustic wave, due to its low propagation speed, has much shorter wavelength than that of the EM waves. For this reason, ultrasound antennas can be created in a very small dimension to form an antenna array to boost the power transfer efficiency [53]. Moreover, the ultrasonic wave can penetrate conductive materials and has small EM interference to the implanted microsystem. The attenuation of the acoustic wave is proportional to the operation frequency and varies for different tissue types. In most of the human tissues, the attenuation coefficient stays in the range of 1–2 dB cm^{-1} MHz^{-1}, for example, the attenuation coefficients in muscle and fat are 1.2 and 0.6 dB cm^{-1} MHz^{-1} [54], respectively. This low attenuation makes it easy to obtain a deep penetration depth of the ultrasonic wave for subcutaneous implantable applications or even for deep-organ implants, such as the wirelessly powered heart pacemaker and drug pumps [55, 56]. However, due to the large attenuation coefficient in bone (22 dB cm^{-1} MHz^{-1}), at a typical operation frequency of 10 MHz, the path loss in skull alone would be more than 100 dB. This considerable attenuation makes the ultrasonic power transfer unlikely an efficient solution for intracranial implantable applications.

4.3.3 Near-Field Capacitive Power Transfer

Near-field capacitive power transfer was initially developed as a WPT scheme for industrial applications. The first exploration of utilizing the capacitive power transfer for implantable applications was reported in [57].

Figure 4.2 illustrates the basic structure of a capacitive power transfer system, which consists of two pairs of capacitive coupled conductor plates, namely the TX plates placed externally on the skin and the RX plates implanted inside the tissue environment. The TX plates are connected to an AC power source, and the power is transferred to the implant through the mutual capacitive coupling between the TX and RX plates in the form of the displacement current across the tissue layer. The operation frequency of the capacitive power transfer system is usually a few megahertz to several hundred megahertz, and the tissue losses (conduction losses and the relaxation losses) are the major factors deteriorating the power transfer efficiency. Since the losses vary with the dielectric properties of the tissue, the operation frequency, and the effective area of the plates, the optimization of the capacitive power transfer system

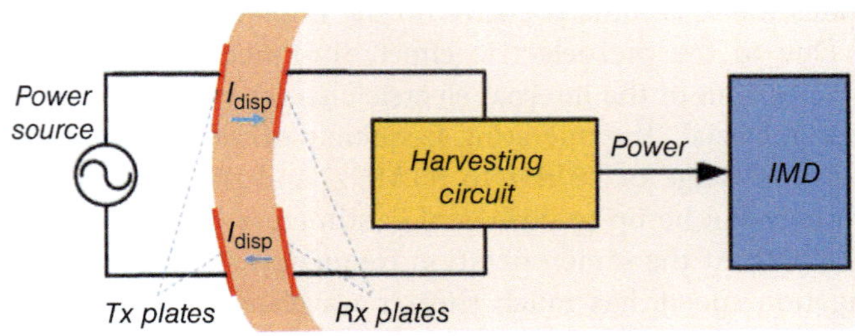

Figure 4.2 Structure of a capacitive power transfer system. (*Source*: Modified from Jegadeesan, R., Agarwal, K., Guo, Y.-X., et al., 2017.)

requires comprehensive case-specific considerations. The authors of [58] give a thorough guideline on the optimization of the capacitive power transfer system by modeling the capacitive power link with an equivalent circuit model. In [58], a flexible subcutaneous capacitive power transfer system is developed. At 98 MHz, with a pair of implanted plates with a size of $20 \times 20\ \text{cm}^2$, the power transfer efficiency reaches more than 70%, and the implant depth is 7 mm. Most recently, the authors of [59] developed an intracranial power transfer system based on the resonant capacitive-coupling approach. The developed power transfer system operates at 6.78 MHz. With a pair of $8 \times 8\ \text{mm}^2$ implantable plates, an implanted intracranial pressure sensor was successfully powered. The maximum implant depth reaches 25 mm, and the power transfer efficiency is 34%. In comparison with the near-field inductive power transfer, the advantage of the capacitive power transfer is its wide operation bandwidth and smaller detuning affect caused by the flexion of the plates. The limitation of the capacitive power transfer is its relative larger implant size due to the necessity of two implanted plates to form the closed current loop.

4.3.4 Far-Field Power Transfer

The principle of the far-field power transfer is the EM radiation. In the free space, when the RX antenna is placed in the far field of the TX antenna, the maximum possible received power by the RX antenna can be calculated with the Friis equation as

$$P_r = \text{PLF} \cdot \frac{P_t G_t G_r \lambda^2}{(4\pi d)^2}, \tag{4.1}$$

where P_t is the output power of the TX antenna, G_t is the gain of the TX antenna, G_r is the gain of the RX antenna, d is the distance between TX and RX antennas, and PLF is the polarization loss factor of the wireless link determined by the polarizations of the antennas and their mutual alignment. In implantable application where the RX antenna is implanted inside the lossy tissue environment, the radiation efficiency (and thereby the gain) of the antenna will be significantly reduced as compared to free space environment. The system level of developing the far-field power transfer system for implantable applications and the relevant safety concerns are presented in [25, 60]. In general, the operation frequency of the far-field power transfer system is in the range of a few hundred megahertz to several gigahertz. The operation distance of the far-field power transfer system can be relative longer (a few decimeters) than that of the inductive- and capacitive-based ones. This longer distance helps communicating with deep implants although the overall link efficiency may not be sufficient for wireless powering of an implant. Moreover, due to the high operation frequency, the RX antenna can be much smaller than that of the near-field-based ones. The limitation of the far-field power transfer is its low power transfer efficiency due to the considerable free space power loss, tissue loss, and the low radiation efficiency of the electrically small antenna. For example, in [25], the authors evaluated a far-field power transfer system for implantable applications, with an operation distance of 0.3 m and the implant depth of 4 mm in the skin. The power transfer efficiency was only 0.01% at 2.4 GHz. This makes the far-field power transfer inapplicable for most of the implantable devices. Recently, with the rapid development of the semiconductor industry, RFID-based ultralow power backscattering microsystems are proposed and evaluated for implantable applications. Without the necessity of the power-consuming active transmitter, the power consumption of the system can be as low as −20 dBm, which opens new possibilities for far-field power transfer in biomedical applications. As a demonstration of this technology, implantable antennas interfaced with a far-field RFID microsystem will be further discussed in Section 4.6.

4.3.5 Computing the Fundamental Performance Indicators of Near-Field WPT Systems Using Two-Port Network Approach

For a WPT system, maximal power transfer efficiency is normally the most decisive performance indicator that directs the design and optimization of the system. In the near-field WPT systems that are the focus of this section, the two antennas that establish the wireless link must be co-optimized and cannot be considered as separate entities as in the far-field WPT. In the biomedical applications, where the wireless link to a medical implant is through the biological tissue and often complex antenna structures with various material types are involved, closed-form formulas for determining the optimal antenna geometries are not available. Thus, the EM optimization of these systems is largely based on the full-wave EM simulations. In this setting, the EM performance parameters characterizing the system and its power efficiency are most conveniently computed from the linear two-port network parameters that model the general relationship between signals at the input and output of the system.

Below, we summarize the computation of some of the most important performance parameters derived from the two-port impedance parameters (Z-parameters) characterizing the WPT system. The analysis could be based on any other network parameter representation, such as scattering parameters (S-parameters), but as compared with most other network parameters, Z-parameters, which map the port voltages to currents, provide a naturalistic connection to circuit analysis. This is beneficial for analyzing impedances, voltages, and currents at nodes of interest within the network.

For further analysis, we consider two sets of Z-parameters as illustrated in Figure 4.3. The first set of the Z-parameters (Z) models the system comprising

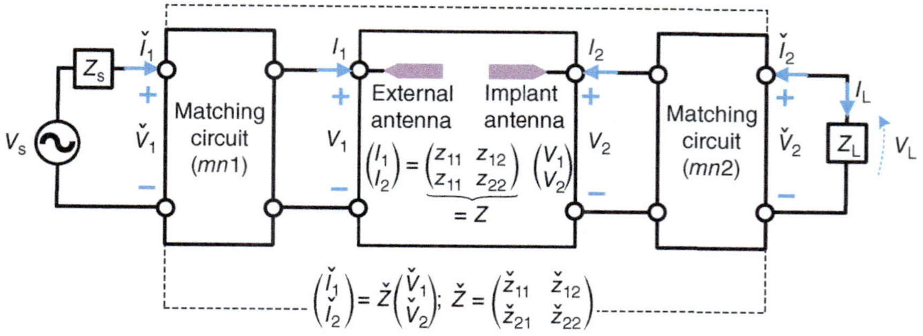

Figure 4.3 Two-port model of a WPT system.

the wireless channel and the antennas only, whereas ($\check{Z}$) models the complete system including the impedance-matching circuits.

In terms of general theory of electronic networks, a WPT system is an unconditionally stable two-port network, because it contains no internal sources of energy. Therefore, it satisfies the following criteria [61, Ch. 2]:

$$\begin{cases} 0 < \mathrm{Re}(z_{11}) \text{ and } 0 < \mathrm{Re}(z_{22}) \\ |z_{12}z_{21}| < 2\mathrm{Re}(z_{11})\mathrm{Re}(z_{22}) - \mathrm{Re}(z_{12}z_{21}) \end{cases}. \tag{4.2}$$

As we consider only regular nonoscillating and unconditionally stable devices acting as the source and load of the system and passive matching circuits, Equation (4.2) implies that the input and output impedances that show up at the external and implant antenna terminals are given by Niknejad [61]

$$Z_{\mathrm{in}} = \frac{V_1}{I_1} = z_{11} - \frac{z_{12}z_{21}}{z_{22} + Z_{mn2}} \quad \text{and} \quad Z_{\mathrm{out}} = \frac{V_2}{I_2} = z_{22} - \frac{z_{12}z_{21}}{z_{11} + Z_{mn1}}, \tag{4.3}$$

where Z_{mn2} and Z_{mn1} denote the impedances seen toward the matching networks from the implant and external antennas, respectively.

The upper bound for the total power efficiency of the system is determined by the link power efficiency that depends on the wireless channel and the antennas only, i.e. the part of the system modeled with **Z** in Figure 4.3. Thus, it is the ratio of the power delivered to the external antenna to the power available from the implant antenna, which is inclusive of the energy dissipation in the biological tissue, link distance, and antenna structures and the related energy dissipation within them and exclusive of the impedance mismatch loss and insertion loss of the matching circuits. The link power efficiency is given by the maximum achievable power gain ($G_{p,\max}$) of the two-port network and computed as [61]

$$G_{p,\max} = \frac{|z_{21}|^2}{q + \sqrt{q^2 - |z_{12}z_{21}|^2}}, \tag{4.4}$$

where $q = 2\text{Re}(z_{11})\text{Re}(z_{22}) - \text{Re}(z_{21}z_{12})$. We note here that the criterion given in Equation (4.3) guarantees that the expression inside the square root will be positive. Overall, the link power efficiency computed from Equation (4.4) is the most crucial performance parameter to be considered in the EM optimization of the antenna structures and to understand the fundamental limit of the total power efficiency of the system.

The total power efficiency is given by the transducer power gain ($\check{G}_t$) of the whole system modeled with ($\check{Z}$) in Figure 4.3. It is the ratio of the power delivered to the load ($Z_L = R_L + jX_L$) to the power available from the source having the internal impedance of $Z_S = R_S + jX_S$ and computed as [61, Ch. 2]

$$\check{G}_t = \frac{4R_S R_L |\check{z}_{21}|^2}{|(Z_S + \check{z}_{11})(Z_L + \check{z}_{22}) - \check{z}_{12}\check{z}_{21}|^2}. \tag{4.5}$$

This quantity is pertinent for the development of the impedance-matching circuits ($mn1$ and $mn2$ in Figure 4.3), following the optimization of the antennas yielding the maximal link power efficiency. The primary target in the circuit development is achieving biconjugate impedance matching for maximizing the total power efficiency. This is achieved by first computing the unique pair of impedances Z_{mS} and Z_{mL}, which once connected to the external and implant antenna terminals, respectively, guarantee simultaneously complex conjugate-matched interfaces between $mn1$ and the external antenna as well as the implant antenna and $mn2$. These optimal antenna terminations are given by Carson [62]

$$Z_{mS/mL} = \frac{\sqrt{q^2 - |z_{12}z_{21}|^2}}{2\text{Re}(z_{22/11})} + j\left(\frac{\text{Im}(z_{12}z_{21})}{2\text{Re}(z_{22/11})} - \text{Im}(z_{11/22})\right), \tag{4.6}$$

where q is as defined in Equation (4.6). Next, the matching circuits for providing the desired impedance transformation for the given source and load impedances of the system are designed. In a weakly coupled system where the factor $Z_{12}Z_{21}$ in Equation (4.6) approaches zero, the approximations $Z_{mS} \approx z_{11}^*$ and $Z_{\text{out}} \approx z_{22}^*$ hold to a good degree of accuracy. In this case, the two matching circuits may be developed independently considering the targets of transforming Z_S to $Z_{mn1} = z_{11}^*$ and Z_L to $Z_{mn2} = z_{22}^*$, which greatly simplifies the circuit development. In both cases, the additional target of the circuit design is using the best practices for component selection and layout design for minimizing the insertion losses of the circuits, so that the total power efficiency ($\check{G}_t$) of the system approaches the link power efficiency ($G_{p,\max}$) at the targeted frequency.

In addition to understanding the power efficiency of the WPT system, for the full assessment, we need to know the power delivered to the load as well as the amplitudes of the load voltage and current. Especially the voltage amplitude is an important parameter for voltage activated circuits, such as rectifiers, that are commonly the frontend stage of a remotely powered microsystem being the load (Z_L) of the WTP system. Given the power available from the source

(P_{avS}), the power delivered to the load is then obtained as $P_L = G_t P_{\text{avS}}$. Finally, Ohm's law ($Z_L = V_L/I_L$) and the fundamental expression [63]

$$P_L = \frac{1}{2}\text{Re}(V_L I_L^*) \tag{4.7}$$

for computing the time-averaged load power from the complex load voltage and current phasors yield the amplitudes of the load voltage and current as follows:

$$|V_L| = \sqrt{\frac{2|Z_L|^2 \breve{G}_t P_{\text{avS}}}{R_L}} \quad \text{and} \quad |I_L| = \sqrt{\frac{2\breve{G}_t P_{\text{avS}}}{R_L}}. \tag{4.8}$$

As an example, we consider a wireless link between a miniature loop antenna formed by metallizing four adjacent faces of a $1 \times 1 \times 1\,\text{mm}^3$-sized cube and a planar circular loop with the inner diameter of 12 mm, which has been developed for a wireless brain–machine interface system [64]. In this application, the cubic loop lies on the cortex harvesting energy for a microsystem that records the electrical activity of the brain. The source of energy is a planar loop placed 5 mm above the scalp. As discussed in [64], due to the miniature size of the implanted antenna and the biological environment, the maximum link power efficiency in this system is attained around 300 MHz, and thus this frequency was considered for further analysis. This result correlates with other works where it has been established that for small implants of the millimeter size and below, the optimum frequency lies in the range from hundreds of megahertz to low-gigahertz range [51, 64, 65], whereas in the WPT systems with centimeter-size and larger implants, the operation frequency is typically lower, in the range of tens of megahertz [66]. The wireless link including the antennas and biological channel was simulated in an anatomical head model of an adult male in ANSYS High-Frequency Structure Simulator (HFSS) for obtaining the impedance parameters **Z** as defined in Figure 4.4. For testing the wireless link, the antennas need to be matched to 50 Ω instruments, and thus we set $Z_S = Z_L = 50\,\Omega$. As expected from the miniature size of the implant, this is a weakly coupled WPT system; thus, as can be seen from Figure 4.5, the approximations $Z_{mS} \approx z_{11}^*$ and $Z_{\text{out}} \approx z_{22}^*$ are valid so that the antenna-matching networks can be designed independently.

Matching circuits made up of two reactive components, also known as L-networks, can transform any complex impedance to a given resistance [63, Ch. 5.1]. Since our source and load are resistive, we followed this simple approach, where the component values and circuit topologies can be determined from closed-form design formulas presented, e.g. [63, Ch. 5.1]. For realizing the matching networks that transform the 50 Ω source and load impedance to $Z_{mn1} = z_{11}^*$ and $Z_{mn2} = z_{22}^*$ at 300 MHz, the following component values were found: $C_{mn1} = 13.0\,\text{pF}$, $L_{mn1} = 1.80\,\text{nH}$, $C_{mn2} = 182\,\text{pF}$, and $L_{mn2} = 0.75\,\text{nH}$. Here, the capacitors are connected in series with the external and implant antennas and are followed by the inductors in parallel. For

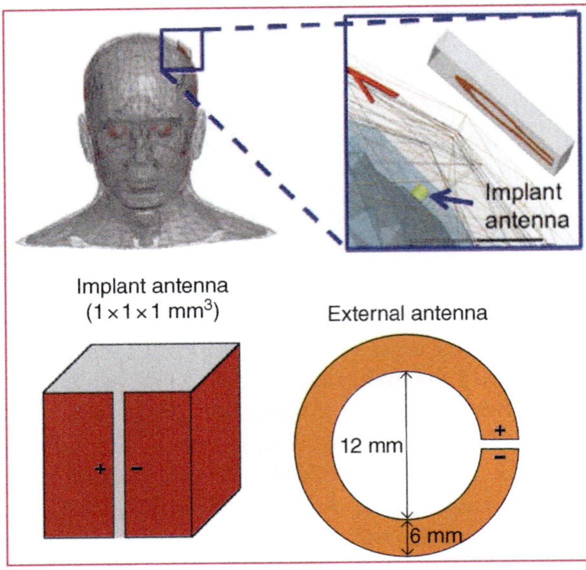

Figure 4.4 Anatomical model with the implant antenna and the external antenna for WPT. (*Source*: Moradi, E., Amendola, S., Björninen, T. et al., 2015. © IEEE.)

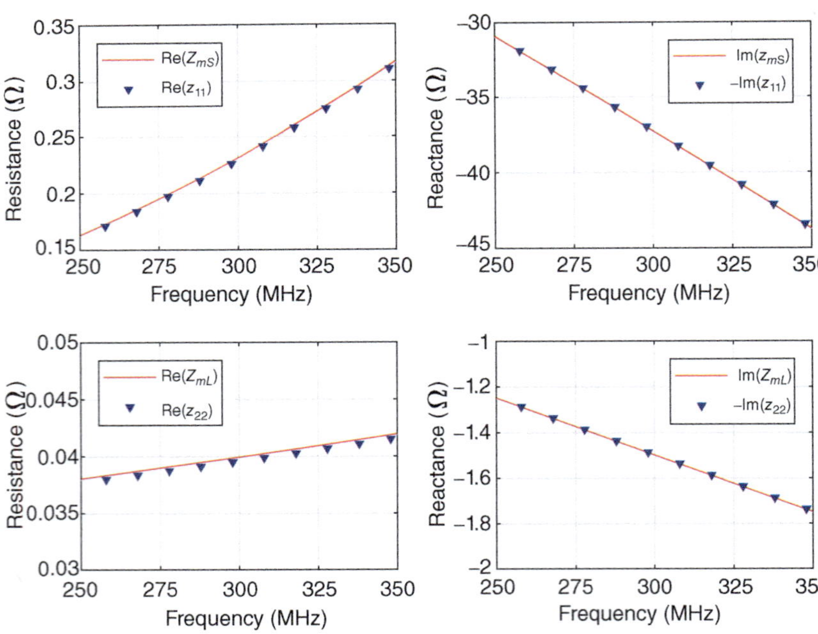

Figure 4.5 Comparison of the exact and approximated optimum antenna terminations.

practical implementations, it should be noted that although the component values are feasible for the targeted frequency, the matching circuits that transform the 50 Ω source and load impedances to impedances with notable low resistance are likely very sensitive toward variability due to, e.g. component tolerances [67], which is a challenge for building robust systems.

The power transfer characteristics of the studied WPT system are summarized in Figures 4.6 and 4.7. The maximum source power for the system is limited by the SAR of the external antenna. In [64], the simulations indicated that under the US FCC safety limit for SAR of 1.6 W kg^{-1} averaged over one gram of tissue, the maximum P_{avS} for the WPT system is 42 mW at 300 MHz.

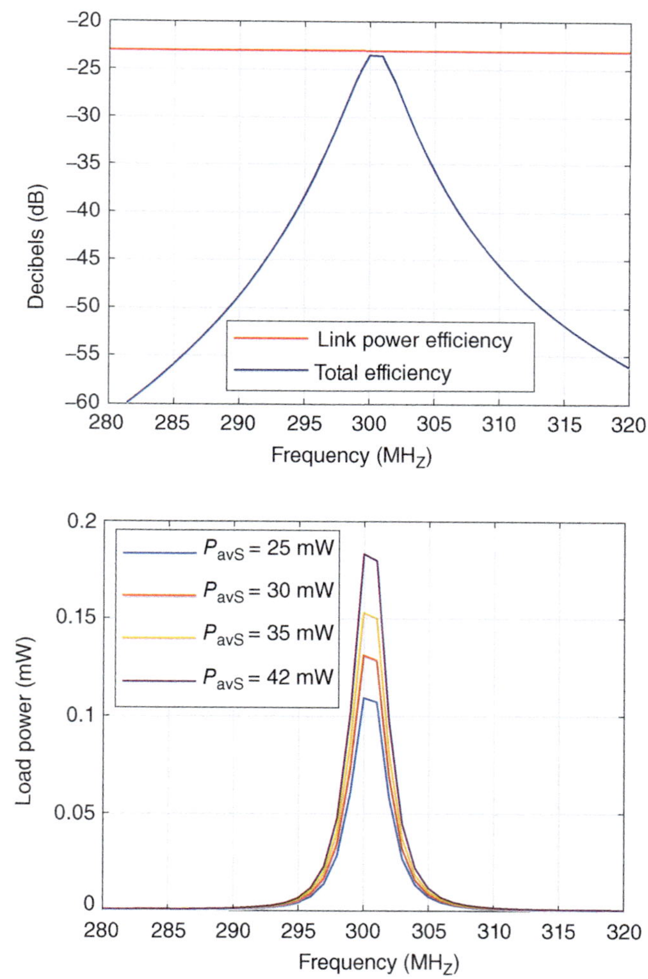

Figure 4.6 Power transfer efficiency and the time-averaged load power of the WPT system.

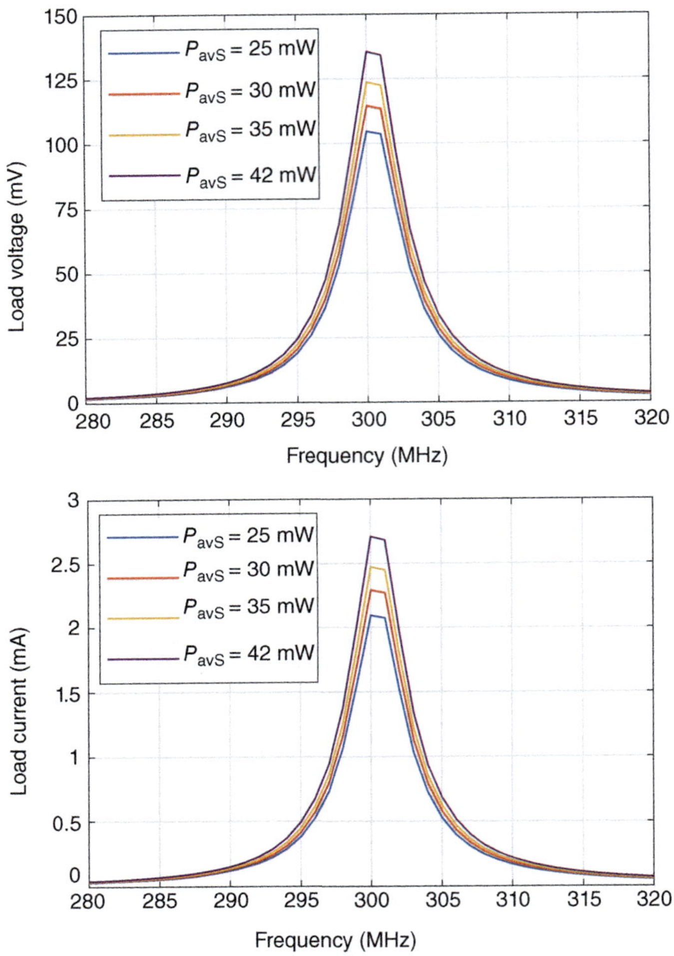

Figure 4.7 Amplitudes of the load voltage and current.

Considering this limit, the maximum load power is 183 mW with the total power efficiency of −23.5 dB at 300 MHz, and the load power remains above 0.1 mW for transmission powers down to 25 mW. Over this range for power transmission, the load voltage and current vary from 100 to 135 mV and from 2 to 2.7 mA. Overall, the data in Figures 4.6 and 4.7 highlights another major challenge for creating biomedical WPT systems with extremely small implants: despite the optimized antennas and operating the system at the frequency of optimal link power efficiency, the power, voltage, and current levels available at the implant are pushing the limits of ultra-low-power circuit design required for the implanted microsystems.

In summary, the two-port network approach offers a computationally simple framework for characterizing near-field coupled biomedical WPT systems. It is compatible with circuit and field simulation software and experiments with vector network analyzer (VNA), which both output the two-port network parameters. It can be applied to both weakly and strongly coupled systems and allows holistic computation of the power efficiency parameters as well as estimation for the absolute load power, voltage, and current, all derived from the network parameters and the given source power.

4.4 Human Body Models for Implantable Antenna Development

In the development of an implantable antenna, computational human body models are indispensable for antenna performance and patient's safety evaluations [68]. On the one hand, the human body models provide the important information on how the surrounding tissues influence the antenna parameters, such as input impedance, radiation efficiency, and directivity. On the other hand, the model reflects the tissue reaction to the EM exposure caused by the antenna radiation. This tissue reaction usually results in the increase of the tissue temperature and may eventually cause tissue damage.

Human body models can be readily made with the computer-aided design (CAD) tools embedded in the EM solvers, such as the finite element method (FEM)-based ANSYS HFSS. The canonical models can be made homogeneously with a single tissue type or with a layered structure including several different tissue types for a better simulation of a specific implant site of the human body. According to the implant sites, the shape of the models can be cubic, cylindrical, or spherical. For example, the seven-layered spherical model with the tissue types of skin, fat, muscle, skull, dura, CSF, and brain is commonly used to mimic the layered structure of the intracranial environment. Table 4.3 lists the five-layered tissue models for mimicking the intracranial environment. The advantage of these homogeneous and layered models is its low computational complexity. When adopted in the full-wave EM solver, it saves the computational resource and increases the simulation speed. Moreover, the favorable deformability of the canonical models gives flexibility to investigate the variations of the tissue structures on the antenna performance. The drawback of these models is the limited anatomical adequacy due to their simplified structure. This inadequacy affects the accuracy of the simulation results, especially when evaluating the antenna far-field parameters, such as the directivity [69].

Apart from the canonical models, the anatomical models based on high-resolution medical imaging (e.g. computerized tomography (CT) and digital magnetic resonance images (MRI)) can be adopted to obtain a more accurate

Table 4.3 Comparison of different human head canonical models.

Refs	Tissue(s)	Shape (volume)
[94]	Skin/tendon/cortical bone	Rectangular ($125 \times 87 \times 12.5\ mm^3$)
[74]	Skin/fat/muscle/skull/dura/CSF/brain	Ellipsoid ($10 \times 10 \times 12.5\ mm^3$)
[89, 95]	Skin/fat/muscle/skull/dura/CSF/gray matter/white matter	Rectangular ($75 \times 35 \times 75\ mm^3$)
[96]	Skin/fat/skull/dura/CSF/brain	Spherical ($\pi \times (200)^2\ mm^3$)
[29]	Skin/fat/skull/brain	Rectangular ($100 \times 100 \times 100\ mm^3$)

Source: Based on Kiourti, A., and Nikita, K. S., 2012.

Table 4.4 FEM-based anatomical human head models.

Refs	Model name	Resolution	Region	Entity/Country
[75]	VHP-female	Variable	Full body	NEVA EM LLC, WPI, USA
[97]	VHP-male	Variable	Full body	NEVA EM LLC, WPI, USA
[98]	BRAIN/SPINAL CORD	$1 \times 1 \times 1\ mm^3$	Head	Universidade de Lisboa, Portugal

Source: Based on Makarov, S. N., Noetscher, G. M., Yanamadala, J., et al. (2017). Virtual human models for electromagnetic studies and their applications. IEEE Reviews in Biomedical Engineering, 10.

estimation of the antenna performance in the tissue environment. Table 4.4 lists three FEM-based anatomical models that can be readily adopted in the HFSS for implantable antenna development. Meanwhile, a thorough and elaborate survey on the most recent anatomical models can be found in [70]. These anatomical models provide the highly detailed structural information of the human tissue. However, the high complexity also makes them computational heavy and consuming more time in the FEM-based EM solvers. Moreover, since each anatomical model reflects the anatomical details of a certain scanned individual, it is generally impossible to adjust the tissue structure to assess the impact of anatomical variability with the anatomical models.

Before any implementation, the human body model must be augmented with the frequency-dependent tissue dielectric properties (e.g. relative permittivity, conductivity, and density). These dispersive dielectric properties can be obtained from the Cole–Cole model or the Debye model. Currently, the IT'IS tissue dielectric database [71], based on the Gabriel's measurements and the four-term Cole–Cole dielectric relaxation model [72, 73], is widely used for the EM modeling of the human body. This database includes the dielectric properties of 45 human tissues in a frequency range from 10 Hz to 100 GHz. Figure 4.8 shows the relative permittivity and conductivity of eight major tissue types of the human head from 1 MHz to 10 GHz.

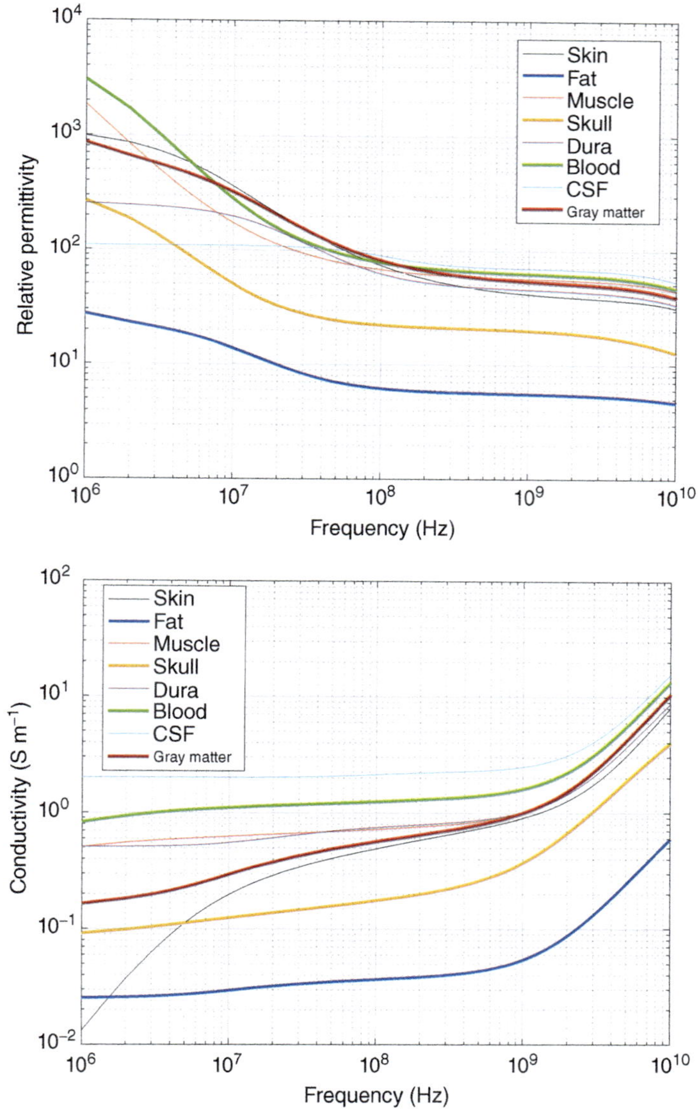

Figure 4.8 Relative permittivity and conductivity of the major tissue types of human head.

4.4.1 Comparison of Human Head Phantoms with Different Complexities for Intracranial Implantable Antenna Development

The selection of human body model influences not only the computation efficiency but more importantly the accuracy of the simulation results. In this section, we evaluate different human head models with an identical implantable antenna. The model complexity and the simulated antenna parameters will be evaluated and compared to provide the reader with a reference of the model selection for implantable antenna development.

The antenna [74] selected in this human head model evaluation is developed for the intracranial RFID backscattering system. Figure 4.9 shows the antenna under test and its dimensions. The antenna consists of wearable and implantable parts. The implant is placed within the CSF, and the wearable part is attached on the scalp concentrically. We used the 2-mm-thick EPDM (Ethylene-Propylene Diene Monomer) ($\varepsilon_r = 1.26$, $\tan\delta = 0.007$ at 915 MHz) as the substrate for the wearable and 50-μm-thick flexible polyethylene ($\varepsilon_r = 2.25$, $\tan\delta = 0.001$ at 915 MHz) for the implantable parts. We made the insulation box with silicone ($\varepsilon_r = 2.2$, $\tan\delta = 0.007$ at 915 MHz) with a thickness of 1 mm. In the simulation, we modeled the RFID microchip with a parallel connection of the resistance and capacitance of 2.85 kΩ and 0.91 pF, respectively. We optimized the antenna impedance to achieve a good complex conjugate matched to the RFID IC in the tissue environment.

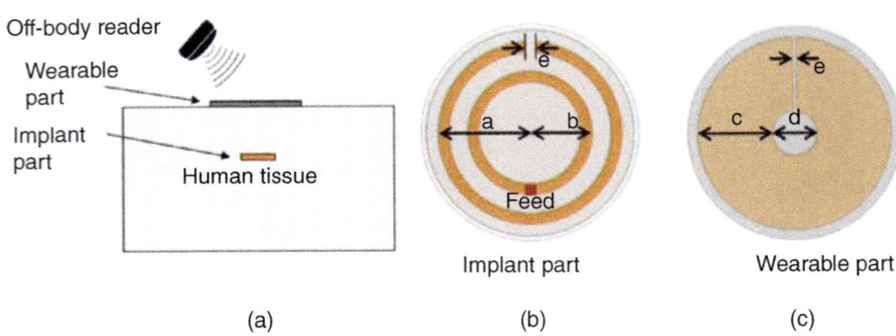

Geometrical parameter (mm)	a	b	c	d	e
	8.6	5.7	20.8	12.6	1.0

Figure 4.9 Implantable antenna with its geometrical dimensions. (*Source*: Modified from Ma, S., Sydänheimo, L., Ukkonen, L., et al., 2018.)

The attainable interrogating distance (d_{tag}) given in Equation (4.9) is the main indicator to evaluate the antenna performance.

$$d_{tag} = \frac{\lambda}{4\pi}\sqrt{\frac{\mathrm{D}e_{r}\tau\mathrm{EIRP}}{\mathrm{P}_{ic0}}}, \quad \text{where } \tau = \frac{4\mathrm{Re}(Z_A)\mathrm{Re}(Z_c)}{|Z_A + Z_C|^2} \tag{4.9}$$

The d_{tag} is inversely proportional to the turn-on power (P_{ic0}) of the IC and proportional to radiation efficiency (e_r), antenna directivity (D), power transfer efficiency (τ), and the equivalent isotropically radiated power limitation (EIRP). The power transfer efficiency evaluates the power transfer efficiency from the antenna to the IC; in another words, it quantifies the goodness of the complex conjugate impedance matching between the antenna and the microchip. Apparently, the d_{tag} is directly influenced by the e_r, D, and τ, and we, respectively, compare these antenna parameters in the four different head models.

Figure 4.10 shows the four human head models in this evaluation. The anatomical head model A is obtained from the open source anatomical VHP-female model [75], which includes 15 individual tissue types and 58 different tissue parts. The model B is a simplified version of the model A. We reduced its complexity by including only six major tissue types: brain, CSF, skull, muscle, fat, and skin. We further reduced the model complexity with the semianatomical model C, where a six-layered ellipsoid is integrated to substitute the VHP model's cranial cavity. The structure of the six-layered ellipsoid was built as ellipsoid shells with an adjustable thickness representing the skin, fat, muscle, skull, CSF, and brain. We set the thickness of each layer according to the measurement from the implant location of the VHP model. The model D is a layered box model with a dimension of $30 \times 30 \times 20\,\mathrm{mm}^3$.

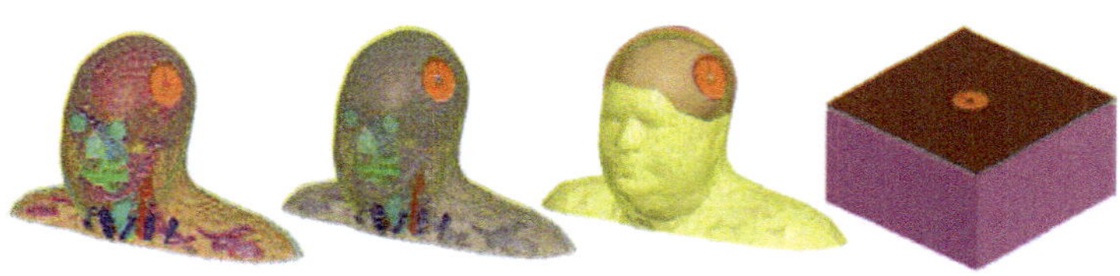

	A	B	C	D
Components	15 individual tissues and 58 seperate tissue parts	Six major tissue layer -skin, fat, muscle, skull, CSF and brain	Six major tissue layer -skin, fat, muscle, skull, CSF and brain	Six major tissue layer skin, fat, muscle, skull, CSF and brain
Layer structure	Original medical image based	Original medical image based	Six-layer ellipsoid replacing the cranial cavity	Six flat block layers 30 × 30 × 20 cm^3

Figure 4.10 Comparison of the evaluated four head models.

The box model has the same six-layered structure as that of the ellipsoid one, but all the layers are in a flat form. The dielectric properties of each tissue type are assigned according to the database from IT'IS foundation [71].

The evaluation is conducted with the full-wave EM solver ANSYS HFSS v.17. The computer that performed the simulations is equipped with Intel i7 X990 at 3.47 GHz with 24 GB of RAM. In the simulation, the change of the simulated τ, e_r, and D in each iteration is monitored. At the sixth iteration, the solution reached the convergence, with the maximum change in τ, e_r, and D being less than 0.01, 0.14, and 0.13%, respectively, between the subsequent mesh adaptation iterations. Figure 4.11 compares the number of solved elements and the simulation time (mesh generation and solving 15 frequency points) in the four head models. The simulation speed of the VHP full model is more than six times slower than that of the ellipsoid and block models. The simplified VHP model also has a noticeable reduction of the model complexity and time consumption.

Figure 4.12 shows the simulated τ, e_r, D, and d_{tag} in the four head models. We considered the results from the VHP full model as the reference model to evaluate the rest models. According to the comparison of the power transfer efficiency τ shown in Figure 4.12a, both the ellipsoid and box models witness a detuning of the peak frequency from 925 to 942 MHz. Contrarily, the simplified VHP model has an inappreciable influence on τ. In the comparison of the e_r in Figure 4.12b, the box model has the worst accuracy with detuning of the peak frequency and more than 50% level underestimation; however, the ellipsoid model estimates the peak frequency correctly with less than 10% overestimation of the efficiency level. Figure 4.12c compares the D; the box model is unable

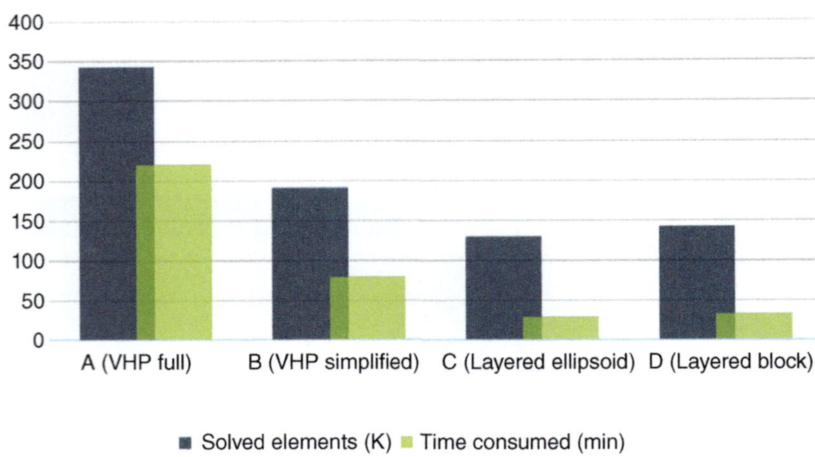

Figure 4.11 Comparison of the solved elements and time consumption of the four head models.

to show its variation with the frequency, and the level estimation is 1.5 dB lower than that from the VHP full model. In contrast, the ellipsoid model reflects the variation of D versus the frequency, and the level estimation is only 0.5 dB than the VHP full model. Finally, the simulated d_{tag} in the four models is compared in Figure 4.12d. Here, although the box model shows a fine agreement with the VHP full model, it should be mentioned that this agreement is only because of its poor estimation of e_r and D compensating each other in the final computation of d_{tag}. Overall, in the estimation of d_{tag}, the simplified VHP model provides nearly the identical results compared with the VHP model, and the ellipsoid model has a minor frequency detuning with a small level shift.

According to the simulation results, the layered box model properly estimates the antenna impedance; however, it fails to provide an accurate estimation of antenna far-field parameters. The layered ellipsoid model not

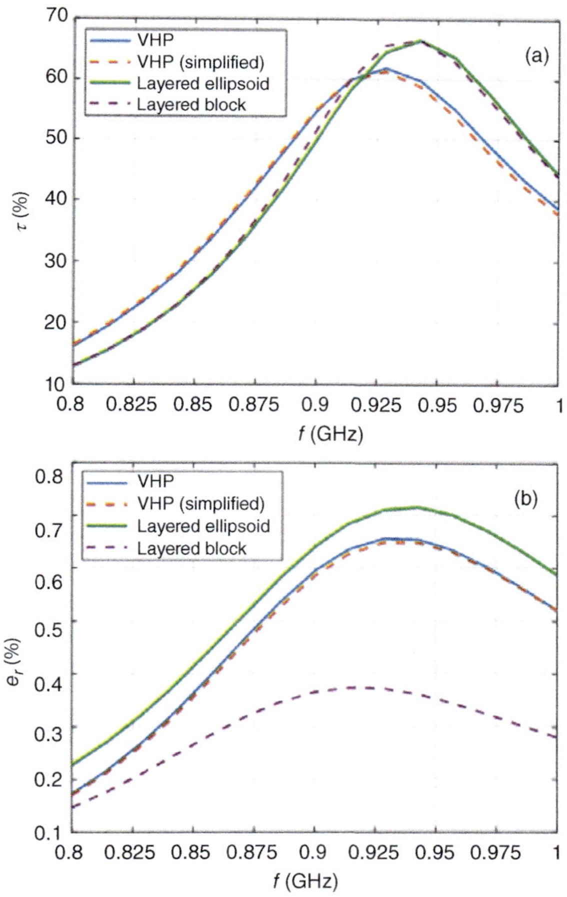

Figure 4.12_1 Comparison of the simulated τ and e_r of the four head models.

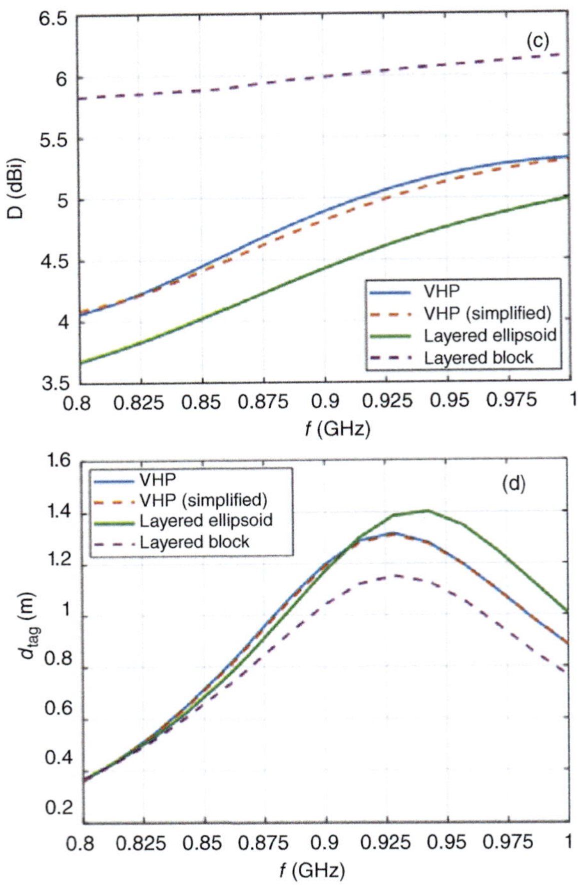

Figure 4.12_2 Comparison of the simulated D and d_{tag} of the four head models.

only accurately predicts the antenna impedance but also estimates the far-field parameters fairly well; moreover, the simulation time with the ellipsoid model is less than the box model. For this reason, the box model is not recommended for intracranial antenna development. The anatomically simplified VHP model predicts nearly the same antenna parameters as that of the VHP full model. Therefore, it is not recommended to use the full anatomical model for its redundant anatomical adequacy. Meanwhile, the inclusion of dominant layer tissues, skin, fat, muscle, skull, CSF, and brain, is enough to obtain accurate results to save the computational resource. Overall, when developing the intracranial implantable antenna, ellipsoid model is recommended for preliminary antenna optimization and robustness studies where the layer thicknesses are variable and the model complexity is simplified. The anatomical models are more suitable for final verifications of the antenna performance.

4.5 Wirelessly Powered Intracranial Pressure Sensing System Integrating Near- and Far-Field Antennas

Intracranial pressure (ICP) is defined as the pressure inside the cranial cavity concealing three major volume components: blood, brain tissue, and CSF. The biological autoregulation of the cerebral blood flow and circulation of CFS maintains the stable ICP below 15 mmHg in adults. The ICP is an important indicator as the dysfunction of autoregulation and/or brain swelling that leads to intracranial hypertension and the increase of the ICP. The excessive ICP impedes the supply of oxygenated blood in the brain and causes brain damage. For this reason, the real-time monitoring of ICP plays a crucial role in the management of various brain diseases and injuries [76]. Currently, for the critically ill patients, the ICP is commonly measured from the ventricular system of the brain through a catheter; this method is accurate, allows on-site recalibration as well as drainage of CSF to manage raised ICP, but is not fit for long-term monitoring due to its invasiveness with the risk of hemorrhage and infection. Therefore, several studies [66, 77–80] focused on the development of wireless implantable sensors for long-term monitoring of ICP are proposed. The authors of [77] present a battery-powered sensor for ICP monitoring at 2.45 GHz. The main limitations of the battery-powered implantable sensors are the large size and limited lifetime of the battery. To address this limitation, passive ICP sensors are proposed in the literature. In [78], a transcranial implant integrated with the antenna and electronics for wireless monitoring of subdural pressures is proposed and demonstrated. To optimize the footprint of the implant and thus minimize the invasiveness, the authors of [79, 80] developed capacitive MEMS-based battery-free ICP sensors. These passive devices are small and flexible; however, they have limited functionality and short operation distance compared with the battery-powered sensors. Alternatively, the batteryless ICP sensors equipped with the wireless power harvester are a potential minimally invasive solution to overcome the lifetime and size limitation of the battery-assisted method and the limited operation distance of the fully passive method. The work in [66] proposes the development of a batteryless wirelessly powered ICP sensor. Figure 4.13 shows the system architecture of the proposed sensor that consists of in-, on-, and off-body units. The in-body unit has four parts including a two-turn coil antenna for wireless powering, a rectifier for RF-to-DC conversion, a piezoresistive pressure sensor, and a data transmission unit. The in-body unit is placed under the skull and powered by the on-body unit through inductive coupling. The piezoresistive pressure sensor has a differential output voltage which is proportional to the change in the pressure. When activated, this output voltage of the pressure sensor is amplified through an amplifier and drives the voltage control oscillator (VCO). Finally, the far-field antenna connected to the VCO output transmits the pressure readout to the off-body unit.

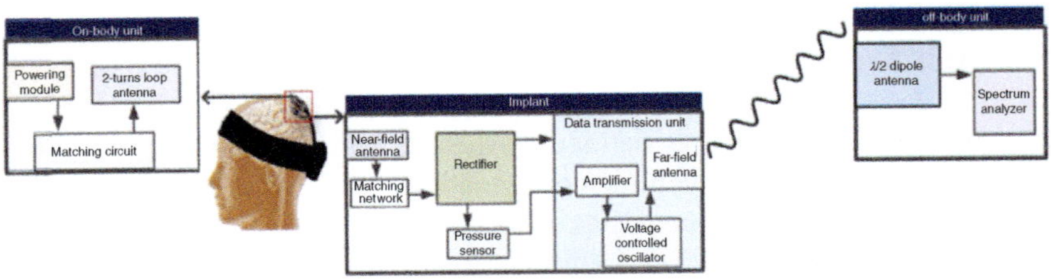

Figure 4.13 System-level description of the pressure sensing system for wireless ICP monitoring.

4.5.1 Far-Field Antenna for Data Transmission

As outlined above, our wirelessly powered ICP sensing system integrates near- and far-field links for the wireless powering and data communication, respectively. Given the application, the development of the whole system is driven by achieving thin and flexible platform with as small as possible overall size. In our case, the size is limited by the size of the inductive loop (discussed in detail in the following section) required for achieving adequate power transfer efficiency. With the aim of not increasing the platform size, the far-field antenna and other electronics must fit within the area of the loop. Stemming from these considerations, the required footprint size of the far-field antenna was limited to $6 \times 5\ \text{mm}^2$. Due to the thinness of the substrate, we considered only planar antennas, and due to the compactness of PIFAs among them, we selected this antenna type for further considerations. As shown in Figure 4.14, we have applied spiral folding on the radiating arm for

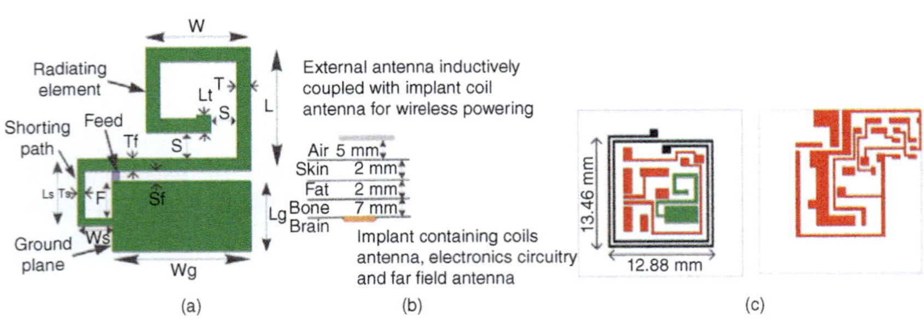

Symbol	L	W	Lg	Wg	Ls	Ws	T	S	Lt	Sf	Tf	F	Ts
Value (mm)	3.55	3	2	4	1.9	1	0.4	0.75	0.5	0.3	0.35	1.05	0.2

Figure 4.14 (a) Top view of the design antenna. (b) Cross-sectional view of the tissue model. (c) Implant front and back side views (red traces represent electronic circuitry, black represents two-turn coil antenna, and green represents far-field antenna). (*Source*: Khan, M. W. A., Moradi, E., et al., 2017. License under CC by 4.0.)

lowering the resonance frequency to 2.45 GHz. The antenna was simulated and optimized in the ANSYS HFSS v15 with the target of maximizing the realized gain pointing outward the brain within the constrained area of $6 \times 5\,\text{mm}^2$. In the simulation, a tissue model with four tissue layers, skin, fat, bone, and brain, was built to represent the intracranial tissue environment.

Figure 4.14b shows the structure of the tissue model. The proposed antenna was placed on the sensor platform together with electronics circuit traces as shown in Figure 4.14c. To isolate the antenna from the tissue environment, a silicone coating was made to cover both sides of the antenna. Figure 4.15a shows the simulated reflection coefficient of the antenna. The −10-dB bandwidth of the proposed antenna in the simulation is 280 MHz (2.21–2.49 GHz), and the antenna reflection ecoefficiency at 2.45 GHz is −14 dB. The simulated 3D antenna gain is demonstrated in Figure 4.15b with peak gain of −19.6 dBi

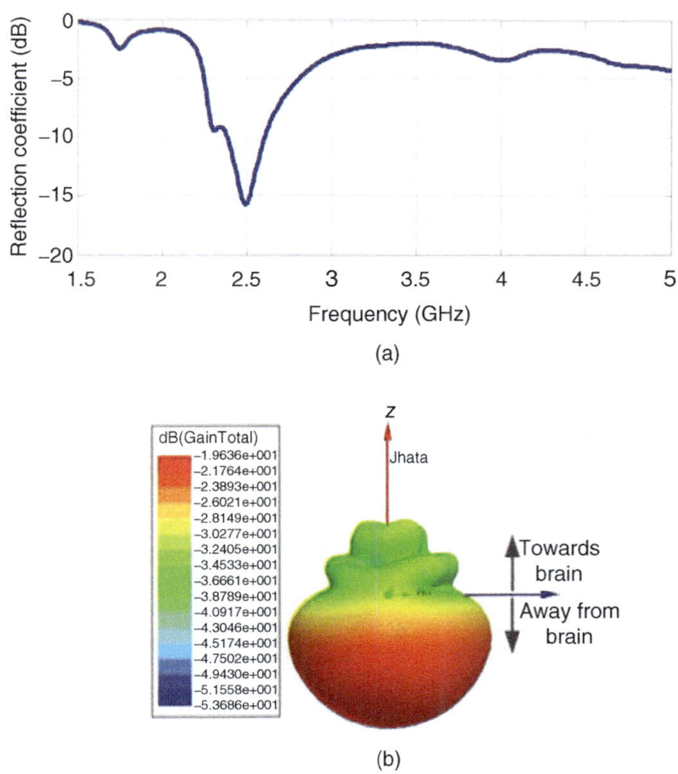

Figure 4.15 (a) Simulated reflection coefficient (dB). (b) Antenna 3D gain pattern at 2.45 GHz. (*Source*: Khan, M. W. A., Moradi, E., Sydänheimo, L., et al., 2017.)

toward the direction away from the brain. The antenna radiation efficiency and directivity at 2.45 GHz are 0.5% and 4.33 dBi, respectively. The SAR estimation of the antenna was conducted using a block phantom ($18.75 \times 18.75 \times 30\,cm^3$) with only brain and bone tissue. The height of the block was set to 30 cm to accommodate two averaging cubes containing approximate 1 g of the brain and bone. Figure 4.16a shows the E-field distribution at 2.45 GHz. The radiating element of the antenna is acting as a $\lambda/2$ resonator at 2.45 GHz. Figure 4.16b

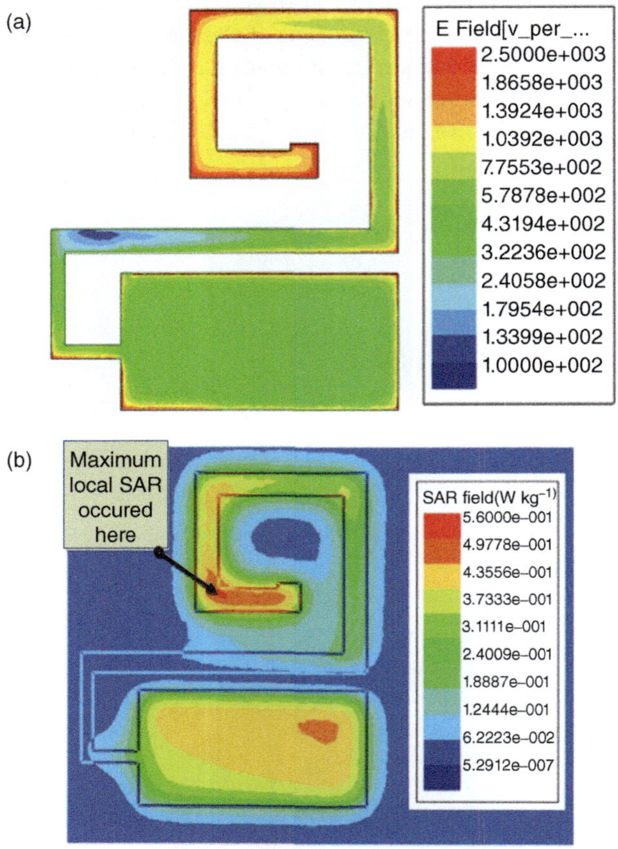

Figure 4.16 (a) E-field ($V\,m^{-1}$) distribution at the antenna surface. (b) Local SAR ($W\,kg^{-1}$) distribution at the bone interface when the input power to antenna is 0.5 mW at 2.45 GHz. (*Source*: Khan, M. W. A., Moradi, E., Sydänheimo, L., et al., 2017.) Miniature coplanar implantable antenna on thin and flexible platform for fully wireless intracranial pressure monitoring system. International Journal of Antennas and Propagation, 1–9. License under CC by 4.0.)

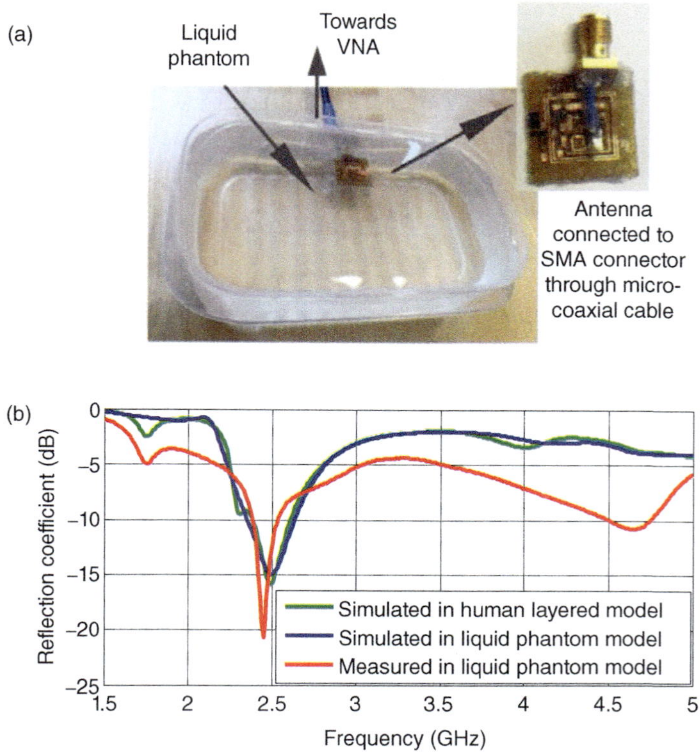

Figure 4.17 (a) Reflection coefficient measurement setup and fabricated antenna. (b) Simulated (both human head and liquid phantom) and measured reflection coefficient (dB). (*Source*: Khan, M. W. A., Moradi, E., Sydänheimo, L., et al., 2017.)

presents the local SAR distribution at the bone interface. The maximum local SAR value is 0.58 W kg^{-1}, and the maximum SAR-compliant transmission power is 5.53 mW.

The antenna was manufactured on the flexible polyimide substrate for the experimental verifications. Figure 4.17a shows the prototype and the measurement setup. The liquid phantom ($\varepsilon_r = 39.2$ and $\sigma = 1.8$ S m^{-1} at 2.45 GHz) made of water, sugar, and salt was used to mimic the human head environment [81]. Figure 4.17b presents the simulated (both human-layered and liquid-phantom models) and measured reflection coefficients. A good agreement can be found between the simulation and measurement results. The measured −10 dB bandwidth is 160 MHz (from 2.38 to 2.54 GHz) with 20.8 dB return loss at 2.45 GHz. The bandwidth is verified to cover the whole range of the ISM band.

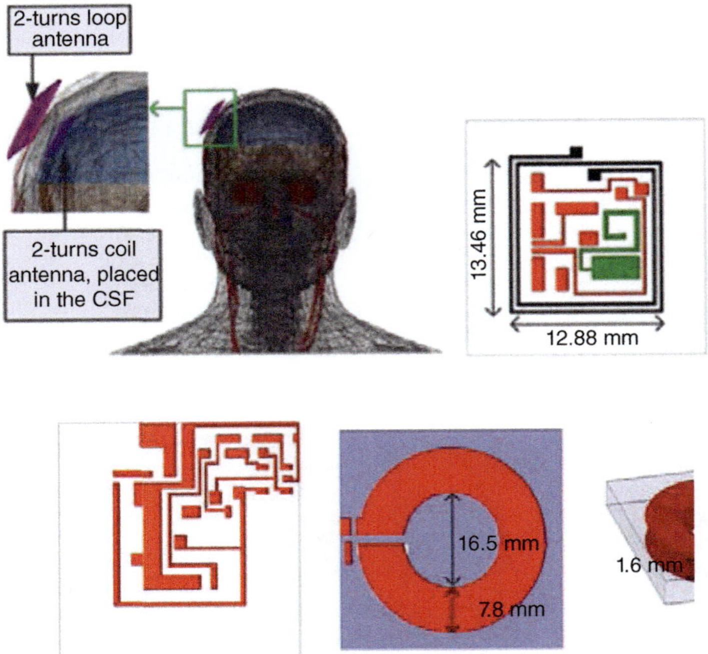

Figure 4.18 (a) Anatomical head model in the simulation for wireless link and antenna modeling. (b) The front side of the implant consists of two-turn coil antenna (black), far-field antenna (green), and traces of other components (red). (c) The backside of the implant consists of traces of electronic components. (d) Top view of the external antenna. (e) Side view of the external antenna.

4.5.2 Antenna for Near-Field Wireless Power Transfer

The WPT link of the proposed ICP sensor is established by two inductively coupled loop antennas. Figure 4.18b and c show the top and bottom sides view of the 2-turn RX loop antenna in the in-body unit, respectively. This antenna is designed on a 50-μm-thick flexible polyimide substrate ($\varepsilon_r = 3.3$ and $\tan\delta = 0.002$ at 15 MHz). For biocompatibility, the implant is encapsulated with silicone and Parylene C coating. Figure 4.18d and e show the two-turn TX loop antenna in the on-body unit. The antenna is designed on FR4 substrate with an inner diameter of 16.5 mm and a trace width of 7.8 mm. The gap between the two loops is 1.6 mm, which is equal to the height of the substrate. As shown in Figure 4.18a, the two-turn TX loop antenna of the on-body unit is placed 5 mm away from the skin. The two-turn RX coil antenna of the in-body unit is placed in the CSF layer. The separation between the two antennas is 16 mm. The two inductively coupled loop antennas can be modeled as a two-port network, and the maximum link power efficiency of the system can be calculated with Equation (4.4). This link power efficiency is determined by the inherent EM properties of the system, and the impedance matching is excluded. The power fed into the TX loop antenna should not exceed the $P_{t,\max}$ that generates $\mathrm{SAR}_{\max}$ (FCC regulation: 1.6 W kg^{-1}) in the closest tissue (skin, in this case). Since the SAR is proportional to the power delivered into the two-turn loop antenna, the $P_{t,\max}$ can be calculated with

$$\frac{\mathrm{SAR}}{\tau P_{\mathrm{test}}} = \frac{\mathrm{SAR}_{\max}}{P_{t,\max}}; \quad \tau = \frac{4 \cdot 50\Omega \cdot \mathrm{Re}(Z_{\mathrm{ext}})}{|50\Omega + Z_{\mathrm{ext}}|^2}, \tag{4.10}$$

where $P_{\mathrm{test}} = 1$ W is the power available from a 50-Ω test source in HFSS, and τ is the power transfer efficiency between the test source and the two-turn loop antenna (impedance: Z_{ext}). Hence, the maximum power available for a load connected to the coil antenna $P_L = P_{t,\max}\, G_{p,\max}$. Figure 4.19 shows the simulated link power efficiency ($G_{p,\max}$), maximum SAR-compliant transmission power ($P_{t,\max}$), and power delivered to the implant antenna load (P_L) under conjugate-matched conditions. The simulation results show that

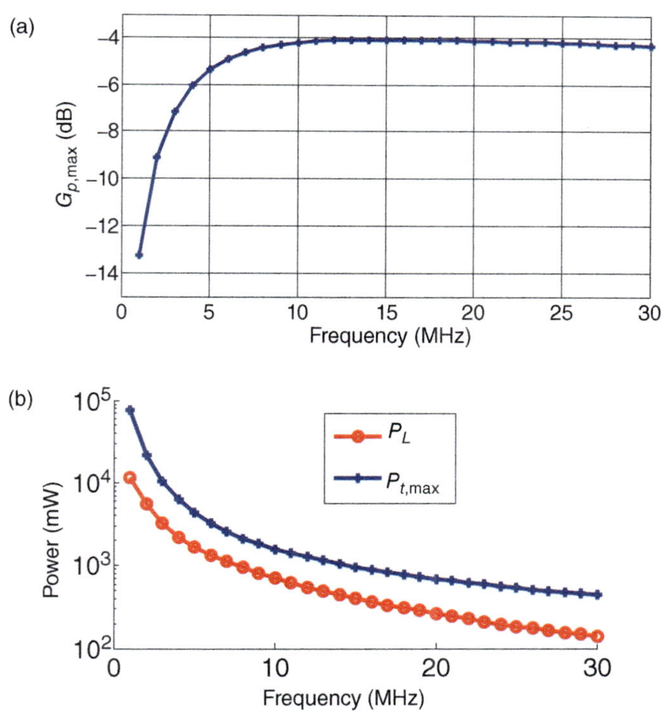

Figure 4.19 (a) Link power efficiency ($G_{p,\max}$). (b) Maximum SAR-compliant transmission power ($P_{t,\max}$) and power delivered to the implant antenna load (P_L) under conjugate-matched conditions.

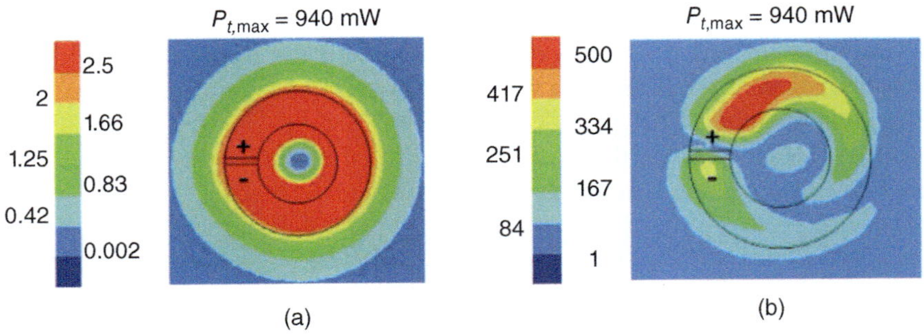

Figure 4.20 (a) Local SAR (W kg^{-1}) distribution on the skin when the maximum allowed power is transmitted at 15 MHz. (b) Local E-field (V m^{-1}) distribution on the skin when the maximum power is transmitted at 15 MHz.

the maximum of $G_{p,max}$ of −4 dB occurs at 15 MHz. Figure 4.20 shows the local SAR and the E-field distribution on the skin when $P_{t,max}$ of 940 mW is transmitted at 15 MHz. In the wireless measurement, the prototyped antennas were fabricated and tested in the tissue-mimicking liquid. The port of the TX loop antenna was connected to the VNA port 1, and the RX coil antenna was connected to the VNA port 2. The two antennas were concentrically aligned with a separation distance of 16 mm. Figure 4.21 shows the measured S-parameters and the power transferred. The measured transmission loss between the antennas is 15.5 dB. The reflection coefficients of the two-turn loop antenna and two-turn coil antenna are −5.3 and −7.3 dB, respectively. With the input power of 31 dBm fed into the on-body unit and S11 of −5.3 dB, the power coupled to the on-body loop antenna is 889 mW, which is under the maximum SAR-compliant transmission power $P_{t,max}$ (940 mW) at 15 MHz. The system power transfer efficiency is 2.81%, and the power delivered to the rectifier is 13.17 dBm.

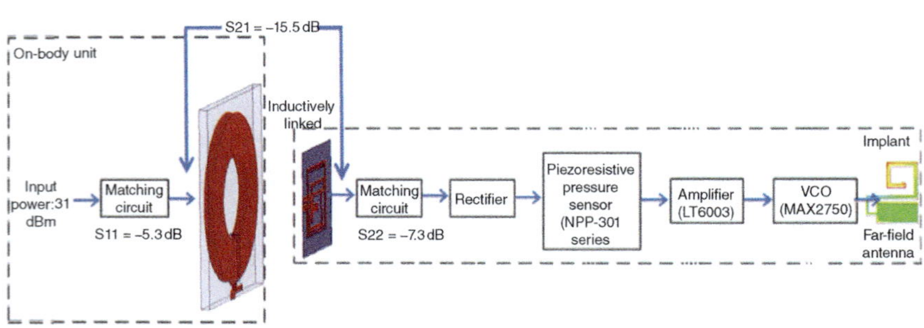

Figure 4.21 Measured S-parameters and power transfer of wireless power transfer system.

4.6 Far-Field RFID Antennas for Intracranial Wireless Communication

In recent years, RFID technique, due to its favorable features such as the low power consumption and simple RF front-end structure, has been considered as a promising strategy in building the wireless data link for biomedical sensing applications. In [82], a tiny RFID sensor tag is proposed for continuous glucose monitoring. The authors of [83] developed the RFID sensor tag equipped with the helix antenna for wireless monitoring of drug dosage. In [84], an RFID-based sensing platform is developed for continuous monitoring of the physiological data of animals. These RFID sensor tags harvest the energy from the reader's carrier wave and use impedance modulation to backscatter the data to the reader. Without the necessity of the battery and the active RF transmitter, the sensor size is significantly minimized. Since the operation of the RFID sensor tag entirely relies on the energy harvested from the incoming EM wave transmitted by the RFID reader, a proper impedance matching between the RFID IC and tag antenna becomes critical for the overall system performance. Unlike the most conventional antennas with a 50-Ω resistance, the RFID antennas need to have an inductive impedance to obtain a proper complex conjugate matching to the RFID IC usually with a large capacitive reactance (for instance −100 to −300 Ω) and a low resistance (for instance 20 to 50 Ω). In this section, we introduce two techniques to develop the miniature implantable RFID antenna with high inductive antenna reactance for intracranial biomedical applications.

4.6.1 Split Ring Resonator-Based Spatially Distributed Implantable Antenna System

Wireless electronic devices targeting for invasive biomedical applications need to meet the strict miniaturization requirement to minimize the invasiveness and reduce the risk of infections. This miniaturization requirement brings considerable challenge to the development of implantable antennas. Antennas with a miniaturized footprint inherently suffer from low radiation efficiency and poor antenna directivity. When implanted in the lossy tissue environment, antenna RF performance becomes even worse. To obtain a proper antenna RF performance while maintaining a small size of the implantable antenna, a spatially distributed implantable RFID antenna system is proposed in [74]. The proposed antenna system has a small implant part carrying the RFID microsystem and an inductively coupled wearable part for antenna gain improvement. Figure 4.22 demonstrates the antenna structure with its geometrical parameters and the implemented position in a layered ellipsoid model. The wearable part of the antenna system is attached on the scalp, and the split ring resonator-based implant part is concentrically implanted in the

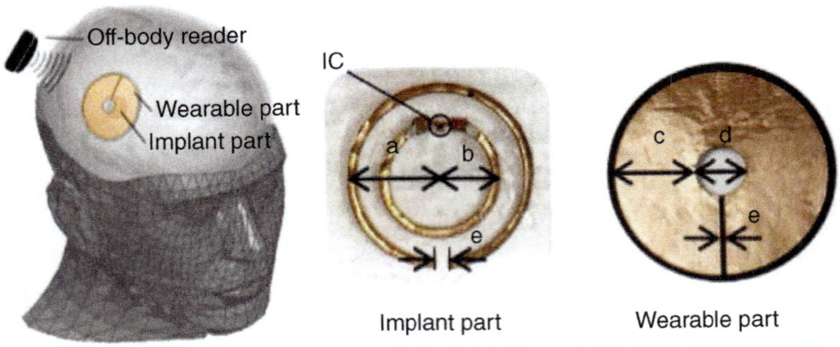

Geometrical parameter (mm)	a	b	c	d	e
	8.6	5.7	20.8	12.6	1.0

Figure 4.22 Anatomical head model and antenna system with its geometrical dimensions. (*Source*: Ma, S., Sydänheimo, L., Ukkonen, L., et al., 2018. © IEEE.)

CSF tissue layer. The implant part is developed on the 50-μm-thick flexible polyimide substrate ($\varepsilon_r = 2.25$, $\tan\delta = 0.001$ at 915 MHz), and the substrate for the wearable part is 2-mm-thick EPDM (Ethylene-Propylene Diene Monomer; $\varepsilon_r = 1.26$, $\tan\delta = 0.007$ at 915 MHz). The NXP UCODE G2iL series RFID IC as the target microsystem was attached to the inner ring split of the implant part using the conductive epoxy—Circuit Works CW2400. The silicone coating ($\varepsilon_r = 2.2$, $\tan\delta = 0.007$ at 915 MHz) with a thickness of 1 mm is used to insulate the antenna from the tissue environment.

The antenna simulation and optimization were conducted with the ANSYS HFSS. In the simulation, the RFID IC is modeled as the parallel connection of the resistance and capacitance of 2.85 kΩ and 0.91 pF, respectively [85]. Meanwhile, the ANSYS anatomical human head model integrated with a seven-layered ellipsoid is built to mimic the human head. Figure 4.23 shows the details of the anatomical head model combined with the layered ellipsoid. All the tissues were assigned with their corresponding relative permittivity and loss tangent according to the database of tissue dialectical properties from IT'IS Foundation [71].

As shown in Figure 4.24, the proposed antenna system has nine geometrical parameters. According to the parametric analysis conducted in [74], the antenna input impedance is dominated by the geometrical structure of the implant part, and the wearable part only influences the antenna directivity. To facilitate the process of antenna optimization, the geometrical parameters of the implant part are first determined. Then the dimension of the wearable part is optimized to maximize the antenna gain.

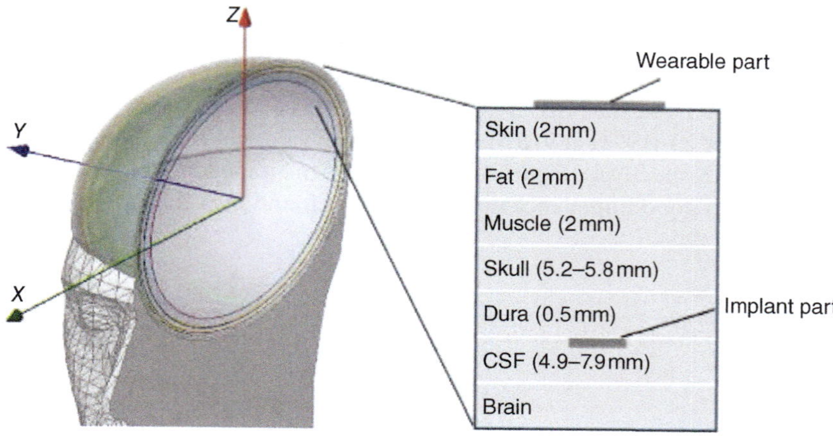

Figure 4.23 Anatomical human head model with the layered ellipsoid. (*Source*: Ma, S., Sydänheimo, L., Ukkonen, L., et al., 2018. © IEEE.)

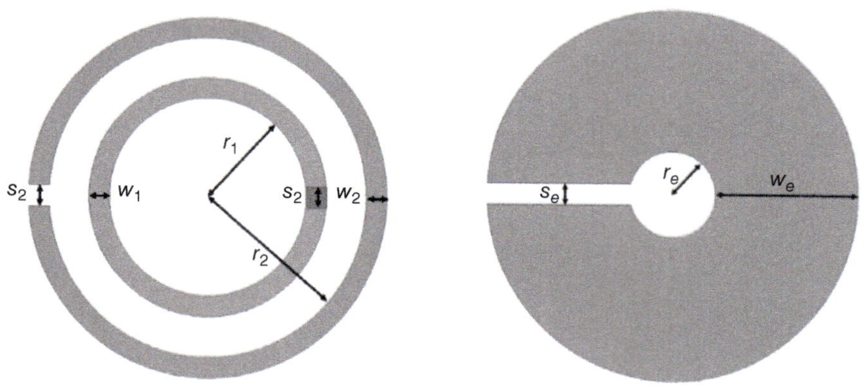

Figure 4.24 Structure and dimensional parameters of the antenna-implantable part and the wearable part.

Among the six geometrical parameters of the implant part, the increase of the inner radius of the inner ring r_1 leads to the increase of the resistance and inductive reactance of the antenna input impedance. The inner radius of the outer ring r_2, on the other hand, is proportional to the resistance of the antenna input impedance, while reversely proportional to the inductive reactance of the antenna input impedance. Both the strip widths of the inner ring and outer ring have a reverse and positive relationship with the antenna resistance and inductive reactance, respectively. The increase of the rings' slit s_1 and s_2 will slightly decrease the antenna resistance; however, it has negligible impact on the antenna reactance. Overall, the inner radius of the inner ring r_1 is for coarse adjustment of the antenna input impedance, and the rest of the parameters can be adjusted to achieve the good complex conjugate impedance matching to the RFID IC. For the NXP UCODE G2iL RFID IC that is modeled with the impedance of 20-j190 Ω at 915 MHz, the optimal values of the r_1 and r_2 are 8.6 and 5.7 mm, respectively. Figure 4.25a compares the impedance of the antenna and the IC. A good impedance matching can be found near the 915 MHz. The

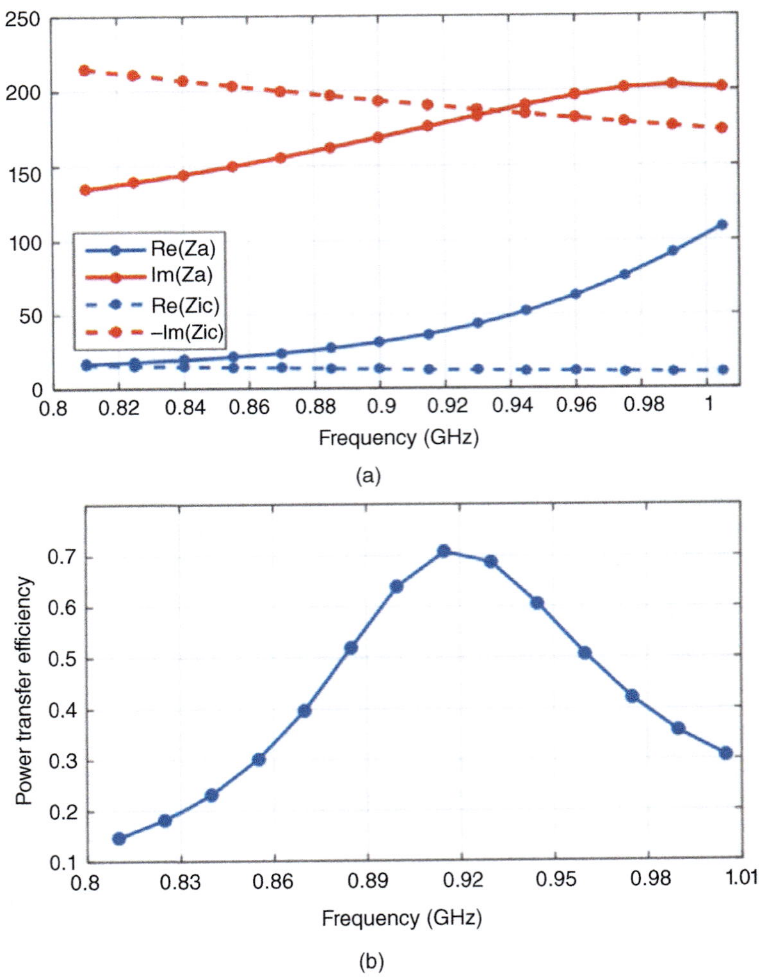

Figure 4.25 (a) Antenna impedance and RFID IC impedance. (b) Simulated power transfer efficiency. (*Source*: Modified from Ma, S., Sydänheimo, L., Ukkonen, L., et al., 2018.)

corresponding power transfer efficiency defined by Equation (4.8) is shown in Figure 4.25b. The maximum power transfer efficiency reaches 70% at 918 MHz.

The implantable part alone has small directivity and low efficiency due to its small size and the lossy human tissue environment. The concentrically placed wearable part is proposed to improve the antenna gain in the far field. As shown in Figure 4.24, the wearable part has three geometrical parameters: the inner radius r_e, the strip width w_e, and the width of the slit s_e. According to the simulation results, with the fixed dimension of the implant part, the three geometrical parameters of the wearable part have a parabolic correlation with the antenna directivity and radiation efficiency. The optimal values of r_e, w_e, and s_e for maximizing the antenna gain are 6.3, 20.8, and 1 mm, respectively. Finally, the wearable part provides more than 8 dB improvement to the antenna directivity (from −4.07 to 4.37 dBi at 915 MHz). Meanwhile, the simulated radiation efficiency is 0.48%. Figure 4.26a shows the radiation efficiency versus the frequency, and the 3D radiation pattern at 915 MHz is shown in Figure 4.26b. In the wireless measurement, the prototyped antenna system was evaluated with the Voyantic Tagformance measurement system in an anechoic chamber. Figure 4.27 demonstrates the measurement setup. The head equivalent liquid mixed with water, sugar, and salt was used to mimic the human tissue environment. In the wireless measurement, the implant part was submerged in the liquid at three different implant depths: 5, 10, and 15 mm. Figure 4.28 shows the comparison between the measured read range and the simulated read ranges from the head model. A good match was found especially in the 5- and 10-mm cases, and the read range with 10 mm implant depth achieves 1.1 m.

4.6.2 LC-Tank-Based Miniature Implantable RFID Antenna

In [86], we proposed the design of an RFID antenna utilizing the coupled resonant LC tank for antenna miniaturization. In the air, the size of the proposed antenna has been reduced to $0.04\lambda \times 0.04\lambda \times 0.02\lambda$ with a maximum read range of more 3 m. In this section, we demonstrate the implementation of this LC-tank-based RFID antenna for intracranial implantable applications. Figure 4.29 shows the structure of the LC-tank-based implantable RFID antenna with an anatomical head model. The proposed antenna is placed in the CSF layer with an implant depth of 16 mm.

The antenna is composed of two concentric copper split rings (IC ring and LC tank ring) with an outer radius of r_1 and r_2, respectively. The antenna port is located at the terminals of the IC ring. The terminals of the LC tank ring are connected with a capacitor. The capacitance of the capacitor in series with the self-inductance from the copper ring together forms the LC tank. The two rings are placed on the top and bottom sides of the 0.04-mm-thick polyethylene ($\varepsilon_r = 2.25$, $\tan\delta = 0.001$ at 915 MHz), respectively. The insulation

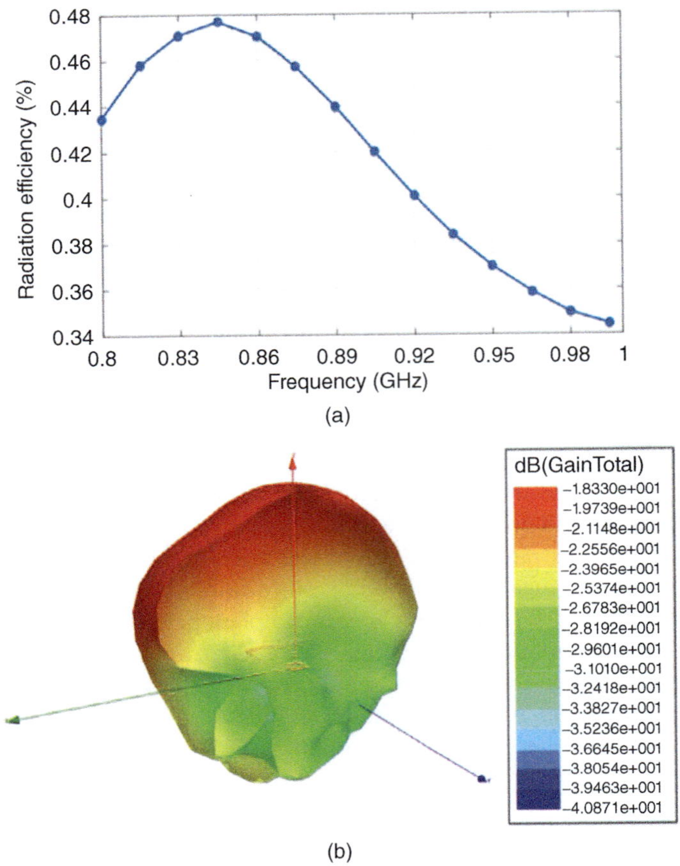

Figure 4.26 (a) Antenna radiation efficiency. (b) Simulated antenna 3D radiation pattern at 915 MHz.

material used in this work is 0.5-mm-thick silicone ($\varepsilon_r = 2.2$, $\tan\delta = 0.007$ at 915 MHz).

The inductive coupling between the two loops can be analyzed with the equivalent circuit model shown in Figure 4.30, where L_1, C_1, and R_1 are the inductance, parasitic capacitance, and parasitic resistance of the IC ring, respectively. L_2, C_2, and R_2 are the inductance, capacitance of the paralleled lumped capacitor and parasitic capacitance, and the parasitic resistance of the LC tank ring. The M stands for the mutual inductance between the two rings. The input impedance from the IC port, Z_{in}, can be calculated using the reflected load theory [87] as

$$Z_{\text{in}} = R_1 + j\omega L_1 + \frac{1}{j\omega C_1} + Z_r, \tag{4.11}$$

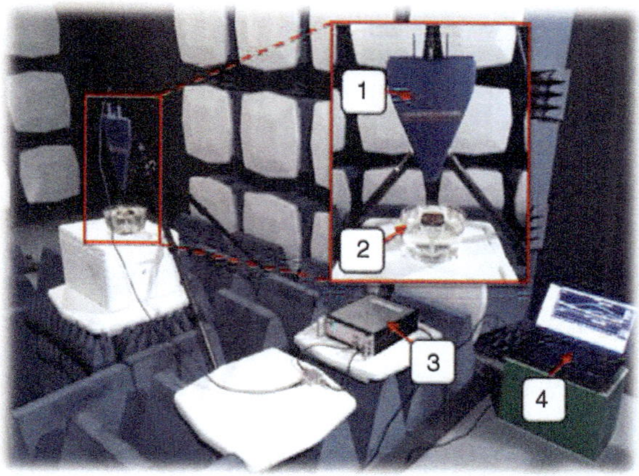

Figure 4.27 Measurement setup: (1) reader antenna, (2) prototyped antenna system with the implantable part submerged in the liquid, (3) Tagformance measurement unit, and (4) Tagformance software. (*Source*: Ma, S., Sydänheimo, L., Ukkonen, L., et al., 2018. Split-ring resonator antenna system with cortical implant and head-worn parts for effective far-field implant communications. IEEE Antennas and Wireless Propagation Letters 17 (4): 710–713. doi: 10.1109/LAWP.2018.2812920.)

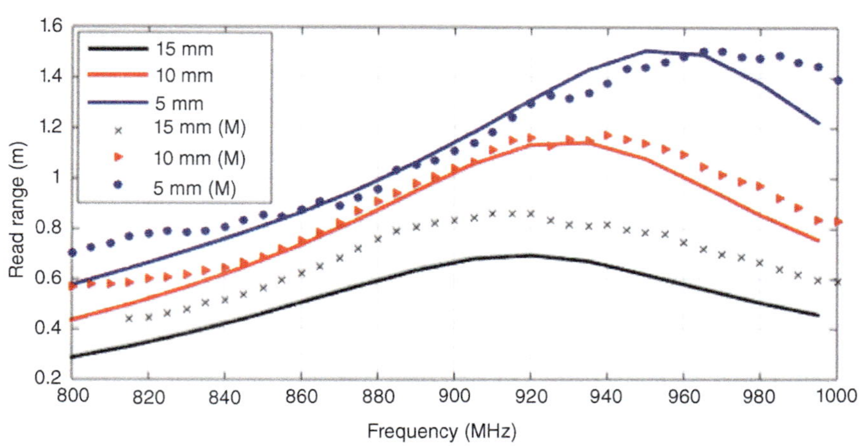

Figure 4.28 Comparison of the simulated and measured attainable read ranges in the human-tissue-like liquid with different implant depths. (*Source*: Ma, S., Sydänheimo, L., Ukkonen, L., et al., 2018. © IEEE.)

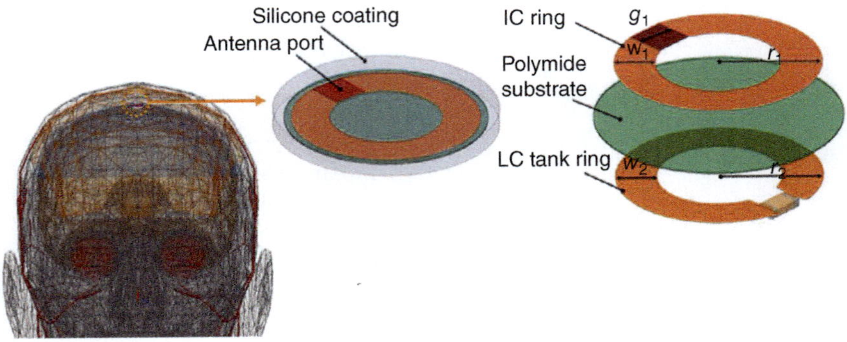

Figure 4.29 Structure of the proposed antenna with the anatomical head model.

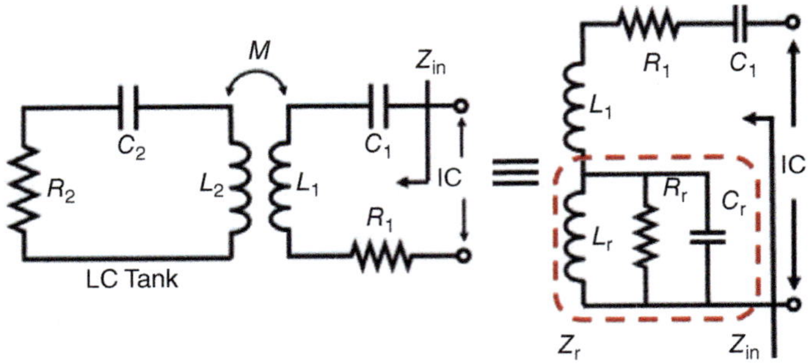

Figure 4.30 Equivalent circuit of the proposed antenna. (*Source*: Modified from Kiani, M., and Ghovanloo, M., 2012.)

where

$$Z_r = \frac{\omega^2 M^2}{j\omega L_2 + \frac{1}{j\omega C_2} + R_2}. \tag{4.12}$$

According to Equation (4.11), the antenna input impedance is not only related to L_1, C_1, and R_1 from the IC ring but also influenced by L_2, C_2, and R_2 of the LC tank ring as well as the mutual inductance M. All of these parameters, except the capacitance from the lumped capacitor, are determined by the geometrical structure of the antenna system. To find out the relationship between the antenna structure and the attainable input impedance of the proposed antenna, we built the antenna model in the ANSYS HFSS and conducted the parametric analysis. In the simulation, the HFSS anatomical head model is adopted to simulate the human head. There are in total six parameters evaluated in the analysis including the capacitance of the lumped capacitor and five geometrical parameters of the antenna which are the outer radius of the two rings r_1 and r_2, trace width of the two rings w_1 and w_2, and the split gap width g_1 of the IC ring. Based on the results of the parametric analysis, the g_1 is found to have negligible effect on the antenna input impedance. On the contrary, the difference between r_1 and r_2 and the capacitance of the lumped capacitor have the dominant influence on the antenna input impedance. Keeping in mind the antenna miniaturization, we fixed the r_1 to 3 mm and gradually increased the r_2 from 3 to 5 mm with a step of 0.25 mm. In each combination of r_1 and r_2, the capacitance of the lumped capacitor swept from 0.5 to 4 pF with a step of 0.1 pF. In this study, the w_1 and w_2 were set to 1 mm.

Figure 4.31 plots the results of the parametric analysis. In Figure 4.31, each dashed line with different colors indicates the impedance value with certain $r_2 - r_1$. Obviously, both the resistance and the reactance of the antenna input impedance are reversely proportional to the increase of the $r_2 - r_1$. When the $r_2 - r_1$ is fixed to a certain value, the antenna input impedance can be further adjusted by changing the capacitance of the lumped capacitor. For instance, the deep blue line represents the range of the antenna input impedance when the r_2 and r_1 are equal to 3 mm. By increasing the capacitance of the lumped capacitor, the antenna input impedance increases along this line. Theoretically, the shadowed area in Figure 4.31 is the range of the attainable antenna input impedance at 915 MHz with different combinations of the r_1, r_2, and the capacitance of the capacitor. This range covers the typical impedance values to achieve the complex conjugate matching to a majority of the RFID ICs.

In this study, we chose the NXP UCODE G2iL series RFID IC as the target microsystem for antenna evaluation and the wireless measurement. This IC has

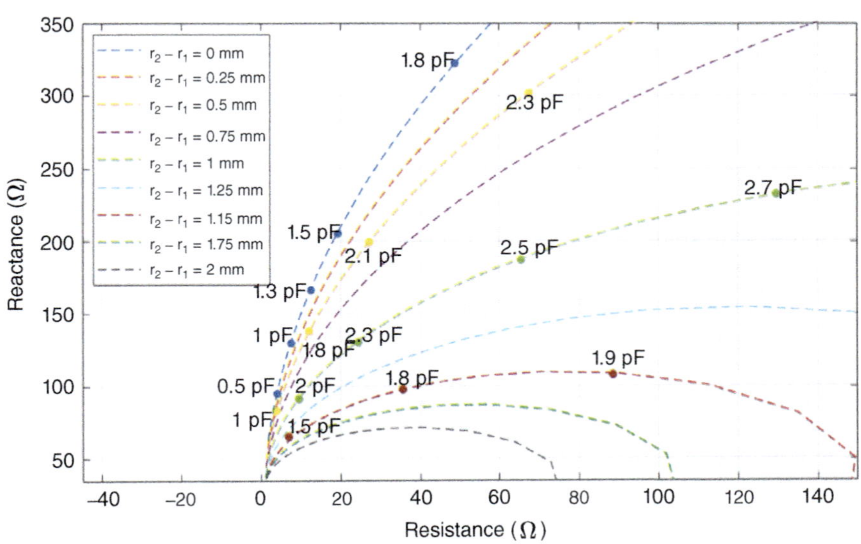

Figure 4.31 Simulated range of the attainable antenna input impedance.

the impedance of 20-j190 Ω at 915 MHz with a wake-up power threshold of −18 dBm. In the simulation, the RFID IC was modeled as the parallel connection of the resistance and capacitance of 2.85 kΩ and 0.91 pF, respectively. The HFSS optimization tool was used to determine the antenna geometrical parameters that optimize the complex conjugate matching to the IC. Figure 4.32a compares the impedance of the IC and the antenna with the r_1, r_2, w_1, and w_2 equal to 3, 3.2, 1, and 1 mm, respectively and the capacitance of the capacitor is 1.5 pF. A good matching can be observed in Figure 4.32b. At 915 MHz, the corresponding power reflection coefficient reaches −12.4 dB.

Figure 4.33a shows the antenna far-field radiation pattern in E and H planes when implemented in the intracranial environment. The proposed antenna has a maximum directivity of 3.6 dBi with a direction outward the human head. Figure 4.33b shows the 3D radiation pattern of the antenna gain with the maximum value of −34.2 dBi.

4.6.3 Antenna Prototype and Wireless Measurement

To evaluate the antenna performance in a realistic tissue environment, we made the prototype and conducted the wireless measurement with the tissue-mimicking liquid and in vivo test in the head of a rat. The antenna was first evaluated in a tissue box model with the size ($50 \times 50 \times 50\ mm^3$) comparable to the dimension of the mouse head. This tissue box was assigned with the dielectric properties of the "averaged head" provided by the FCC. In the simulation, the proposed antenna maintains a good complex conjugate matching with the IC at 915 MHz, while the antenna gain, due to the reduced dimensions of the tissue box compared with the human head model, improved to −15.4 dBi. Then, the prototyped antenna was evaluated with the tissue-mimicking liquid with the relative permittivity of 45.74 and conductivity $0.77\ S\ m^{-1}$ at 915 MHz.

Figure 4.34a shows the fabricated antenna with the silicone coating wrapping the two split rings and the polyimide substrate. The RFID IC and the ceramic capacitor were soldered to the terminals of the upper and lower rings, respectively. The measurement setup is shown in Figure 4.34b and c where the antenna was immersed inside the liquid, and the Voyantic Tagformance RFID evaluation system with a linear polarized patching reader antenna was used to read the response from the IC.

Following the evaluation with the liquid, an in vivo test was conducted with a rat. Figure 4.35a demonstrates the implementation of the antenna inside the rat cranial cavity. The antenna was implanted under the rat skull with an implant depth around 6 mm. Figure 4.35b demonstrates the measurement setup for the in vivo test. The distance between the reader antenna and the rat with the implanted antenna is 30 cm.

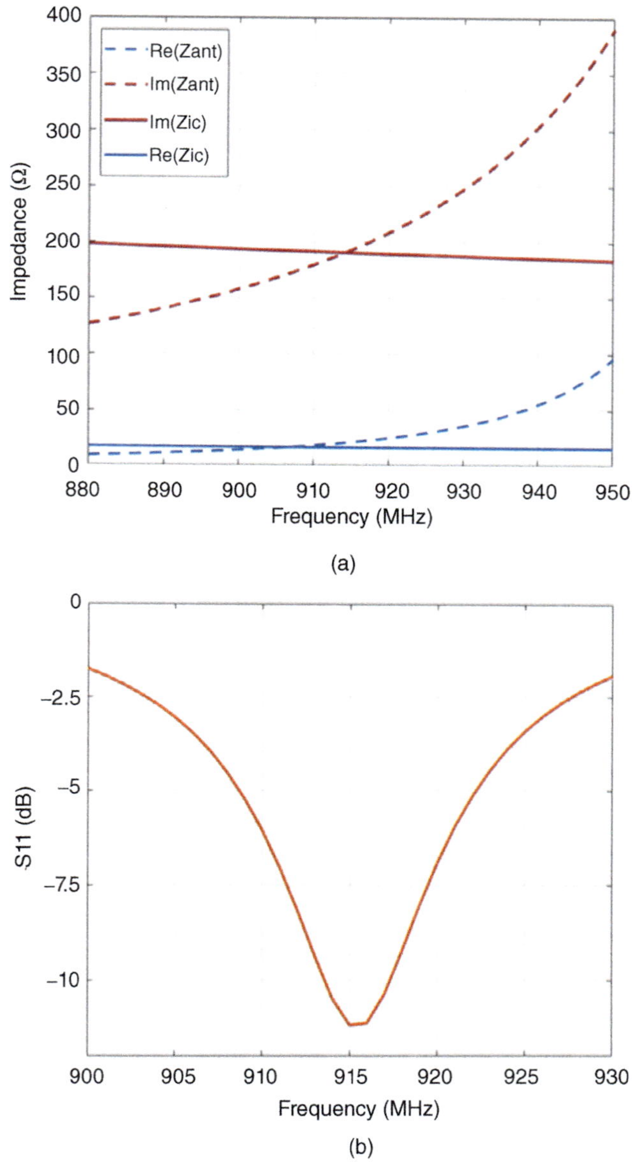

Figure 4.32 (a) Comparison of the simulated antenna impedance and the IC impedance. (b) Simulated antenna power reflection coefficient.

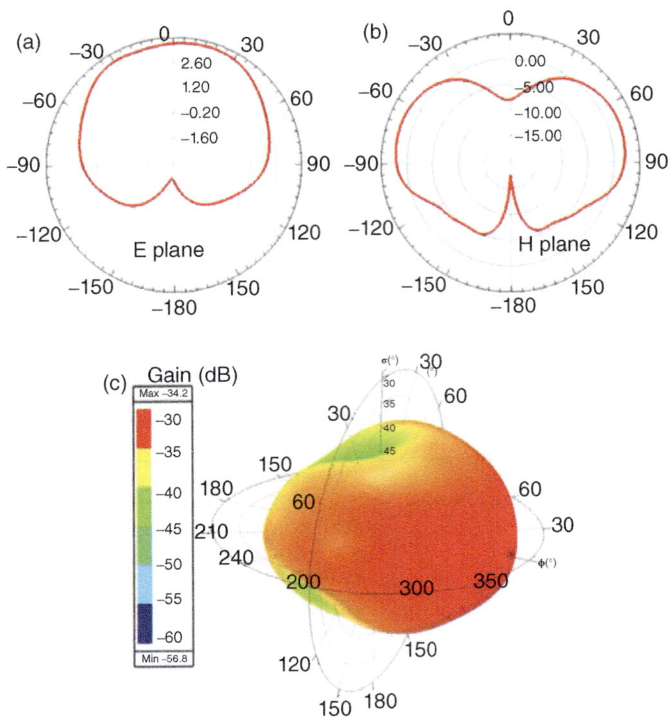

Figure 4.33 (a) Antenna radiation pattern in E-plane. (b) Antenna radiation pattern in H-plane. (c) 3D radiation pattern of the proposed antenna.

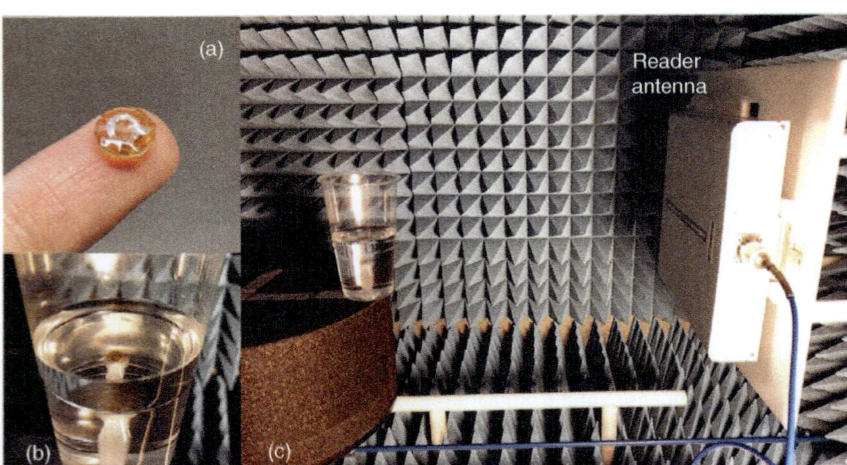

Figure 4.34 (a) Prototyped antenna. (b) Prototyped antenna with the tissue-mimicking liquid. (c) Setup for the wireless measurement with the tissue-mimicking liquid.

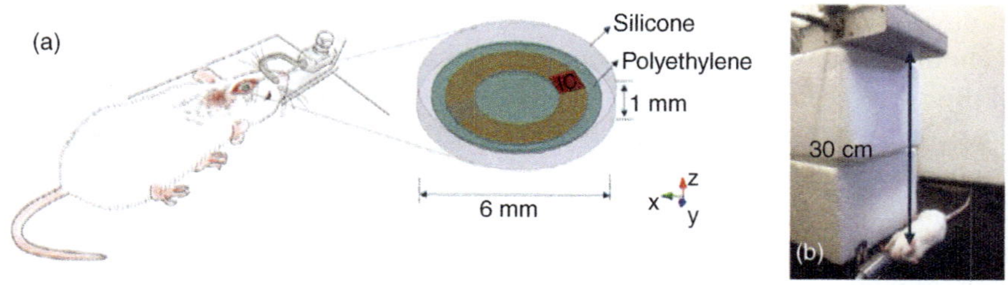

Figure 4.35 (a) Implementation of the proposed antenna in rat head. (b) Measurement setup for the in vivo test.

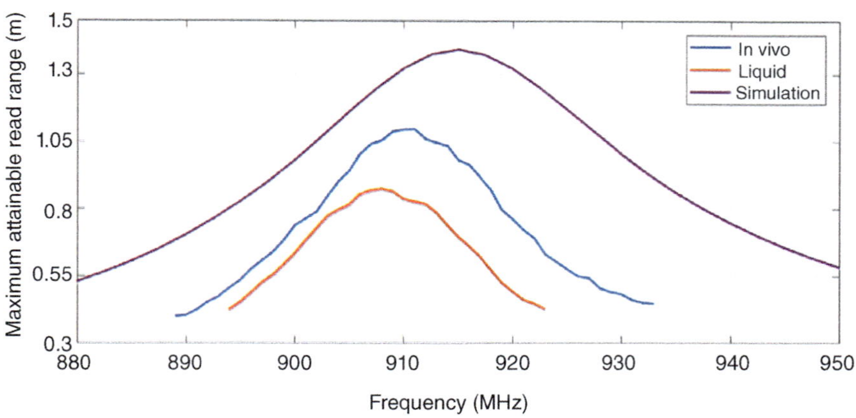

Figure 4.36 The measured and simulated read ranges of the prototyped antenna.

Figure 4.36 compares the read ranges of the wireless measurement in the tissue-mimicking liquid, the in vivo test with the rat, and the simulation with the tissue box model. The result from the in vivo test has a good agreement with that from the liquid test and better performance than that in the simulation. According to the red line in Figure 4.36, the estimated maximum attainable read range of the proposed antenna reaches 1 m when implanted 6 mm in the rat's cranial cavity.

4.7 Conclusion

Wireless intracranial implantable devices are believed to potentially innovate the management of brain disorders and the treatment of neurological diseases. Over the past few years, various implantable antennas and WPT techniques have been proposed to establish the wireless through-body radio link for biomedical applications. In this chapter, we briefly discussed the challenges in developing the intracranial implantable antennas and compared different techniques for WPT in the presence of human body tissues. A brief summary of the most recent miniature implantable antennas and inductive power transfer systems for implantable applications is provided. Next, we discussed and compared the merits of different methodologies to build the computational head models for implantable antenna development. A thorough comparison of the human head models with different complexity is provided. Then, the development and the performance of a wirelessly powered ICP sensing system integrating near- and far-field antennas were elaborately discussed in the human head environment. Additionally, two far-field RFID antennas for intracranial wireless communication were demonstrated and evaluated. The antenna performance and the tuning parameters were discussed through a parametric analysis.

References

1 Zago, S., Ferrucci, R., Fregni, F. et al. (2008). Bartholow, Sciamanna, Alberti: Pioneers in the electrical stimulation of the exposed human cerebral cortex. *History of Neuroscience* 14 (5): 521–528.

2 Lebedev, M.A. and Nicolelis, M.A.L. (2006). Brain–machine interfaces: past, present and future. *Trends in Neurosciences* 29: 536–546.

3 Chapin, J.K., Moxon, K., Markowitz, R. et al. (1999). Real-time control of a robot arm using simultaneously recorded neurons in the motor cortex. *Nature Neuroscience* 2: 664–670.

4 Nicolelis, M. (2001). Actions from thoughts. *Nature* 409: 403–407.

5 Flora, E.D., Perera, C.L., Cameron, A.L., and Maddern, G.J. (2010). Deep brain stimulation for essential tremor: a systematic review. *Movement Disorders* 25: 1550–1559.

6 Shaeri, M.A. and Sodagar, A.M. (2015). A method for compression of intra-cortically-recorded neural signals dedicated to implantable brain–machine interfaces. *IEEE Transactions on Neural Systems and Rehabilitation Engineering* 23 (3): 485–497.

7 Pazzini, L., Polese, D., Weinert, J.F. et al. (2018). An ultra-compact integrated system for brain activity recording and stimulation validated over cortical slow oscillations in vivo and in vitro. *Scientific Reports* 8: 16717.

8 Chen, R., Canales, A., and Anikeeva, P. (2017). Neural recording and modulation technologies. *Nature Reviews Materials* 2: 16093.

9 Khan, M.W.A., Rizwan, M., Sydänheimo, L. et al. (2017). Characterization of 3-D loop antenna to overcome the impact of small lateral misalignment in wirelessly powered intracranial pressure monitoring system. *IEEE Transactions on Antennas and Propagation* 65 (12): 7405–7410.

10 Wang, J., Xie, H., Chung, T. et al. (2017). Neural probes with integrated temperature sensors for monitoring retina and brain implantation and stimulation. *IEEE Transactions on Neural Systems and Rehabilitation Engineering* 25 (9): 1663–1673.

11 Lee, C.W., Kiourti, A., Chae, J., and Volakis, J.L. (2015). A high-sensitivity fully passive neurosensing system for wireless brain signal monitoring. *IEEE Transactions on Microwave Theory and Techniques* 63 (6): 2060–2068.

12 Pena, C., Bowsher, K., Costello, A. et al. (2007). An overview of FDA medical device regulation as it relates to deep brain stimulation devices. *IEEE Transactions on Neural Systems and Rehabilitation Engineering* 15 (3): 421–424.

13 Oluigbo, C.O., Salma, A., and Rezai, A.R. (2012). Deep brain stimulation for neurological disorders. *IEEE Reviews in Biomedical Engineering* 5: 88–99.

14 Mohammed, A., Zamani, M., Bayford, R., and Demosthenous, A. (2017). Toward on-demand deep brain stimulation using online Parkinson's disease prediction driven by dynamic detection. *IEEE Transactions on Neural Systems and Rehabilitation Engineering* 25 (12): 2441–2452.

15 Kim, H., Hirayama, H., Kim, S. et al. (2017). Review of near-field wireless power and communication for biomedical applications. *IEEE Access* 5: 21264–21285.

16 Zeng, F.G., Rebscher, S., Harrison, W. et al. (2008). Cochlear implants: system design, integration, and evaluation. *IEEE Reviews in Biomedical Engineering* 1 (1): 115–142.

17 Hendry, M. (2014). *Near Field Communications Technology and Applications*. Cambridge: Cambridge University Press.

18 Shah, S.A.A. and Yoo, H. (2018). Scalp-implantable antenna systems for intracranial pressure monitoring. *IEEE Transactions on Antennas and Propagation* 66 (4): 2170–2173.

19 Das, S. and Mitra, D. (2018). A compact wideband flexible implantable slot antenna design with enhanced gain. *IEEE Transactions on Antennas and Propagation* 66 (8): 4309–4314.

20 Zhang, Y., Liu, C., Liu, X. et al. (2018). A wideband circularly polarized implantable antenna for 915 MHz ISM-band biotelemetry devices. *IEEE Antennas and Wireless Propagation Letters* 17 (8): 1473–1477.

21 Liu, X.Y., Wu, Z.T., Fan, Y., and Tentzeris, E.M. (2017). A miniaturized CSRR loaded wide-beamwidth circularly polarized implantable antenna for subcutaneous real-time glucose monitoring. *IEEE Antennas and Wireless Propagation Letters* 16: 577–580.

22 Xu, L., Guo, Y., and Wu, W. (2015). Miniaturized circularly polarized loop antenna for biomedical applications. *IEEE Transactions on Antennas and Propagation* 63 (3): 922–930.

23 Liu, C., Guo, Y., and Xiao, S. (2014). Capacitively loaded circularly polarized implantable patch antenna for ISM band biomedical applications. *IEEE Transactions on Antennas and Propagation* 62 (5): 2407–2417.
24 Kim, J. and Rahmat-Samii, Y. (2006). Planar inverted-F antennas on implantable medical devices: meandered type versus spiral type. *Microwave and Optical Technology Letters* 48: 567–572.
25 Liu, C., Guo, Y., Sun, H., and Xiao, S. (2014). Design and safety considerations of an implantable rectenna for far-field wireless power transfer. *IEEE Transactions on Antennas and Propagation* 62 (11): 5798–5806.
26 Elloian, J.M., Noetscher, G.M., Makarov, S.N., and Pascual-Leone, A. (2014). Continuous wave simulations on the propagation of electromagnetic fields through the human head. *IEEE Transactions on Biomedical Engineering* 61 (6): 1676–1683.
27 Collin, R.E. and Zucker, F.J. (1969). *Antenna Theory*. New York, NY, USA: McGraw-Hill.
28 Manoufali, M., Bialkowski, K., Mohammed, B. et al. (2019). Compact implantable antennas for cerebrospinal fluid monitoring. *IEEE Transactions on Antennas and Propagation* 67 (8): 4955–4967.
29 Sharma, A., Kampianakis, E., and Reynolds, M.S. (2017). A dual-band HF and UHF antenna system for implanted neural recording and stimulation devices. *IEEE Antennas and Wireless Propagation Letters* 16: 493–496.
30 Jiang, Z., Wang, Z., Leach, M. et al. (2019). Wideband loop antenna with split-ring resonators for wireless medical telemetry. *IEEE Antennas and Wireless Propagation Letters* 18 (7): 1415–1419.
31 Zargham, M. and Gulak, P.G. (2012). Maximum achievable efficiency in near-field coupled power-transfer systems. *IEEE Transactions on Biomedical Circuits and Systems* 6 (3): 228–245.
32 Galbraith, D.C. (1984). An implantable multichannel neural stimulator, Ph.D. dissertation, Electrical Engineering, Stanford University, Stanford, CA, USA, December 1984.
33 Heetderks, W.J. (1988). RF powering of millimeter- and submillimeter-sized neural prosthetic implants. *IEEE Transactions on Biomedical Engineering* 35 (5): 323–327.
34 Schormans, M., Valente, V., and Demosthenous, A. (2018). Practical inductive link design for biomedical wireless power transfer: a tutorial. *IEEE Transactions on Biomedical Circuits and Systems* 12 (5): 1112–1130.
35 Flack, F.C., James, E.D., and Schlapp, D.M. (1971). Mutual inductance of air-cored coils: effect on design of radio-frequency coupled implants. *Medical & Biological Engineering* 9 (2): 79–85.
36 Ko, W.H., Liang, S.P., and Fung, C.D. (1977). Design of radio-frequency powered coils for implant instruments. *Medical & Biological Engineering & Computing* 15: 634–640.

37 Soma, M., Galbraith, D.C., and White, R.L. (1987). Radio-frequency coils in implantable devices: misalignment analysis and design procedure. *IEEE Transactions on Biomedical Engineering* BME-34 (4): 276–282.

38 Jow, U. and Ghovanloo, M. (2007). Design and optimization of printed spiral coils for efficient transcutaneous inductive power transmission. *IEEE Transactions on Biomedical Circuits and Systems* 1 (3): 193–202.

39 Ho, J.S., Yeh, A.J., Neofytou, E. et al. (2014). Wireless power transfer to deep-tissue microimplant. *Proceedings of the National Academy of Sciences of the United States of America* 111 (22): 7974–7979.

40 Xu, Q., Hu, D., Duan, B., and He, J. (2015). A fully implantable stimulator with wireless power and data transmission for experimental investigation of epidural spinal cord stimulation. *IEEE Transactions on Neural Systems and Rehabilitation Engineering* 23 (4): 683–692.

41 Soltani, N., Aliroteh, M.S., Salam, M.T. et al. (2016). Low-radiation cellular inductive powering of rodent wireless brain interfaces: methodology and design guide. *IEEE Transactions on Biomedical Circuits and Systems* 10 (4): 920–932.

42 Ibrahim, A. and Kiani, M. (2016). A figure-of-merit for design and optimization of inductive power transmission links for millimeter-sized biomedical implants. *IEEE Transactions on Biomedical Circuits and Systems* 10 (6): 1100–1111.

43 Ahn, D. and Ghovanloo, M. (2016). Optimal design of wireless power transmission links for millimeter-sized biomedical implants. *IEEE Transactions on Biomedical Circuits and Systems* 10 (1): 125–137.

44 Jiang, D., Cirmirakis, D., Schormans, M. et al. (2017). An integrated passive phase-shift keying modulator for biomedical implants with power telemetry over a single inductive link. *IEEE Transactions on Biomedical Circuits and Systems* 11 (1): 64–77.

45 Mirbozorgi, S.A., Yeon, P., and Ghovanloo, M. (2017). Robust wireless power transmission to mm-sized free-floating distributed implants. *IEEE Transactions on Biomedical Circuits and Systems* 11 (3): 692–702.

46 Moradi, E., Sydänheimo, L., Bova, G.S., and Ukkonen, L. (2017). Measurement of wireless power transfer to deep-tissue RFID-based implants using wireless repeater node. *IEEE Antennas and Wireless Propagation Letters* 16: 2171–2174.

47 Manoufali, M., Bialkowski, K., Mohammed, B., and Abbosh, A. (2018). Wireless power link based on inductive coupling for brain implantable medical devices. *IEEE Antennas and Wireless Propagation Letters* 17 (1): 160–163.

48 Aldaoud, A., Redoute, J.M., Ganesan, K. et al. (2018). Near-field wireless power transfer to stent-based biomedical implants. *IEEE Journal of Electromagnetics, RF and Microwaves in Medicine and Biology* 2 (3): 193–200.

49 Machnoor, M., Gámez Rodríguez, E.S., Kosta, P. et al. (2019). Analysis and design of a 3-coil wireless power transmission system for biomedical applications. *IEEE Transactions on Antennas and Propagation* 67 (8): 5012–5024.

50 Khan, W., Jia, Y., Madi, F. et al. (2019). Inductively coupled, mm-sized, single channel optical neuro-stimulator with intensity enhancer. *Microsystems & Nanoengineering* 5: 23.

51 Poon, A.S.Y., O'Driscoll, S., and Meng, T.H. (2010). Optimal frequency for wireless power transmission over dispersive tissue. *IEEE Transactions on Antennas and Propagation* 58 (5): 1739–1749.

52 Taalla, R.V., Arefin, M.S., Kaynak, A., and Kouzani, A.Z. (2019). A review on miniaturized ultrasonic wireless power transfer to implantable medical devices. *IEEE Access* 7: 2092–2106.

53 Mazzilli, F., Lafon, C., and Dehollain, C. (2014). A 10.5 cm ultrasound link for deep implanted medical devices. *IEEE Transactions on Biomedical Circuits and Systems* 8 (5): 738–750.

54 Hendee, W.R. (2002). *Medical Imaging Physics*, 4e. Wiley-Liss.

55 Fowler, A.G. and Moheimani, S.O.R. (2016). A 4-DOF MEMS energy harvester using ultrasonic excitation. *IEEE Sensors Journal* 16 (21): 7774–7783.

56 Kawanabe, H., Katane, T., Saotome, H. et al. (2001). Power and information transmission to implanted medical device using ultrasonic. *Japanese Journal of Applied Physics* 40 (5): 3600–3603.

57 Sodagar, A.M. and Amiri, P. (2009). Capacitive coupling for power and data telemetry to implantable biomedical microsystems. Proceedings of the IEEE 4th International Conference on Neural Engineering, 411–414.

58 Jegadeesan, R., Agarwal, K., Guo, Y.X. et al. (2017). Wireless power delivery to flexible subcutaneous implants using capacitive coupling. *IEEE Transactions on Microwave Theory and Techniques* 65 (280): 1–292.

59 Narayanamoorthi, R. (2019). Modeling of capacitive resonant wireless power and data transfer to deep biomedical implants. *IEEE Transactions on Components, Packaging and Manufacturing Technology* 9 (7): 1253–1263.

60 Bercich, R., Duffy, D.R., and Irazoqui, P.P. (2013). Far-field RF powering of implantable devices: safety considerations. *IEEE Transactions on Biomedical Engineering* 60 (8): 2107–2112.

61 Niknejad, A.M. (2007). *Electromagnetics for High-Speed Analog and Digital Communication Circuits*. Cambridge University Press.

62 Carson, R.S. (1982). *High-Frequency Amplifiers*. Wiley.

63 Pozar, D.M. (2012). *Microwave Engineering*. Hoboken: Wiley.

64 Moradi, E., Amendola, S., Björninen, T. et al. (2015). Backscattering neural tags for wireless brain-machine interface systems. *IEEE Transactions on Antennas and Propagation* 63 (2): 719–726.

65 Rabaey, J.M., M. Mark, D. Chen, C. Sutardja, T. Chongxuan, S. Gowda, M. Wagner, and D. Werthimer (2011). Powering and communicating with

mm-size implants. Design, Automation and Test in Europe Conference and Exhibition, Conference Proceedings, Grenoble, 2011, 1–6.
66 Khan, M.W.A., Sydänheimo, L., Ukkonen, L., and Björninen, T. (2017). Inductively powered pressure sensing system integrating a far-field data transmitter for monitoring of intracranial pressure. *IEEE Sensors Journal* 17 (7): 2191–2197.
67 Björninen, T. (2018). Extrema of transducer power gain and voltage gain of two-port network under varying terminations: semi-analytical method and application to biotelemetry system. *Applied Computational Electromagnetics Society Journal* 33 (6): 561–568.
68 Kim, J. and Rahmat-Samii, Y. (2004). Implanted antennas inside a human body: simulations, designs, and characterizations. *IEEE Transactions on Microwave Theory and Techniques* 52 (8): 1934–1943.
69 Kiourti, A. and Nikita, K.S. (2012). A review of implantable patch antennas for biomedical telemetry: challenges and solutions [wireless corner]. *IEEE Antennas and Propagation Magazine* 54 (3): 210–228.
70 Makarov, S.N., Noetscher, G.M., Yanamadala, J. et al. (2017). Virtual human models for electromagnetic studies and their applications. *IEEE Reviews in Biomedical Engineering* 10: 95–121.
71 Hasgall, P.A., Di Gennaro F, Baumgartner C, Neufeld E, Lloyd B, Gosselin MC, Payne D, Klingenböck A, Kuster N (2018). IT'IS database for thermal and electromagnetic parameters of biological tissues, Version 3.0. www.itis.ethz.ch/database (accessed July 2020).
72 Gabriel, S., Lau, R.W., and Gabriel, C. (1996). The dielectric properties of biological tissues: II. Measurements in the frequency range 10Hz to 20 GHz. *Physics in Medicine and Biology* 41 (11): 2251–2269.
73 Gabriel, S., Lau, R.W., and Gabriel, C. (1996). The dielectric properties of biological tissues: Part III. Parametric models for the dielectric spectrum of tissues. *Physics in Medicine and Biology* 41 (11): 2271–2293.
74 Ma, S., Sydänheimo, L., Ukkonen, L., and Björninen, T. (2018). Split-ring resonator antenna system with cortical implant and head-worn parts for effective far-field implant communications. *IEEE Antennas and Wireless Propagation Letters* 17 (4): 710–713.
75 Yanamadala, J., Noetscher GM, Rathi VK et al. (2015). New VHP-female V.2.0 full-body computational phantom and its performance metrics using FEM simulator ANSYS HFSS. Proceedings of the 37th Annual International Conference of the IEEE Engineering in Medicine and Biology Society, Milano, Italy (August 2015), 3237–3241.
76 Raboel, P.H., Bartek, J. Jr., Andresen, M. et al. (2012). Intracranial pressure monitoring: invasive versus non-invasive methods – a review. *Critical Care Research and Practice* 2012, article ID: 950393.

77 Kawoos, U., Tofighi, M.-R., Warty, R. et al. (2008). In-vitro and in-vivo trans-scalp evaluation of an intracranial pressure implant at 2.4 GHz. *IEEE Transactions on Microwave Theory and Techniques* 56 (10): 2356–2365.

78 Hu, P., You, Y.W., Chen, F.Y.B. et al. (2016). Wireless power supply for ICP devices with hybrid supercapacitor and battery storage. *IEEE Journal of Emerging and Selected Topics in Power Electronics* 4 (1): 273–279.

79 Chen, L.Y., Tee, B.C.K., Bao, Z. et al. (2014). Continuous wireless pressure monitoring and mapping with ultra-small passive sensors for health monitoring and critical care. *Nature Communications* 5, article 5028.

80 Behfar, M.H., Moradi, E., Björninen, T. et al. (2015). Biotelemetric wireless intracranial pressure monitoring: an in vitro study. *International Journal of Antennas and Propagation* 2015, article ID 918698, 10 pages.

81 Khan, M.W.A., Moradi, E., Sydänheimo, L. et al. (2017). Miniature co-planar implantable antenna on thin and flexible platform for fully wireless intracranial pressure monitoring system. *International Journal of Antennas and Propagation*, Article ID: 9161083, 9 pages.

82 Xiao, Z., Tan, X., Chen, X. et al. (2015). An implantable RFID sensor tag toward continuous glucose monitoring. *IEEE Journal of Biomedical and Health Informatics* 19 (3): 910–919.

83 Huang, H., Zhao, P., Chen, P.Y. et al. (2014). RFID tag helix antenna sensors for wireless drug dosage monitoring. *IEEE Journal of Translational Engineering in Health and Medicine* 2: 1–8, Art no. 1700108.

84 Volk, T., Gorbey, S., Bhattacharyya, M. et al. (2015). RFID technology for continuous monitoring of physiological signals in small animals. *IEEE Transactions on Biomedical Engineering* 62 (2): 618–626.

85 Björninen, T., Sydänheimo, L., and Ukkonen, L. (2012). Development and validation of an equivalent circuit model for UHF RFID IC based on wireless tag measurements. AMTA Symposium, Bellevue, WA, USA.

86 Ma, S., Sydänheimo, L., Ukkonen, L., and Björninen, T. (2019). Electrically small UHF RFID tag antenna based on inductively coupled resonant LC tank. Asia-Pacific Microwave Conference 2019, Singapore.

87 Kiani, M. and Ghovanloo, M. (2012). The circuit theory behind coupled-mode magnetic resonance-based wireless power transmission. *IEEE Transactions on Circuits and Systems I: Regular Papers* 59 (9): 2065–2074.

88 Chen, Z., Sun, H., and Geyi, W. (2017). Maximum wireless power transfer to the implantable device in the radiative near field. *IEEE Antennas and Wireless Propagation Letters* 16: 1780–1783.

89 Rana, B., Shim, J., and Chung, J. (2019). An implantable antenna with broadside radiation for a brain–machine interface. *IEEE Sensors Journal* 19 (20): 9200–9205.

90 Karacolak, T., Hood, A.Z., and Topsakal, E. (2008). Design of a dual-band implantable antenna and development of skin mimicking gels for

continuous glucose monitoring. *IEEE Transactions on Microwave Theory and Techniques* 56 (4): 1001–1008.

91 Duan, Z., Guo, Y., Je, M., and Kwong, D. (2014). Design and in vitro test of a differentially fed dual-band implantable antenna operating at MICS and ISM bands. *IEEE Transactions on Antennas and Propagation* 62 (5): 2430–2439.

92 Li, H., Guo, Y., Liu, C. et al. (2015). A miniature-implantable antenna for MedRadio-band biomedical telemetry. *IEEE Antennas and Wireless Propagation Letters* 14: 1176–1179.

93 Abdi, A. and Aliakbarian, H. (2019). A miniaturized UHF-band rectenna for power transmission to deep-body implantable devices. *IEEE Journal of Translational Engineering in Health and Medicine* 7: 1–11.

94 See, T.S.P., Qing, X., Liu, W., and Chen, Z.N. (2015). A wideband ultra-thin differential loop-fed patch antenna for head implants. *IEEE Transactions on Antennas and Propagation* 63 (7): 3244–3248.

95 Rana, B., Shim, J., and Chung, J. (2018). Implant communication for future leadless cardiac pacemakers. *IEEE Transactions on Biomedical Engineering* 65 (12): 2798–2807.

96 Song, L. and Rahmat-Samii, Y. (2017). An end-to-end implanted brain–machine interface antenna system performance characterizations and development. *IEEE Transactions on Antennas and Propagation* 65 (7): 3399–3408.

97 Noetscher, G.M., Htet, A.T., Maino, N., and Lacroix, P. (2017). The visible human project male CAD based computational phantom and its use in bio-electromagnetic simulations. Proceedings of the 39th Annual International Conference of the IEEE Engineering in Medicine and Biology Society, Jeju Island, South Korea, July 11–15, 2017.

98 Wenger, C., Salvador, R., Basser, P.J., and Miranda, P.C. (2015). The electric field distribution in the brain during TTFields therapy and its dependence on tissue dielectric properties and anatomy: a computational study. *Physics in Medicine and Biology* 60 (18): 7339–7357.

5

In Vitro and In Vivo Testing of Implantable Antennas

Ryan B. Green[1], *Mary V. Smith*[2] *and Erdem Topsakal*[3]

[1] *Department of Electrical and Computer Engineering, Mississippi State University, Mississippi State, MS, USA*
[2] *VERO Biotech, LLC, Atlanta, GA*
[3] *Department of Electrical and Computer Engineering, Virginia Commonwealth University, Richmond, VA, USA*

5.1 Introduction

After the initial design phase for implantable antennas, the next steps should be the construction and testing of the device. While a traditional antenna is meant to operate in either free space or low loss dielectrics, implantable antennas are required to operate within more conductive and higher permittivity environments than free space. The environment an implantable antenna must operate is dynamic and hostile. The body seeks to encapsulate, isolate, and neutralize foreign objects. As a result, the antenna design must be adapted to the environment because the body will absorb certain materials that can pose a health risk. Antenna engineers must account for these biological effects in the design in order to validate antenna performance in a living being. In another aspect, the high-permittivity surrounding allows for antenna miniaturization, but certain material choices negate these miniaturization effects. Different conductive materials, commonly used in nonmedical antenna fabrication, are absorbed and metabolized by the body. Some pose health risks to the host, resulting in low dielectric medical grade silicones and epoxies which shield the body from the potentially toxic materials. This containment strategy, however, counteracts the miniaturization effects of the tissue. An understanding of materials, biocompatibility, and miniaturization is necessary.

Design considerations aside, a major aspect in developing implantable antennas is the validation of the designs after simulation. There are two major phases in this validation: in vivo and in vitro testing. In vitro testing is a process where tissues are either grown or mimicked outside of the context of a living being in order to test a device. In vivo testing corresponds to testing within a

Antenna and Sensor Technologies in Modern Medical Applications,
First Edition. Edited by Yahya Rahmat-Samii and Erdem Topsakal.

living model. In both cases, testing antenna performance has some challenges, spanning the regulatory and the technical aspects.

This chapter is organized to discuss the commonly used implantable antenna materials, in vitro, and in vivo testing. Common conductors, their health effects, and alternate conductors are discussed in conjunction with biocompatibility and miniaturization techniques. Bench top testing discusses the mixture and measurement of in vitro gels, and common tests are performed on the bench top. An overview of in vivo testing is given, including different animal test models compared to a human test subject, dielectric mismatches between the dielectric properties of tissues seen in the literature and the tissues seen in the surgery room, and some practical testing considerations to perform antenna testing in a hospital or medical research facility.

5.2 Antenna Materials

Before an antenna can move from the design stage to the testing stage, the material needs to be considered in the context of biocompatibility and footprint. In the context of biocompatibility, the design will be composed of materials that may not be compatible with the human body, and therefore consideration of minimal adverse effects is necessary. From a sizing context, the design needs to incorporate antenna placement and how this will be placed and how this antenna will affect the efficacy of the design as well as the comfort of the patient. Additionally, these considerations each must answer questions of longevity: How much time will the device designed need to be inside the body? If the antenna is designed to operate only for a few hours, the answers to the biocompatibility and sizing questions could be different from that of an antenna needed to last six months or even longer. The method the antenna is administered is another application-dependent consideration that can affect the sizing question. If the antenna will be administered through a small tube or through an outpatient procedure drastically changes the bounds of what is needed for size or topology. This section discusses some of the common design considerations necessary in the design of implantable antennas. This includes the materials used in antennas (both commonly used and some alternatives) and some miniaturization techniques in order for an antenna to operate in the body.

5.2.1 Biocompatibility

There are many aspects in the design and fabrication of implantable antennas. Depending on the intended use of the antenna, the answers to design questions may differ. One major consideration is reducing the exposure of the body to bioincompatible materials. In Table 5.1, a list of conductive elements commonly used in the development of antennas or other electronics (as a radiating element or soldering agent) is given. The table shows the element name, the health effect summary (implantation or ingestion), and the conductivity of the

Table 5.1 Conductive elements, common health effects, and conductivity.

Elements	Health effect summary	Conductivity ($S\ m^{-1}$)
Aluminum	Some studies show that aluminum has links to Alzheimer's disease in humans and nervous system damage in laboratory animals [1]. Bone diseases have been seen in children who take medicine containing aluminum, caused by aluminum preventing the absorption of phosphate in the stomach [1]	3.5×10^7
Copper	Copper is an essential metal (in low doses not toxic) [2]. In high doses and long exposure, copper can cause headaches, dizziness, nausea, and diarrhea. In some cases, high doses can cause kidney damage, liver damage, and, in some cases, death [3]	5.8×10^7
Gold	No adverse effects expected for ingestion. However, if inhaled, irritation is expected [4]	4.10×10^7
Iron	Iron is an essential component of every living being [5]. However, in extremely high doses (hundreds of milligrams and above), iron can lead to organ failure, convulsions, comas, and even death. The upper daily intake limit for adults aged 19 years and older is 45 mg [6]	1.00×10^7
Lead	Lead poisoning has long been linked to various health problems. Lead has been linked with neurological diseases, cardiovascular disorders, and reproductive effects. The Environmental Protection Agency has also classified inorganic lead compounds as a probable human carcinogen [7]	4.55×10^6
Nickel	The most common health effect of nickel is allergic reaction, often through jewelry that has direct contact on the skin. Exposure to incredibly high amounts of nickel (100,000 times larger than the amount usually found in drinking water) can cause stomach aches, blood effects, and kidney effects [8]	1.43×10^7
Silver	Silver compounds can cause skin coloration (blue gray) called argyria. However, no studies of cancer or birth defects in animals from eating, drinking, or breathing in silver compounds have been found. Long-term exposure to moderately high levels of silver nitrate may have a slight effect of brain activity [9]	6.30×10^7
Titanium	Titanium and other titanium compounds (titanium dioxide and titanium nitride) are low-risk materials for toxicity. Titanium is not carcinogenic [10]	2.38×10^6
Zinc	Mild toxicity of zinc (over 40 mg but below 150 mg) can cause nausea, vomiting, loss of appetite, diarrhea, and headaches. Chronic toxicity (80 mg daily exposure for six years or more) has affected urinary physiology [11]	1.69×10^7

material. Some of these elements are lethal when ingested or absorbed into the human body, while others commonly cause some allergic reactions or are safe for implantation.

Depending on the end application, there are different ways to minimize exposure. In the case of a limited, short-term implantation (such as microwave ablation therapy), picking a material such as copper may be an adequate conductive material. However, for long-term implantation, elements such as copper, zinc, and iron are poor choices for direct contact due to their absorption and potential health risks. A very common method is to encapsulate a long-term implant antenna in a medical grade epoxy or silicone. This method allows for a design to be made using conventional methods (milling machine or chemical etch), using conventional materials (copper clad FR-4 or Rogers substrates). This method also allows for a rapid turnaround between design, fabrication, test, and redesign. There is one adverse effect to the design: frequency shifts. If designed to operate in a high-permittivity tissue, frequency shifts will be present between a design intended for uncovered implantation and the same design coated in medical grade silicone. Figure 5.1 shows an example design to show these frequency shifts. A patch antenna is designed to operate on the 2.4-GHz Industrial Scientific and Medical (ISM) band without a layer surrounding the antenna. The antenna is designed on a Rogers 6010

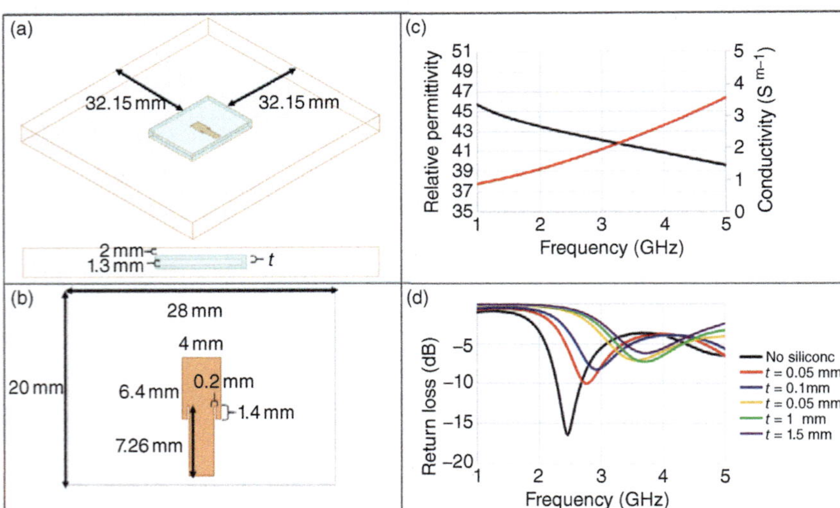

Figure 5.1 Simulation of resonance shifts due to silicone coating. (a) Simulation setup for 2.4 GHz implantable antenna with 2 mm of skin above and below the antenna. A silicone thickness of *t* coats the antenna. (b) The physical dimensions of patch antenna on a 1.3-mm-thick substrate of Rogers 6010. (c) Dielectric properties (relative permittivity and conductivity) of human skin between 1 and 5 GHz. (d) Simulated return loss for implanted patch antenna for silicone thicknesses up to 1.5 mm.

substrate ($\varepsilon_r = 10.2$) of thickness 1.3 mm. The antenna design dimensions can be seen in Figure 5.1a,b. The antenna is designed to operate in a thin-section skin (2 mm on each side sandwiching the antenna coated in silicone). The dielectric properties, permittivity and conductivity, can be seen in Figure 5.1c. The bare antenna simulated return loss can be seen in Figure 5.1d. As silicone ($\varepsilon_r = 3.5$ and $\sigma = 0\,\mathrm{S\,m^{-1}}$) is introduced around the antenna substrate the frequency resonance shifts to higher and higher frequencies, requiring a redesigned antenna to increase in size. As a result, it is necessary to employ some degree of antenna miniaturization, not just to make the implantable antenna feasible for implantation in general but also to counter the effects of low-permittivity coating.

5.2.2 Miniaturization

Implantable antenna miniaturization has been explored in various different methods. One common method is the use of high-permittivity materials for substrates and superstrates. A substrate is the dielectric material that supports printed circuit boards or antennas. In the context of a patch antenna, a substrate is the dielectric material between the patch and the ground plane. The superstrate is a dielectric material placed on top of the radiating element. This method takes advantage of the high permittivity reducing the phase velocity ($u = c/\sqrt{\varepsilon_r}$), and thus reducing the wavelength of the operating antenna ($\lambda = u/f = \lambda_0/\sqrt{\varepsilon_r}$). While this method does allow for some miniaturization, depending on the material used and the tissue implanted in, the superstrate still acts as a lower permittivity isolator from the surrounding tissue, yielding a similar issue seen in Figure 5.1.

Another method for miniaturization is to alter the current-flow path on the antenna, allowing for longer current paths while remaining compact in size. Some of the techniques to lengthen the electrical size of the antenna include meandering, spiraling, and waffling [12] (Figure 5.2).

Yet another miniaturization method technique includes inserting shorting pins between the radiating element and the ground plane or layering patch elements. Ultimately, the goal of all miniaturization techniques is to electrically

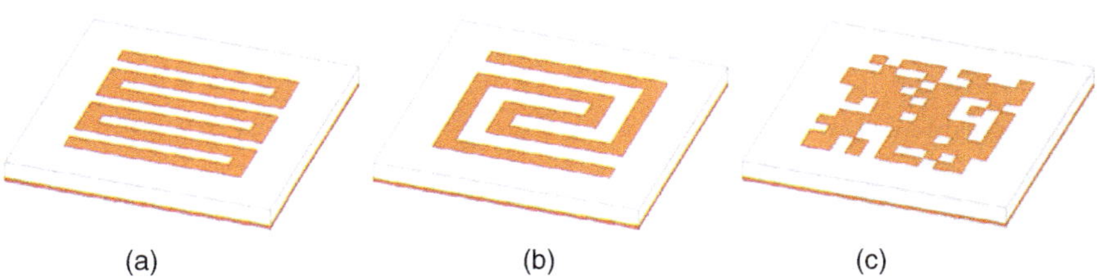

Figure 5.2 Different path lengthening schemes for miniaturization. (a) Meandering line, (b) spiraling line, and (c) waffling patch.

lengthen the current path while reducing the footprint. While these methods are effective for reducing the footprint of the implantable antenna, they do require a more complex fabrication process to consider multiple layers and shorting pin soldering. While stacking patches would reduce the footprint, such a technique would necessarily increase the thickness of the antenna, making a sizing trade-off between the footprint and the height.

5.2.3 Biocompatible Conductors and Thin Films

In any case of miniaturization, if bioincompatible materials are chosen, they must be coated, yielding a frequency shift as seen in Figure 5.1. As a result, there must be a method that takes advantage of the high permittivity of human tissues while not poisoning the patient. Another method to forgo bioincompatibility and larger antennas for implant is to use biocompatible conductor. In addition to the elements shown previously in Table 5.1, some biocompatible, conductive compounds are shown in Table 5.2. There are numerous biocompatible conductive materials being researched and explored, but only a snapshot of them is shown.

While these materials will be an exquisite alternative to traditional conductors, there is a major aspect of these materials to consider when using them for an implantable antenna. Antenna efficiency is lower in a material fabricated using these thin films as opposed to thicker traditional conductors. The antenna efficiency is a function of film thickness and film conductivity. An antenna designed with a perfect conductor assumes no added resistance due to

Table 5.2 Conductive biocompatible materials and conductivity.

Conductors	Conductivity ($S\,m^{-1}$)
AgNWs [13]	8.13×10^5
Carbon nanotubes [14]	5.96×10^4
Elgan ink [15]	4.80×10^5
ELCOAT Silver Paste [16]	1.50×10^5
GZO [17, 18]	3.00×10^5
Graphene [19]	2.62×10^4
PEDOT:PSS [20]	9.00×10^4
Poly(p-phenylene) [21]	1.00×10^3
Poly(p-phenylenevinylene) [21]	5.00×10^3
Polyacetylene [21]	1.70×10^5
Polypyrrole [21]	7.50×10^3
Polythiophene [21]	1.00×10^3
Titanium nitride (TiN) [22]	3.70×10^5

Figure 5.3 Thin-film geometry including the length, the width that varies along the path of current flow, and the thickness of the film.

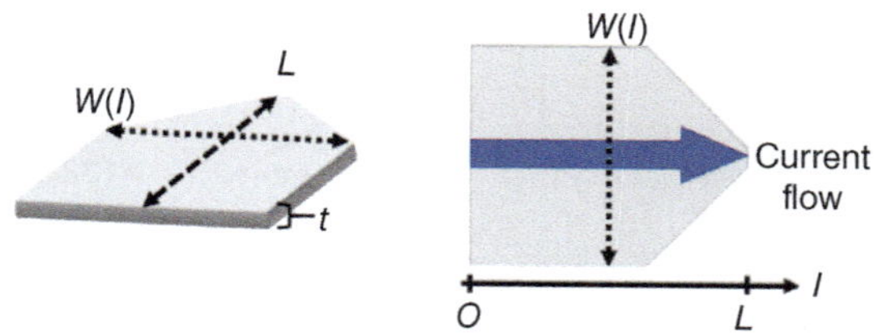

conductive losses. However, the finite conductivity and small film thicknesses add these conductive losses that can be represented with a resistance R, calculated using Equation (5.1),

$$R = R_s \int_0^L \frac{dl}{W(l)}, \tag{5.1}$$

where L is the total length of the conductor, $W(l)$ is the width of the conductor along the current path (see Figure 5.3), and R_s is the sheet resistance of the film. The sheet resistance is calculated in Equation (5.2) [23],

$$R_s = \frac{1}{\sigma\delta\left(1 - e^{-\frac{t}{2\delta}}\right)}, \tag{5.2}$$

where σ is the conductivity of the film, t is the film thickness, and δ is the skin depth of the film ($\delta = \sqrt{2/(\omega\mu_0\sigma)}$, where $\omega = 2\pi f$ and $\mu_0 = 4\pi \times 10^{-7}$ F m^{-1}). If the antenna has a rectangular conductor, the resistance of the thin film simplifies to $R = R_s(L/W)$.

This added resistance due to film thickness affects the impedance of the antenna, thus affecting the return loss and antenna gain. Gain G is a function of the antenna directivity D and the antenna efficiency *eff* ($G = D{*}eff$). The directivity and efficiency will vary between different antenna topologies, but the efficiency will also vary with film thickness. In Figure 5.4, the simulated effects of film thickness are shown. For this comparison, two different styles of simulations were conducted in ANSYS High Frequency Simulation System (HFSS). The first simulation was setting the patch and the ground plane to "finite conductivity" boundaries with a conductivity value of 3.70×10^5 S m^{-1}. "Finite conductivity" boundary conditions are used when a material is assumed to be thick enough compared to the skin depth to not add a sufficient amount of resistance due to material thickness. The simulated maximum gain for the antenna shown in Figure 5.4a and b is −15 dBi, and the simulated return loss is shown in Figure 5.4c. The second method of simulation considers the film thickness. The patch and the ground plane were set to "layered impedance" boundaries, with a conductivity value of 3.7×10^5 S m^{-1}, for titanium nitride [22], and a film thickness that is swept from 100 nm to 50 μm. In both the return loss and antenna gain, the thin-film performance approaches the performance of the finite conductivity performance when the film thickness is

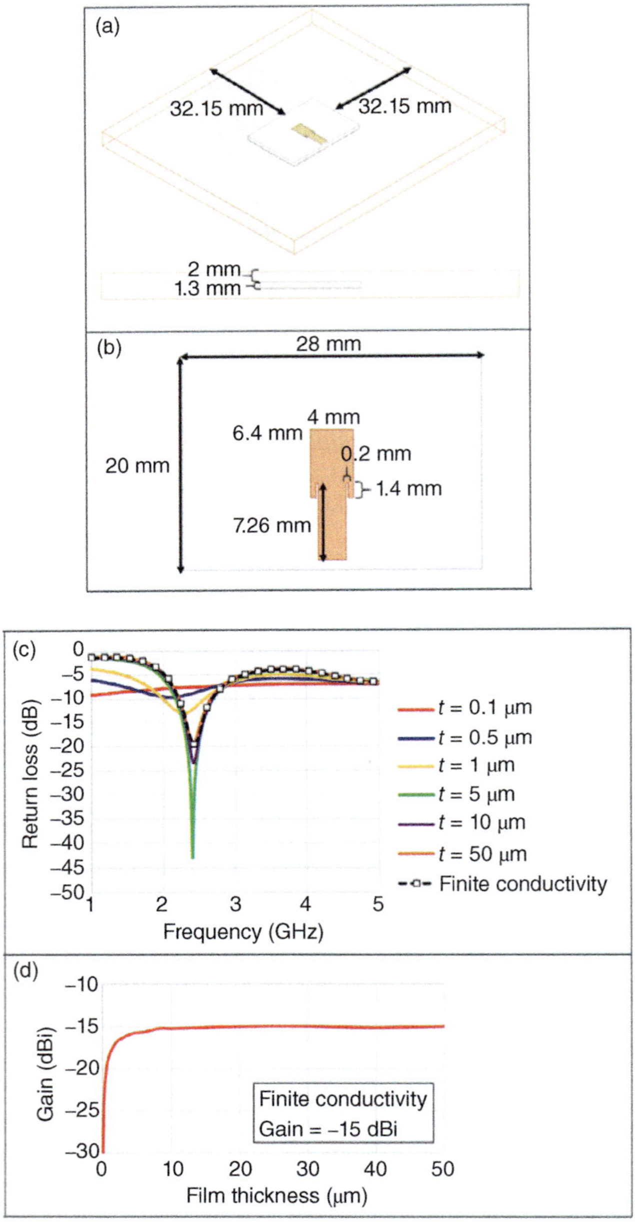

Figure 5.4 Simulation of resonance shifts due to silicone coating. (a) Simulation setup for 2.4 GHz implantable antenna with 2 mm of skin above and below the antenna. A silicone thickness of *t* coats the antenna. (b) The physical dimensions of patch antenna on a 1.3-mm-thick substrate of Rogers 6010. (c) Simulated return loss for implanted patch antenna for silicone thicknesses up to 1.5 mm. (d) Simulated antenna gain for various film thicknesses.

approximately 10 μm. In terms of return loss, there is small frequency shifts, but it is small compared to the reduction in magnitude of the return loss at 2.45 GHz.

5.2.4 Ports and Cables

Another, incredibly important aspect to consider in design is how the antenna will be fed (by a network analyzer, spectrum analyzer, or signal generator) in the testing stage. Depending on the antenna design, the feed on the port of the antenna could be a traditional coaxial jack that is hand soldered or specialty conductor electrically connected either through mechanical pressure or solder. However, what is necessary to consider is the how the material properties of the antenna (either conductor or dielectric) come into play when determining how to apply the ports and cables. For example, if the antenna is designed in tandem to a transmission line for a short-term implantation (e.g. an ablation probe manufactured with a coaxial line intended to come out of the body), the port connecting the out-of-body amplifier or signal generator may not need to be coated in medical grade silicone.

If, however, the antenna is designed to operate with an implantable communication system, and the antenna is to be tested separately from an implantable communication system, there must be a bridge between the implant and the out of the body. Often this bridge is a coaxial cable. RF connectors are often made from materials such as brass, which are not biocompatible. Solder and conductive epoxies also are not biocompatible. Therefore, it is necessary to isolate the brass and solder from the body and incorporate these into the design. Figure 5.5 shows an example of this. In this figure, a titanium nitride antenna is fabricated on a sapphire substrate. The antenna is fed via a surface mount, coplanar U.Fl connector, adhered to the titanium nitride with silver epoxy. The U.Fl connector is then connected to a three-inch coaxial transmission line and terminated with a SubMiniature version A (SMA) connector. The connector, silver epoxy, transmission line, and portions of the SMA connector are coated in silicone in order to biologically isolate the incompatible materials from the implantation site.

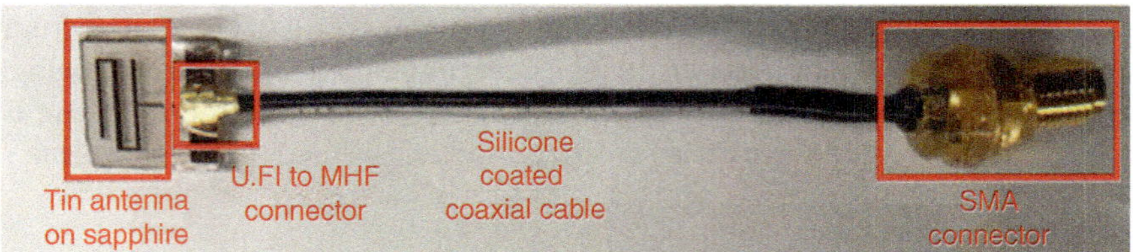

Figure 5.5 Fabricated titanium nitride antenna to silicone-coated U.Fl surface mount connector and MHF to SMA coaxial cable [24, 25].

5.3 Bench Top Testing

After the device is developed and sealed to prevent toxic exposure, a next critical step in the development is the guaranteeing function within the environment it was designed. Because testing these devices in the human body is not practical during the design phase, an alternative method for testing implantable antennas is necessary. One method is to use an animal test model. This method, however, is expensive and highly regulated. Entering live testing should be pursued as the last stage of development of an implantable antenna. As a result, having a bench top testing method for an implantable antenna is paramount. There are two major methods to validate an implantable antenna before live testing: ex vivo and in vitro testing.

5.3.1 Ex Vivo Tissues

Ex vivo is Latin for "Out of the Living." In the context of this chapter, ex vivo means using tissues extracted from living beings, either animals or people, to test the implantable antenna. Ex vivo tissues for animal models can be garnered in a couple of ways. One method is to euthanize laboratory animal models and extract the tissues needed for the study. Another method is to purchase the tissue from a butchery or slaughterhouse. In either case, make sure to use the tissues collected for ex vivo testing very soon after extraction. Also make sure that the tissues are stored and transported in sterile and appropriate areas (labeled refrigerators or ice chests).

The ex vivo testing methodology has numerous benefits. Extracted tissues can be used to validate antenna performance using common antenna measurements. The common tests performed for ex vivo (and in vivo) tests are discussed later in this chapter.

While ex vivo tissues can validate the basic antenna performance, this method does have some limitations. Because the tissues are separated from the animal model, the tissues begin decaying as soon as they are extracted. As a result, there is a very short window (hours) where the tissues can model a living animal. Ex vivo tissues cannot model long-term performance of the antenna due to the change in dielectric properties. Additionally, long-term performance cannot be explored because the tissues have been severed from an immune system. Whenever an object is implanted into a living being, a healthy immune system will attack and try to isolate it. When a tissue is severed from an immune system, no attack and encapsulation can take place.

5.3.2 In Vitro Gels

An alternative to ex vivo tissues is an in vitro material to validate the antenna. In vitro, Latin phrase for "in glass," means that the tissue is artificially developed outside of the body (animal or otherwise) and within a laboratory. For our purposes, in vitro means using dielectrically similar tissue-mimicking phantoms.

Much like ex vivo tissues, in vitro phantoms also have some benefits and drawbacks. Much like ex vivo, the gels can be used to measure the basic antenna performance. Extracted tissues can be used to validate the antenna performance using common antenna measurements. The common antenna tests are discussed later in the chapter. Much like ex vivo tissues, the biomimicking gel cannot validate biological responses of an implanted device. As a result, long-term performance and bioencapsulation effects cannot be measured using in vitro gels.

Unlike ex vivo tissues, however, biomimicking gels only mimic the dielectric properties of the corresponding biological tissue, not the thermal, biological, or mechanical properties. As a result, biomimicking gels cannot validate ablation zone or temperature effects. While biological tissues tend to cook during the ablation process, biomimicking gels tend to melt when heat is applied. There is, however, a major difference between ex vivo tissues and in vitro gels that gives the gels an advantage: shelf life. While the decaying process is relatively quick for biological tissues, the gels have a relatively long shelf life (months versus hours) comparatively. As a result, in vitro gels can be used and reused in testing over the design and development period, making them researcher and student friendly.

In the past, different tissue-mimicking phantom materials have been synthesized and used throughout several studies as an alternative to testing electromagnetic equipment on human subjects [26–30]. The core ingredient varies with each phantom causing the material to acquire three different forms: liquid, solid, and semisolid. Most liquid phantoms are composed of saline mixtures or similar body fluid equivalent materials. They have been used on several applications regarding antenna and RF equipment to simulate and measure the specific absorption rate (SAR) of the tissue once exposed to electromagnetic radiation [26–30]. Because the liquid phantoms form a state, there are limitations on their use by prohibiting the creation of complex phantoms. Liquid phantoms are required to be kept in a container and therefore cannot be implemented to create a phantom that mimics a complex biological construct with multiple tissue layers and a dynamic shape. For this reason, the tissue-mimicking material needs to be in a solid or semisolid form to acquire realistic tissue equivalent models. In addition, testing the device in liquids can be messy and quite cumbersome. The solid phantoms synthesized in previous research consisted of plastics, polyethylene powder and saline, silicon rubber, ceramic powder and resin, and strontium titanate powder and resin [31–37]. Solid body phantoms have been used throughout several studies to measure SAR at radio frequencies [35–39]. The solid phantoms are intended for mimicking the average dielectric properties among various tissues rather than of each individual tissue. Consequently, phantoms with multiple layers of tissue cannot be synthesized. The solution to this is the implementation of semisolid mimicking materials. The core ingredients for tissue-mimicking semisolid phantoms that other researchers have used are polyacrylamide, TX-150, cryogel, and gelatin [40–49].

In this chapter, we concentrate on gelatin-based semisolid tissue-mimicking phantoms for the purpose of in vitro testing. The advantages of using a gelatin-based material include the following: very few ingredients, no elaborative steps and expensive facilities to be characterized, composed of inexpensive materials, and is a quick process when compared to in vivo testing. Materials have been characterized that mimic the electrical properties of the following human tissues: skin, adipose tissue, muscle, malignant and nonmalignant fibroglandular tissue that contains 0–30% adipose tissue, malignant and nonmalignant fibroglandular tissue that contains 31–84% adipose tissue, liver, pancreas, and kidney. These materials are characterized to be applied to implantable medical telemetry, breast cancer detection system, and microwave hyperthermia.

5.3.2.1 Mixture and Characterization of Skin-Mimicking Material

The skin-mimicking material is characterized by mixing deionized water, vegetable oil, Gelatin A, Ultra Ivory® hand soap, polyethylene glycol mono phenyl ether (Triton X-100), and sodium chloride (salt). Pink food coloring is added for color. An investigation of the electrical properties of each ingredient showed that vegetable oil has the lowest electrical properties among all ingredients, while deionized water holds the highest. Varying the proportions of these two ingredients allows the mimicking of both low and high water content human soft tissues. Salt is used to increase the conductivity of the material while decreasing the relative permittivity. Salt also causes the permittivity to decrease rapidly from 500 MHz to 1 GHz and then slowly decrease from 1 to 20 GHz. Gelatin A, Triton-X, food coloring, and hand soap all have small effects on the electrical properties of the material because of the composition of the material or its small content within the total mixture. Each human soft tissue-mimicking material is characterized based on these facts. Table 5.3 shows the list of ingredients along with their percent volume, while Figure 5.6 shows the equipment that is used during the process.

First, salt is mixed in a beaker with the total required amount of deionized water. The beaker is covered with plastic cling wrap and placed in an 80°C water bath until all of the salt granules are dissolved in the water. In a separate beaker, Triton X-100 and Gelatin A are mixed until the gelatin granules are covered. Gelatin A is a gelling agent used to solidify the mixture. Once the salt is dissolved in the water, the saline solution is poured into the beaker that contains the Gelatin A compound. While stirring, pink food coloring is added to the mixture. The beaker is then covered with plastic cling wrap and placed in an 80°C water bath for 20 minutes. Gelatin A is soluble in water at high temperatures

Table 5.3 Recipe for skin-mimicking material.

Ingredients	Percent volume
Deionized water	68.33
Vegetable oil	20.68
Gelatin A	8.99 ($\rho = 1.2\,g\,mL^{-1}$)
Ultra Ivory soap	0.899
Triton X-100	0.899
Sodium chloride	0.166 ($\rho = 2.165\,g\,mL^{-1}$)
Pink food coloring	0.037 (1 drop = 0.042 mL)

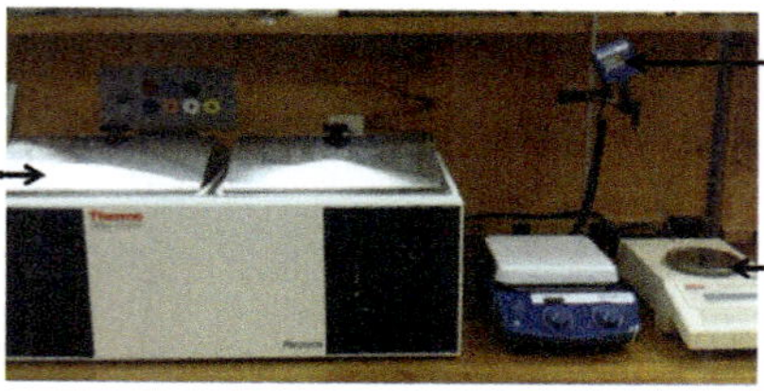

Figure 5.6 Equipment for characterization of tissue-mimicking material.

and sets as a gel at or above room temperature. The total required amount of vegetable oil is poured in a separate beaker, covered with plastic cling wrap, and placed in an 80°C water bath for 20 minutes. The oil needs to be at the same temperature as the Gelatin A compound when they are mixed together so that the gelatin does not prematurely form before the mixture is thoroughly mixed. Once the gelatin and oil mixtures have both reached 80°C, the vegetable oil and Gelatin mixtures are mixed with Ultra Ivory hand soap in a 500-mL Whip Mix Vac-U-Mixer. The hand soap acts as a surfactant that allows the oil to mix into the water. Once the lid is sealed, the mixer's drive nut is inserted into the Whip-Mix Combination Vacuum Mixer Unit's drive chuck. The gel should be mixed for 15 seconds. Figure 5.7 shows the equipment used in the mixing process.

Mixing a gel without air bubbles is vital to achieve accurate dielectric properties measurement. The vacuum mixer should mitigate air bubbles during the mixing process. Pour the mixture into a beaker and set to form in a refrigerator for 30 minutes. Air bubbles may form while pouring the mixture into this beaker. Figure 5.8 shows the skin-mimicking material once it is completely formed. Any air bubbles that are within the material rise to the top of the mixture during the forming process. To obtain a mixture with absolutely no air bubbles, approximately 1 cm of the top of the gel is cut off.

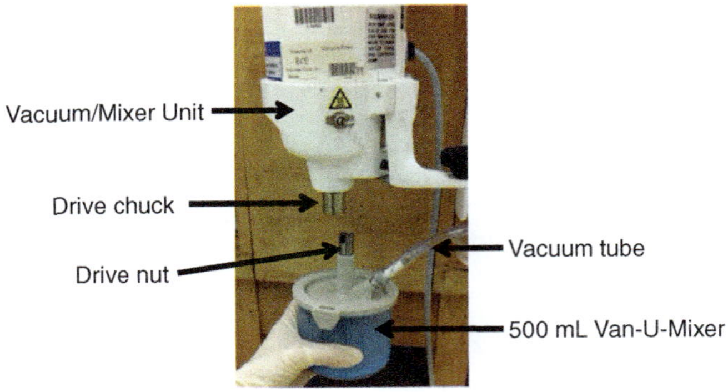

Figure 5.7 Whip Mix Combination Vacuum Mixer Unit and Vac-U-Mixer.

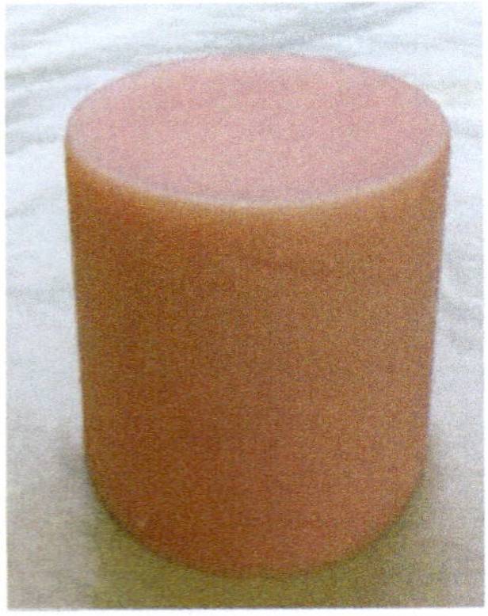

Figure 5.8 Characterized skin-mimicking material.

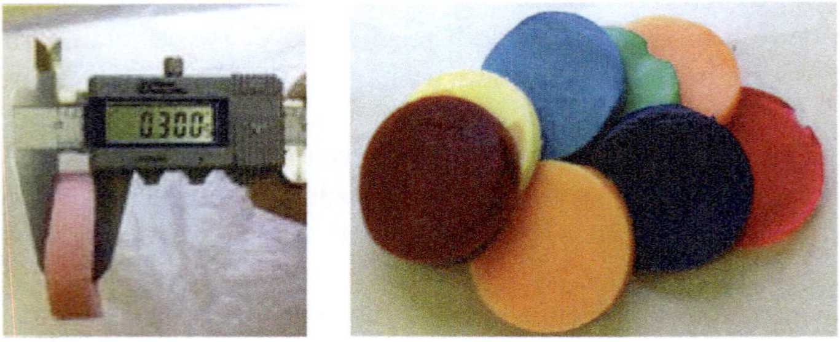

Figure 5.9 Top slices of gels to avoid air bubbles.

As shown in Figure 5.9, this procedure is done for all of the tissue-mimicking gels characterized.

Once the skin-mimicking material has gelatinized, the relative permittivity and conductivity are measured from 500 MHz to 20 GHz using Agilent

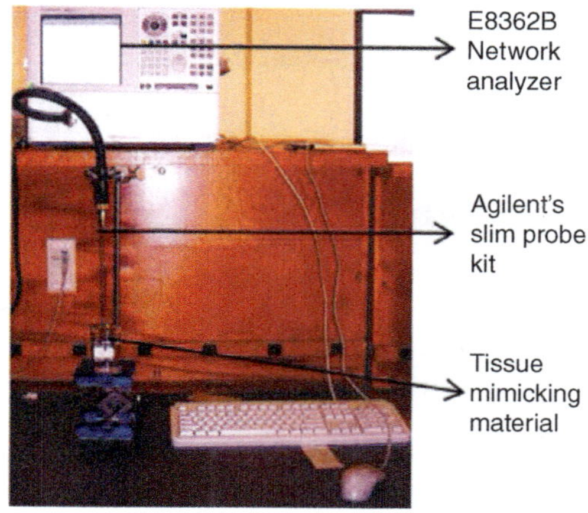

Figure 5.10 Dielectric probe measurement setup.

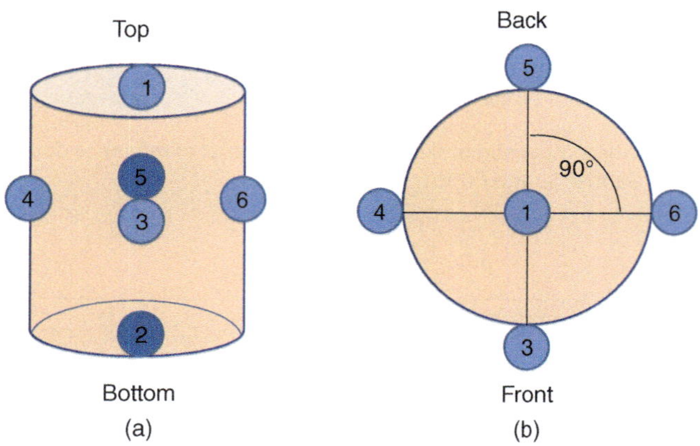

Figure 5.11 Points of measurements: (a) the side view and (b) the top view of the material.

Technologies® E8362B PNA Network Analyzer and Agilent Technologies 85070E Dielectric Slim Probe Kit. The experimental setup for the electrical property measurements is demonstrated in Figure 5.10.

To ensure data reliability, six different points on the material are measured with the Agilent slim probe: one on the top, one on the bottom, and four on the side where each measurement is at a 90° angle from the previous measurement. Figure 5.11 shows a diagram of the areas in which the measurements are taken.

The relative permittivity and conductivity are shown in Figures 5.12 and 5.13. The average of the six sets of measured properties is compared with the human wet skin reference data obtained from [50, 51]. In [50], a comprehensive literature survey of previously measured dielectric properties of different tissues either excised from humans or animals is provided. In [51], the dielectric property measurements of different tissues from 10 Hz to 20 GHz are given. The

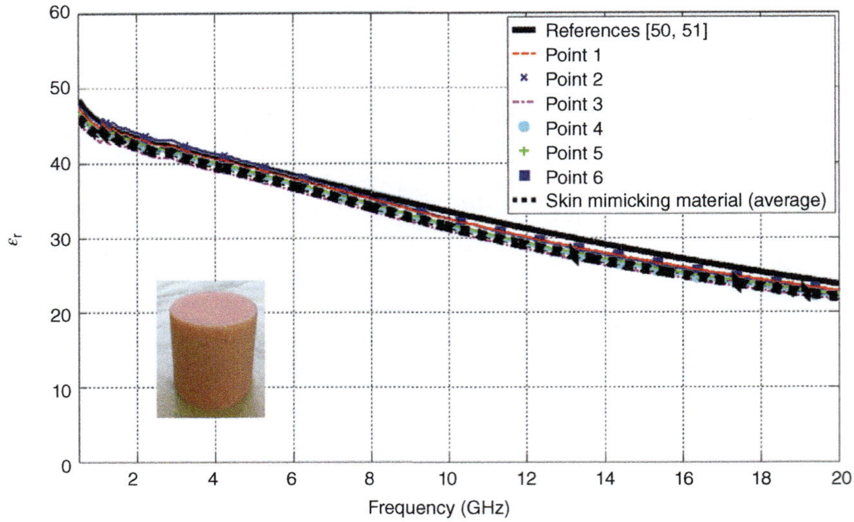

Figure 5.12 Relative permittivity comparison of skin-mimicking material to reference data. (*Source*: Based on Gabriel, C., Gabriel, S., and Corthout, E., 1996.)

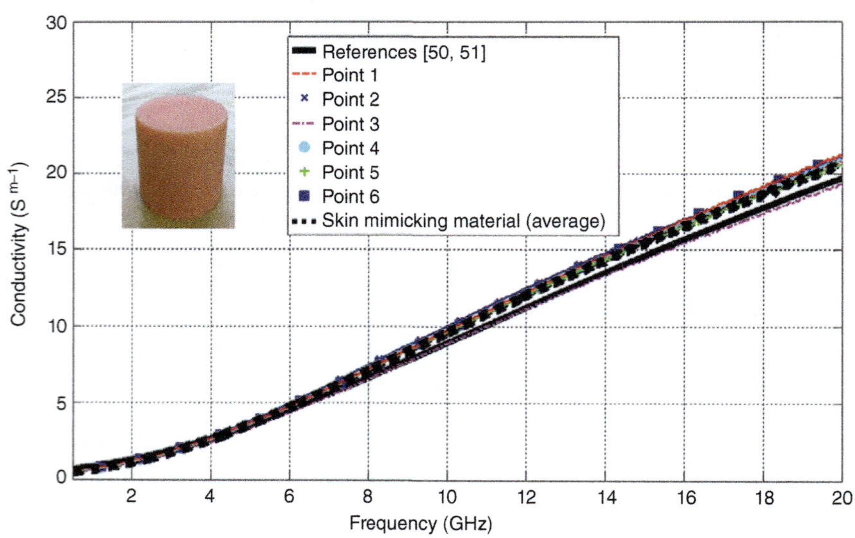

Figure 5.13 Conductivity comparison of skin-mimicking material to reference data. (*Source*: Based on Gabriel, S., Lau, R. W., and Gabriel, C., 1996.)

measurements are taken from (i) excised animal tissue mostly from freshly killed ovine and some porcine; (ii) human autopsy materials; and (iii) human skin and tongue in vivo. The human tissues are obtained 24–48 hours after death, while the animal tissues are measured two hours after death. Figures 5.12 and 5.13 show a graphical comparison between the skin's relative permittivity and conductivity of each point of measurements, the average of the six points, and reference data in [50, 51], respectively.

As shown in the figures, a consistent agreement is obtained between the reference data in [50, 51] and the measurements of the skin-mimicking material. It is important to obtain a maximum deviation that is less than 10% of the data found in [50, 51]at a set frequency. The characterized skin-mimicking gel maximum deviation from the reference data from 500 MHz to 20 GHz is

$$\max \Delta\varepsilon_r = \max(\varepsilon_{r_{\text{reference}}} - \varepsilon_{r_{\text{material}}}) = 2.35 \tag{5.3}$$

for relative permittivity and

$$\max \Delta\sigma = \max(\sigma_{\text{referece}} - \sigma_{\text{material}}) = 1.02 \tag{5.4}$$

for conductivity.

The maximum deviation falls under 10% of the data given in the literature; thus, the material can be used to accurately investigate the interaction between the electromagnetic waves and the skin tissue at 500 MHz to 20 GHz. This comparison is performed during the characterization process of all of the tissue-mimicking materials until a desirable recipe is reached.

Once the skin-mimicking gel is characterized, the shelf life of the material is studied for a period of eight weeks. Two identical skin-mimicking gel samples are created and kept covered in plastic cling wrap to study the effects refrigeration has on the electrical properties of the mimicking material. One of the samples is kept in the refrigerator during the eight-week study, while the other sample is kept at room temperature. Every week the relative permittivity and conductivity are measured at room temperature from 500 MHz to 20 GHz using a Keysight® E8362B PNA Network Analyzer and Agilent Technologies 85070E Dielectric Slim Probe Kit. Approximately 1 cm of the top of the gel is cut off each week to obtain the electrical properties within layers of the gel. Six measurements are made at different locations as shown in Figure 5.11. Figures 5.14–5.17 show the dielectric properties of the refrigerated and nonrefrigerated materials.

After week 2, the unrefrigerated skin-mimicking material becomes moldy. Because of this, the measurements on the nonrefrigerated sample are not performed for the weeks following. Figure 5.18 shows the appearance of the nonrefrigerated skin-mimicking material at week 0 and week 3, respectively. The refrigerated gel does not spoil during the eight-week period, and the dielectric properties are consistent.

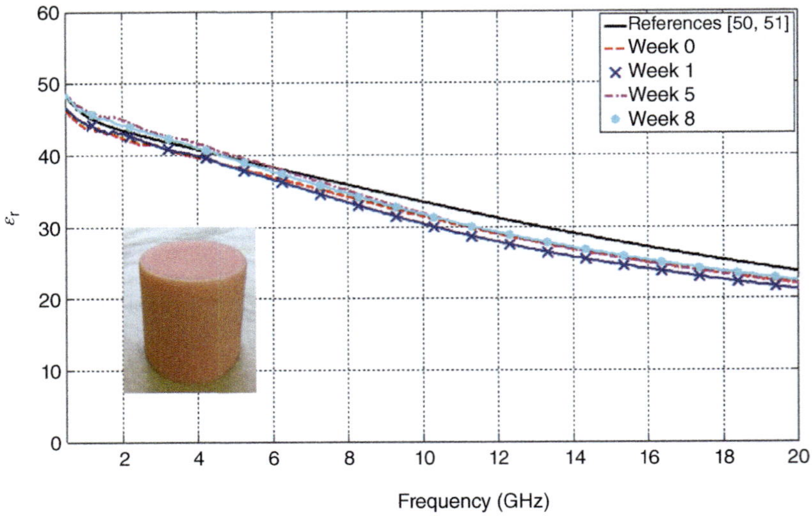

Figure 5.14 Relative permittivity of refrigerated skin-mimicking material.

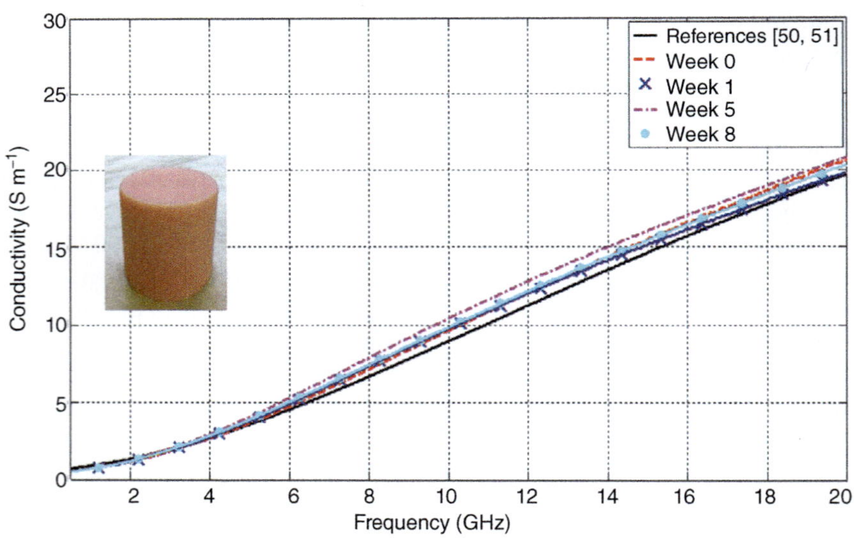

Figure 5.15 Conductivity of refrigerated skin-mimicking material.

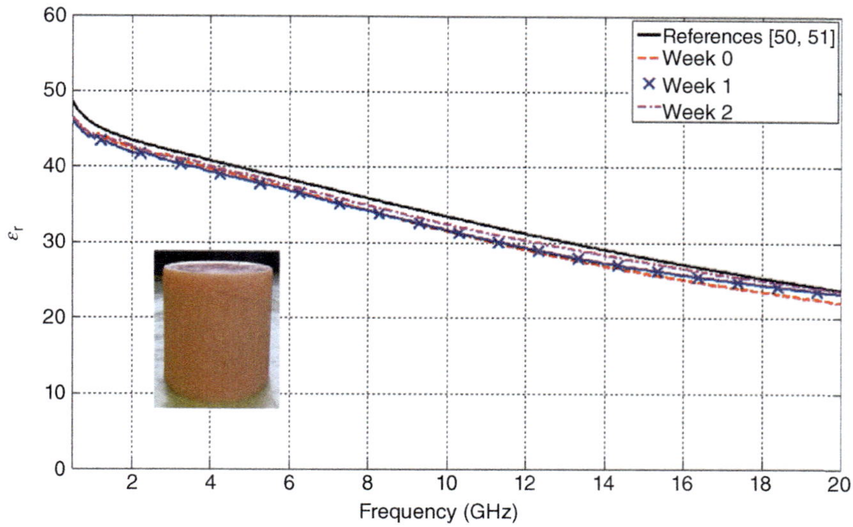

Figure 5.16 Relative permittivity of nonrefrigerated skin-mimicking material.

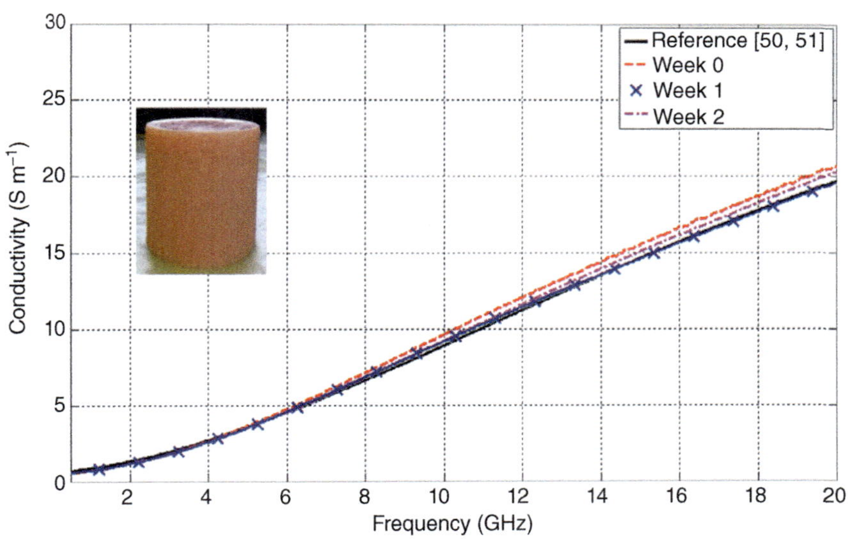

Figure 5.17 Conductivity of nonrefrigerated skin-mimicking material.

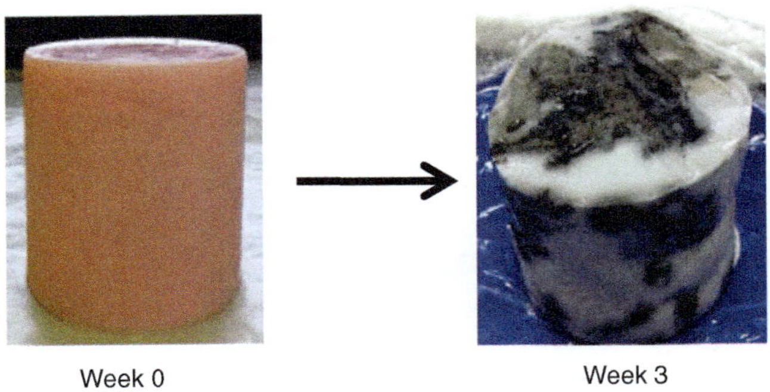

Figure 5.18 Molding of the nonrefrigerated material.

Table 5.4 Recipe for adipose-mimicking material.

Ingredients	Percent volume
Deionized water	11.39
Vegetable oil	83.44
Gelatin B	2.84 ($\rho = 1.2\,\text{g mL}^{-1}$)
Ultra Ivory soap	1.52
Triton X-100	0.76
Yellow food coloring	0.06 (1 drop = 0.0417 mL)

5.3.2.2 Mixture and Characterization of Adipose-Mimicking Material

An adipose tissue-mimicking material is made by mixing deionized water, vegetable oil, Ultra Ivory hand soap, Gelatin B, Triton X-100, and yellow food coloring. Gelatin B is a gelling agent used to solidify the mixture. Table 5.4 shows the list of ingredients with their percent volume of the mixture.

In a beaker, the Gelatin B granules are coated with Triton X-100. Then, the required amounts of deionized water and food coloring are stirred into the mixture. This beaker is covered with plastic cling wrap and placed at 80°C water bath for 20 minutes. The total required amount of vegetable oil is placed in a separate beaker, covered with plastic cling wrap, and put in an 80°C water bath for 20 minutes. The Gelatin B mixture along with Ultra Ivory hand soap is poured into a bowl and the material stirred by hand. As the material is mixing, the oil is slowly poured into the mixture. Lastly, the homogeneous mixture is poured into a beaker and set to form in the refrigerator for 30 minutes. A formed adipose tissue-mimicking gel is shown in Figure 5.19.

Once the adipose tissue-mimicking material has formed, the relative permittivity and conductivity are measured from 500 MHz to 20 GHz using Agilent

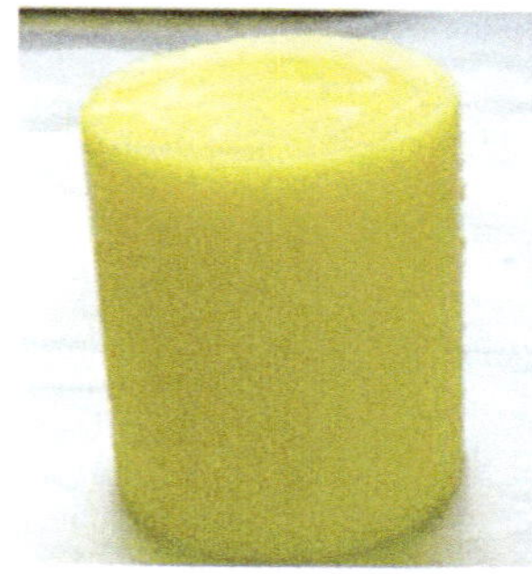

Figure 5.19 Characterized adipose tissue-mimicking gel.

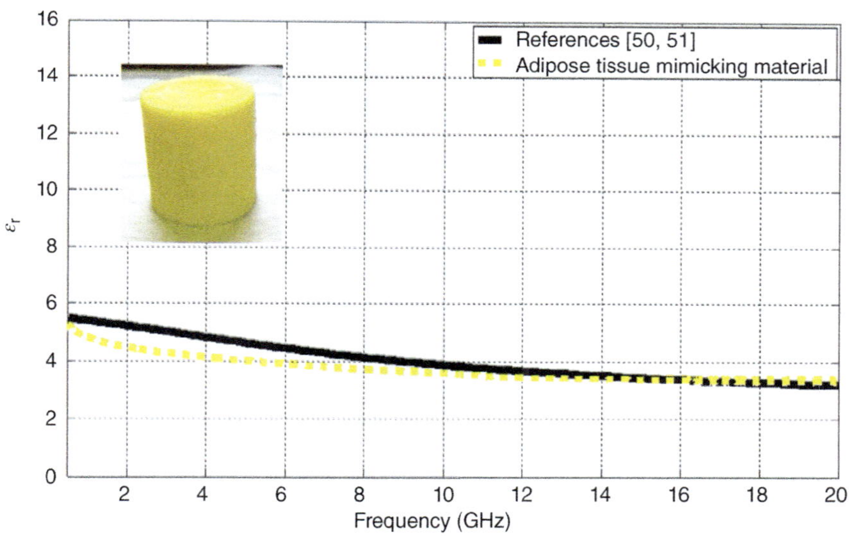

Figure 5.20 Relative permittivity comparison of adipose tissue-mimicking material to reference data.

Technologies E8362B PNA Network Analyzer and Agilent Technologies 85070E Dielectric Slim Probe Kit. Similar to the skin-mimicking gel, six different points on the material are measured with the Agilent slim probe (see Figure 5.11). The average of the obtained measurements is compared with the human breast fat reference data obtained from [50, 51]. Figures 5.20 and 5.21 show a graphical comparison between an adipose tissue's relative permittivity and conductivity of measured and reference data [50, 51], respectively.

The graph shows that a consistent agreement is obtained between the reference data in [50, 51] and measurements of the adipose tissue-mimicking material. The characterized adipose tissue-mimicking gel maximum deviation from

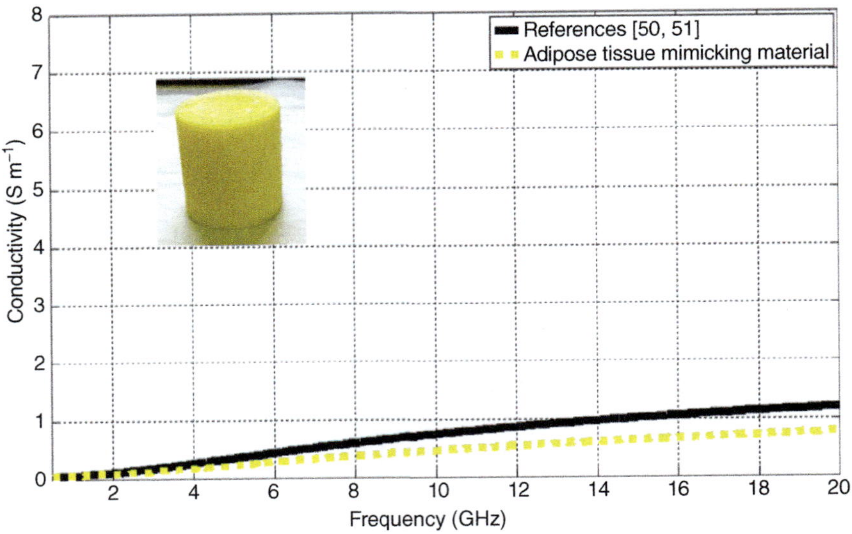

Figure 5.21 Conductivity comparison of adipose tissue-mimicking material to reference data.

the reference data from 500 MHz to 20 GHz is 0.82 for the relative permittivity and 0.44 S m^{-1} for conductivity.

The shelf life of the adipose tissue-mimicking material is studied for a period of eight weeks. The steps previously described for the skin is applied to the two adipose tissue-mimicking materials to investigate the material's shelf life and the effects refrigeration has on the dielectric properties of the characterized adipose tissue-mimicking material. Figures 5.22–5.25 show the dielectric properties throughout the eight-week study of both the refrigerated and nonrefrigerated materials, respectively.

After week 1, the nonrefrigerated adipose tissue-mimicking material gets spoiled. Because of this, the measurements on the nonrefrigerated sample are not performed for the weeks following. Figure 5.26 shows the appearance of the nonrefrigerated adipose tissue-mimicking material at week 0 and week 2.

5.3.2.3 Mixture and Characterization of Muscle-Mimicking Material

A muscle-mimicking material is made by mixing deionized water, vegetable oil, Ultra Ivory hand soap, Gelatin A, Triton X-100, salt, and red food coloring. Table 5.5 shows the list of ingredients and their percent volume. The steps described for skin are followed to characterize the muscle-mimicking material. The formed muscle-mimicking gel is shown in Figure 5.27.

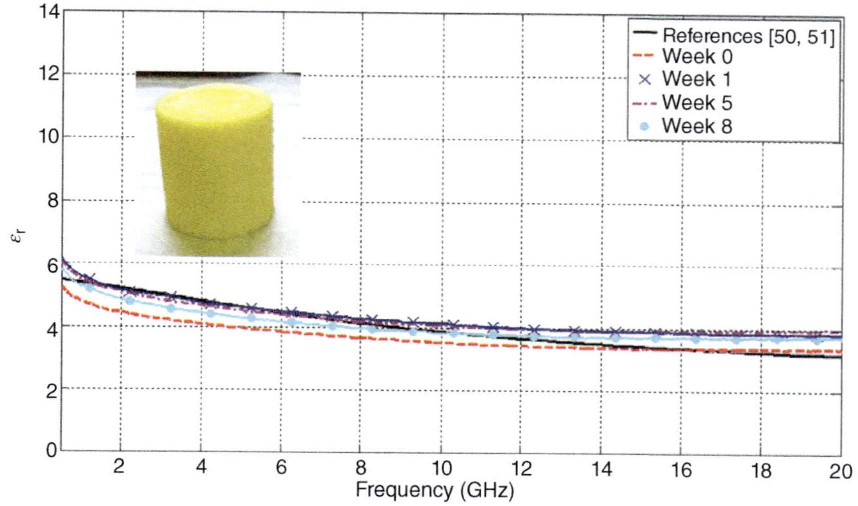

Figure 5.22 Relative permittivity of refrigerated adipose tissue-mimicking material.

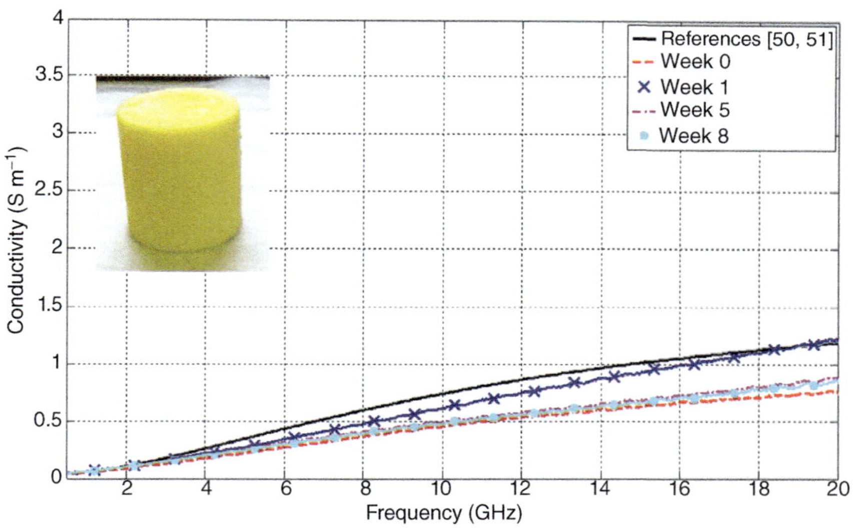

Figure 5.23 Conductivity of refrigerated adipose tissue-mimicking material.

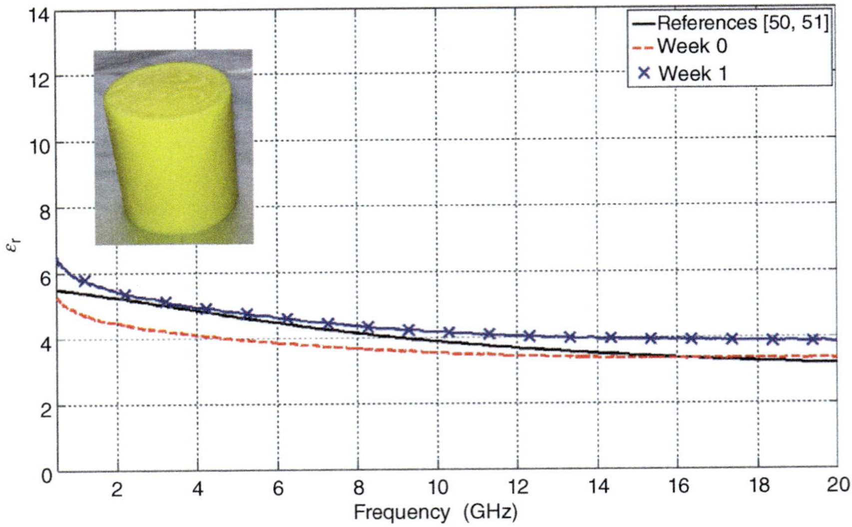

Figure 5.24 Relative permittivity of nonrefrigerated adipose tissue-mimicking material.

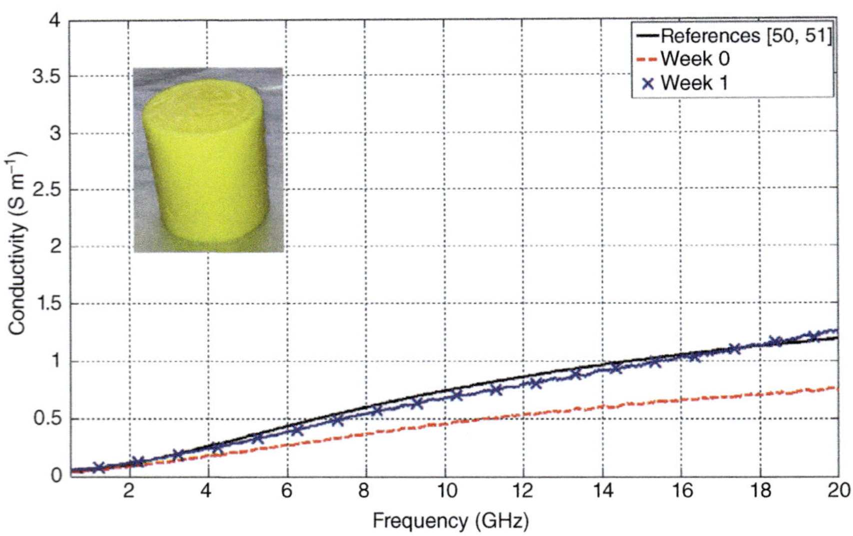

Figure 5.25 Conductivity of nonrefrigerated adipose tissue-mimicking material.

Figure 5.26 Spoiling of the nonrefrigerated material.

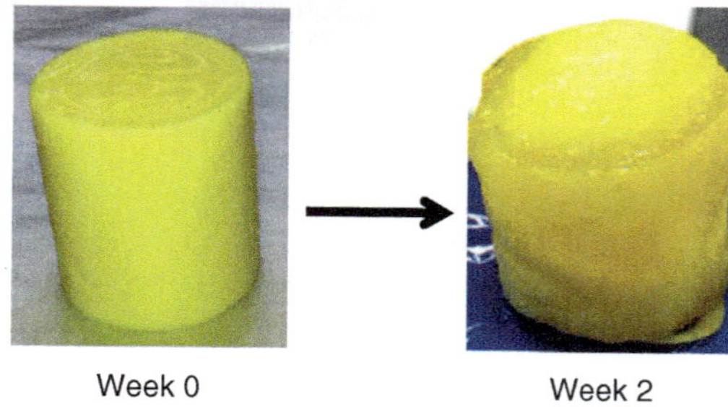

Table 5.5 Recipe for muscle-mimicking material.

Ingredients	Percent volume
Deionized water	72.47
Vegetable oil	13.59
Gelatin A	9.06 ($\rho = 1.2\,\mathrm{g\,mL^{-1}}$)
Ultra Ivory soap	2.72
Triton X-100	0.91
Sodium chloride	0.13 ($\rho = 2.165\,\mathrm{g\,mL^{-1}}$)
Red food coloring	1.13 (1 drop = 0.042 mL)

Figure 5.27 Characterized muscle-mimicking material.

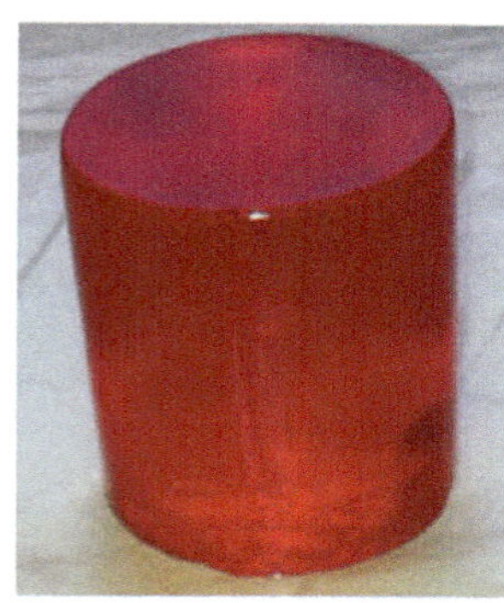

The relative permittivity and conductivity are measured from 500 MHz to 20 GHz. As described in the skin gel section, six different points on the material are measured with the Agilent slim probe. The average of the obtained measurements is compared with the human muscle reference data obtained from [50, 51]. Figures 5.28 and 5.29 show a graphical comparison between a muscle's relative permittivity and conductivity of the measured and reference data in [50, 51], respectively.

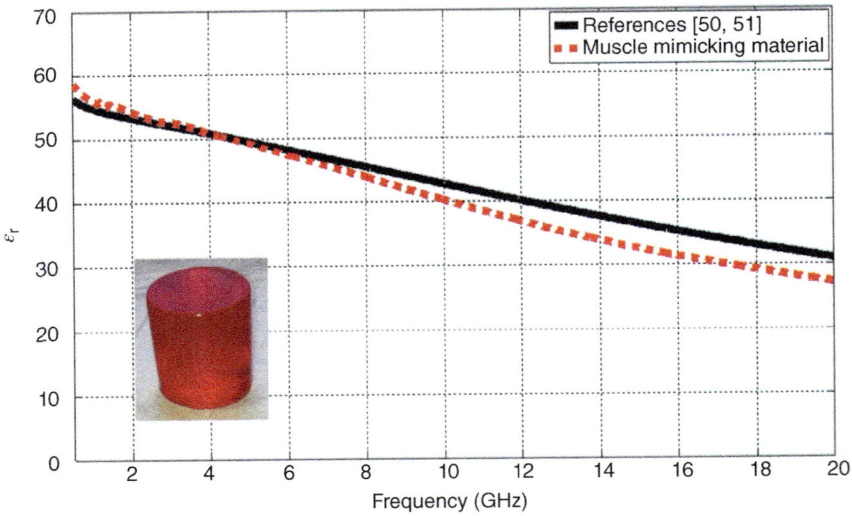

Figure 5.28 Relative permittivity comparison of muscle-mimicking material to reference data.

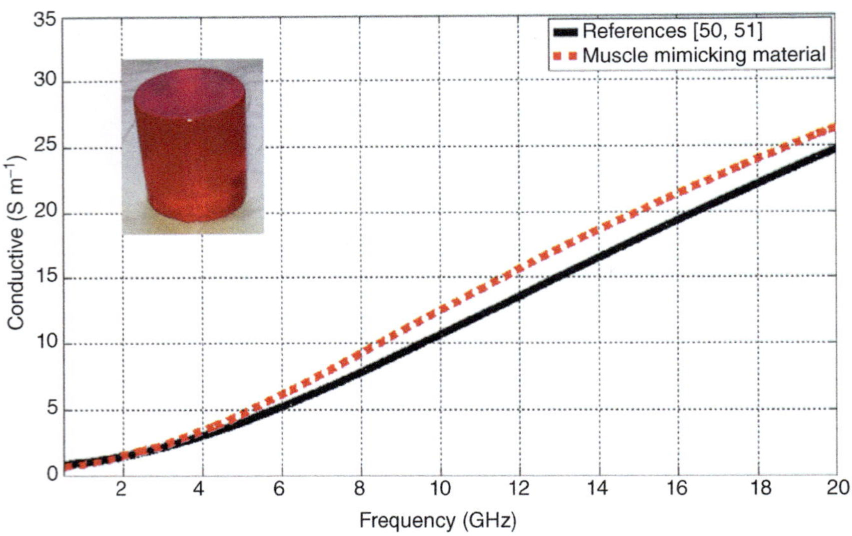

Figure 5.29 Conductivity comparison of muscle-mimicking material to reference data.

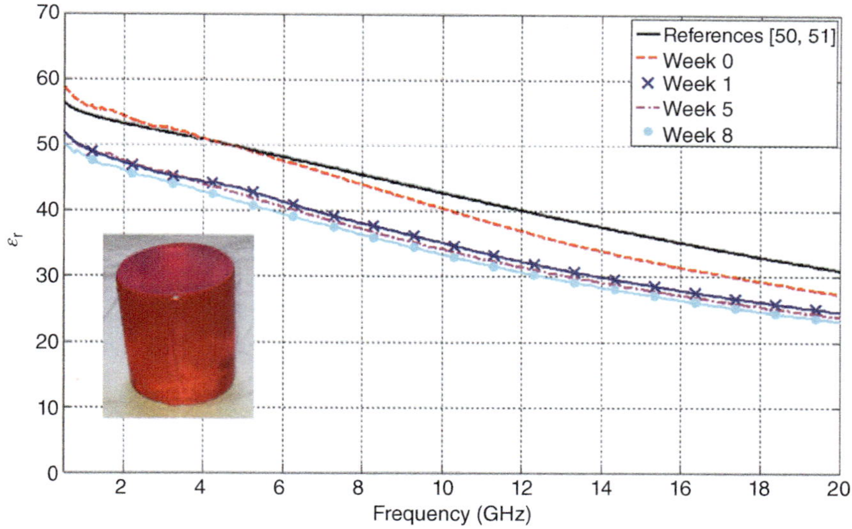

Figure 5.30 Relative permittivity of refrigerated muscle-mimicking material.

A good agreement is obtained between the reference data in [50, 51] and the measurements of the muscle-mimicking material. The characterized muscle-mimicking material maximum deviation from the reference data from 500 MHz to 20 GHz is 3.94 for the relative permittivity and 0.57 S m^{-1} for conductivity.

The shelf life of the muscle-mimicking material is studied for a period of eight weeks. The steps previously described for skin are applied to two muscle-mimicking materials to investigate the material's shelf life and the effects refrigeration has on the electrical properties of the tissue-mimicking material. Figures 5.30–5.33 show the electrical properties throughout the eight-week study of both the refrigerated and nonrefrigerated materials, respectively.

After week 1, the nonrefrigerated muscle-mimicking material gets spoiled. Because of this, the measurements on the nonrefrigerated sample are not performed for the weeks following. Figure 5.34 shows the appearance of the nonrefrigerated muscle-mimicking gel at week 0 and week 2.

5.4 In Vivo Testing

While the in vitro and ex vivo testing can provide usable and necessary data for an implantable system, there are some aspects that are still lacking. In terms of a tissue-mimicking gel, the inability to show temperature effects from the

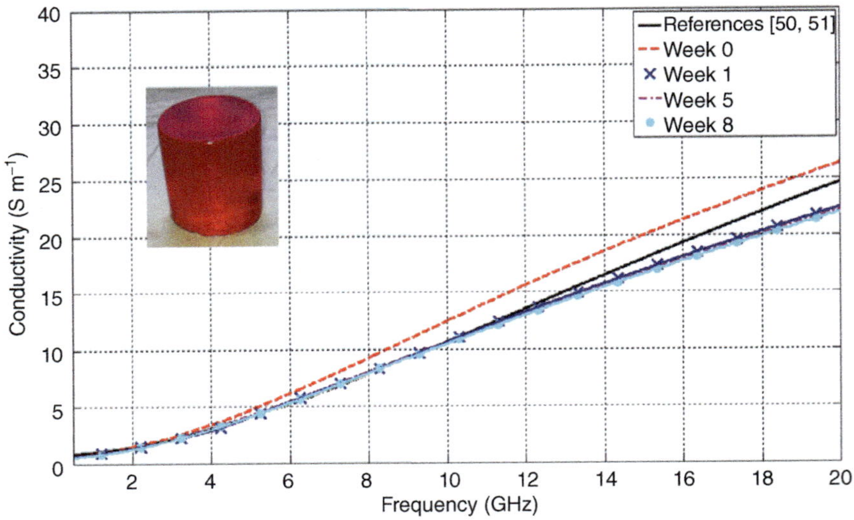

Figure 5.31 Conductivity of refrigerated muscle-mimicking material.

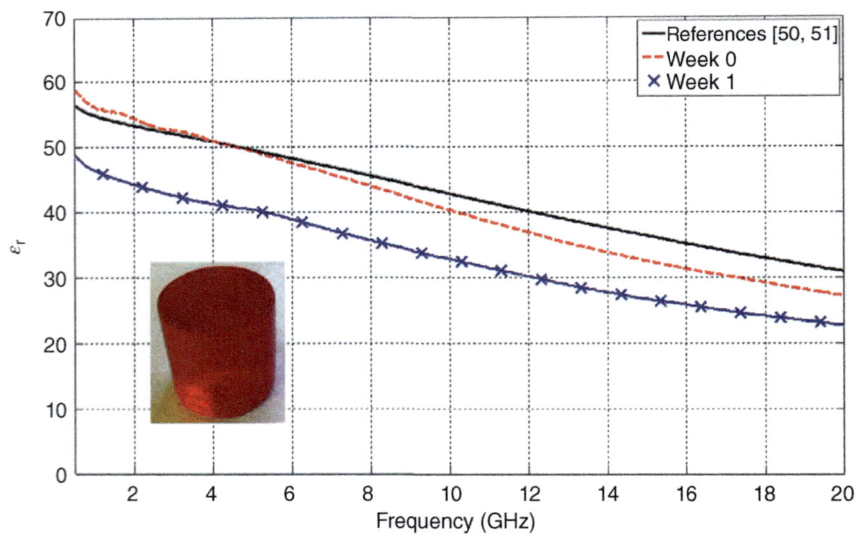

Figure 5.32 Relative permittivity of nonrefrigerated muscle-mimicking material.

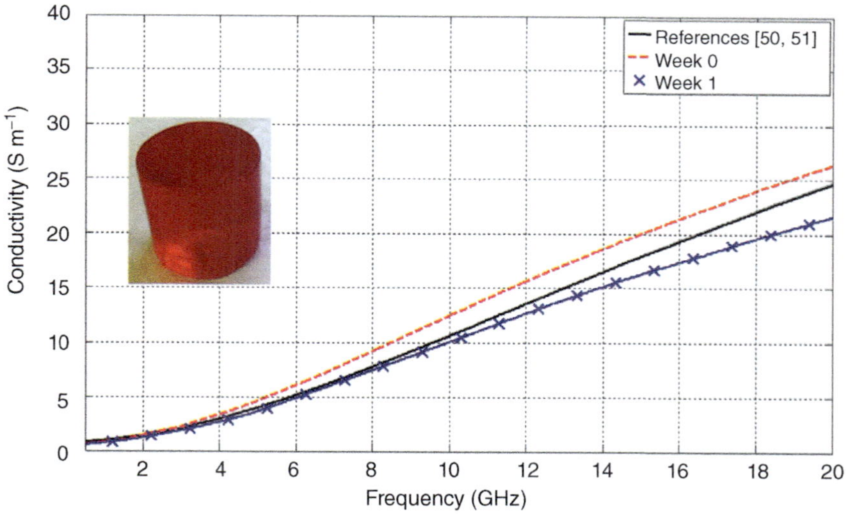

Figure 5.33 Conductivity of nonrefrigerated muscle-mimicking material.

Figure 5.34 Spoiling of the nonrefrigerated material.

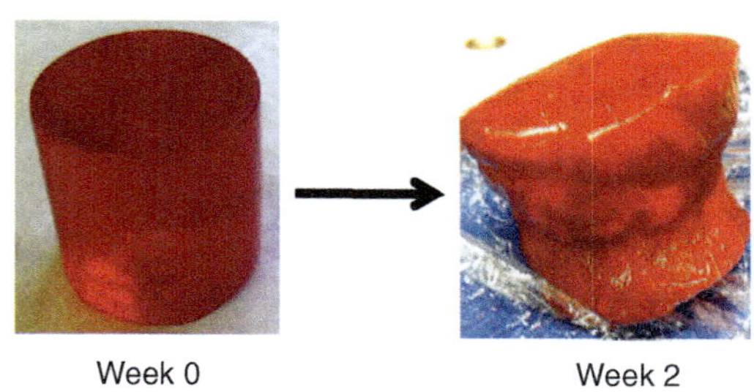

implanted antenna. Ex vivo tissues have short shelf lives, not only making a long-term study impossible but put extra strain on a short-term study. Neither method can show biological reaction to the implanted device. In order to round out the performance validation of an implantable device, it is necessary to move on to an in vivo testing method.

In vivo is Latin for "in the living." In a testing perspective, in vivo means testing a device on or within a living being. There are some similarities between a bench top test and an in vivo test. The first similarity is that the basic antenna performance can be evaluated in the same way. Return loss, link budget, and gain can be validated using the exact same setup as mentioned in the previous section. Additionally, an ablation zone can be validated in the same way as a bench top test; however, this test often will have to result in the extraction of the cooked tissue for analysis. This process, depending on the animal model used, could result in the euthanasia of the animal model.

There are many differences between the two steps. For instance, an in vivo test can validate long-term performance of the implanted device. Because a live animal model possesses an immune system, encapsulation is expected as the white blood cells attack and isolate the "threatening" implanted device. Similar, to this, after a long-term test has been performed, tissues can be extracted for histography or other tests to validate the biocompatibility of the implanted device. A major difference between a bench-top test and an in vivo test involves the approval and regulation surrounding the tests themselves. For example, in the United States, an Institutional Animal Care and Use Committee (IACUC) is such a regulatory agency that approves the use, facilitation, and care for animals used in scientific studies. Additionally, IACUC performs inspections and examinations of institutions in the care for animals in studies. Additionally, in the United States, an implantable device needs approval from other regulatory agencies, such as the Food and Drug Administration (FDA).

The rest of this section discusses the differences between human tissue and two common animal test models, porcine and rodent. This section also discusses some practical testing concerns for testing in vivo.

5.4.1 Different Animal Models for Different Frequency Bands

Depending on the frequency of operation and the tissue environment, different animal models may be used to validate similar performance for antennas in vivo similar to that of human tests. The cole–cole model is common when modeling the frequency-dependent dielectric properties (relative permittivity ε_r and conductivity σ). Equation (5.5) shows the multipole cole–cole model,

$$\varepsilon_c(\omega) = \varepsilon_\infty + \left(\sum_{i=1}^{N} \left(\frac{\varepsilon_{si} - \varepsilon_\infty}{1 + (j\omega\tau_i)^{1-\alpha_i}} \right) \right) + \frac{\sigma_s}{j\omega\varepsilon_0} = \varepsilon_0\varepsilon_r(\omega) - j\frac{\sigma(\omega)}{\omega}, \quad (5.5)$$

where ε_c is the frequency (ω)-dependent complex permittivity, ε_∞ is the permittivity at very high frequencies, ε_{si} is the permittivity at low frequencies per pole i, τ_i is a time constant associated with pole i, α_i is the exponential parameter per pole, σ_s is the static frequency conductivity, and ε_0 is the free space permittivity ($8.85 \times 10^{-12}\ \mathrm{F\,m^{-1}}$). Table 5.6 shows the cole–cole parameters for human, porcine, and rodent tissues (skin, adipose, muscle, fibroglandular, and liver). The separated frequency-dependent relative permittivity (ε_r) and frequency-dependent conductivity (σ) are shown in Figure 5.35.

There are a couple of conclusions that can be drawn from this comparison of human tissue to animal model tissues. The first conclusion is that different frequency bands of operation may cause a researcher to choose one animal model over the other. For example, if the antenna is designed for subcutaneous implantation, using a porcine animal model would make sense at frequencies lower

Table 5.6 Cole–Cole model parameters for human, rodent, and porcine animal model tissues.

Models	ε_∞	σ_{si}	ε_{s1}	ε_{s2}	ε_{s3}	ε_{s4}	α_1	α_2	α_3	α_4	τ_1 (ps)	τ_2 (ns)	τ_3 (µs)	τ_4 (ms)
Skin														
Rodent [52]	3	0.079	36.35	—	—	—	0.24	—	—	—	9.44	—	—	—
Porcine [53]	3	0.57	47.23	—	—	—	0.3	—	—	—	8.84	—	—	—
Human [54]	4	0	43	284	30,004	30,004	0.1	0.0	0.16	0.2	7.958	79.557	1.592	1.592
Adipose														
Rodent [55]	3.05	0.123	12.004	—	—	—	0.169	—	—	—	9.015	—	—	—
Porcine [53]	3	0.17	13.33	—	—	—	0.19	—	—	—	10.02	—	—	—
Human [54]	2.5	0.035	11.5	37.5	30,002.5	10,000,002.5	0.2	0.1	0.05	0.01	7.958	15.915	159.155	15.915
Muscle														
Rodent [52]	3	0.119	52.33	—	—	—	0.21	—	—	—	10	—	—	—
Porcine [56]	3	0.109	49.64	—	—	—	0.1	—	—	—	12.21	—	—	—
Human [54]	4	0.2	54	7004	1,200,004	25,000,004	0.1	0.1	0.1	0.0	7.234	353.678	318.31	2.274
Fibro glandular														
Rodent [57]	2.5	0.8825	76.31	—	—	—	0.6087	—	—	—	35.10	—	—	—
Porcine[53]	3	0.77	47.84	—	—	—	0.22	—	—	—	8.05	—	—	—
Human [58]	7.821	0.713	49.301	—	—	—	0.047	—	—	—	10.66	—	—	—
Liver														
Rodent [55]	3	0.009	47.10	—	—	—	0.17	—	—	—	9.14	—	—	—
Porcine [59]	4	0.02	43.00	—	—	—	0.1	—	—	—	8.84	—	—	—
Human [54]	4	0.02	43	6004	50,004	30,000,004	0.1	0.2	0.2	0.05	8.842	530.5165	22.736	15.915

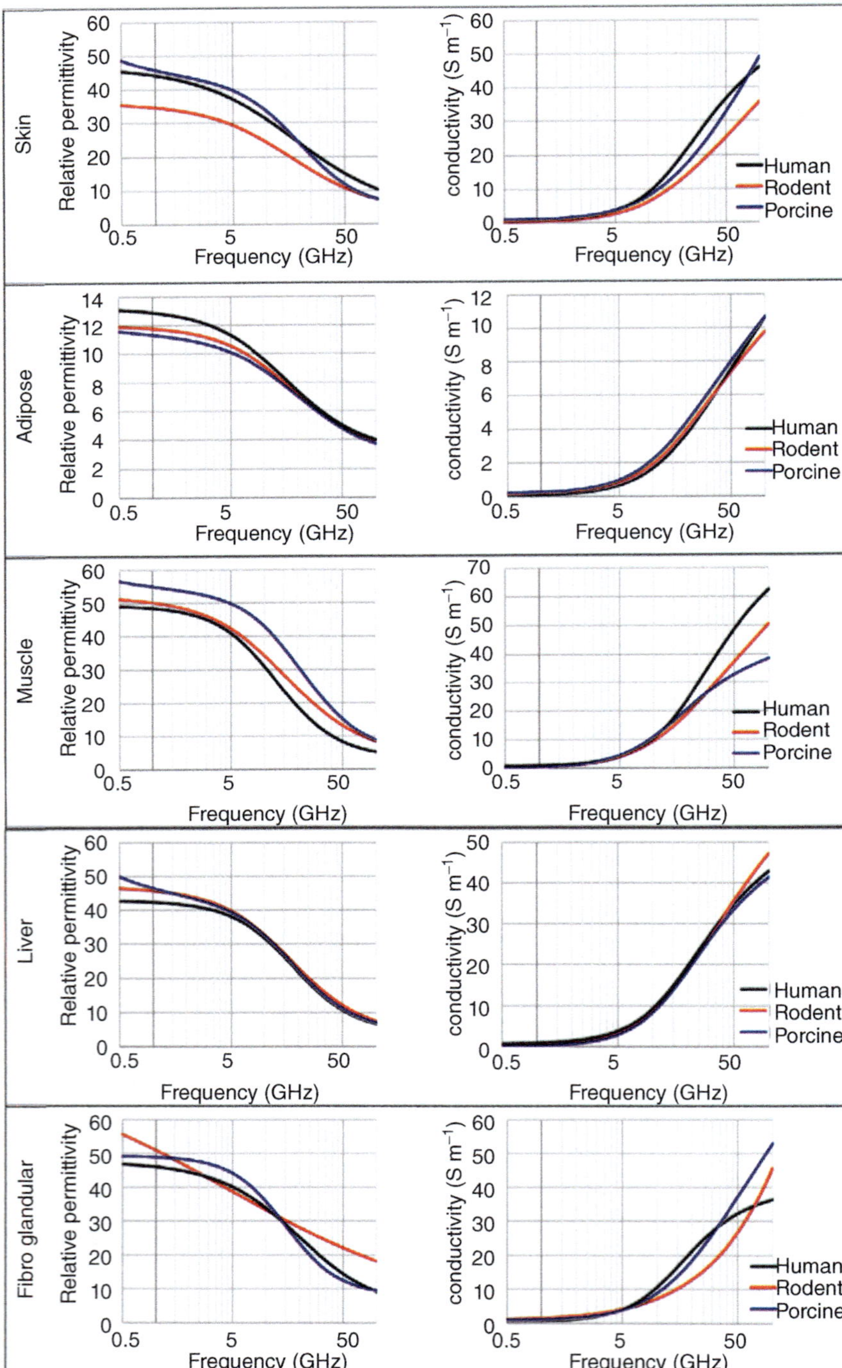

Figure 5.35 Dielectric properties (relative permittivity and conductivity) of skin, adipose, muscle, liver, and fibroglandular tissue for human, porcine, and rodent animal models.

than 40 GHz, as the dielectric properties of skin between humans and pigs are relatively similar. However, if the antenna is to be placed deeper than subcutaneous at these same frequencies of operation (further into the fatty adipose tissues or into the muscle), a rodent animal model may be a better fit for a direct comparison to human performance.

The second conclusion that can be drawn is that conductivity differences are more prevalent at higher frequencies (40 GHz) and above. At the MedRadio bands (approximately 400 MHz) and ISM bands (2.4, 5.8, or 24 GHz bands), these conductivity values are comparable to that of a human specimen. However, at higher frequencies the conductivity differences are more profound than the permittivity differences in some tissues over others. While the liver and adipose show strong correlation between the three at 50 GHz, muscle and skin show significant difference.

5.4.2 Dielectric Mismatch

Differences in dielectric properties are not just inherent between different test models. In many circumstances, the environment encountered in vivo will not match the tissues presented in the cole–cole models. This dielectric mismatch, when a material does not match the averaged or theoretical dielectric properties, can result in frequency shifts and attenuation. Figures 5.36 and 5.37 show this reality. Figure 5.36 presents a dual-band copper antenna [60] that is designed to operate on both the Wireless Medical Telemetry System (WMTS) and the 2.4 GHz ISM bands. The antenna designed was adapted from the design developed by Karacolak and Topsakal [61–63]. Two antennas were milled, assembled, coated in silicone, sterilized, and implanted in a porcine animal model. The simulated return loss of the antenna shows three resonances: 1.4, 2, and 2.44 GHz. Antenna 1, implanted on the upper back of a porcine animal model, shows frequency shifts from 1.4 to 1.45 GHz (3.6% shift), 2 to 2.3 GHz (15% shift), and 2.44 to 2.6 GHz (6% shift). The return loss for the 2.4 GHz resonance increased from −22.58 dB at 2.44 GHz to −10.37 dB at 2.6 GHz. These shifts indicate that the dielectric properties of the surrounding tissue are lower than the simulation. A similar study performed with a titanium nitride antenna for the 2.4 GHz ISM band is shown in Figure 5.37 [25, 64, 65]. The antenna is grown and etched on a sapphire substrate, connected to a coaxial cable via a UMCX connector, and coated in silicone on the connector and the coaxial cable (leaving the radiating element exposed). The antenna is then implanted into the upper back, in the same location as Antenna 1 in Figure 5.36, only on a different pig. The return loss sees a resonance shift that is more prevalent than the antenna-coated entirely in silicone. This suggests that not only could the silicone act as an isolator from the surrounding tissue, but also that the tissues differ between the two animals. These two practical

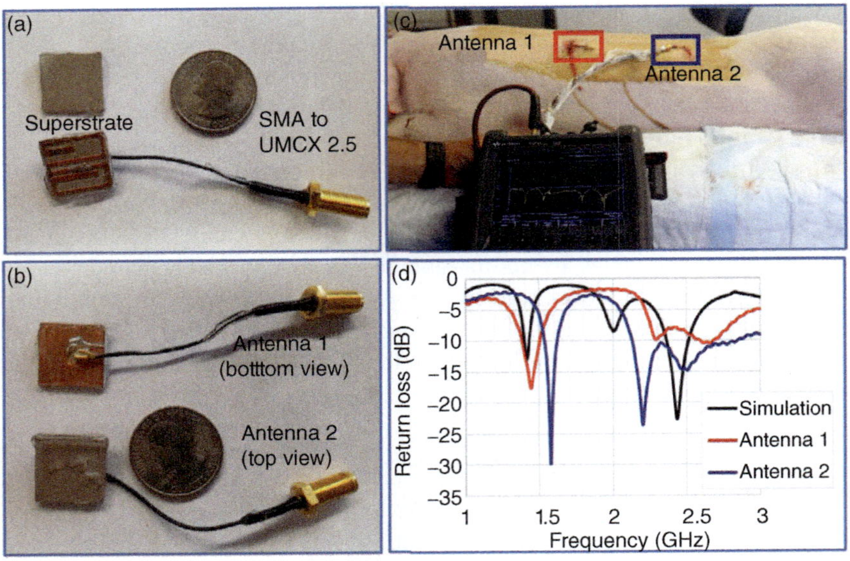

Figure 5.36 Dual-band antenna made for WMTS (1.4 GHz) and ISM (2.4 GHz) [60]. (a) Antenna with superstrate connected to SMA to UMCX cable. (b) Two fully assembled antennas and coated in medical grade silicone. (c) Implanted antennas into porcine animal model. One antenna is implanted in the upper back and the other is implanted into the lower back. (d) Simulated and measured return loss. (*Source*: Green, R.B., Hays, M., and Topsakal, E., 2018.)

examples show how dielectric mismatch can affect implanted electronics, but leaves a major question: What causes dielectric mismatch?

Living beings are not a static system dielectrically. Biological tissues change with various different factors including age [66–68], temperature [69–72], water content [51, 73], and even blood chemistry [74–79]. It is important to remember that the cole–cole parameters for tissues are best fit models for the average values for large numbers of individual measurements over several different specimens at particular snapshots in time and circumstance. Variations are expected. These variations between individual subjects in the same animal model, and even from hour to hour, lead to a dielectric mismatch between the antenna and the surrounding tissue. This dielectric mismatch is due to several different factors. The first factor discussed is how temperature affects the dielectric properties of tissues. As the temperature of the material is increased, especially in an ablation context, it is expected that the water content of the tissue will decrease due to evaporation. As a result, it is also expected that the relative permittivity of the tissue decreases at lower frequencies (Figure 5.38).

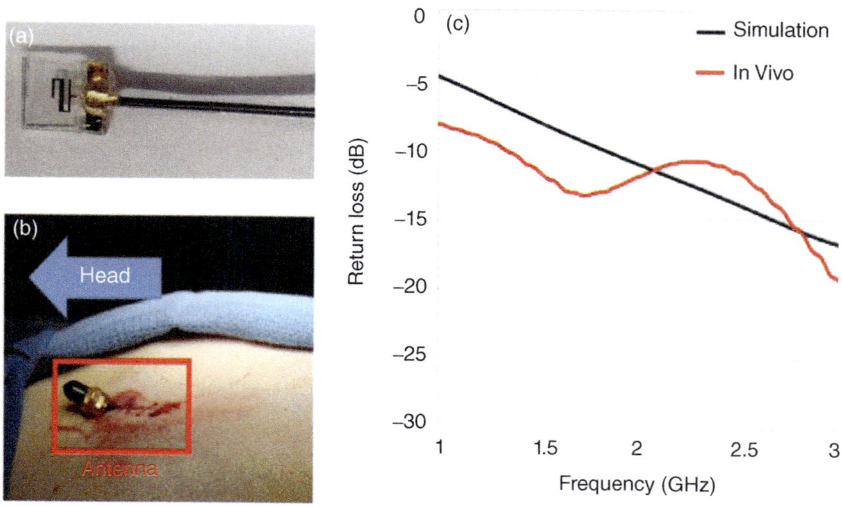

Figure 5.37 Titanium nitride antenna for 2.4 GHz [25, 64]. (a) Antenna fabricated on sapphire wafer. (b) Antenna implanted into upper back of porcine animal model. (c) Simulated and measured return loss. (*Source*: Green, R.B, and Topsakal, E., 2019.)

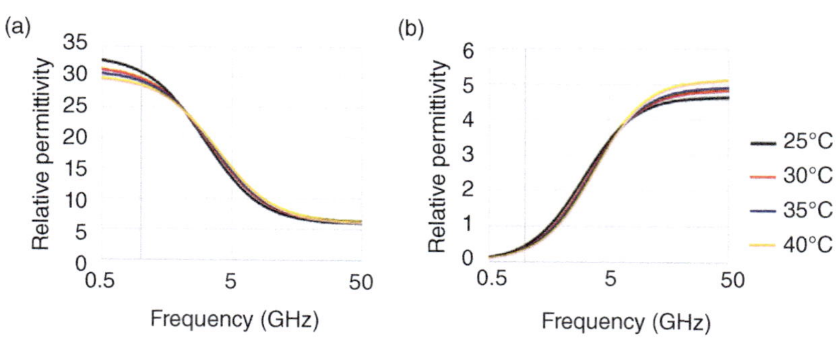

Figure 5.38 Dielectric properties of porcine muscle over frequency for various temperatures: (a) relative permittivity and (b) conductivity [56]. (*Source*: Based on Abdilla, L., Sammut, C.V., and Mangion, L.Z., 2013.)

Another factor in dielectric mismatch is the age of the subject. Peyman et al. [52] performed a study on rat tissues until the age of 70 days. The relative permittivity and conductivity are shown from this study for the rodent tissues of skin, muscle, and liver. The study shows that, in general, tissues tend to decrease both permittivity and conductivity with age. Skin sees a significant decrease in permittivity and increase in conductivity as age increases. As the specimen ages, different tissues mature and age much faster than others, seeing different

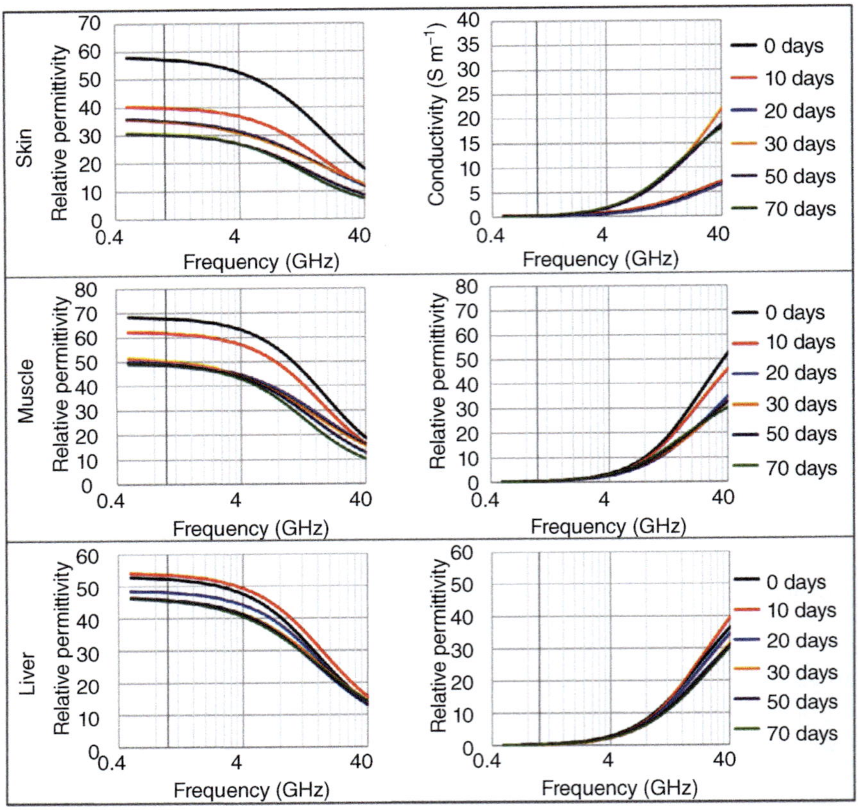

Figure 5.39 Dielectric properties of rodent tissue over frequency for various ages [52]. (*Source*: Based on Peyman, A., Rezazadeh, A.A., and Gabriel, C., 2002.)

rates of changes in dielectric properties per tissue [52]. The presence of free or bound water content in the tissues contributes to these changes (Figure 5.39).

Dielectric mismatch can also mean that there are other biological tissues or liquids not considered in simulation. This kind of mismatch is very common for subcutaneous implantation. When a device is surgically placed just below the surface of the skin, there are a couple of things that can cause immediate dielectric mismatch between the antenna and the skin. During surgery, an adequate separation between the skin and adipose or muscle will not separate the dermis (skin) from the hypodermis (an interstitial linking material). As a result, as seen in Figure 5.40, there may be some adipose on the top of the antenna not accounted for in simulation. Additionally, blood in the surgical pocket could affect the resonance of the antenna. As blood is introduced into the incision

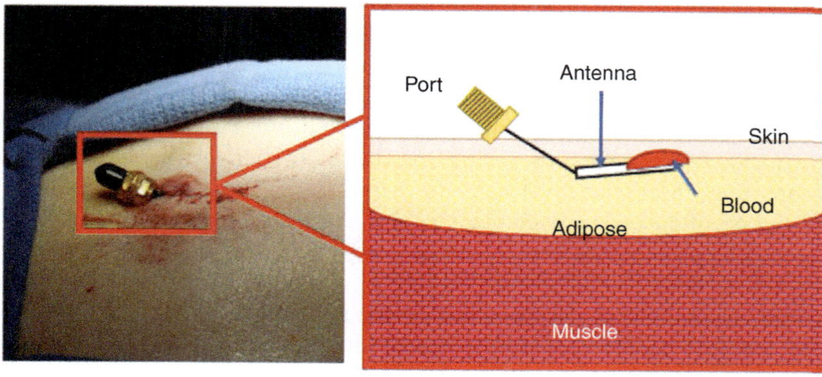

Figure 5.40 Cross section of implanted device.

point, the effective medium is altered in proportion to the amount of blood around the antenna, causing attenuation and frequency shifts. Another form of dielectric mismatch is the amount of adipose and muscle tissue present at the incision point. Different parts of the body accumulate fat in higher amounts than others. The presence of a lower dielectric in more abundance around the implanted antenna may present resonance shifts between the simulated and the measured results. Furthermore, in a long-term context, the body will encapsulate the foreign object over time, resulting in a dielectric mismatch that develops over weeks and months after implantation.

5.4.3 Practical Testing Concerns

With the knowledge of what animal model is needed and the possible dielectric mismatches that are present in in vivo testing, there are some practical testing concerns a researcher must be aware of before testing. The first concern is timing and scheduling. In order to perform in vivo tests, a veterinary expert will need to be on site. This expert will be responsible for the housing, feeding, and anesthesia of the test subject. In terms of anesthesia, an estimate for the amount of time needed for the study is paramount, because anesthesia often is administered in doses and not continuously. Additionally, keep in mind that scheduling time with surgeons, researchers, handlers, veterinary experts, and students can cause mismatched schedules.

Another concern is the protection of the subject from undue pain, disease, or infection. Due to this, the implanted devices, surgical equipment, and those in the room participating in the research must be sterile, or wearing the proper protective equipment to avoid infection to either the subject or the researcher. One commonly overlooked aspect in the in vivo stage is the sterilization process of the antenna. Not all sterilization processes are the same. Some require high temperatures, while others are a chemical sterilization. As a result, keep the fabricated antenna in mind to prevent damage of the antenna during the sterilization process. For example, if the port to the antenna is adhered with silver epoxy, the heat in the sterilization process could break the antenna through the expansion of the metal, severing the connection between the port and the antenna. Sometimes this severing of the connection is not noticeable, especially by members of the research team not trained in electronics development. Additionally, keep in mind the length the antenna will have to be implanted before the study is completed. This will also have an effect on what animal model you may chose for the study. For example, if the study performed requires weeks of the antenna being implanted, a rodent animal model will not be the best choice. This is not due to any electromagnetic or dielectric reason but based on the anatomy of the rodent. While a porcine animal model can crush or destroy the implanted device, rodents have fingers and will remove any source of aggravation if it can be reached. If a porcine animal model is used, make sure that the port on the outside of the animal is adequately protected.

Finally, the differences in the testing environment may have an effect on how the measurements are taken. For example, surgery rooms are often not equipped with network analyzers and other test equipment. It may be the case that the engineering laboratory where bench top tests were completed is physically separated from the surgery room by a significant distance. A rack-mounted network analyzer may not be the optimum solution. A portable network analyzer may be the solution. Additionally, the presence of an anechoic chamber in a research hospital or animal hospital may not be possible. As a result, measuring the radiation pattern becomes a challenge in logistics (transportation of the test subject or administration of anesthesia). As a result, a link budget analysis may be the closest a researcher can get to measuring gain or radiation pattern with an in vivo test.

5.5 Conclusion

The in vitro and in vivo testing steps in the development are crucial. Through these steps an implantable device's performance can be validated and readied to move to the clinical testing phase. The in vitro testing phase of development helps validate antenna performance, including impedance, radiation pattern, and gain. In vitro ought to be the first testing phase in testing an implantable antenna to validate not only operation but to measure a radiation pattern due to the cost and challenges associated with in vivo test models. In general, the impedance of an implantable antenna can be evaluated in either a small phantom or small animal model. However, challenges with live animal model testing, including anesthesia and device protection, can affect the ease of radiation pattern measurement. The radiation pattern may be affected by the size and shape of the animal model used. Additionally, in vitro is an optimal stage to fine-tune the device parameters and explore alternate materials and topologies. Before moving from in vitro to in vivo, several design challenges, including miniaturization and biocompatibility must be addressed. From a biocompatibility standpoint, a common way to isolate the antenna from the body is to encapsulate the antenna in a medical grade silicone or epoxy. Another method is to use biocompatible materials (such as titanium nitride) to allow the antenna design to take advantage of the high permittivity of some biological tissues to assist in the miniaturization.

In vivo can validate basic antenna performance as well as physiological effects of the implanted device. For long-term implantation, understanding how the body reacts and encapsulates the foreign object, as well as verifying nontoxicity is paramount. While necessary, in vivo has many challenges including dielectric mismatch, device damage, and subject safety. In some cases, the medical grade epoxy can act as a mechanical fortifier and a biological isolator. Other challenges include long-term implantation. The rodent animal model is not an optimum animal model for long-term implantation due to their dexterity, allowing them to remove the device after surgery. However, the porcine animal model does not possess the dexterity to remove implanted devices implanted in the upper back. However, the pig will tend to crush the device if not adequately protected. Moving forward, researches will have to address device protection and dielectric mismatch at the bench top testing stage to make in vivo testing less of a challenge.

Acknowledgment

The authors of this chapter want to thank Umit Ozgur, Vitaliy Avrutin, and Hadis Morkoc for their help in the fabrication of the Titanium Nitride antenna in this work.

References

1 Center of Disease ControlAgency for Toxic Substances and Disease Registry (21 January 2015). Toxic substances portal - aluminum [Online]. https://www.atsdr.cdc.gov/phs/phs.asp?id=1076&tid=34 (accessed 16 December 2019).

2 National Institutes of HealthOffice of Dietary Supplements (19 July 2019). Copper: fact sheet for health professionals [Online]. https://ods.od.nih.gov/factsheets/Copper-HealthProfessional/#h4 (accessed 16 December 2019).

3 Center of Disease ControlAgency for Toxic Substances and Disease Registry (21 January 2015). Toxic substances portal - copper [Online]. https://www.atsdr.cdc.gov/phs/phs.asp?id=204&tid=37 (accessed 16 December 2019).
4 Gold, Lenntech (2019). Chemical properties of gold - health effects of gold - environmental effects of gold [Online]. https://www.lenntech.com/periodic/elements/au.htm (accessed 16 December 2019).
5 National Institutes of Health Office of Dietary Supplements (16 October 2019). Iron: fact sheet for health professionals [Online]. https://ods.od.nih.gov/factsheets/Iron-HealthProfessional (accessed 16 December 2019).
6 National Institutes of Health Office of Dietary Supplements (10 December 2019). Iron: fact sheet for consumers [Online]. https://ods.od.nih.gov/factsheets/Iron-Consumer (accessed 16 December 2019).
7 Center for Disease Control Agency for Toxic Substance and Disease Registry (12 June 2019). Lead toxicity: what are possible health effects from lead exposure [Online]. https://www.atsdr.cdc.gov/csem/csem.asp?csem=34&po=10 (accessed 16 December 2019).
8 Center for Disease Control Agency for Toxic Substance and Disease Registry (August 2005). Public health statement for nickel [Online]. https://www.atsdr.cdc.gov/phs/phs.asp?id=243&tid=44 (accessed 16 December 2019).
9 Center for Disease Control Agency for Toxic Substances and Disease Registry (December 1990). Toxic substances portal - silver [Online]. https://www.atsdr.cdc.gov/phs/phs.asp?id=537&tid=97 (accessed 16 December 2019).
10 Lenntech (2019). Titanium - Ti chemical properties of titanium - health effects of titanium - environmental effects of titanium [Online]. https://www.lenntech.com/periodic/elements/ti.htm (accessed 16 December 2019).
11 National Institutes of Health Office of Dietary Supplements (10 July 2019). Zinc: fact sheet for health professionals [Online]. https://ods.od.nih.gov/factsheets/Zinc-HealthProfessional (accessed 16 December 2019).
12 Kiourti, A. and Nikita, K.S. (2012). A review of implantable patch antennas for biomedical telemetry: challenges and solutions. *IEEE Antennas and Propagation Magazine* 54 (3): 210–228.
13 Xu, F. and Zhu, Y. (2012). Highly conductive and stretchable silver nanowire conductors. *Advanced Materials* 24 (37): 5117–5122.
14 Lipomi, D.J., Vosgueritchian, M., Tee, B. et al. (2011). Skin-line pressure and strain sensors basd on transparent elastic films of carbon nanotubes. *Nature Nanotechnology* 6 (12): 788–792.
15 Li, X., Li, M., Zong, L. et al. (2018). Liquid metal droplets wrapped with polysaccharide microgel as biocompatible aqueous ink for flexible conductive devices. *Wiley Advanced Functional Materials* 28 (39): 1–8.

16 Chrysler, A., Furse, C., and Chung, Y. (2016). Biocompatible, implantable UHF RFID antenna made from conductive ink. 2016 IEEE International Symposium on Antennas and Propagation, Fajardo, 2016.

17 Topsakal, E. (2017). Long-term implantable medical wireless telemetry. 2017 International Conference on Electromagnetics in Advanced Applications (ICEAA), Verona, 2017.

18 Green, R.B., Toporkov, M., Ullah, M.B. et al. (2017). An alternative material for transparent antennas for commercial and medical applications. *Wiley Microwave and Optical Technology Letters* 59 (4): 773–777.

19 Rogers, J.A., Someya, T., and Huang, Y. (2010). Materials and mechanics of stretchable electronics. *Science* 327 (5973): 1603–1607.

20 Vosgueritchian, M., Lipomi, D.J., and Bao, Z. (2012). Highly conductive and transparent PEDOT:PSS films with a fluorosurficant for stretchable and flexible transparent electrodes. *Advanced Functional Materials* 22 (2): 421–428.

21 Balint, R., Cassidy, N.J., and Cartmell, S.H. (2014). Conductive polymers: towards a smart biomaterial for tissue engineering. *Acta Biomaterialia* 10 (6): 2341–2353.

22 Igasaki, Y., Mitsuhashi, H., Azuma, K., and Muto, T. (1978). Structure and electrical properties of titanium nitride films. *Japanese Journal of Applied Physics* 17 (1): 85–96.

23 Saberin, J.R. (2010). *Optically Transparent Antennas for Small Satellites.* Salt Lake City: Department of Electrical and Computer Engineering, University of Utah.

24 Green, R.B., Dyke, J., Hays, M. et al. (2018). Dual band biocompatible titanium nitrite antennas for implantable wireless telemetry. International Symposium on Antennas and Propagation and USNC-URSI National Radio Science Meeting (IEEE AP-S/USNC-URSI-2018), Boston, 2018.

25 Green, R.B. and Topsakal, E. (2019). Telemetry for implantable biosensors. 2019 IEEE 69th Electronic Components and Technology Conference (ECTC), Las Vegas, 2019.

26 Ballen, M., Kanda, M., Chou, C., and Balzano, Q. (2001). Formulation and characterization of tissue simulating liquids used for SAR measurement. Procedures 23rd Annual Bioelectromagnetic Society Meeting, 2001, vol. 14 (issue 3), 80.

27 Peyman, A. and Gabriel, C. (2002). Tissue equivalent liquids for SAR measurement at microwave frequencies. Procedures 24th Annual Bioelectromagnetics Society Meeting, 2002, vol. P (issue 53), 184–185.

28 Fukunaga, K., Watanabe, S., and Yamanaka, Y. (2004). Dielectric properties of tissue equivalent liquids and their effects on specific absorption rate. *IEEE Transactions on Electromagnetic Compatibility* 46 (1): 126–129.

29 Fukunaga, K., Watanabe, S., Asou, H., and Sato, K. (2005). Dielectric properties of non-toxic tissue-equivalent liquids for radiowave safety tests. IEEE International Conference on Dielectric Liquids, Coimbra, 2005.

30 Kim, J. and Rahmat-Samii, Y. (2004). Implanted antennas inside a human body: simulations, designs, and characterizations. *IEEE Transactions on Microwave Theory and Thechniques* 52 (8): 1934–1943.

31 Chang, J.T., Fanning, M.W., Meaney, P.M., and Paulsen, K.D. (2000). A conductive plastic for simulating biological tissue at microwave frequencies. *IEEE Transactions on Electromagnetic Compatibility* 42 (1): 78–81.

32 Guy, A.W. (1971). Analysis of electromagnetic fields induced in biological tissue by thermographic studies on equivalent phantom models. *IEEE Transactions on Microwave Compatibility* 19 (2): 205–214.

33 Maggi, L.E., vonKruger, M.A., Pereira, W., and Monteiro, E. (2009). Development on silicon-based materials for ultrasound biological phantoms. 2009 IEEE International Ultrasonics Symposium, Rome, 2009.

34 Chio, H., Shim, H., Lee, C.H. et al. (1999). Electromagnetic and electromagnetic wave-absorbing properties of the SrTi03-epoxy composite. *Journal of Applied Polymer Science* 72: 75–83.

35 Nikawa, Y., Chino, M., and Kikuchi, K. (1996). Soft and dry phantom modeling material using silicone rubber with carbon fibre. *IEEE Transactions on Microwave Theory and Techniques* 44 (10): 1949–1953.

36 Gabriel, C. (2007). Tissue equivalent material for hand phantoms. *Physics in Medicine and Biology* 52 (14): 4205–4210.

37 Kobayashi, T., Nojima, T., Yamada, K., and Uebayashi, S. (1993). Dry phantom composed of ceramics and its application to SAR estimation. *IEEE Transactions on Microwave Theory and Techniques* 41 (1): 136–140.

38 Stuchly, S.S. (1987). Specific absorption rate distributions in heterogeneous model of the human body at radio frequencies. Environmental Protection Agency Project Summary, 1987, 89.

39 Stuchly, S.S., Kraszewski, A., Stuchly, M.A. et al. (1987). RF energy deposition in heterogeneous model of man: far-field exposures. *IEEE Transactions in Biomedical Engineering* 34 (12): 951–957.

40 Davidson, S. and Sherar, M. (2003). Measurement of the thermal conductivity of plyacrylamide tissue-equivalent meterial. *International Journal on Hyperthermia* 19 (5): 551–562.

41 Surowiec, A., Shrivastava, P.N., Astrahan, M., and Petrovich, Z. (1992). Utilization of a multilayer plyacrylamide phantom for evaluation of hyperthermia applicators. *International Journal on Hyperthermia* 8: 795–807.

42 Chou, C.K., Chen, G.W., Guy, A.W., and Luk, K.H. (1984). Formulas for preparing phantom muscle tissue at various radiofrequencies. *Bioelectromagnetics* 5 (4): 435–441.

43 Ito, K., Furuya, K., Okano, Y., and Hamada, L. (2001). Development and characteristics of a biological tissue-equivalent phantom for microwaves.

Electronics and Communications in Japan (Part I: Communications) 84 (4): 67–77.

44 Groch, M.W., Urbon, J.A., Erwin, W.D., and Al-Doohan, S. (1991). An MRI tissue equivalent lesoin phantom using a novel polysaccharide material. *Magnetic Resonance Imaging* 9 (3): 417–421.

45 Surry, K.J., Austin, H.B., Fenster, A., and Peters, T.M. (2004). Poly(vinyl alcohol) cryogel phantoms for use in ultrasound and MR imaging. *Physics in Medicine and Biology* 49: 5529–5546.

46 Marchal, C., Nadi, M., Tosser, A.J. et al. (1989). Dielectric properties of gelatin phantoms used for simulations of biological tissues between 10 and 50 MHz. *International Journal on Hyperthermia* 5: 725–732.

47 Sunaga, T., Ikehira, H., Furukawa, S. et al. (2003). Development of a dielectric equivalent gel for better impedance matching for human skin. *Bioelectromagnetics* 24: 725–732.

48 Lazebnik, M., Madsen, E.L., Frank, G.R., and Hagness, S.C. (2005). Tissue mimicking phantom materials for narrowband and ultrawideband microwave applications. *Physics in Medicine and Biology* 50: 4245–4258.

49 Madsen, E.L., Zagzebski, J.A., and Frank, G.R. (1982). Oil-in-gelatin dispersions for use as ultrasonically tissue-mimicking materials. *Ultrasound in Medicine and Biology* 8 (3): 277–287.

50 Gabriel, C., Gabriel, S., and Corthout, E. (1996). The dielectric properties of biological tissues: I. Literature survey. *Physics in Medicine and Biology* 41: 2231–2249.

51 Gabriel, S., Lau, R.W., and Gabriel, C. (1996). The dielectric properties of biological tissues: II. Measurement in frequency range 10 Hz to 20 GHz. *Physics in Medicine and Biology* 41: 2251–2269.

52 Peyman, A., Rezazadeh, A.A., and Gabriel, C. (2001). Changes in dielectric properties of rat tissue as a function of age at microwave frequencies. *Physics in Medicine and Biology* 46: 1617–1629.

53 Peyman, A. and Gabriel, C. (2010). Cole-cole parameters for the dielectric properties of porcine tissues as a function of age at microwave frequencies. *Physics in Medicine and Biology* 55 (15): N413–N419.

54 Andreuccetti, D., Fossi, R., and Petrucci, C. (1997). An Internet resource for the calculation of the dielectric properties of body tissues in the frequency range of 10 Hz - 100 GHz, Florence, Italy, 1997.

55 Rodrigues, D.R., Stauffer, P.R., Colebeck, E. et al. (2016). Dielectric properties measurement of brown and white adipose tissue in rats from 0.5 to 10 GHz. *Biomedical Physics and Engineering Express* 2: 025005.

56 Abdilla, L., Sammut, C.V., and Mangion, L.Z. (2013). Dielectric properties of muscle and liver from 500 MHz - 40 GHz. *Electromagnetic Biology and Medicine* 32 (2): 244–252.

57 Kim, T.H. and Pack, J.K. (2012). Measurement of electrical characteristics of female breast tissues for the development of the breast cancer detector. *Progress in Electromagnetics Research C* 30: 189–199.
58 Lazebnik, M., McCartney, L., Popovic, D. et al. (2007). A large-scale study of the ultrawideband microwave dielectric properties of normal breast tissue obtained from reduction surgeries. *Physics in Medicine and Biology* 52 (10): 2637–2656.
59 Lazebnik, M., Converse, M.C., Booske, J.H., and Hagness, S.C. (2006). Ultrawideband temperature-dependent dielectric properties of liver tissue in microwave frequency range. *Physics in Medicine and Biology* 51 (7): 1941–1955.
60 Green, R.B., Hays, M., and Topsakal, E. (2018). A dual band implantable antenna for wireless medical telemetry service (WMTS) and ISM band communication. 2018 National Radio Science Meeting, Boulder, 2018.
61 Topsakal, E. (2009). Antennas for medical applications: Ongoing research and future challenges. 2009 International Conference on Electromagnetics in Advanced Applications, Torino, 2009.
62 Karacolak, T., Hood, A.Z., and Topsakal, E. (2008). Design of a dual-band implantable antenna and development of skin mimicking gels for continuous glucose monitoring. *IEEE Transactions on Microwave Theory and Techniques* 56 (4): 1001–1008.
63 Karacolak, T., Cooper, R., Butler, J. et al. (2010). In vivo verification of implantable antennas using rats as animal models. *IEEE Antennas and Wireless Propagation Letters* 9: 334–337.
64 Green, R.B., Shaffer, J., Hays, M., and Topsakal, E. (2019). Short range titanium nitrite antenna for subcutaneous implant. 2019 National Radio Science Meeting, Boulder, 2019.
65 Green, R.B. and Topsakal, E. (2019). Biocompatible antennas for implantable biosensor systems. 2019 International Workshop on Antenna Technology (iWAT), Miami, 2019.
66 Sabouni, A., Hahn, C., Noghanian, S. et al. (2013). Study of the effects of changing physiological conditions on dielectric properties of breast tissues. *ISRN Biomedical Imaging* 2013: 1–5.
67 Peyman, A., Gabriel, C., Grant, E., and Martens, L. (2010). Variations of the dielectric properties of tissues with age: the effects on the values of SAR in children when exposed to walkie-talkie devices. *Physics in Medicine and Biology* 54 (2): 227–241.
68 Karacolak, T. and Topsakal, E. (2008). Electrical properties of nude rat skin and design of implantable antennas for wireless data telemetry. IEEE MTT-S International Microwave Symposium Digest, Atlanta, 2008.
69 Colebeck, E., Asili, M., Green, R.B., and Topsakal, E. (2013). The effects of temperature on the microwave dielectric properties of porcine liver, lung, and heart. 2013 National Radio Science Meeting, Boulder, 2013.

70 Asili, M., Colebeck, E., Green, R.B., and Topsakal, E. (2013). The effects of temperature on antenna return loss for microwave ablation antennas. 2013 National Radio Science Meeting, Boulder, 2013.
71 Colebeck, E. and Topsakal, E. (2013). Ultra-wideband microwave ablation therapy (UMAT). IEEE MTT-S International Microwave Symposium Digest (MTT), Seattle, 2013.
72 Topsakal, E., Colebeck, E., Asili, M., and Green, R.B. (2013). Ultrawide-band microwave ablation therapy (UMAT0). 2013 National Radio Science Meeting, Boulder, 2013.
73 Schepps, J.L. and Foster, K.R. (1980). The UHF and microwave dielectric properties of normal and tumor tissues: variation in dielectric properties with tissue water content. *Physics in Medicine and Biology* 25 (6): 1149–1159.
74 Nusrat, N., Hays, M., Secondo, L. et al. (2019). Microwave dielectric properties characterization of rat plasma over various glucose concentrations. 2019 National Radio Science Meeting, Boulder, 2019.
75 Topsakal, E., Karacolak, T., and Moreland, E.C. (2011). Glucose-dependent dielectric properties of blood plasma. 2011 XXXth URSI General Assembly and Scientific Symposium, Istanbul, 2011.
76 Topsakal, E., Karacolak, T., and Moreland, E. (2011). Glucose-dependent dielectric properties of blood plasma. 2011 National Radio Science Meeting, Boulder, 2011.
77 Topsakal, E., Asili, M., Chen, P., and Demirci, U. (2014). Lab-on-a-chip: continuous glucose monitoring antenna sensors. 2014 National Radio Science Meeting, Boulder, 2014.
78 Karacolak, T., Moreland, E.C., and Topsakal, E. (2013). Cole-cole model for glucose-dependent dielectric properties of blood plasma for continuous glucose monitoring. *Wiley Microwave and Optical Technology Letters* 55 (5): 1160–1164.
79 Topsakal, E., Moreland, E.C., Karacolak, T., and Acar, M. (2008). The impact of glucose concentration in blood plasma on relative dielectric constant and conductivity. 2008 National Radio Science Meeting, Boulder, 2008.

6

Wireless Localization for a Capsule Endoscopy: Techniques and Solutions

Yongxin Guo and Guoliang Shao

Department of Electrical and Computer Engineering, National University of Singapore, Singapore

6.1 Introduction

A wireless capsule endoscopy is a noninvasive medical device designed for human gastrointestinal (GI) tract diagnosis. The idea of wireless capsule endoscopy was first proposed in [1] and published in Nature [2] for relieving the patient from the discomfort of digestive diagnosis and providing an image diagnosis for the entire small bowel as shown in Figure 6.1. Different from the traditional fiber-optical endoscopy, the capsule endoscopy is designed to be easily swallowed and propelled by GI tract peristalsis only. During the mouth-to-evacuation period, the capsule endoscopy transmits all the captured images wirelessly using ultra-high frequency (UHF)-band radio frequency to a data recorder, which will be carried by the patient portably. The invention of the wireless capsule endoscopy brings a painless diagnosis for the entire internal GI tract, which will greatly promote the screening of digestive diseases [4, 5].

Since the original capsule endoscopy structure was proposed in [6] and approved by the US Food and Drug Administration (FDA) in 2001, the wireless capsule endoscopyhas been widely used in hospitals and clinics. There are several commercially available capsule endoscopies in 2019 as listed in Table 6.1. Without any wire connection, a capsule endoscopy is powered by an embedded battery to provide a low frame rate screening within a period of over eight hours, which generally covers the entire inspection of small bowel and limited inspection of esophagus, stomach, and cecum (Figure 6.2). Although the wireless capsule endoscopy has been proved effective in the diagnosis of digestive bleeding and tumor, there are some risks from the clinical perspective:

- *Blurred images*: propelled by the peristalsis of the digestive tract, the movement of the wireless capsule endoscopy is highly unstable, i.e. moving fast

Antenna and Sensor Technologies in Modern Medical Applications,
First Edition. Edited by Yahya Rahmat-Samii and Erdem Topsakal.

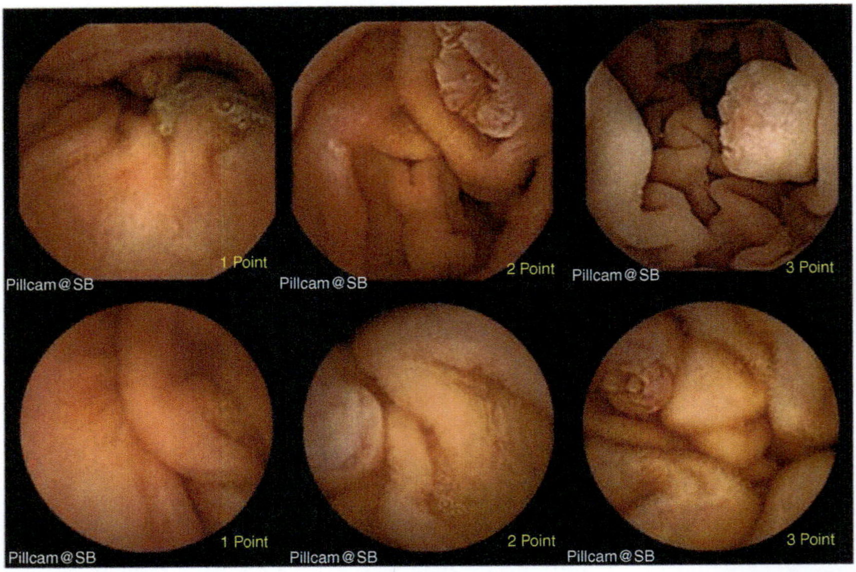

Figure 6.1 Representative images captured by PillCam SB [3]. (*Source*: Park, S., Chun, H.J., Keum, B. et al., 2012.)

during the muscle contraction and moving slow during the muscle relaxation. The unstable movement can result in the blurred images which will influence the diagnosis procedure [11].

- *Missed inspection:* in order to provide a longer inspection period, the capsule endoscopy adopts a low frame rate for image capturing. The low frame rate reduces the power consumption of the camera and the number of redundant images; on the other hand, the number of images capturing the lesion area is also limited, where the missed inspection may occur [12, 13].
- *Retention within the digestive tract:* although the capsule endoscopy is small enough to be swallowed and move smoothly within the GI tract, the clinical study [14] shows a retention occur rate of ~3.1%. The retention of the capsule endoscopy may not be predicted from prescanning, and the risk of retention is increased when patients are with motility disorders, suspected small bowel ulcers, or malignancies.

In order to address the aforementioned risks, researchers started to work on the wireless charging function and the wireless localization function designed for a capsule endoscopy during the past decades [16–18]. The localization function of the capsule provides a real-time monitoring on the capsule movement, which can detect the retention at an early stage. Besides, labeling each captured

Table 6.1 Typical parameters of commercially used wireless capsule endoscopy.

Capsule endoscopy	Manufacturer	Size	Weight	Frame rate	Field of view	Battery duration
PillCam SB3 [7]	Medtronic	Length: 26.2 mm	3.0 g	2 fps or 2–6 fps	156°	≥8 h
		Diameter: 11.4 mm				
EndoCapsule EC-S10 [8]	Olympus	Length: 26 mm	3.3 g	2 fps	160°	8–12 h
		Diameter: 11 mm				
MiroCam MC1600 [9]	IntroMedic	Length: 30.1 mm	3.5 g	6 fps	170°	12 h
		Diameter: 10.8 mm				
CapsoCam Plus [10]	Capsule Vision	Length: 30.5 mm	3.75 g	3–5 fps	162°	15 h
		Diameter: 11.3 mm				

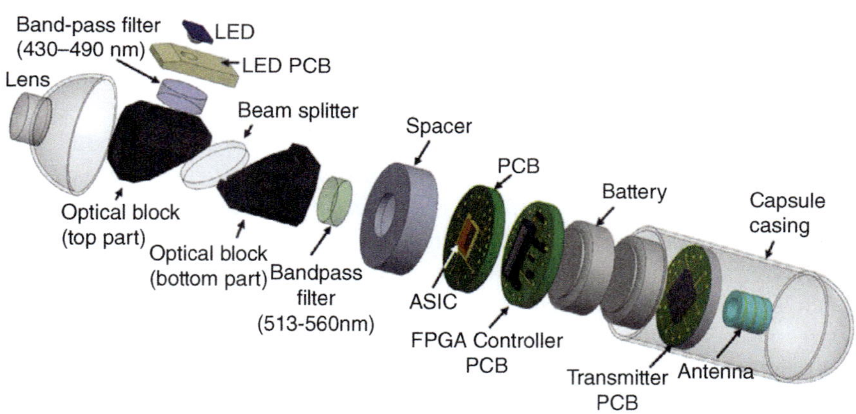

Figure 6.2 An exploded 3D structure of a typical wireless capsule endoscopy [15]. (*Source:* Al-Rawhani, M. A., Beeley, J., and Cumming, D. R. S., 2015.)

image with a corresponding piece of location information can support the accurate diagnosis and treatment for the entire digestive tract, i.e. support the GI laparoscopic surgery. Compared to the wireless charging function, a real-time wireless positioning system is more complicated due to the complex electromagnetic environment within a human body. Different in-body localization methods for a capsule endoscopy have been researched and developed since 2006.

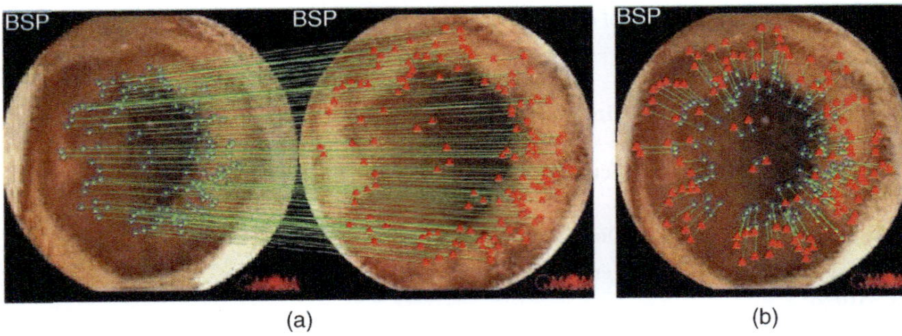

Figure 6.3 Features matching between captured images [19]. (a) Matching points between consecutive images. (b) Motion vectors between the corresponding points. The matching points are used to reconstruct the inner structure of bowel for localization purpose. (*Source*: Bao, G., Pahlavan, K., and Mi, L., 2014. © IEEE.)

6.1.1 Visual-based Localization Method

Visual odometry is a process to retrieve the position and the orientation of a robot solely from image information which has been used extensively in robotics and computer vision. Without involving external or internal sensors, the consecutive images captured are used to trace and retrieve the pose of the camera. The projection model of the camera establishes a transformation from the 3D point in the space to the 2D point on the image. Under a different camera pose, the projected 2D point locates at a different coordinate on the captured image. The relationship of the different camera poses viewing the same 3D point in the space is expressed as the epipolar geometry in computer vision. By matching 2D points with similar feature on consecutive images, which represent the same point in the 3D space, the relative movement between the two consecutive images can be retrieved from the epipolar geometry (Figure 6.3). Besides, the matched feature points can be reconstructed in the 3D space as well. All the detected feature points can be stored in a 3D point cloud, which represents the environment structure. The localization performance can be optimized by minimizing the reprojection error between the 3D point cloud and a series of captured frames. The visual odometry and the environment reconstruction contribute to the well-known technology "simultaneously localization and mapping" (SLAM) as shown in Figure 6.4.

A direct and dense visual SLAM system structure was adopted in [20] to perform the localization for wireless capsule endoscopy on a nonrigid, realistic surgical esophagogastroduodenoscopy simulator. A video stream containing over 10,000 frames within 15 minutes is used to reconstruct the stomach simulator, and an average trajectory error of 10% was reported for this work. A

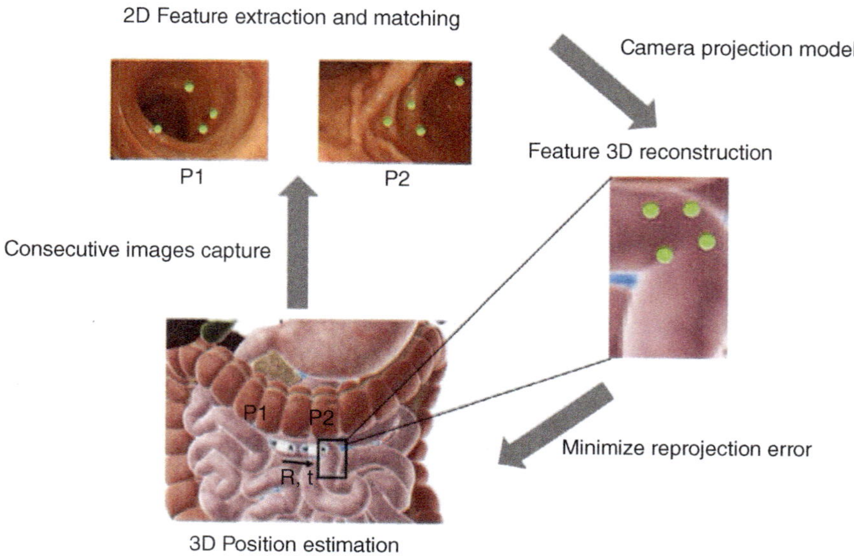

Figure 6.4 Typical SLAM structure for capsule endoscopy localization. Two consecutive images captured by the same WCE with relative motion of *R* and *t*. The feature points representing the same physical point are matched (marking green) to reconstruct the 3D structure of the digestive tube through the camera projection model. By minimizing the reprojection error of the second image, the relative motion R and t can be precisely estimated.

speed estimation based on the similar structure was proposed in [21], which reported an average accuracy of 2.71 cm based on over 5000 artificial frames generated from the virtual test bed. The speed estimation is further used to perform data fusion based on localization with RF sensors in [19], which reported a stable average positioning error of 2.3 cm based on the data collected from the emulation test. An image classification-based landmarking method combined with magnetic localizationperformed within a real stomach of an animal was proposed in [22], in which a trajectory error of 6% was reported.

Visual-based localization has the advantages that it does not require any attached hardware on the current capsule endoscopy system, and the performance is relatively stable under a stable image stream. On the other hand, it is difficult to validate the localization performance based on the real image dataset, because once the capsule is swallowed, the ground truth position of the capsule may not be obtained at the current stage. Moreover, with an extremely low frame rate (around 2 frame per second), the matched features between consecutive frames can be very limited, which may lead to the tracking-lost problem.

6.1.2 Radio-frequency Localization

Radio-frequency (RF) localization is a traditional localization method widely used in normal life. The basic theory of RF localization is to use the propagation characteristic of the electromagnetic (EM) wave to calculate the distance and estimate the position based on triangulation. The typical distance-calculation method includes the calculation of the time of flight, the power attenuation, and the propagation direction. Generally, RF localization gives a good position estimation in an open space, i.e. global positioning system (GPS), and ultra wideband (UWB) localization. However, reflections and diffractions on the objects construct a multipath environment which makes it difficult to perform the non-line-of-sight localization. When implementing the RF localization for capsule endoscopy localization, the nonnegligible problem is the lossy human tissue. As a mixture of many materials with different conductivity and dielectric property, human tissue has a huge influence not only on the speed but also on the attenuation, even the propagation direction of the EM wave. Due to the constrained distance within the body area, the majority of RF localization research for capsule endoscopy uses the received signal strength (RSS), time of arrival (TOA), and direction of arrival (DOA) to estimate the position, as shown in Figure 6.5.

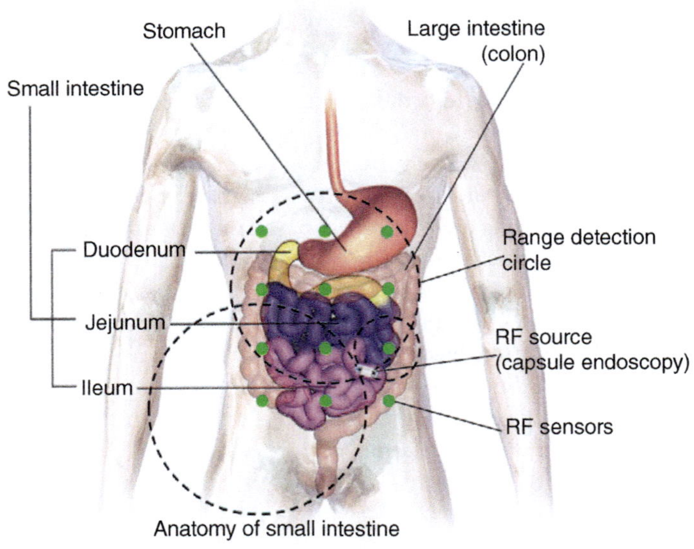

Figure 6.5 Typical structure of RF localization for wireless capsule endoscopy. Each RF sensor estimates the range to the target RF source from TOA, RSSI, or DOA information. The intersection point with highest possibility is the estimated position of the target capsule endoscopy.

A localization system structure extracting the RSS and DOA information from the RF source of the capsule endoscopy inside a simulated phantom was proposed in [23] to address the difficulties in simulating the in-body environment, in which multiple RF sensors were placed on the simulated body surface to evaluate the strength attenuation in the full-wave simulation. A positioning accuracy of 5 cm with 32 RF sensors implemented was reported in this work. Another RSS-based capsule endoscopy localization algorithm based on spatial sparsity was proposed in [24], in which the location of the capsule was directly estimated from the RSS information. A root-mean-square (RMS) positioning error of 8.8 mm was reported using a binary phase shift keying (BPSK) modulation signal with a bandwidth of 300 kHz at 406 MHz under the simulation. The fundamental localization accuracy based on the posterior Cramer–Rao lower bound for a hybrid method using RF localization and image processing was derived in [25]. This work concluded that on the condition where the position estimation from the image processing method was high enough and the number of RF sensors evaluating the RSS was large enough, the localization error can be restricted to 3 cm. A localization system integrating TOA, DOA, and inertial measurement unit (IMU) information by the extended Kalman filter (EKF) was proposed in [26], and an average positioning error of 1 cm along each axis was reported. A performance comparison between the RSS-based localization and the TOA-based localization for WCE was conducted in [27]. The comparison showed that the RSS-based localization method was expected to present an average positioning error of 5 cm, while the TOA-based localization method was expected to present a lower average positioning error of 1.5 cm. An RSS-based in vivo localization at UWB frequency from 3.1 to 5.1 GHz was conducted in [28]. Considering the multipath propagation inside the human body, a modified propagation attenuation model was adopted. The experiment verification conducted on the human body showed a positioning error of around 0.8 cm with an ideal SNR. Moreover, the number of sensors mounted on the body surface and the sensors placement played an important role in the achieved positioning error [29]. Generally, 32 RF sensors were required to achieve the aforementioned positioning error. Apart from using the propagation information, the RF radiation pattern can be used for capsule localization as well. A 3D positioning algorithm based on the RF radiation pattern from radio-frequency identification (RFID) was proposed in [30]. Implementing a receiver array around the human body to detect the symmetrical radiation pattern from the RFID tag embedded in the capsule, the proposed system achieved a good positioning error within a small area. Another RFID-based tracking system using the phased difference data collected from multiple receivers was proposed in [31] in which a sufficient positioning error of 2 mm for biomedical applications was reported. Recently, several studies reveal that obtaining orientation information could increase the positioning accuracy and enlarge the detection area. A comparison study on sensor fusion techniques with DOA-based localization for WCE conducted in [32] showed that the DOA algorithm had the capability of directly estimating the target orientation and reducing the misalignment, which was beneficial to the system design with limited receiving antennas. A study on estimating the target orientation based on the RSS information collected from the UWB frequency range showed that orientation of the capsule endoscopy can be calculated from the correlation coefficient between each receiver antenna and the transmitting antenna [33].

Similar to the visual-based localization, the advantages of RF localization are few extra hardware required on the capsule endoscopy and the acceptable power consumption of the external sensors. Compared to the visual-based localization, each position estimated in RF localization is independent, which avoids the occurrence of the tracking-lost problem. However, due to the complex EM wave propagation characteristic inside the human body, the positioning accuracy of RF-based method is relatively high. Theoretically, fused with image processing, RF localization is suitable for situations with a relatively undemanding requirement on positioning accuracy but a demanding requirement on the simplicity of the system configuration, i.e. requiring a wearable system design, and the limitations of the hardware implementation on the capsule endoscopy, i.e. the size, the weight, and the power consumption of the added hardware occupied inside the capsule endoscopy.

6.1.3 Microwave Imaging

Microwave imaging has been successfully applied in breast cancer diagnosis [34]. The essential idea of microwave imaging is to solve the inverse problembased on the induction field and scattering field reflected by different materials [35]. The system structure of microwave imaging consists of one or more transmitting antennas illuminating the area of interest and multiple receiving antennas collecting the scattering EM wave reflected on the surface between different materials. In other words, if the area of interest is made of homogeneous material, no scattering wave will be reflected. Therefore, instead of obtaining a detailed image of the body like X-ray, microwave imaging constructs the EM model of the body which can be used for the localization of different objects. By solving the maximum likelihood estimation of the scattering field on a grid-based search, the position of the interested object can be obtained.

A microwave imaging-based capsule endoscopy localization structure was proposed in [36], in which simulation results with a human phantom were provided. In this work, a finite-difference-time-domain (FDTD) field simulation was performed using an RF source of 403.5 MHz. An average positioning error of 9 mm was reported from the 2D phantom simulated data. Using the similar simulation structure, a sparse reconstruction model was calculated for an implanted device inside the human body in [37]. Under a high-SNRand a large grid scenario, a positioning accuracy of 1 cm was reported for the implantable device in this work. The advantage of microwave imaging is the capability of achieving a high positioning accuracy. However, the high positioning accuracy brings a high computational cost which makes it difficult to perform the real-time localization of capsule endoscopy. Moreover, the microwave imaging method requires multiple antennas to perform the microwave illumination and scattering field measurement, which makes it difficult to achieve a portable external system.

6.1.4 Magnetic Localization

Different from the complex EM wave propagation environment that occurred in the RF-based localization, the magnetic permeability of a human body is approximately the same as that of the vacuum. This common assumption makes the magnetic localization a practicable method to perform the in-body localization. According to the magnetic source types, the magnetic localization can be divided into two categories: the static method and the inductive method. In the static method, a permanent magnet, which is usually put inside the capsule endoscopy, performs as the magnetic source, and multiple sensors are mounted on the body surface to measure the magnetic field generated by the embedded magnet (Figure 6.6). In the inductive method, the coils driven by the alternating current, which are usually put externally, perform as the magnetic source, and the receiving coils along three orthogonal directions are put inside the capsule endoscopy. Stimulated by the alternating current, the magnetic field generated by the external coils is alternating, and the 3D coils embedded inside the capsule endoscopy detect the field strength through the Faraday's law of EM induction. Both the methods apply the maximum likelihood estimation to solve the inverse problem, where the theoretical field distribution at the estimated target position well fits the actual measured field distribution.

The static magnetic localizationwas first proposed in [38], within a static volume of 200 mm by 200 mm by 200 mm; an average positioning error of around 6 mm was reported with 16 magnetic sensors covered. A calibration method for the magnetic sensors array was proposed in [39] based on the same structure; the average positioning error was improved from 3.84 to 1.5 mm after the calibration of sensors array. A linear approximation was adopted in [40] where the inverse problem was transformed to accelerate the numerical calculation. An average positioning error of 3.72 mm was reported from the linear approximation, while the average positioning error calculated from the nonlinear optimization algorithm was reported as 1.82 mm with a longer calculation time. A Jacobian-based iterative method was proposed to avoid using the magnetic dipole (MD) model in [41], in which an average positioning error of 7 mm with a refresh rate of 7 ms was reported under a close-loop magnetic control.

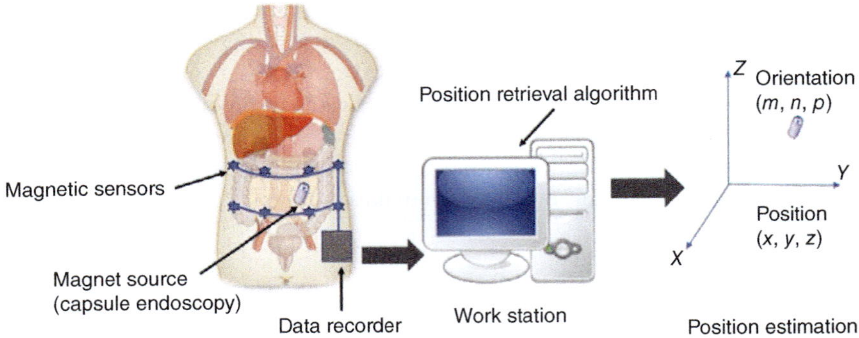

Figure 6.6 The typical structure of static magnetic localization. The magnetic field stimulated by the permanent magnet is sampled by multiple magnetic sensors and processed with the position retrieval algorithm.

An annular magnet model was selected in [42] to provide a 6-D localization for the target. The average positioning error of 0.003 mm was reported from the simulation results within a volume of 360 mm by 370 mm by 300 mm. The possible optimal sensors distribution based on grid optimization was proposed in [43], which further increased the positioning accuracy to 1.4 mm within a 2D area of 200 mm by 200 mm.

One of the inductive magnetic localization methods applying three 3D transmitting coils and two 3D receiving coils was published in [44]. Using the signal amplitude and phase information detected by the sensor coils, the nonlinear inverse problem was formulated and optimized to estimate the target position and orientation. An average positioning accuracy of 0.87 mm and an average orientation accuracy of 0.64°were reported covering the volume of 500 mm by 400 mm by 400 mm. However, the receiver coils selected in this work were too big to be embedded inside the capsule endoscopy. Another inductive magnetic localization example applying a set of closed-form formulas to optimize the inverse tracking problem was proposed in [45], in which an RMS positioning error of 1.29 mm was reported with a sufficient refreshing period of 0.143 ms.

Different from RF localization, the human tissue hardly influences the magnetic field distribution, which greatly simplifies the physical model. Besides, the static magnetic localization system requires little power consumption, and it is easy to transform the system structure into a wearable system for capsule endoscopy. However, magnetic localization suffers from many kinds of magnetic noises such as the geomagnetic field, the magnetic field from ferromagnetic materials, and surrounding currents, which may influence the final positioning accuracy without a careful calibration.

Regarding to the localization system for capsule endoscopy, the selection of localization methods should follow the requirements of the system, for instance, the requirements on hardware configuration and positioning accuracy. Considering the working condition of capsule endoscopy, the localization system should satisfy the following requirements:

- The localization system should be a wearable system to support a working period of around 8 hours.
- The hardware added inside the capsule endoscopy should be as small in size and light in weight as possible.
- The positioning accuracy should achieve a subcentimeter level, and the estimation accuracy should be stable within the whole volume of the abdominal cavity.
- The power consumption of the internal hardware should be as low as possible.

Comparing the aforementioned four localization methods, magnetic localization is the most promising method to achieve the above four requirements. The following content will focus on the principles and possible improvements for magnetic localization. Challenges of static magnetic localization will be discussed, and corresponding solutions will be proposed. An innovative inductive magnetic localization combined with inductive charging techniques will be proposed to address the weight problem caused by the permanent magnet.

6.2 Static Magnetic Localization

Static magnetic localization is a localization system retrieving a target magnet position from multiple magnetic field measurements. The target magnet is a permanent magnet to be embedded inside a capsule endoscopy. The magnetic field intensity is sampled by multiple magnetic sensors. The system structure of static magnetic localization is shown in Figure 6.7, where the position of the target magnet is (x, y, z), the orientation vector M_0 of the target magnet is (m, n, p), the position of the ith magnetic sensor is (x_i, y_i, z_i), the distance vector between the target and the ith magnetic sensor P_i is $(x_i - x, y_i - y, z_i - z)$, and the measured magnetic field by each magnetic sensor is a vector B_{meas} representing the field components along x, y, and z axes. The magnetic field measured by each magnetic sensor is a static magnetic field, which consists of the magnetic field stimulated from the target magnet, geomagnetic field, and magnetic noise from ferromagnetic materials and very low-frequency currents.

The position retrieval algorithm of static magnetic localization is essentially a maximum likelihood estimation. The position retrieval consists of modeling the theoretical magnetic field distribution stimulated by the target magnet, which is the direct problem, and finding the estimated position of the target best aligned with the measured magnetic field distribution, which is the inverse problem. Specifically, with the position of each magnetic sensor fixed, the theoretical

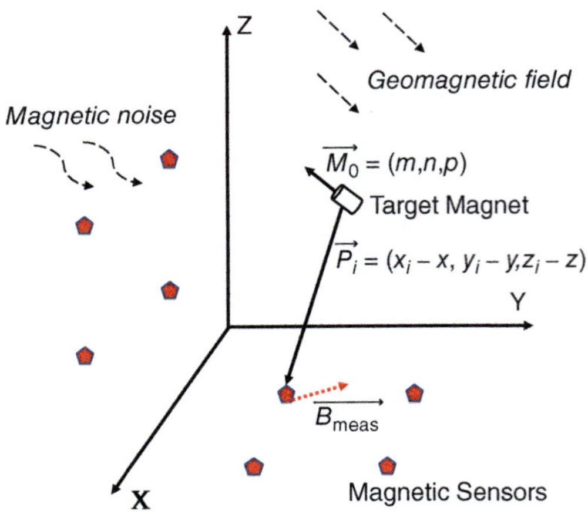

Figure 6.7 The schematic of magnetic dipole model and magnetic field measurement [46]. (*Source*: Shao, G. and Guo, Y.-X., et al., 2019. © IEEE.)

magnetic field stimulated at each magnetic sensor's position by the target can be calculated in the direct problem, given the position of the target magnet. In the inverse problem, given a set of measurements by all of the magnetic sensors, the algorithm adjusts the estimated target position to find the position whose theoretical field distribution best aligned with the measurements. Implementing a function $\mathbf{T}(\mathbf{X})$ to describe the direct problem, where $\mathbf{X}$ denotes the position and orientation vector of the target magnet, the position retrieval algorithm is defined as

$$\hat{\mathbf{X}} = \arg\min_{\mathbf{x}} \sum_{i=1}^{N} \|\mathbf{B_{mi}} - \mathbf{T_i}(\mathbf{X})\|_2, \tag{6.1}$$

where $\mathbf{B_{mi}}$ denotes the measurement from the ith sensor, and $\mathbf{T_i}(\mathbf{X})$ denotes the theoretical field intensity measured by the ith sensor when the target is placed at $\mathbf{X}$.

In order to obtain a good positioning accuracy, several challenges should be considered and addressed when the system is realized from algorithm to reality. Four aspects of challenges and corresponding solutions will be discussed in the following sections including the model of the target magnet, the adaptive noise cancellation, the calculation of the position retrieval algorithm, and the impact of the placement of sensors.

6.2.1 Model of the Target Magnet

The formulation of the direct problem$\mathbf{T}(\mathbf{X})$ is closely related to the field model of the target magnet. With a different selection of target magnet, a different field model should be adopted correspondingly. The target magnet should be compatible with the size of the capsule endoscopy, and the far-field model of the target magnet should be focused on because the target–sensor distance is generally larger than the linear dimension of the magnet.

The commonly used magnet is a cylindrical permanent magnet, which can be modeled as a MD. Following the notations in Figure 6.7, the MD is expressed as

$$\mathbf{B}_\mathrm{i} = B_\mathrm{T}\left(\frac{3(\mathbf{M}_0 \cdot \mathbf{P}_\mathrm{i})\mathbf{P}_\mathrm{i}}{R_i^{\,5}} - \frac{\mathbf{M}_0}{R_i^3}\right) \quad (i = 1, 2, 3\ ,\ \ldots,\ N), \tag{6.2}$$

where $\mathbf{M}_0$ is the orientation vector of the target magnet, $\mathbf{P}_\mathrm{i}$ is the distance vector pointing from the target to the ith sensor, R_i denotes the norm of the distance vector $\mathbf{P}_\mathrm{i}$, and B_T denotes the constant related to the magnetization of the target magnet. B_T can be written as [47]

$$B_\mathrm{T} = \frac{\mu_\mathrm{r}\mu_0\pi r^2 L H_0}{4\pi}, \tag{6.3}$$

where μ_r is the relative permeability of the medium, μ_0 is the constant permeability of vacuum ($4\pi \times 10^{-7}$ T m A^{-1}), r and L represent the radius and length of the target magnet, respectively, and H_0 is the surface magnetization of the target magnet which can be measured by a Tesla meter.

The MD modelis a simple and effective field model for a cylindrical permanent magnet; however, the cylindrical magnet only provides a 5 degree-of-freedom (DOF) localization. If the magnet is selected as an annular shape or with other texture, a MD model would no longer be effective. The distributed multipole model(DMP) was proposed in [48] to address the field modeling for magnets with complex shapes. Instead of using one MD to model the permanent magnet, the DMP model uses a multidipole to fit the analytical magnetic field distribution outside the magnet. In DMP, the magnetic flux density of the target magnet was modeled as

$$\mathbf{B} = \sum_{j=0}^{k}\sum_{i=0}^{n} m_{ji}\beta_{ji} = \boldsymbol{B}^T\boldsymbol{m}, \tag{6.4}$$

where m_{ji} is the strength of the ith dipole distributed in the jth loop, and β_{ji} is the field model of the corresponding dipole with the source and sink length of ℓ_{ji}. The configuration of the dipole strength matrix and the dipole size was calculated by minimizing the field difference between the model and the analytical measurements. The comparison between the DMP model and the single MD is plotted in Figure 6.8. From the figure, it can be concluded that the DMP model fits the actual field density within the near-field area better than the single magnetic dipole model, where the distance R is less than 2 dipole length ℓ.

A field model for an axisymmetric permanent magnet based on the artificial neural network(ANN) was proposed in [49] to enhance the localization accuracy of the near-field area of the permanent magnet. The input of the ANN

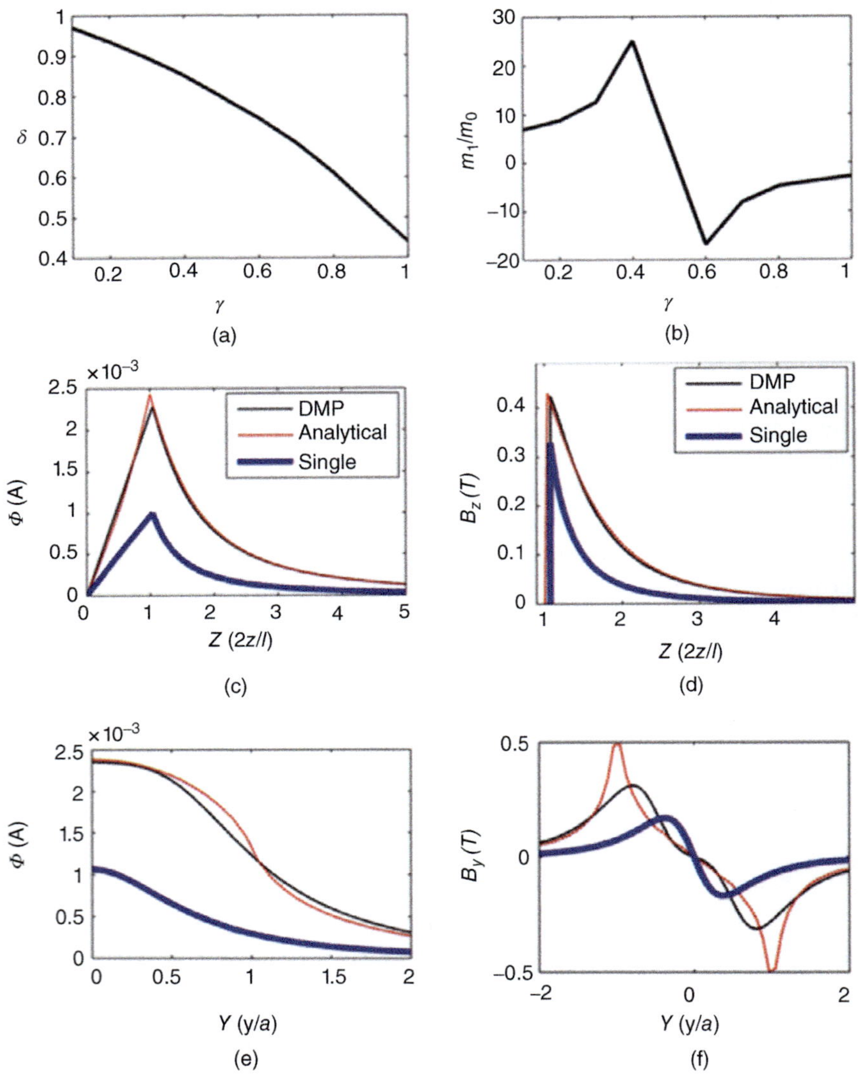

Figure 6.8 The field comparison between the analytical value, single magnetic dipole model, and the DMP model [48]. As the graph shows, the DMP model has a higher accuracy than the single dipole model within the near field of the magnet. The strength within the far-field area of the DMP model and the single dipole model has smaller difference. (*Source:* Lee, K.-M. and Son, H., 2007. © IEEE.)

Table 6.2 Positioning error comparison between different models [49].

Magnet model	MD	DMP	ANN
Average position error on XY-plane (mm)	1.72	2.51	0.43
Average position error on XZ-plane (mm)	1.74	0.93	2.14

Source: Data from Wu, F., Robert, N. M., Frey, D. D., and Foong, S. (2013). Enhanced magnetic localization with artificial neural network field models. 2013 IEEE International Conference on Robotics and Automation.

model is the coordinates of the permanent magnet, and the output of the ANN model is the theoretical magnetic field intensity. A simple ANN structure with one hidden layer containing 20 nodes was selected to map the magnetic field. The ANN model was trained over a dataset of 40,000 pairs of magnet position and actual magnetic field. Within a cylindrical area of radius (ρ) of 30 mm and height (z) of 12 mm, the root mean square of the tracking error comparisons among the MD model, the DMP model, and the ANN model are listed in Table 6.2. However, the ANN model requires plenty of data for training, which may not be suitable for field estimation within a large area.

From the aforementioned analysis, the model accuracy shows little difference between the single dipole model and the multipole model when the region of interest is related to the far field of the target magnet. On the other hand, the single dipole model shows a large field intensity error when the measuring point is within the near field of the target magnet. From the localization of the capsule endoscopy point of view, the measuring sensors are to be mounted on the body surface, where the majority of the sensors would be in the far-field area of the target magnet. Therefore, the MD model is simple and acceptable for providing a magnetic field estimation, while the DMP model would provide a more accurate magnetic field estimation. For simplicity, the MD model will be selected to demonstrate the magnetic localization in the following sections.

6.2.2 Noise Cancellation and Sensor Calibration

The magnetic field measured by magnetic sensors is the combination of field stimulated by the target magnet and the magnetic noise in the environment [50]. The magnetic noise consists of the geomagnetic field, the magnetic interference from the ferromagnetic materials, and the noises generated by the surrounding current. In order to obtain a good positioning accuracy, the desired magnetic field measured by sensors should have a good signal-to-noise ratio (SNR) to avoid the drifting effect when the error function is evaluated. Therefore, implementing a noise cancellation module in the system is critical to the

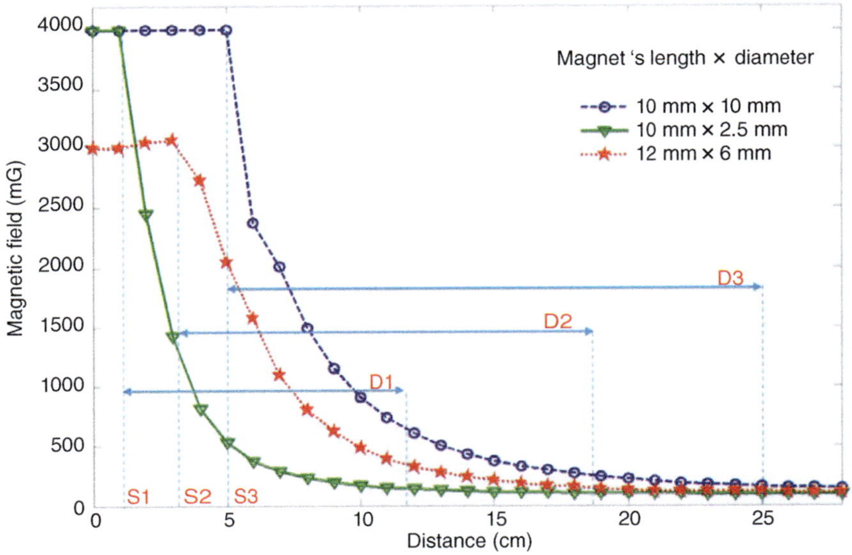

Figure 6.9 Field intensity attenuation vs. the distance under different cylindrical magnets [52]. The distance *D* represents the corresponding effective distance. (*Source*: Pham, D. and Aziz, S. M., 2014.)

localization performance. The location of the target to be estimated is under the body coordinate system. As the human body moves, the magnetic noise added on the magnetic sensor, which keeps static with the body, changes accordingly. Therefore, the major challenge of noise cancellation is to adaptively estimate the noise existing in the environment.

Adaptive noise cancellation can be simply achieved by implementing extra magnetic sensors for the environmental noise measurement [51], which are called noise-evaluation sensors. Generally, the environmental noise added on each sensor is similar. The difference between the localization sensors and the noise-evaluation sensors is the detected magnetic field stimulated from the target magnet. Knowing the fact that the magnetic field attenuates quickly as the distance increases, the noise-evaluation sensors should be placed at a certain distance away from the area of interest. In [51], a magnet of grade N52 with length of 10 mm and diameter of 10 mm is selected as the target. Evaluating the measured magnetic field intensity with respect to the target–sensor distance, the measured field intensity gradually reaches to the environmental noise level as the target–sensor distance increases. A similar comparison of the magnetic field intensity with magnets of different size is conducted in [52] as shown in Figure 6.9. Therefore, the environmental noise can be carefully estimated when the distance to the target is over the effective distance.

Apart from the sensing noise, the calibration of the magnetic sensors is another engineering problem to be addressed. The calibration of the sensors includes the measurement sensitivity calibration and the assembly orientation calibration for the sensors. The measurement sensitivity calibration is involved when the selected magnetic sensor is analog and additional ADC is involved [53]. Digital magnetic sensors are usually embedded with a fixed sensitivity calibration during the manufacturing. However, both analog and digital sensors require the orientation calibration. Measured by a three-axis magnetic sensor, the magnetic field is divided into three orthogonal components under each sensor's coordinate system. The inevitable assembly error of the magnetic sensor usually leads to a performance reduction. The sensor calibration process was proposed in [53, 54], and a simultaneous calibration on the localization sensors array and the actuation system is proposed in [55] under a different application scenario. The rotation matrix R_T between the body coordinate system and the sensor coordinate system can be calibrated through minimizing the following error function:

$$E = \sum_{i=1}^{N} \|R_{Ti} \cdot \boldsymbol{B}_{mi} - \boldsymbol{B}_{ei}\|_2,$$
$$\text{s.t.} \|R_{Ti}\|_2 = 1 \quad (i = 1,\ 2,\ \dots,\ N). \tag{6.5}$$

where $\boldsymbol{B}_{mi}$ refers to the measurements from the ith sensor with an orientation deviation R_{Ti} from the body coordinate system, and $\boldsymbol{B}_{ei}$ denotes the expected field measurement along the three axes of the body coordinate system. The rotation matrix R_{Ti} is a 3-by-3 matrix but with only 3 DOF. Therefore, instead of directly optimizing the nine elements in R_{Ti}, a three-dimensional vector (pitch, roll, and yaw) is introduced as the parameters to be optimized for each sensor rotation matrix in [51] to avoid involving additional optimization constraints. In [56], a magnetocardiography system is established to calibrate the biomedical magnetic sensors array following the similar principle to obtain the effective position, orientation, and sensitivity of each sensor using multiple current coils.

6.2.3 Solving the Inverse Problem

By selecting the field model as the MD, the position retrieval algorithm can be specifically expressed as

$$(a, b, c, m, n, p) = \underset{(a,b,c,m,n,p)}{\arg\min} \sum_{i=1}^{N} \|\boldsymbol{B}_{mi} - \boldsymbol{B}_{ti}\|_2, \tag{6.6}$$

$$\|\boldsymbol{B}_{mi} - \boldsymbol{B}_{ti}\|_2 = \sqrt{(B_{mxi} - B_{txi})^2 + (B_{myi} - B_{tyi})^2 + (B_{mzi} - B_{tzi})^2}, \tag{6.7}$$

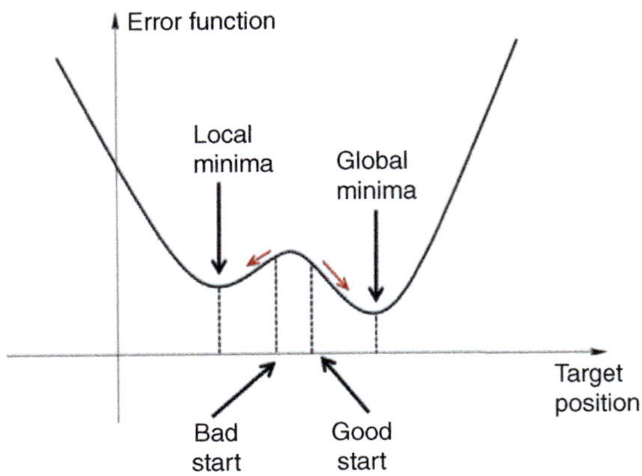

Figure 6.10 Simplified gradient-based optimization process of nonlinear problem.

where (a, b, c) and (m, n, p) represent the position vector and the orientation vector of the target magnet under the body coordinate system, respectively. $\boldsymbol{B}_{mi} = (B_{mxi}, B_{myi}, B_{mzi})$ and $\boldsymbol{B}_{ti} = (B_{txi}, B_{tyi}, B_{tzi})$ denote the measured field vector and the theoretical field vector stimulated by the target magnet, respectively.

The aforementioned position retrieval algorithm is a nonlinear and nonconvex problem. The typical method of solving a nonlinear optimization equation is the gradient descent method[57], in which the optimal solutions are calculated numerically. The calculation process starts from an initial point and finds the direction which gives a descending gradient for each iteration. The optimal solution is obtained when the process reaches a point with a gradient nearly close to zero. The gradient descent method is a reliable method when solving the nonlinear problem, while it may take a lot of iterations to get the optimal solution. However, a nonconvex problem may have multiple local minimal solutions, and each of the local minima has a gradient close to zero [58]. The gradient descent method may be trapped within one of the local minima during the optimization process if a bad start point is selected as shown in Figure 6.10. The local minima generally leads to a large estimation error, which downgrades the localization performance. Therefore, the challenge of solving the inverse problem is to make full use of the sensor's information and reduce the drifting effect caused by the local minima.

An improved linear algorithm was proposed in [40, 59] to address the possible singular solution calculated from the iterations and provide a possible way to find the initial guess for the nonlinear optimization. Instead of directly solving the least-square error function, a linear constraint is derived from the MD model (6.2) for each sensor measurement as

$$(\boldsymbol{B}_i \times \boldsymbol{P}_i) \cdot \boldsymbol{M}_0 = 0(i = 1, 2, \dots, N). \tag{6.8}$$

The above equation can be extended as a six-order linear form:

$$[B_{xi}\ B_{yi}\ B_{zi}\ B_{zi}y_i - B_{yi}z_i\ B_{xi}z_i - B_{zi}x_i\ B_{yi}x_i - B_{xi}y_i].\begin{bmatrix} bp - cn \\ cm - ap \\ an - bm \\ m \\ n \\ p \end{bmatrix} = 0, \quad (6.9)$$

where (x_i, y_i, z_i) and (B_{xi}, B_{yi}, B_{zi}) represent the position and the measured field vector of the *i*th sensor. The six-order linear equation requires at least six sensor measurements to calculate the position (a, b, c) and the orientation (m, n, p) of the target magnet. With the measurement noise existing, a least-square error is formed from N $(N > 6)$ equations. The optimal solution is obtained by solving the first-order linear approximation of the least-square error. The experimental results showed that compared to the aforementioned nonlinear optimization, the linear algorithm gave fewer singular solutions, which is more robust than the nonlinear optimization; however, the average positioning error of the linear algorithm is larger than that of the nonlinear optimization despite the existence of the singular solution. Therefore, the linear algorithm can be used in situations where the computational time is limited and the positioning accuracy is less demanding. Moreover, the linear algorithm can provide a good estimation of the initial guess for the nonlinear optimization process to avoid being trapped in the local minima. The results in [40] showed that the positioning accuracy calculated from the nonlinear iteration method could be improved using the initial guess obtained from the linear algorithm.

The genetic algorithm (GA) and the particle swarm optimization (PSO) are popular bionic algorithms to find the global minima of the nonlinear problem [60]. Instead of strictly following the descending gradient direction, the search direction of the GA and the PSO is randomly distributed within the solution space from the initial start point. Within each iteration, the GA and the PSO will search multiple directions and decide to proceed with the next iteration along the direction which gives the highest possibility of finding the global minima. The solution is obtained when all the searching directions converge. In [61], the aforementioned position retrieval algorithm was solved using the PSO algorithm. Compared to the gradient descent method, the experimental results in [61] showed that the average positioning accuracy was increased when the PSO algorithm was applied, but the execution time for each solution was also increased. Given that the PSO algorithm has the capability of finding the correct direction toward the global minima, the inverse problem can be solved by first obtaining a good initial guess from the PSO algorithm and then drives the optimization toward the final solution using the gradient descent algorithm. An artificial bee colony algorithm was also used to find the optimal solution of the error function in [62], which showed a superior performance than Levenberg–Marquardt method when the environment noise exists.

A novel method of finding the initial guess for this specific inverse problem was proposed in [63] by deriving the trust region of each sensor measurement. Evaluating the magnetic field intensity of the MD model, the following relationship can be derived:

$$\boldsymbol{B}_i = \frac{B_{\mathrm{T}}}{R_i^3}(3\cos\ \theta\widehat{\boldsymbol{P}}_i - \boldsymbol{M}_0),\quad \widehat{\boldsymbol{P}}_i = \frac{\boldsymbol{P}_i}{\|\boldsymbol{P}_i\|_2}, \tag{6.10}$$

where θ is the angle between $\widehat{\boldsymbol{P}}_{\mathrm{i}}$ and $\boldsymbol{M}_0$. With a fixed position and orientation of the target magnet, the upper and lower bounds of the field intensity can be derived as

$$\|\boldsymbol{B}_i\|_2 = \frac{B_{\mathrm{T}}}{R_i^3}\sqrt{3\cos^2\theta + 1} \in \left[\frac{B_{\mathrm{T}}}{R_i^3}, 2\frac{B_{\mathrm{T}}}{R_i^3}\right]. \tag{6.11}$$

The measurement data and the theoretical upper and lower bounds of the field intensity are plotted in Figure 6.11. As the figure shows, for each sensor measurement, the target is contained within the spherical shell with the radius of the corresponding upper and lower target–sensor distance. The intersection area of multiple spherical shell performs as the trust region, where the sensor gives a high-SNR measurement. As such, the initial guess of the target position in [63] was selected as the center point of the trust region, where the target had the highest possibility to appear. Compared to the GA and PSO algorithms, this method provides an efficient procedure to find a good initial guess for this specific problem with fewer computation iterations.

Apart from the initial guess, the measurement SNR is another aspect influencing the positioning accuracy [64]. As shown in Figure 6.11b, the random noise of a small field intensity still exists despite the implementation of the adaptive noise cancellation, which consists of the measurement noise from sensors and the regional environment noise. As such, with a different target–sensor distance, each sensor will provide a different SNR measurement. When the field intensity stimulated from the target magnet equals the random noise intensity, the measurement SNR is 0. In [63], a sensor measurement was recognized as a high-SNR measurement when the deviation of the estimated target–sensor distance from the real distance was under 10%. An SNR threshold of 6 dB was calculated and proved with experiments to divide multiple sensor measurements into the high- and low-SNR categories. When the error function defined in (6.6) is evaluated, the error contribution from each sensor is treated equally. As a result, the optimal solution obtained from a measurement set containing multiple low-SNR measurements may be drifted from the real target position. In order to reduce the influence caused by this drifting effect, a weighted error function was introduced to emphasize

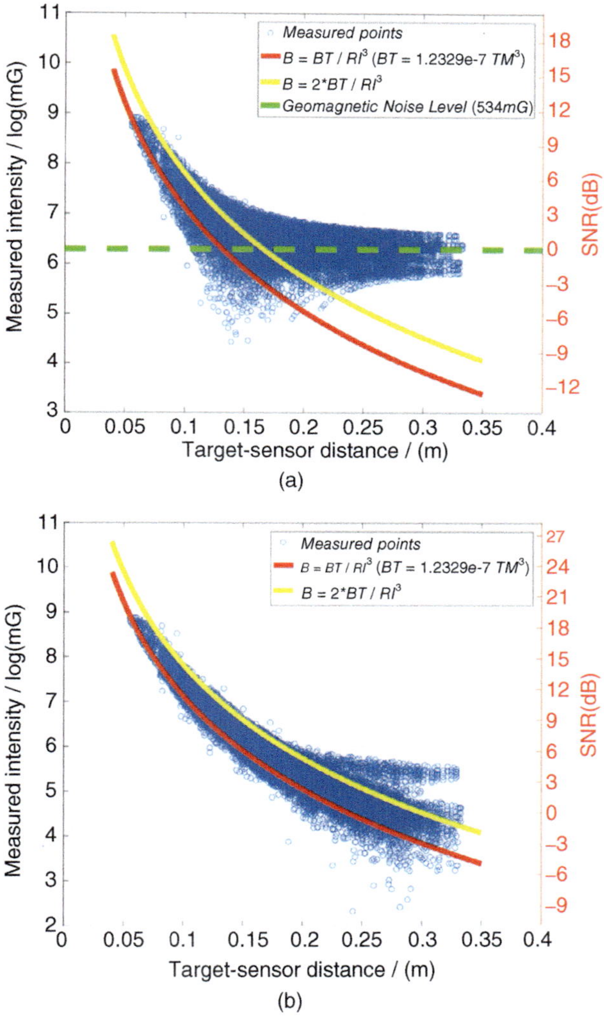

Figure 6.11 Comparison between the actual measurements and the derived upper and lower bounds. (a) The actual measurements before geo-noise cancellation. (b) The actual measurements after geo-noise cancellation. From the graph, a 6-dB SNR is expected to obtain a measurement align within the range [46]. (*Source*: Shao, G. and Guo, Y.-X., et al., 2019. © IEEE.)

the effect of high-SNR sensors. The weighted error function and the weight selection for two categories are shown as

$$E = \sum_{i=1}^{N} w_i \|\boldsymbol{B}'_{mi} - \boldsymbol{B}_{ti}\|_2, \tag{6.12}$$

where

$$w_i = \begin{cases} 1.2 & \text{SNR} \geq 6\ \text{dB} \\ (N_\text{s} - 1.2 \times N_\text{h})/N_\text{l}, & \text{SNR} < 6\ \text{dB} \end{cases}. \tag{6.13}$$

In the weighted error function, each sensor measurement is assigned to a weight w_i based on the measurement SNR. $\boldsymbol{B}'_{mi}$ represents the sensor measurement after the sensors orientation calibration, and $\boldsymbol{B}_{ti}$ represents the theoretical field intensity from the magnetic model. N_s is the total number of sensors, and N_h and N_l are the number of sensors recognized as high SNR and low SNR, respectively.

Implementing the adaptive environment noise cancellation, sensors orientation calibration, initial guess estimation, and weighted error function, the optimal position retrieval algorithm-based SNR evaluation was proposed in [63]. The flow chart of the algorithm is plotted in Figure 6.12. Compared to other systems, a stable positioning accuracy and less iterations performed for each position calculation are reported in the aforementioned algorithm.

6.2.4 Sensors Distribution

The performance of the localization system is determined by not only the algorithm but also the input information. In the static magnetic localization, the distribution of the sensors determines the "quality" of the input information. On one hand, the information delivered to the algorithm will benefit from an increasing number of sensors. On the other hand, too many sensors will increase the computation complexity and introduce an overwhelmed low-SNR measurement. Moreover, from the wearable system design perspective, the number of sensors implemented should be limited. As such, the distribution of the limited number of sensors is another aspect to be considered for an optimal system.

Following the aforementioned analysis, the sensor measurement will be greatly influenced by a larger target–sensor distance, and a small target–sensor distance usually leads to a high-SNR sensor measurement. Given the region of interest for the capsule endoscopy, which is the abdominal cavity, a careful sensor arrangement outside the region of interest will increase the high-SNR coverage. An optimization for the sensor arrangement was proposed in [59, 65]. In the experiment setup in [65], magnetic sensors were arranged uniformly on a plane and placed in the region of interest above the sensors plane. The experiment results showed that the localization error was reduced as the number

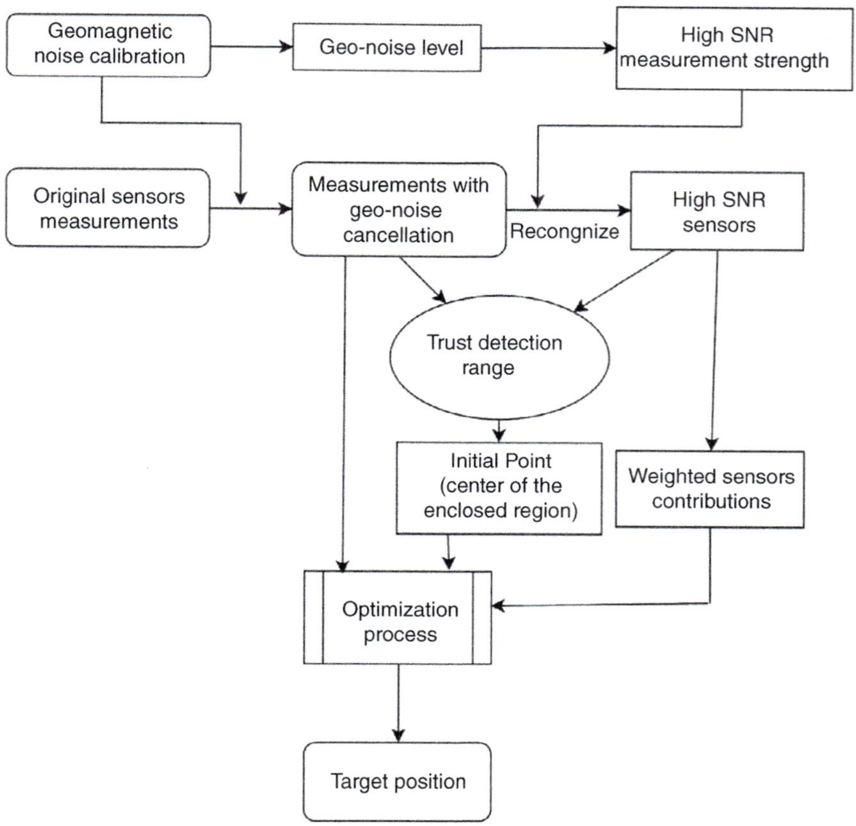

Figure 6.12 Flowchart of the position-estimation process proposed in [63]. (*Source*: Shao, G. and Guo, Y.-X., 2019. © IEEE.)

of sensors increased. Besides, the localization error is generally small when the target is close to the sensors plane as shown in Figure 6.13. As such, two sensor planes with 25 sensors on each plane were adopted in the experiment to reduce the overall target–sensor distance within the region of interest.

An arrangement optimization for a limited number of sensors on one plane was proposed in [43]. Different from the uniform distribution of sensors in [65], only eight sensors were placed at the designed grids on one plane. The localization performance was evaluated over seven sensor placement patterns. The experiment results showed that the pattern of largest coverage area gave the lowest localization error. Similarly, a grid-based sensor arrangement conducted in [66] gave the lowest positioning error, in which a smaller grid was applied and a generic algorithm was used to find the optimal arrangements.

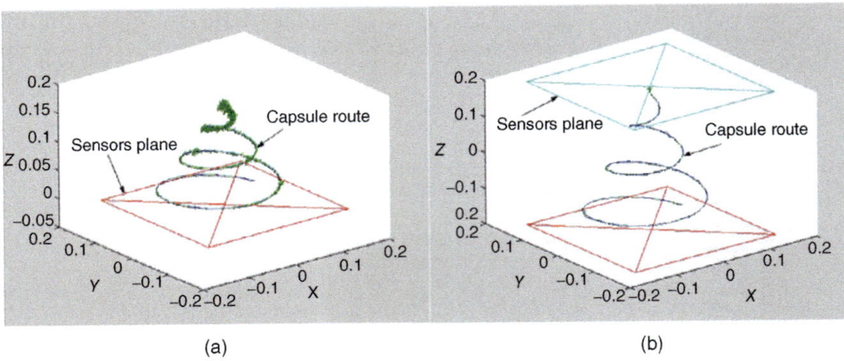

Figure 6.13 Sensors plane arrangements comparison in [65]. (a) The positioning error under single sensors plane configuration. (b) The positioning error under two sensors planes configuration. (*Source*: Hu, C., Ma, T., and Meng, M. Q.-H., 2007. © IEEE.)

Assigning a trust region for each sensor in the grid patterns, it can be found that the grid pattern establishing the largest trust region coverage of the localization area had the lowest positioning error. Therefore, an optimal sensor arrangement strategy was proposed in [63].

The principle of the optimal sensor arrangement is to provide the algorithm with as much target information as possible. The quality of the target information can be evaluated from two aspects: SNR and redundancy. For the first aspect, from the aforementioned analysis, different measurement SNR corresponds to different trust regions, as such, evaluating the overall SNR of the measurement setup can be transformed to evaluate the trust region coverage of the localization area. For the second aspect, the variance of the sensor measurements should be as large as possible to reduce the information redundancy, because the information provided from two sensors placed adjacently is similar to the information obtained from one. In [63], instead of applying the grid method to determine the placement of sensors, the sensors' coordinates were determined by the following strategies:

- Each point within the localization area should be covered within the trust region of at least three sensors;
- Sensors should be separated as far as possible to avoid providing redundant field measurements;
- With a limited number of sensors, the peripheral localization region should be considered preferentially.

In [63], the localization area of 380 mm by 240 mm by 270 mm was monitored by 16 sensors mounted on four side planes, with each plane having 4 sensors. Applying the proposed sensor arrangement strategies, it was reported that the high-SNR measurement coverage was increased from 80% under the uniform arrangement to 85%, the RMSE positioning error was reduced from 0.0529 mm under the uniform arrangement to 0.0364 mm, and the RMSE orientation error was reduced from 17.3° under the uniform arrangement to 13.7°.

6.2.5 Conclusion of the Static Magnetic Localization

The static magnetic localization is a simple but effective solution for capsule endoscopy localization. Experiencing less interference from human tissue, a high positioning accuracy can be achieved by the static magnetic localization compared to the RF-based method. The performance of the typical static magnetic localization system can be improved from both the hardware and the algorithm perspectives. From the hardware perspective, the localization performance can be improved by implementing the environment noise cancellation, sensors assembly error calibration, and sensors optimal arrangements. From the algorithm perspective, the positioning accuracy can benefit from a better target magnet model; besides, a carefully designed position retrieval process could reduce the localization error and computation complexity. However, the static magnetic localization is still facing some challenges under certain cases, for example, the size and weight of the target magnet. In order to obtain a high measurement SNR, a relatively large magnet with a strong magnetism is usually selected, which will increase the overall weight of the capsule endoscopy. Moreover, embedding a magnet inside the capsule endoscopy could bring certain difficulties to the design of other components, for instance, the miniaturized antenna inside the capsule.

6.3 Modulated Magnetic Localization

The DC signal (static magnetic field) measured in the static magnetic localization suffers from the static noise interference in the environment. One of the methods to avoid DC interference is to modulate the information to a certain frequency, where the alternating magnetic field is adopted. Generally, the alternating magnetic field can be obtained from the periodic movement of the static field or the conductor driven by the alternating current.

6.3.1 Static Field Modulation

A prototype implementing the static field modulation method was proposed in [67, 68] in which a permanent magnet was periodically driven by a robotic arm at 5 Hz. Six Hall sensors were installed inside the capsule and monitor the modulated field intensity at 200 Hz as shown in Figure 6.14. The orientation of the capsule was first calculated from the maximum and minimum detected field intensities, and the position of the capsule was solved from the estimated orientation. A positioning error of 2 mm and an orientation error of 5° were reported from the proposed setup when the distance between the driven magnet and the sensor capsule was around 138 mm. Modulating the static field on a certain frequency, the prototype reduces the interference from most of the environment noise; on the other hand, the position-updated frequency is highly related to the rotation frequency of the driven magnet and the sampling frequency of the embedded sensors, because at least one full period measurement is required to retrieve the target position.

6.3.2 Inductive-based Magnetic Localization

Another field modulation method is to generate the magnetic field using alternating current, which involves the magnetic field induction. Inductive-based magnetic localizationis one type of EM tracking methods which uses the magnetic field induction to localize the target. Different from the aforementioned static field modulation method, the inductive-based magnetic localization uses coils to generate the alternating magnetic field within the localization area. The alternating field distribution is detected by the receiving coils from the magnetic induction. Similar to the static field modulation method, the alternating signal modulates the field information to a certain frequency, which avoids the complex static noise inference from the environment. The modulated frequency can reach from kilohertz to megahertz as the modulation is driven by the alternating current rather than the mechanical movement of the motor.

An inductive-based magnetic localization system implementing a single receiving coil and a large 2D-transmitting coils array was proposed in [69] as shown in Figure 6.15. The tracking algorithm in [69] formulated an optimization equation similar to the static magnetic localization. Each transmitting coil was treated as an alternating MD, while the receiving coil detected the combination alternating field stimulated by the 64 coils in the 2D coils array. The equation was solved using the Levenberg–Marquardt algorithm. Facing the similar problem of selecting the good initial point, a subarray containing eight coils within the 2D array was activated sequentially to find a good stage to start the optimization. The transmitting coils array was driven by an alternating current of 1 A amplitude and 50 kHz frequency, and the activated power on each transmitting coil was less than 1 W. A positioning accuracy of 1 mm and an orientation accuracy of 0.6° were reported when the receiving coil was placed 200 mm over the transmitting array. Regarding the assembly error of each transmitting coil, a calibration method procedure was proposed for this prototype in [70].

Another prototype implementing a 2D coil array was proposed in [71–73] as shown in Figure 6.16, where the localization theory is similar to the microwave imaging method. The prototype included a square exciting coil of the side

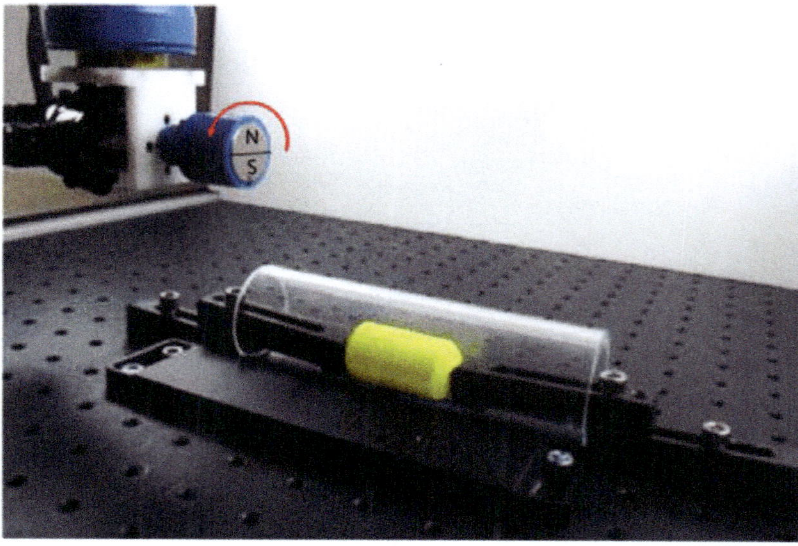

(a)

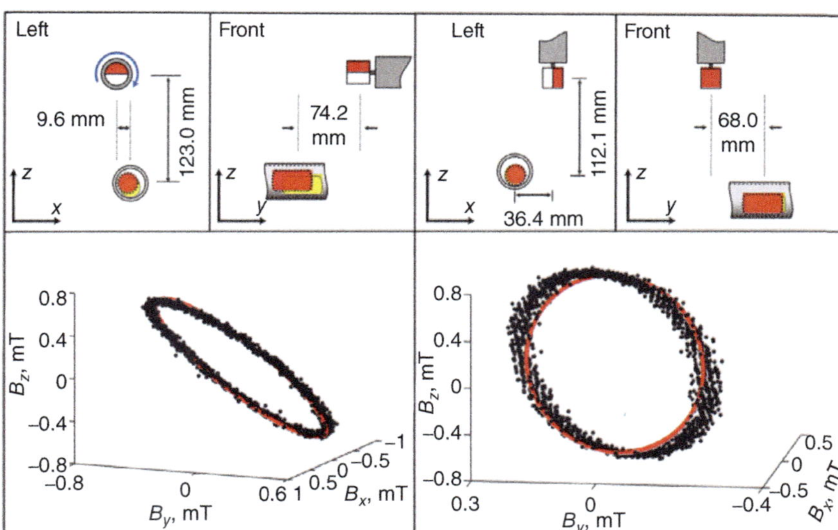

(b)

Figure 6.14 Mechanical static field modulation proposed in [67]. (a) The experiment setup. (b) The localization results. (*Source*: Popek, K. M., Mahoney, A. W., and Abbott, J. J., 2013. © IEEE.)

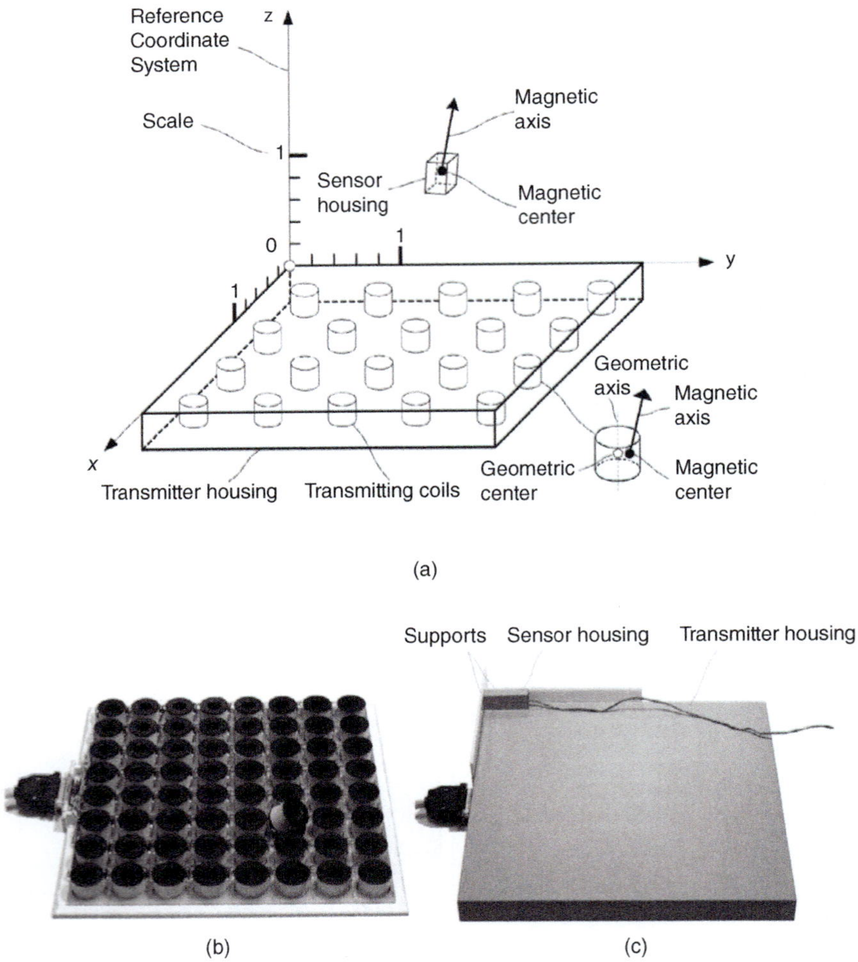

Figure 6.15 The 2D transmitting coils array proposed in [69, 70]. (*Source*: Plotkin, A., Kucher, V., Horen, Y., et al., 2008. © IEEE.)

length of 390 mm. The target was an LC resonant circuit located between the exciting coil and the 2D coil array, which was used as a marker. Instead of being used as the transmitter, the 2D coil array constructed a pickup array to receive the magnetic flux generated from the exciting coil. The target LC circuit had the same resonant frequency as the exciting coil, as a result, the target LC marker was excited by the alternating magnetic flux. An inverse problem was constructed to retrieve the target position by evaluating the detected magnetic

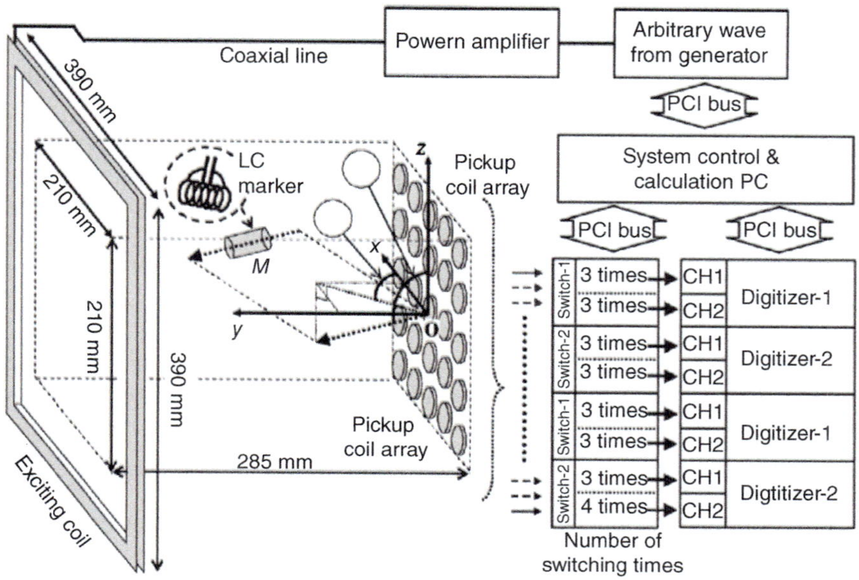

Figure 6.16 The structure schematic with one exciting coil and a 2D pickup coils array proposed in [72]. (*Source*: Hashi, S., Yabukami, S., Kanetaka, H., et al., 2011. © IEEE.)

flux on the pickup coils array. Without the orientation estimation for the target LC marker, a submillimeter positioning error was reported when the distance between the target and the pickup array was less than 120 mm, and the positioning error slightly increased to 2 mm when the distance was over 130 mm.

The aforementioned methods implementing coils array in the localization system achieve good positioning accuracy, while the complexity of the system configuration is increased. From the localization of wireless capsule endoscopy perspective, these two methods are only suitable for situations where patients are required to be stationary. A simple system design implementing a 3D transmitting coil and a single uniaxial coil was first proposed in [74] and realized in [64, 75] to reduce the system complexity. The 3D transmitting coil was excited by three independent alternating currents of three different frequencies. The transmitting coil along each axis can be treated as a MD generating an alternating magnetic field. The single coil transformed the magnetic induction into the alternating voltage signal of the corresponding frequency. The rotation angle of the single receiving coil was obtained from a two-step rotation method. Using two electrical motors, the orientation vector of the single receiving coil was aligned with the orientation vector of one of the transmitting coils by monitoring the maximum output voltage. The DC component of the detected maximum voltage is proportional to the cube of the distance between the transmitting coil and the receiving coil, where the coordinates of the receiving coil can be estimated from the distance and the rotation angle. An average distance error of 0.46 mm and an average rotation angle error of around 1.5° were reported. To avoid rotating the receiving coil, an improved configuration using the same transmitting coil structure but with a three-axis receiving coil was proposed in [44, 76, 77]. Processing the detected output of different frequencies along each axis of the receiving coils, the distance between the transmitting coil and the receiving coil can be calculated analytically, and the orientation of the receiving coils can be determined from the calculated rotation matrix. An average positioning error of 0.7 mm and an average orientation error of 2.4° were reported for the improved configuration. Instead of implementing a nonlinear optimization process to obtain the estimated position, this method directly calculates the position and orientation from the amplitude and phase of the induced voltage, which can be processed within one period of excitation (Figure 6.17).

The aforementioned EM tracking system using the alternating magnetic field is used extensively in the localization and control system, for example, biomedical devices. Similar to the static magnetic localization, the generated alternating magnetic field attenuates drastically as the distance increases, which brings limitations to the effective range of the tracking system [72, 78]. With a limited transmitter power, an optimization method for the transmitter coil design was proposed in [79] to make the receiving coil get the maximum induced voltage. By optimizing the radius, the length, the maximum width, the number of turns, and the number of layers of the three-axis orthogonal transmitting coils, the effective measurement range was increased. A 37% improvement in the measurement range was reported with an example transmitting coil configuration of 39 mm radius, 20 mm length, 4 mm width, and 60 turns in four layers using 0.9-mm-diameter wire. Correspondingly, the careful tuning for the resonant receiving coil was conducted in [80] to increase the induced voltage detected by the receiving coil in the EM tracking system as shown in Figure 6.18. Compared to the conventional EM tracking system, a 300-mm effective detection range was reported, and the positioning error and orientation error were reported as 14.9 mm and 5.9°, respectively. A miniaturized 3D cross-type receiver coil was proposed to be implanted inside the capsule endoscopy in [81] with a diameter of 8 mm for a better matching with the transmitting coil.

The tracking system established in [76, 79] implemented a 3D receiving coil to detect the magnetic field strength generated by the transmitting coils, which is a typical application of Faraday's law of EM induction similar to the inductive wireless charging[82]. The differences between the inductive wireless positioning and the inductive wireless charging appear in two aspects: the distribution of the magnetic field and the receiving circuit. From the

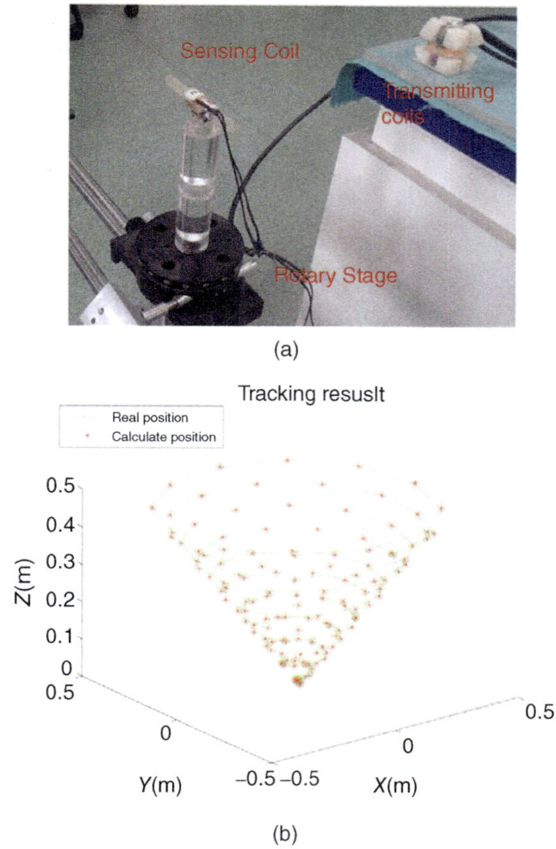

Figure 6.17 The inductive localization using a 3D transmitting coil and a sensing coil proposed in [75]. (a) The experiment setup. (b) The localization result of the proposed setup. (*Source*: Song, S., Qiao, W., Li, B., et al., 2013. © IEEE.)

field distribution perspective, in order to obtain a stable charging ability, the magnetic flux detected by the receiving coil is expected to be stable within the whole charging area, which indicates a uniform amplitude of alternating magnetic field[83]. Conversely, a nonuniform field distribution is required to distinguish different target positions under both static and inductive-based magnetic localization. From the receiver perspective, different aspects are focused on the received AC signals with respect to charging and positioning functions. When applying the wireless charging function, a rectifier circuit is connected to the receiving coil to convert the energy from AC to DC [84]. On the contrary, when applying the positioning function, the amplitude of the AC signals, even the phase information, is focused to retrieve the received position. As a result, the receiver circuit connected to the receiving coil is usually selected as an envelope detection circuit, an analog-to-digital converter (ADC), or an oscilloscope to directly analyze the induced AC voltage.

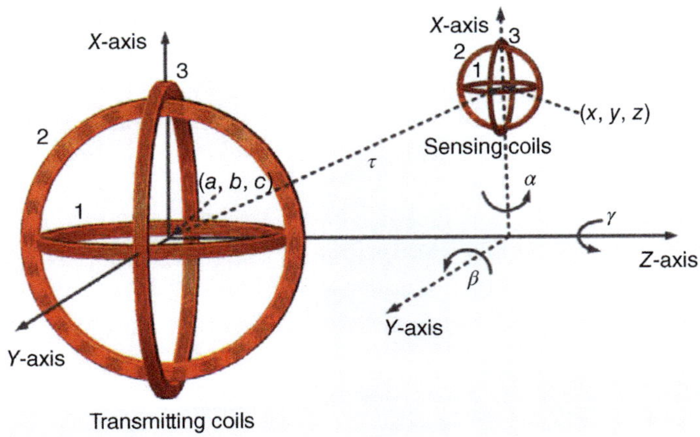

Figure 6.18 The 6-DOF inductive-based localization system with an extended detection range [79]. (*Source*: Islam, M. N. and Fleming, A. J., 2017. © IEEE.)

Both wireless charging and wireless positioning are critical technical challenges and progressive tendencies in the next-generation design of wireless capsule endoscopy[84, 85]. While developing two individual systems for wireless charging and wireless positioning can be space consuming and complexity increasing, using the same transmitting and receiving structure to achieve both functions can be a solution for the compact design inside the capsule endoscopy. A hybrid system for wireless charging and wireless positioning based on Helmholtz coils was proposed in [46].

Helmholtz coils are used extensively in a wireless charging system for biomedical applications [86, 87], in which a uniform field distribution is produced within the region of interest when two coils are excited with zero phase difference. On the other hand, a pair of fine-tuned Helmholtz coils can be used to generate an one-dimensional static gradient magnetic field distribution in a simple MRI structure where the coils are not excited synchronously [88]. The gradient field causes a spin frequency deviation of the protons which encodes the position information of the protons along the gradient direction [89]. Implementing a switch to change the excitation mode of the Helmholtz coils, a hybrid system was proposed in [46, 90], where the alternating magnetic field was switched between the uniform distribution and the gradient distribution, to provide the basis of wireless charging and wireless positioning. The different field distributions under different coil excitation mode can be found in Figure 6.19.

As shown in Figure 6.20, the Helmholtz coils performed as the two-port inductance in the LC oscillator from the transmitter perspective. When the switch connected the same end of the two coils, respectively, the Helmholtz coils were excited by the in-phase current, which generated a uniform

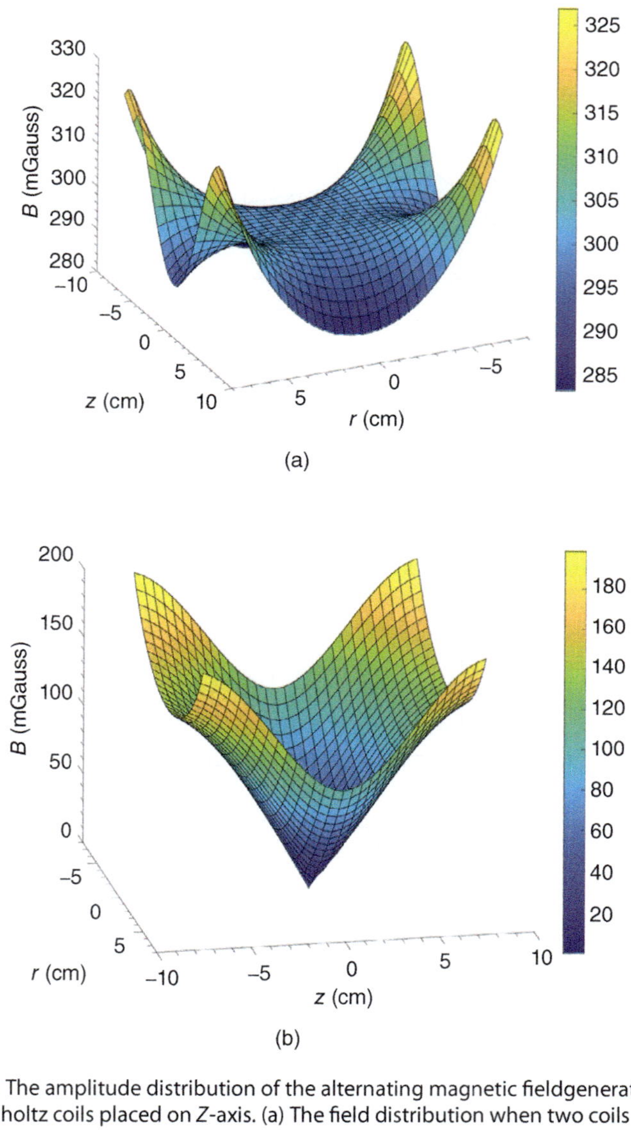

Figure 6.19 The amplitude distribution of the alternating magnetic fieldgenerated from a pair of Helmholtz coils placed on *Z*-axis. (a) The field distribution when two coils are excited by in-phase current. (b) The field distribution when two coils are excited by out-of-phase current [90]. (*Source:* Shao, G., and Guo, Y.-X., 2020. © IEEE.)

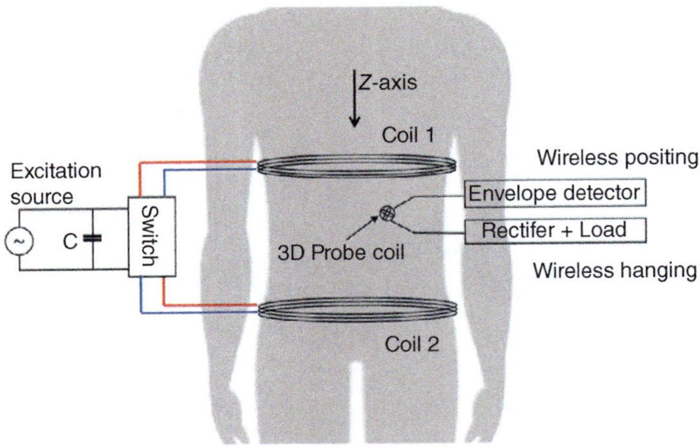

Figure 6.20 Structure schematic of the hybrid wireless charging and wireless positioning system [90]. (*Source*: Shao, G., and Guo, Y.-X., 2020. © IEEE.)

distributed alternating magnetic fieldfor wireless charging function. When the switch connected the anisotropic end of two coils, respectively, the Helmholtz coils were excited by the out-of-phase current, which generated a gradient distributed alternating magnetic field for wireless positioning function. The equivalent inductance of the Helmholtz coils is determined by the self-inductance of the individual coils and the mutual inductance of the coil pair. Changing the connection of two coils will modify the equivalent inductance of the LC oscillator, which results in a different oscillating frequency under different functions. By detecting the frequency of the induced voltage on the receiving coils, the untethered capsule could identify the function performed currently. The rectifier circuit and the envelope detection circuit were connected to the 3D receiving coils through another switch inside the capsule. Upon detecting the current function, the switch at the receiver side would connect the corresponding circuit to the receiving coils to perform either wireless charging or wireless positioning (Figure 6.21).

The uniformity and linearity of the generated field distribution directly influence the performance of wireless charging and wireless positioning, respectively. Besides, the detection sensitivity of the induced voltage influences the theoretical resolution of the positioning function. A careful transmitting and receiving coils design for both transmitter and receiver will balance the performance trade-off between the wireless charging and wireless positioning functions and improve the positioning accuracy [83, 91, 92]. A millimeter-level positioning accuracy along one axis can be achieved using the hybrid structure proposed in [46]. Although the inductive-based localization could eliminate the magnetic noise, the safety issue of illuminating the RF magnetic field to the

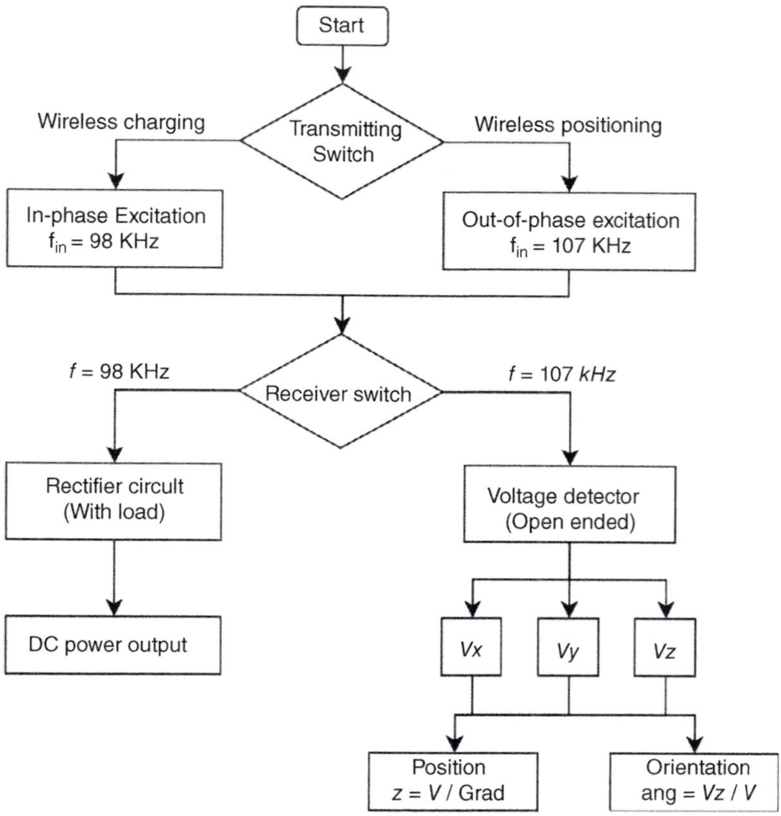

Figure 6.21 Work flowchart of the hybrid charging and positioning system [90]. (*Source:* Shao, G., and Guo, Y.-X., 2020. © IEEE.)

human tissue is a critical aspect. According to the exposure guidelines for the magnetic field [93, 94], inappropriate alternating field exposure could cause the effects on the human nervous system and the heating effects on human tissue. Therefore, a trade-off balance between the system performance and a safe field density should be conducted during the system design.

6.4 Conclusion

The prescreening and precise diagnosis are widely promoted in the modern medical system. The wireless capsule endoscopy plays an important role in the early diagnosis of digestive diseases. Apart from the basic image screening function, the wireless charging, the wireless positioning, and possible mechanical functions are demanded in the next-generation design of the capsule endoscopy. The localization for wireless capsule endoscopy is a challenging but worth exploring problem. Over the past decades, four major research directions are explored to find the possible solutions and techniques to increase the positioning accuracy while making the system compactable in the capsule endoscopy. The visual-based localization method has the highest positioning accuracy of around 0.001 mm and the lowest system configuration. However, a low frame rate and unstable image quality provided by the current capsule endoscopy make the visual-based method fail to perform a long-term and robust localization. The RF-based localization method has a simple system configuration to perform the wireless localization, but the complex EM environment inside the human body results in the lowest positioning accuracy of around 6–80 mm. Generally, the RF-based method will be integrated with the visual-based method to increase the positioning accuracy. The microwave imaging method is also a possible method to obtain a good positioning accuracy of around 3–10 mm under the cost of heavy system configuration and complicated algorithm design. Compared to the other three methods, the magnetic localization provides a trade-off solution between the positioning accuracy and the system configuration. The challenges and possible solutions of the magnetic localization are discussed in detail in this chapter.

The static magnetic localization implements a simple field sampling configuration to achieve a sub-centimeter positioning accuracy while suffering from the environmental magnetic noises. Embedding a permanent magnet inside the capsule endoscopy, the static magnetic localization requires no power supply from the capsule endoscopy; on the other hand, the magnet takes space inside the capsule and increases the overall weight. Improvements on the static magnetic localization including selecting different field models, performing adaptive noise cancellation, modifying the optimization equation, and adopting an optimal sensor placement are introduced with examples. The inductive-based magnetic localization modulates the field information on a certain frequency, which eliminates the environment noise to a certain extent. Based on the similar optimization equation as used in the static method, the inductive-based localization improves the positioning accuracy with less noise interference. Compared with the embedded permanent magnet, both the size and the weight of the receiving coil inside the capsule are much smaller for a compact design. Finding the similarity and difference between the inductive-based localization and the wireless charging, the hybrid system for achieving both charging and positioning functions is introduced. However, the transmitting coils placed outside the human body can consume huge power to generate the required alternating magnetic field, and the effective range is also related to the driving current. Moreover, the exposure limits of the time-varying magnetic field should also be considered in the inductive-based method.

With different requirements on system performance and configurations, a trade-off between different methods should be considered. Not restricted in the application of wireless capsule endoscopy, the introduced localization methods can also be used in other related biomedical applications with appropriate adjustment.

References

1 Swain, C., Gong, F., and Mills, T. (1997). Wireless transmission of a colour television moving image from the stomach using a miniature CCD camera, light source and microwave transmitter. *Gastrointestinal Endoscopy* 45 (4): AB40.

2 Iddan, G., Meron, G., Glukhovsky, A., and Swain, P. (2000). Wireless capsule endoscopy. *Nature* 405 (6785): 417.

3 Park, S., Chun, H.J., Keum, B. et al. (2012). Capsule endoscopy to detect normally positioned duodenal papilla: performance comparison of SB and SB2. *Gastroenterology Research and Practice* 2012 https://doi.org/10.1155/2012/202935.

4 Flemming, J. and Cameron, S. (2018). Small bowel capsule endoscopy: indications, results, and clinical benefit in a University environment. *Medicine* 97 (14).

5 Karargyris, A. and Koulaouzidis, A. (2014). OdoCapsule: next-generation wireless capsule endoscopy with accurate lesion localization and video stabilization capabilities. *IEEE Transactions on Biomedical Engineering* 62 (1): 352–360.

6 Gong, F., Swain, P., and Mills, T. (2000). Wireless endoscopy. *Gastrointestinal Endoscopy* 51 (6): 725–729.

7 U. F. a. D. Administration (2017). FDA approval of PillCam SBC capsule endoscopy system. [Online]. https://www.accessdata.fda.gov/cdrh_docs/pdf17/K170210.pdf (accessed on 15 November 2019).

8 U. F. a. D. Administration (2018). FDA approval of OLYMPUS SMALL INTESTINAL CAPSULE ENDOSCOPE SYSTEM. [Online]. https://www.accessdata.fda.gov/cdrh_docs/pdf17/K173459.pdf (accessed on 15 November 2019).

9 U. F. a. D. Administration (2018). FDA approval of MiroCam® Capsule Endoscope System. [Online]. https://www.accessdata.fda.gov/cdrh_docs/pdf17/K170438.pdf (accessed on 15 November 2019).

10 U. F. a. D. Administration (2016). FDA approval of Capsocam Plus. [Online]. https://www.accessdata.fda.gov/cdrh_docs/pdf16/K161773.pdf (accessed on 15 November 2019).

11 Fireman, Z., Paz, D., and Kopelman, Y. (2005). Capsule endoscopy: improving transit time and image view. *World Journal of Gastroenterology: WJG* 11 (37): 5863.

12 Chong, A.K., Chin, B.W., and Meredith, C.G. (2006). Clinically significant small-bowel pathology identified by double-balloon enteroscopy but missed by capsule endoscopy. *Gastrointestinal Endoscopy* 64 (3): 445–449.
13 Adler, S.N. and Metzger, Y.C. (2011). PillCam COLON capsule endoscopy: recent advances and new insights. *Therapeutic Advances in Gastroenterology* 4 (4): 265–268.
14 Ormeci, A.C., Akyuz, F., Baran, B. et al. (2016). Retention during capsule endoscopy: Is it a real problem in routine practice? *Journal of International Medical Research* 44 (4): 968–975.
15 Al-Rawhani, M.A., Beeley, J., and Cumming, D.R. (2015). Wireless fluorescence capsule for endoscopy using single photon-based detection. *Scientific Reports* 5: 18591.
16 Moglia, A., Menciassi, A., Schurr, M.O., and Dario, P. (2007). Wireless capsule endoscopy: from diagnostic devices to multipurpose robotic systems. *Biomedical Microdevices* 9 (2): 235–243.
17 Basar, M.R., Malek, F., Juni, K.M. et al. (2012). Ingestible wireless capsule technology: A review of development and future indication. *International Journal of Antennas and Propagation* 2012 https://doi.org/10.1155/2012/807165.
18 Mateen, H., Basar, R., Ahmed, A.U., and Ahmad, M.Y. (2017). Localization of wireless capsule endoscope: A systematic review. *IEEE Sensors Journal* 17 (5): 1197–1206.
19 Bao, G., Pahlavan, K., and Mi, L. (2014). Hybrid localization of microrobotic endoscopic capsule inside small intestine by data fusion of vision and RF sensors. *IEEE Sensors Journal* 15 (5): 2669–2678.
20 Turan, M., Almalioglu, Y., Araujo, H. et al. (2017). A non-rigid map fusion-based direct SLAM method for endoscopic capsule robots. *International Journal of Intelligent Robotics and Applications* 1 (4): 399–409.
21 Bao, G., Mi, L., Geng, Y., and Pahlavan, K. (2014). A computer vision based speed estimation technique for localizing the wireless capsule endoscope inside small intestine. 36th Annual International Conference of the IEEE Engineering in Medicine and Biology Society (EMBC), vol. 123.
22 Turan, M., Shabbir, J., Araujo, H. et al. (2017). A deep learning based fusion of RGB camera information and magnetic localization information for endoscopic capsule robots. *International Journal of Intelligent Robotics and Applications* 1 (4): 442–450.
23 Pahlavan, K., Bao, G., Ye, Y. et al. (2012). RF localization for wireless video capsule endoscopy. *International Journal of Wireless Information Networks* 19 (4): 326–340.
24 Pourhomayoun, M., Jin, Z., and Fowler, M.L. (2013). Accurate localization of in-body medical implants based on spatial sparsity. *IEEE Transactions on Biomedical Engineering* 61 (2): 590–597.

25 Geng, Y. and Pahlavan, K. (2015). On the accuracy of rf and image processing based hybrid localization for wireless capsule endoscopy. IEEE Wireless Communications and Networking Conference (WCNC), 452–457.

26 Nafchi, A.R., Goh, S.T., and Zekavat, S.A.R. (2014). Circular arrays and inertial measurement unit for DOA/TOA/TDOA-based endoscopy capsule localization: Performance and complexity investigation. *IEEE Sensors Journal* 14 (11): 3791–3799.

27 Ye, Y., Pahlavan, K., Bao, G. et al. (2014). Comparative performance evaluation of RF localization for wireless capsule endoscopy applications. *International Journal of Wireless Information Networks* 21 (3): 208–222.

28 Barbi, M., Garcia-Pardo, C., Nevárez, A. et al. (2019). UWB RSS-based localization for capsule endoscopy using a multilayer phantom and in vivo measurements. *IEEE Transactions on Antennas and Propagation* 67 (8): 5035–5043.

29 Barbi, M., Garcia-Pardo, C., Cardona, N. et al. (2018). Impact of receivers location on the accuracy of capsule endoscope localization. 2018 IEEE 29th Annual International Symposium on Personal, Indoor and Mobile Radio Communications (PIMRC), 340–344.

30 Zhang, L., Zhu, Y., Mo, T. et al. (2010). Design and implementation of 3D positioning algorithms based on RF signal radiation patterns for in vivo micro-robot. 2010 IEEE International Conference on Body Sensor Networks, 255–260.

31 Wille, A., Broll, M., and Winter, S. (2011). Phase difference based RFID navigation for medical applications. 2011 IEEE International Conference on RFID, 98–105.

32 Dey, N., Ashour, A.S., Shi, F., and Sherratt, R.S. (2017). Wireless capsule gastrointestinal endoscopy: direction-of-arrival estimation based localization survey. *IEEE Reviews in Biomedical Engineering* 10: 2–11.

33 Krhac, K., Sayrafian, K., Alasti, M. et al. (2018). A study of capsule endoscopy orientation estimation using received signal strength. 2018 IEEE 29th Annual International Symposium on Personal, Indoor and Mobile Radio Communications (PIMRC), 345–349.

34 Meaney, P.M., Fanning, M.W., Li, D. et al. (2000). A clinical prototype for active microwave imaging of the breast. *IEEE Transactions on Microwave Theory and Techniques* 48 (11): 1841–1853.

35 Pastorino, M. (2010). *Microwave Imaging*. Wiley.

36 Chandra, R., Johansson, A.J., Gustafsson, M., and Tufvesson, F. (2014). A microwave imaging-based technique to localize an in-body RF source for biomedical applications. *IEEE Transactions on Biomedical Engineering* 62 (5): 1231–1241.

37 Ito, T., Iida, T., Anzai, D., and Wang, J. (2016). An EM imaging-based localization method with sparse reconstruction for implant devices. 2016 38th

Annual International Conference of the IEEE Engineering in Medicine and Biology Society (EMBC), 239–242.

38 Hu, C., Meng, M.Q.-H., and Mandal, M. (2005). Efficient magnetic localization and orientation technique for capsule endoscopy. *International Journal of Information Acquisition* 2 (01): 23–36.

39 Li, M., Song, S., Hu, C. et al. (2009). A new calibration method for magnetic sensor array for tracking capsule endoscope. 2009 IEEE International Conference on Robotics and Biomimetics (ROBIO), 1561–1566.

40 Hu, C., Yang, W., Chen, D. et al. (2008). An improved magnetic localization and orientation algorithm for wireless capsule endoscope. 2008 30th Annual International Conference of the IEEE Engineering in Medicine and Biology Society, 2055–2058.

41 Di Natali, C., Beccani, M., Simaan, N., and Valdastri, P. (2016). Jacobian-based iterative method for magnetic localization in robotic capsule endoscopy. *IEEE Transactions on Robotics* 32 (2): 327–338.

42 Song, S., Li, B., Qiao, W. et al. (2014). 6-D magnetic localization and orientation method for an annular magnet based on a closed-form analytical model. *IEEE Transactions on Magnetics* 50 (9): 1–11.

43 Song, S., Qiu, X., Wang, J., and Meng, M.Q.-H. (2017). Design and optimization strategy of sensor array layout for magnetic localization system. *IEEE Sensors Journal* 17 (6): 1849–1857.

44 Hu, C., Song, S., Wang, X. et al. (2012). A novel positioning and orientation system based on three-axis magnetic coils. *IEEE Transactions on Magnetics* 48 (7): 2211–2219.

45 Kim, W., Song, J., and Park, F.C. (2017). Closed-form position and orientation estimation for a three-axis electromagnetic tracking system. *IEEE Transactions on Industrial Electronics* 65 (5): 4331–4337.

46 Shao, G. and Guo, Y.-X. (2019). Switched magnetic field for hybrid wireless positioning and wireless charging using Helmholtz coils. 2019 IEEE MTT-S International Wireless Symposium (IWS), 1–3.

47 Su, S., Yang, W., Dai, H. et al. (2017). Investigation of the relationship between tracking accuracy and tracking distance of a novel magnetic tracking system. *IEEE Sensors Journal* 17 (15): 4928–4937.

48 Lee, K.-M. and Son, H. (2007). Distributed multipole model for design of permanent-magnet-based actuators. *IEEE Transactions on Magnetics* 43 (10): 3904–3913.

49 Wu, F., Robert, N.M., Frey, D.D., and Foong, S. (2013). Enhanced magnetic localization with artificial neural network field models. 2013 IEEE International Conference on Robotics and Automation, 1560–1565, 2013.

50 Aziz, S.M., Grcic, M., and Vaithianathan, T. (2008). A real-time tracking system for an endoscopic capsule using multiple magnetic sensors. In: *Smart Sensors and Sensing Technology*, 201–218. Springer.

51 Shao, G., Tang, Y., Tang, L. et al. (2019). A novel passive magnetic localization wearable system for wireless capsule endoscopy. *IEEE Sensors Journal* 19 (9): 3462–3472.

52 Pham, D. and Aziz, S.M. (2014). A real-time localization system for an endoscopic capsule using magnetic sensors. *Sensors* 14 (11): 20910–20929.

53 Hu, C., Meng, M.Q.-H., and Mandal, M. (2006). The calibration of 3-axis magnetic sensor array system for tracking wireless capsule endoscope. 2006 IEEE/RSJ International Conference on Intelligent Robots and Systems, 162–167.

54 Shen, H.-M., Hu, L., and Qin, L.-H. (2015). Real-time orientation-invariant magnetic localization and sensor calibration based on closed-form models. *IEEE Magnetics Letters* 6: 1–4.

55 Son, D., Dong, X., and Sitti, M. (2018). A simultaneous calibration method for magnetic robot localization and actuation systems. *IEEE Transactions on Robotics* 35 (2): 343–352.

56 Adachi, Y., Oyama, D., Terazono, Y. et al. (2019). Calibration of room temperature magnetic sensor array for biomagnetic measurement. *IEEE Transactions on Magnetics* 55 (7): 1–6.

57 Ruder, S. (2016). An overview of gradient descent optimization algorithms. arXiv preprint arXiv:1609.04747.

58 Boyd, S. and Vandenberghe, L. (2004). *Convex Optimization*. Cambridge University Press.

59 Hu, C., Li, M., Song, S. et al. (2010). A cubic 3-axis magnetic sensor array for wirelessly tracking magnet position and orientation. *IEEE Sensors Journal* 10 (5): 903–913.

60 Abd-El-Wahed, W., Mousa, A., and El-Shorbagy, M. (2011). Integrating particle swarm optimization with genetic algorithms for solving nonlinear optimization problems. *Journal of Computational and Applied Mathematics* 235 (5): 1446–1453.

61 Hu, C., Meng, M.Q.-H., Song, S., and Dai, H. (2009). A six-dimensional magnetic localization algorithm for a rectangular magnet objective based on a particle swarm optimizer. *IEEE Transactions on Magnetics* 45 (8): 3092–3099.

62 Suveren, M. and Kanaan, M. (2019). 5D magnetic localization for wireless capsule endoscopy using the Levenberg-Marquardt method and artificial bee colony algorithm. 2019 IEEE 30th International Symposium on Personal, Indoor and Mobile Radio Communications (PIMRC Workshops), 1–6.

63 Shao, G. and Guo, Y.-X. (2020). An optimal design for passive magnetic localization system based on SNR evaluation. *IEEE Transactions on Instrumentation and Measurement* 69 (7): 4324–4333. https://doi.org/10.1109/TIM.2019.2947173.

64 Li, M., Song, S., Hu, C. et al. (2010). A novel method of 6-DoF electromagnetic navigation system for surgical robot. 2010 8th IEEE World Congress on Intelligent Control and Automation, 2163–2167.

65 Hu, C., Ma, T., and Meng, M.Q.-H. (2007). Sensor arrangement optimization of magnetic localization and orientation system. 2007 IEEE International Conference on Integration Technology, 311–315.

66 Maréchal, L., Foong, S., Ding, S. et al. (2014). Optimal spatial design of non-invasive magnetic field-based localization systems. 2014 IEEE International Conference on Robotics and Automation (ICRA), 3510–3516.

67 Popek, K.M., Mahoney, A.W., and Abbott, J.J. (2013). Localization method for a magnetic capsule endoscope propelled by a rotating magnetic dipole field. 2013 IEEE International Conference on Robotics and Automation, 5348–5353.

68 Popek, K. and Abbott, J. (2015). 6-d localization of a magnetic capsule endoscope using a stationary rotating magnetic dipole field. Hamlyn Symposium on Medical Robotics, 47–48.

69 Plotkin, A. and Paperno, E. (2003). 3-D magnetic tracking of a single subminiature coil with a large 2-D array of uniaxial transmitters. *IEEE Transactions on Magnetics* 39 (5): 3295–3297.

70 Plotkin, A., Kucher, V., Horen, Y., and Paperno, E. (2008). A new calibration procedure for magnetic tracking systems. *IEEE Transactions on Magnetics* 44 (11): 4525–4528.

71 Yabukami, S. et al. (2005). Development of a position-sensing system for a wireless magnetic marker using a differential pickup coil. *Journal of the Magnetics Society of Japan* 29 (2): 146–152.

72 Hashi, S., Yabukami, S., Kanetaka, H. et al. (2011). Wireless magnetic position-sensing system using optimized pickup coils for higher accuracy. *IEEE Transactions on Magnetics* 47 (10): 3542–3545.

73 Hashi, S., Yabukami, S., Kanetaka, H. et al. (2009). Numerical study on the improvement of detection accuracy for a wireless motion capture system. *IEEE Transactions on Magnetics* 45 (6): 2736–2739.

74 Paperno, E., Sasada, I., and Leonovich, E. (2001). A new method for magnetic position and orientation tracking. *IEEE Transactions on Magnetics* 37 (4): 1938–1940.

75 Song, S., Qiao, W., Li, B. et al. (2013). An efficient magnetic tracking method using uniaxial sensing coil. *IEEE Transactions on Magnetics* 50 (1): 1–7.

76 Song, S., Hu, C., Li, B. et al. (2012). An electromagnetic localization and orientation method based on rotating magnetic dipole. *IEEE Transactions on Magnetics* 49 (3): 1274–1277.

77 Song, S., Ren, H., and Yu, H. (2014). An improved magnetic tracking method using rotating uniaxial coil with sparse points and closed form analytic solution. *IEEE Sensors Journal* 14 (10): 3585–3592.

78 Guo, X.-d., Yan, G.-z., and Jiang, P.-p. (2008). Feasibility of localizing in vivo micro-devices with electromagnetic methods. *Journal of Shanghai Jiaotong University (Science)* 13 (5): 559–561.

79 Islam, M.N. and Fleming, A.J. (2017). An algorithm for transmitter optimization in electromagnetic tracking systems. *IEEE Transactions on Magnetics* 53 (8): 1–8.

80 Islam, M.N. (2018). *Real Time Endoscope Capsule Localization Using the Electromagnetic Field Method*. University of Newcastle.

81 Khan, S.R., Pavuluri, S.K., Cummins, G., and Desmulliez, M.P. (2019). Miniaturized 3-D cross-type receiver for wirelessly powered capsule endoscopy. *IEEE Transactions on Microwave Theory and Techniques* 67 (5): 1985–1993.

82 Ryu, M., Kim, J.D., Chin, H.U. et al. (2007). Three-dimensional power receiver for in vivo robotic capsules. *Medical and Biological Engineering and Computing* 45 (10): 997–1002.

83 Basar, M.R., Ahmad, M.Y., Cho, J., and Ibrahim, F. (2016). Stable and high-efficiency wireless power transfer system for robotic capsule using a modified Helmholtz coil. *IEEE Transactions on Industrial Electronics* 64 (2): 1113–1122.

84 Pan, G. and Wang, L. (2012). Swallowable wireless capsule endoscopy: progress and technical challenges. *Gastroenterology Research and Practice* 2012.

85 Ciuti, G., Menciassi, A., and Dario, P. (2011). Capsule endoscopy: from current achievements to open challenges. *IEEE Reviews in Biomedical Engineering* 4: 59–72.

86 RamRakhyani, A.K., Mirabbasi, S., and Chiao, M. (2010). Design and optimization of resonance-based efficient wireless power delivery systems for biomedical implants. *IEEE Transactions on Biomedical Circuits and Systems* 5 (1): 48–63.

87 Kiani, M., Jow, U.-M., and Ghovanloo, M. (2011). Design and optimization of a 3-coil inductive link for efficient wireless power transmission. *IEEE Transactions on Biomedical Circuits and Systems* 5 (6): 579–591.

88 Kauczor, H.U., Ebert, M., Kreitner, K.-F.J. et al. (1997). Imaging of the lungs using 3He MRI: preliminary clinical experience in 18 patients with and without lung disease. *Journal of Magnetic Resonance Imaging* 7 (3): 538–543.

89 Plewes, D.B. and Kucharczyk, W. (2012). Physics of MRI: a primer. *Journal of Magnetic Resonance Imaging* 35 (5): 1038–1054.

90 Shao, G. and Guo, Y. (2020). Hybrid wireless positioning and charging with switched field Helmholtz coils for wireless capsule endoscopy. *IEEE Transactions on Microwave Theory and Techniques*: 1–10. https://doi.org/10.1109/TMTT.2019.2959762.

91 Lee, Y.U., Kim, J.D., Ryu, M., and Kim, J. (2006). In vivo robotic capsules: determination of the number of turns of its power receiving coil. *Medical and Biological Engineering and Computing* 44 (12): 1121–1125.

92 Kurschner, D., Rathge, C., and Jumar, U. (2011). Design methodology for high efficient inductive power transfer systems with high coil positioning flexibility. *IEEE Transactions on Industrial Electronics* 60 (1): 372–381.

93 International Commission on Non-Ionizing Radiation Protection (2010). Guidelines for limiting exposure to time-varying electric and magnetic fields (1 Hz to 100 kHz). *Health Physics* 99 (6): 818–836.

94 Guideline, I. (1998). Guidelines for limiting exposure to time-varying electric, magnetic, and electromagnetic fields (up to 300 GHz). *Health Physics* 74 (4): 494–522.

7

Study on Channel Characteristics and Performance of Liver-Implanted Wireless Communications

Pongphan Leelatien[1], Koichi Ito[2] and Kazuyuki Saito[2]

[1] *Department of Electrical and Computer Engineering, Faculty of Engineering, Thammasat University, Pathumthani, Thailand*
[2] *Center for Frontier Medical Engineering, Chiba University, Chiba, Japan*

7.1 Introduction

Recently, many studies on wireless communications for in-body scenarios have been presented because of their various potential applications especially for medical telemetry [1–18]. The wireless implanted devices for medical telemetry, which allow the measurement of body parameters from a distance, are viewed to be a promising solution to accommodate the need for the healthcare system improvements [19, 20]. These implanted devices have functions of monitoring, processing, and transmitting a person's or a patient's physiological data to an exterior monitoring or control device at the medical centers, contributing to the advances of medical diagnoses and treatments. One attractive application of wireless medical telemetry using implanted devices is the transplanted organs monitoring.

Transplantation of organs has now become a typical part of medical procedures, and the most commonly transplanted organs include liver, heart, and kidney [21]. Particularly, due to the progress in the medical area, liver transplantation has been widely accepted to be an effective therapy for end-stage liver diseases [22–26]. Nevertheless, even though liver transplant is being performed increasingly more than before, the availability of donated organs is still limited. Consequently, minimizing the rate of liver transplantation failure is very crucial as it is reported that the failure rate is highest within the two weeks immediately after operation [21]. Currently, the standard methods for posttransplant monitoring, for instance, daily blood test and tissue biopsy examinations, do not enable immediate interventions and prompt complication detections [27]. A liver-implanted wireless monitoring system can be a practical approach to this issue by allowing efficient monitoring in

Antenna and Sensor Technologies in Modern Medical Applications,
First Edition. Edited by Yahya Rahmat-Samii and Erdem Topsakal.

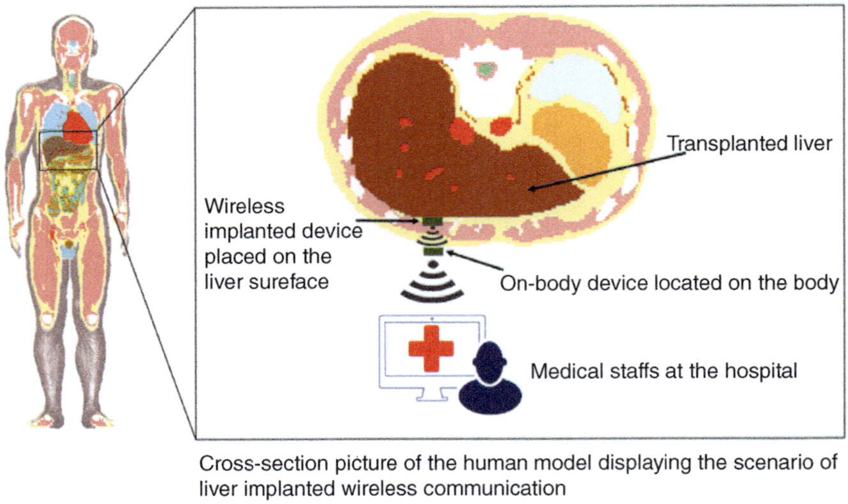

Figure 7.1 An overview of the liver-implanted wireless monitoring system.

a real-time and continuous manner, which leads to timely detections before serious damage occurs to the graft, which can contribute to reductions of organ failure and mortality [27]. In addition, the need to remove implanted devices will become unnecessary due to the use of biodegradable materials in the future. This eventually reduces the risk of the user.

Figure 7.1 presents an overview of a wireless monitoring system for liver implant in a use-case scenario. An in-body wireless device is placed on the graft surface. This application permits the monitoring of physiological conditions such as hepatic perfusion and oxygenation levels, the risk indicators of a transplanted liver [27], and the data transmission from an implantable/in-body device to an on-body/exterior device. Acting as a transmission hub, this on-body/exterior device then wirelessly transfers the data to devices of patients and medical staff and servers of healthcare service providers. This application can offer monitoring that reports the physiological state of a patient to medical staff in a real-time manner [21].

To design such wireless implanted telemetry systems, it is important to consider the operating frequency band for facilitating the telemetry link between the implanted device and the exterior hub. This type of communication commonly utilizes medical implant communication service (MICS) and industrial, scientific, and medical (ISM) radio bands, for example [28–30]. The MICS band is allocated for implanted communication and operates in a frequency range from 402 to 405 MHz in many countries [31–34]. Compared with other higher frequency bands, this frequency band has lower signal attenuation. Nevertheless, to alleviate interferences in this same frequency band, it has to transmit at a very low maximum transmit power as 25 μW equivalent isotropic radiated power (EIRP). Its maximum bandwidth including both the uplink and downlink bandwidths is 300 kHz; thus, it is difficult to transmit at a high data rate.

The ISM band is widely used for ISM purposes as its name suggests [35–41]. For body area network communications, the band consists of the 430-MHz and the 2.4-GHz bands. This band accommodates high data rate applications and can be used globally. While it is subjected to local authorizations, licenses are not required for the ISM band at power levels of up to 1 W. Nonetheless, possible interferences cannot be ignored because despite its original frequency allocation, many other wireless technologies, for instance, Bluetooth, Wi-Fi, and wireless local area network (WLAN), operate at ISM band in recent years, leading to transmission problems such as false activation, link unavailability, and data corruption, subsequently making them less attractive for medical applications requiring high fidelity [20].

Ultra-wideband (UWB) technology is considered by many pieces of research as a favorable option for in-body wireless communication [28, 42–46]. This band allocates the frequency between 3.1 and 10.6 GHz. As, at present, the data rate of wireless medical devices for implanted applications is very low compared with those of other wireless communication systems, various works have reported the feasibility to use UWB technology which offers transmissions at a high data rate [47]. Not only for medical telemetry applications, but its potential high data rate transmission can also encourage many applications in the medical domain including implantable drug delivery [48] and microrobots for in-body biopsy and treatment procedures [49]. Additionally, because of the high-frequency level, the size of an antenna can be considerably reduced. Its wide available bandwidth allows a transmission at high data rate and also a good time resolution which is fit for healthcare monitoring [50]. With the combination of the recent progress in electronic circuits, the low complexity of UWB system can further enhance device miniaturization [42, 51–53]. Furthermore, device longevity can be increased due to its low power consumption feature. Besides, UWB signal is noise-like because the transmitted signal has low energy density and pseudorandom characteristics. Subsequently, the transmission using UWB technology does not introduce severe interference to other communication systems [54]. Although these characteristics of UWB are appealing for WBAN applications, its signal is susceptible to a strong attenuation for an in-body communication scenario. This consequently leads to system performance degradation, and accomplishing effective in-body wireless communications at UWB frequency range becomes difficult. Therefore, a comprehensive knowledge of the channel characteristics at the UWB range is important to implement reliable wireless communication links.

Modeling the in-body communication channel is extremely challenging because of the involvement of different tissues and organs inside the human body having different dielectric properties, the lossy environment, and the non-line-of-sight propagation condition [20]. The characteristics of the in-body propagation channel greatly depend on the implant location since channels involve different organs and tissues, thus causing variations in the channel characteristics. Channel characteristics for the in-body scenario at UWB range in different locations have been reported in various researches, for instance, in the chest [55], brain [56], and torso [53, 57]. Nevertheless, to the best of the authors' knowledge, no report of liver-to-skin propagation channels at UWB range is presented in the open literature.

In this study, the liver-implanted channel characteristics at UWB range are presented with path loss (PL) models and also the assessment of system performance. To begin with, as the first attempt to gain understanding of the liver-implanted channel, measurements and simulations were performed using simplified multilayer semisolid phantoms. We present and discuss frequency-dependent channel characteristics for the in-body communication case scenario to analyze the attenuation characteristics of the liver-implanted channel. Then, numerical investigations on the liver-implanted channel characteristics were carried out via simulations using two digital human models, male and female, taking into account of various factors, for example, the influence of organ movements due to human breathing, the effect of body size and composition, the misalignment of antennas, and communications in off-body scenarios. Numerical results including PL data and PL model will be derived and analyzed accordingly. Subsequently, based on the obtained PL information, the performance of the communication system will be evaluated for two common in-body communication scenarios, i.e. in-body to on-body (IN2ON) and in-body to off-body (IN2OFF) scenarios, by means of link budget evaluation considering various parameters such as system margins, communication distance, and data rate.

7.2 Study of In-Body Communications at Liver Area Using Simplified Multilayer Phantoms

In this part of our study, measurements and simulations were performed using simplified multilayer human-equivalent semisolid phantoms at UWB range as a first step to characterize liver-implanted channel [58]. We derived frequency-dependent attenuation characteristics as well as evaluated the possibility of liver-implanted wireless communications at the UWB frequency range. For this, we developed simplified multilayer human-equivalent semisolid phantoms that consisted of fat, muscle, and liver to represent a part of the internal structure of the human body for the study of wireless communications for in-body scenario via both experimental measurements and simulations.

7.2.1 UWB Antenna

In our investigation of the liver-implanted channels, both measurements and simulations were conducted at 4.5–6.5 GHz using a compact and lightweight tapered-slot UWB antenna which is 1.25-mm thick [59] as in- and on-body antennas. This antenna was fabricated in the Antenna Measurement Laboratory at Queen Mary University of London.

7.2.2 Measurement Setup

For the in-body communication scenario, a body can be viewed approximately as a multilayer structure. Consequently, a simplified multilayer phantom model is deployed to mimick a part of the human internal structure. These human-equivalent semisolid UWB phantoms consisted of fat, muscle, and liver tissues, the main tissues and organs involving in the propagation path as shown in Figure 7.2. Skin tissue was neglected for simplicity, because, as discussed in [60], using a homogeneous phantom can accomplish similar results of antenna performances to that of using multilayer phantoms. The overall phantom size was roughly 180 mm × 120 mm × 90 mm. The thicknesses of the fat, muscle, and liver layers of the phantom were 20, 25, and 45 mm, respectively. The compositions of fat, muscle, and liver phantoms are provided in Tables 7.1–7.3, respectively. The dielectric properties of the measurement phantoms are shown in Figures 7.3 and 7.4. It can be observed that there are good agreements with the values reported in [61] over the considered frequency range. The measurement setup consisted of the two UWB antennas, a vector network analyzer (VNA), two coaxial cables connecting each antenna to Port 1 and Port 2 of the VNA, and the human-equivalent semisolid UWB phantom. The output power of the VNA was set to 10 dBm. Measurements were performed within 3–10 GHz, with $N = 12\,602$ frequency points. The presented results are within 4.5–6.5 GHz. The resolution bandwidth was 20 kHz. The noise level was −100 dB. Consequently, S-parameter results were recorded for different separation gaps between both the antennas. The in-body antenna was placed on the liver surface under the muscle layer at a fixed position, and the location of the on-body antenna placed directly on the fat layer was changed from its beginning position (0 mm) along the x-axis up to the ending position (80 mm) in steps of 20 mm for each measurement.

7.2.3 Simulation Setup

Simulations were done in order to validate the measured results. The simulation model of a simplified human-equivalent flat phantom consisting of fat, muscle, and liver tissues was developed as seen in Figure 7.5. The dielectric properties of the tissues derived from the CST Microwave Studio Material

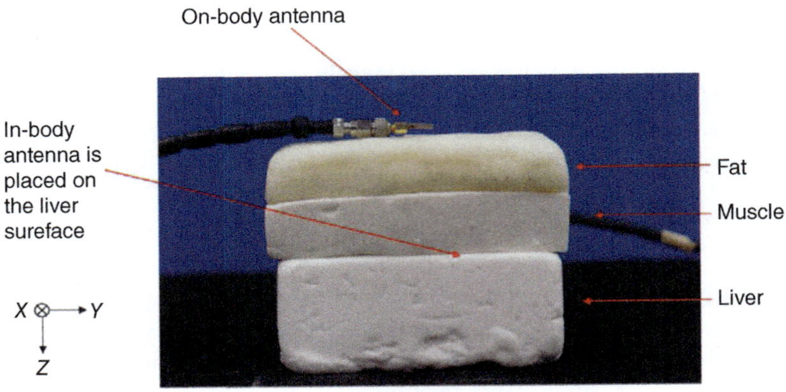

Figure 7.2 Measurement setup with the on-body antenna, the in-body antenna, and the multilayer phantom consisting of fat, muscle, and liver layers.

Table 7.1 Recipe for the fat phantom.

Ingredient	Amount (g)
Deionized water	40
Agar	27
Glycerin	40
Oil	300
Silicone	200
Polyethylene powder	400

Table 7.2 Recipe for the muscle phantom.

Ingredient	Amount (g)
Deionized water	3375.0
Agar	104.6
Sodium chloride (NaCl)	16.3
Sodium dehydroacetate	2.0
TX-151	83.3
Polyethylene powder	337.5

Table 7.3 Recipe for the liver phantom.

Ingredient	Amount (g)
Deionized water	3375.0
Agar	104.6
Sodium chloride (NaCl)	27.2
Sodium dehydroacetate	2.0
TX-151	45.6
Polyethylene powder	675

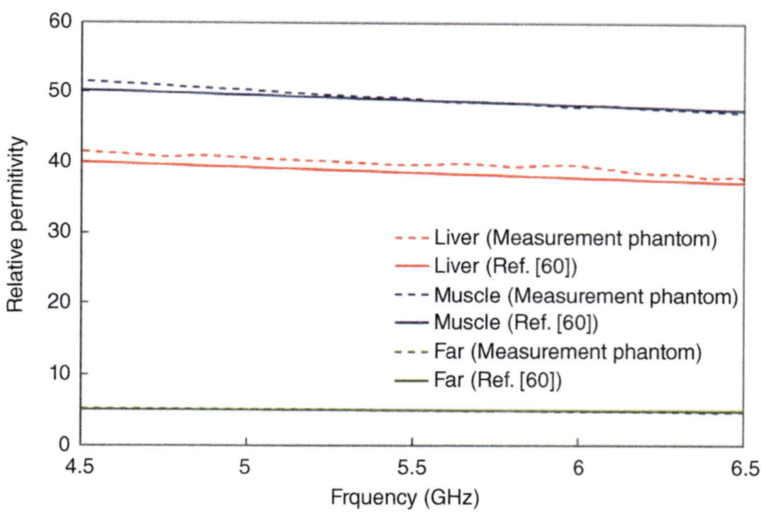

Figure 7.3 Permittivity of human tissues (muscle, liver, and fat) [61] and phantoms used in the measurements. (*Source*: Leelatien, P., Ito, K., Saito, K., et al., 2018. © IEEE.)

Library corresponded with the precise values of the tissues based on the work of Gabriel [61]. The skin layer was also neglected here for simplicity purposes. The overall phantom size was 180 mm × 120 mm × 70 mm. For the reduction of the computation time, the thickness of the liver tissue in the simulations was reduced from 45 mm used for the measurements to 20 mm, because this thickness difference did not lead to any major change in the simulated results. Furthermore, the thickness of the muscle layer in the simulation was set to 30 mm in order to accomplish the same 45 mm separation between the in-body antenna and the surface of the fat layer as in the measurement setup. Then, *S*-parameter results for various gaps between the antennas were obtained. The same approach as in the measurements was adopted here, i.e. the antenna (referred to as the in-body antenna) was kept fixed on the liver surface inside

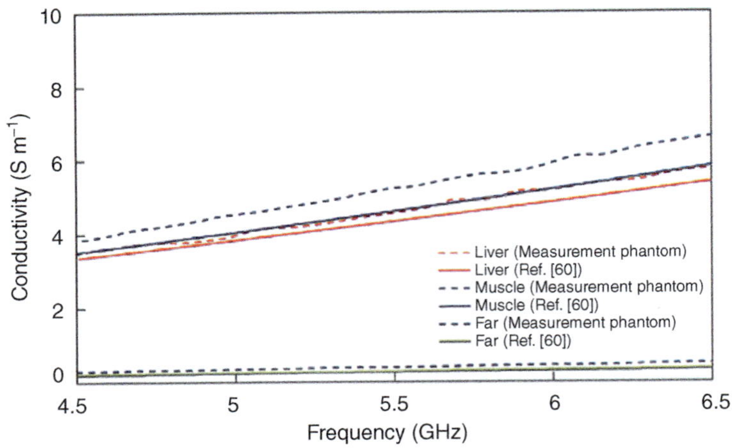

Figure 7.4 Conductivity of human tissues (muscle, liver, and fat) [61] and phantoms used in the measurements. (*Source*: Leelatien, P., Ito, K., Saito, K., et al., 2018. © IEEE.)

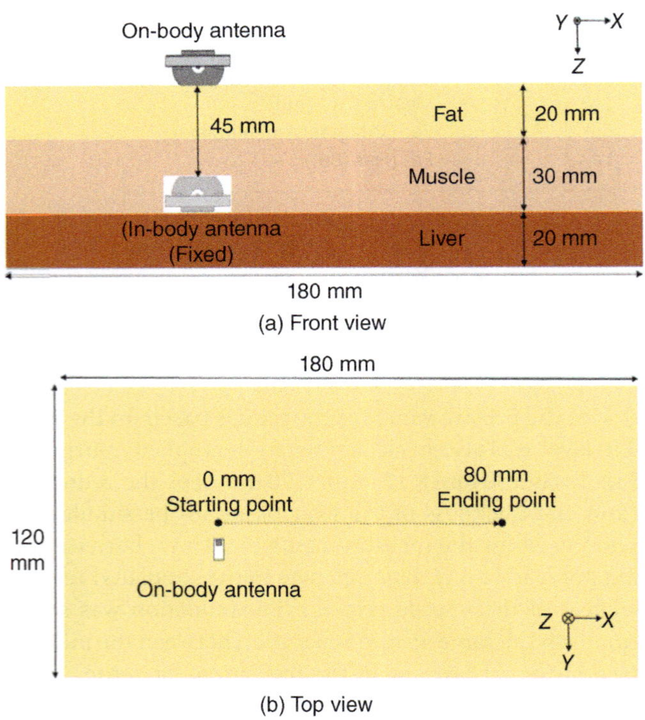

Figure 7.5 Simulation setup with the on-body antenna, the in-body antenna, and the multilayer phantom consisted of fat, muscle, and liver layers. (*Source*: Leelatien, P., Ito, K., Saito, K., et al., 2018. © IEEE.)

the muscle layer, and the antenna (referred to as the on-body antenna) placed directly on the fat layer was moved along the x-axis from its initial position (0 mm) by 20 mm up to the last position (80 mm). Both the antennas were aligned in a face-to-face direction as illustrated in Figure 7.5.

7.2.4 Experimental and Numerical Results

7.2.4.1 S_{11} and S_{22} Results

S_{11} results of the on-body antenna and S_{22} results of the in-body antenna were obtained within 4.5 and 6.5 GHz band as illustrated in Figure 7.6. It can be noticed that both the antennas exhibited acceptable performances, i.e. S_{11} and S_{22} were approximately below −10 dB over the considered band. It should be pointed out that when using inside the phantom in the experiment, since the antennas were designed for the on-body use case, there could be a mismatch in the antenna impedance and the cables.

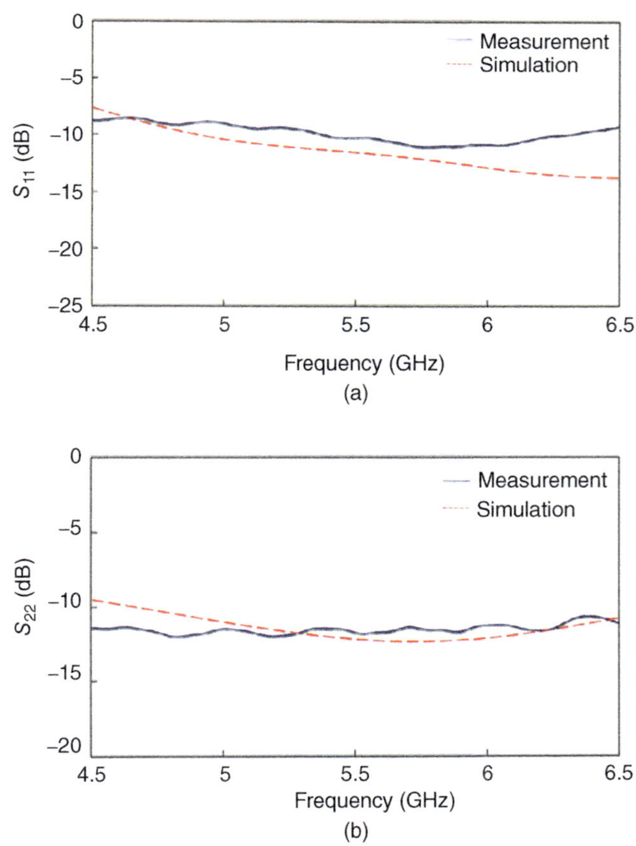

Figure 7.6 (a) S_{11} results of the on-body antenna and (b) S_{22} results of the in-body antenna within the 4.5–6.5 GHz band. (*Source*: Leelatien, P., Ito, K., Saito, K., et al., 2018. © IEEE.)

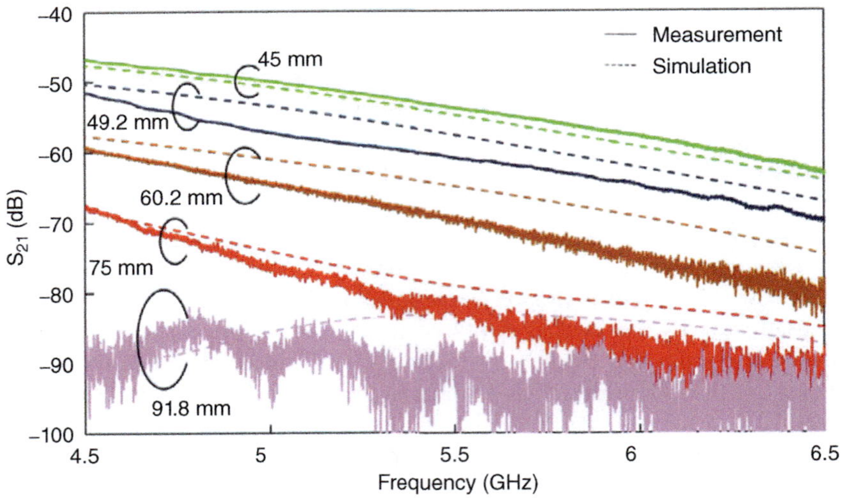

Figure 7.7 Measured and simulated S_{21} results for various separation gaps between the in- and on-body antennas within the 4.5–6.5 GHz range. (*Source*: Leelatien, P., Ito, K., Saito, K., et al., 2018. © IEEE.)

7.2.4.2 S_{21} Results

To investigate the characteristics of signal attenuation inside the human body, the S_{21} results are displayed in Figure 7.7 versus frequency for various separation distances between the on- and in-body antennas. The attenuation varied roughly between −50 and −100 dB within the 4.5–6.5 GHz frequency band. The results suggest that despite the separation distances, the magnitude of S_{21} decreases with the increase in frequency. In addition, it is observed that the S_{21} decays nearly linearly as the frequency increases, for the distance up to 75 mm. Moreover, as reported in [43], it can be observed that the S_{21} decays at an increasing rate when the antenna separation distance is increased. For example, considering the measured results at the 45-mm distance, the S_{21} decays approximately from −47 dB at 4.5 GHz to −64 dB at 6.5 GHz. This equals attenuation of 17 dB. Likewise, considering the S_{21} at the 60.2-mm distance, it decays from roughly −60 dB at 4.5 GHz to −81 dB at 6.5 GHz, representing 21 dB of attenuation.

7.3 Numerical Study of Liver-Implanted Channel Characteristics Using Digital Human Models

Channel model depends on many aspects, for example, size and shape of the human body, propagation environments, and antenna configurations. Hence, our objective in this part is to gain understanding of the liver-implanted channel characteristics at UWB frequency band for wireless communications taking into account various aspects including the influence of the movements of internal organs caused by human breathing [58, 62], human individuality [62], and antenna alignments under more realistic environments. Here, we used two digital human models of male and female named Taro (height: 173.2 cm, weight: 65 kg, body mass index: 21.7) and Hanako (height: 160.8 cm, weight: 53 kg, body mass index: 20.4) developed by the National Institute of Information and Communication Technology (NICT) [63]. The frequency range considered here was from 4.5 to 6.5 GHz. The simulations were carried out utilizing CST Microwave Studio software.

7.3.1 Simulation Setup

The same UWB antenna developed by Queen Mary University of London [59] and used in the previous section was also used as in- and on-body antennas here. The antenna was put in a rectangular case to have part of the antenna covered in the liver tissue-equivalent material as displayed in Figure 7.8 for the improvement of the impedance-matching characteristics of the antenna. The dimensions of this case were 14.9 mm × 23.4 mm × 10.7 mm. Its thickness was 0.5 mm.

As seen in Figure 7.9, the location of the in-body antenna was set on the liver surface at 31.5 mm from the front skin surface and 44 mm from the left-side skin surface in the Taro male model. For the Hanako female model case, the in-body antenna was kept at the fixed location on the liver surface, 24 mm from the front skin surface and 74 mm from the left side skin surface as presented in Figure 7.10. Subsequently, for both model case scenarios, with the in-body antenna remained in the same position, the on-body antenna (placed on the skin surface) was relocated horizontally by 20 mm along the reference line to the endpoint at the 80-mm distance. Consequently, we collected S-parameter

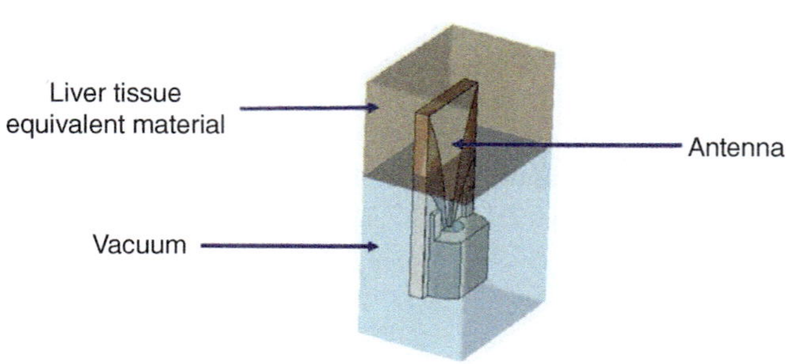

Figure 7.8 The UWB antenna covered by a material mimicking liver tissue inserted in a rectangular case. (*Source:* Based on Sharma, M., Parini, C. G., and Alomainy, A., 2014.)

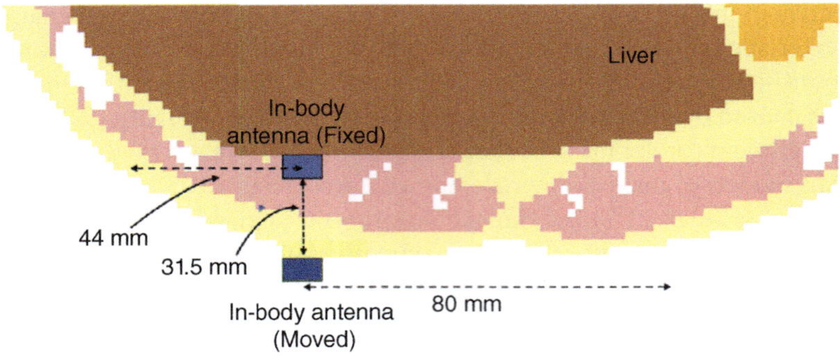

Figure 7.9 Cross-sectional view of the Taro model sliced at a height of 1170 mm (as shown in Figure 7.11), displaying locations of the on- and in-body antennas in the simulation setup. (*Source*: Leelatien, P., Ito, K., Saito, K., et al., 2018. © IEEE.)

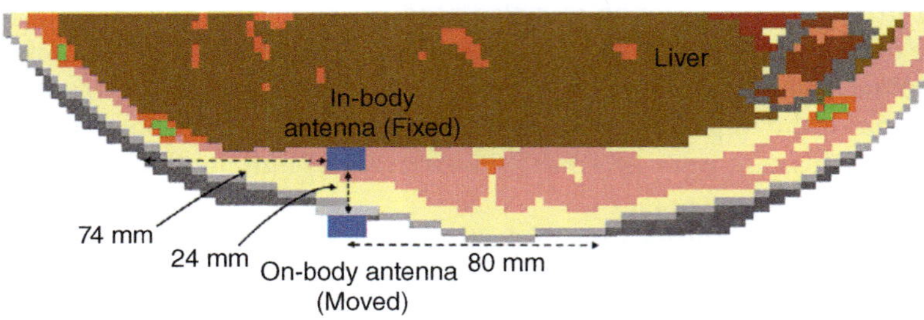

Figure 7.10 Cross-sectional view of the Hanako model sliced at a height of 1116 mm (as shown in Figure 7.12), displaying locations of the on- and in-body antennas in the simulation setup.

results at various separation distances between the two antennas. The liver movement during normal breathing is found to be approximately 40 mm at maximum in the craniocaudal direction [64]. Thus, to study the impact of the internal organ movement, the same methods were repeated up to the 40-mm distance above and below the reference line in vertical direction. Numerical S-parameter results were obtained for both horizontal and vertical orientations of the in- and on-body antennas. A total of 25 locations of the on-body antenna considered here are displayed in Figures 7.11 and 7.12 for the Taro and Hanako models, respectively.

7.3.2 Return Loss Results

The return loss curves of the in- and on-body antennas for both Taro and Hanako case scenarios are shown in Figures 7.13 and 7.14, respectively, within

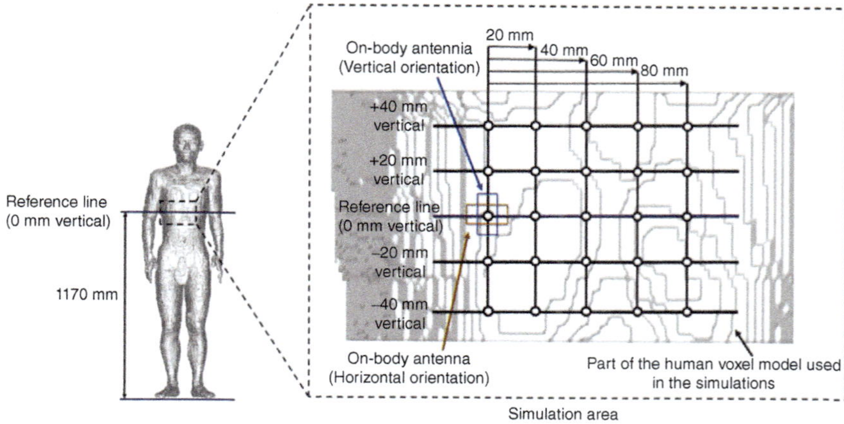

Figure 7.11 3-D model of Taro displaying simulation area and all on-body antenna locations.

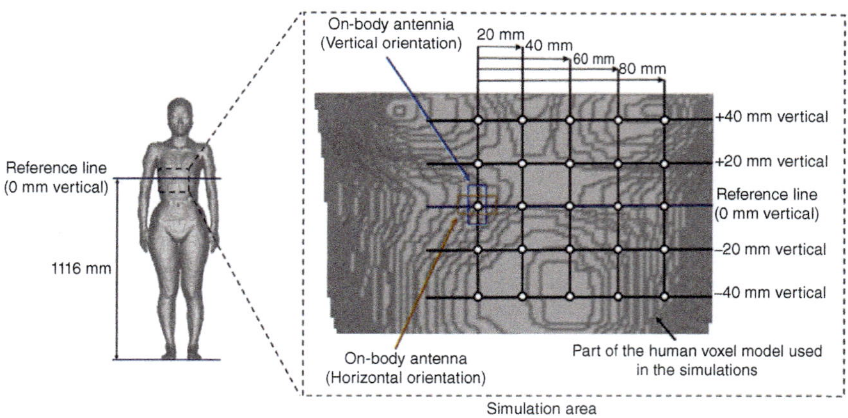

Figure 7.12 3-D model of Hanako displaying simulation area and all on-body antenna locations.

the 4.5–6.5 GHz band. It is noticed that even though the return loss curves of the antennas are different for each model, both antennas still have good performances in the considered band. The discrepancies in the results in the case of the in-body antennas could be due to the diversity of the surrounding tissues. In the on-body antenna case, the variations of the results could be because of the shape differences between the male and female bodies considering that the body of female has more curvatures compared to the male body.

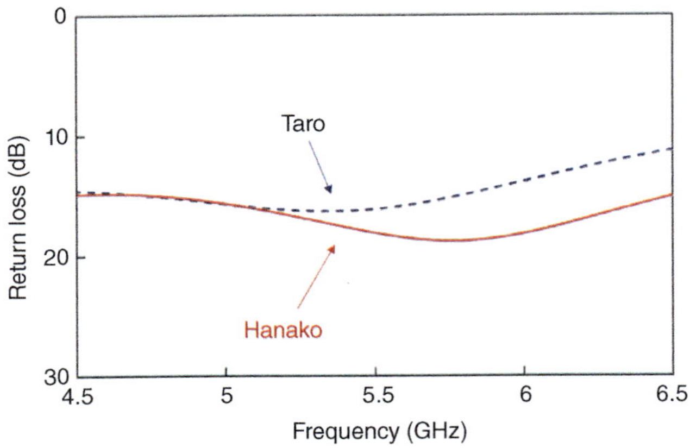

Figure 7.13 Return loss results of the in-body antennas within the 4.5–6.5 GHz band for the Taro and Hanako models.

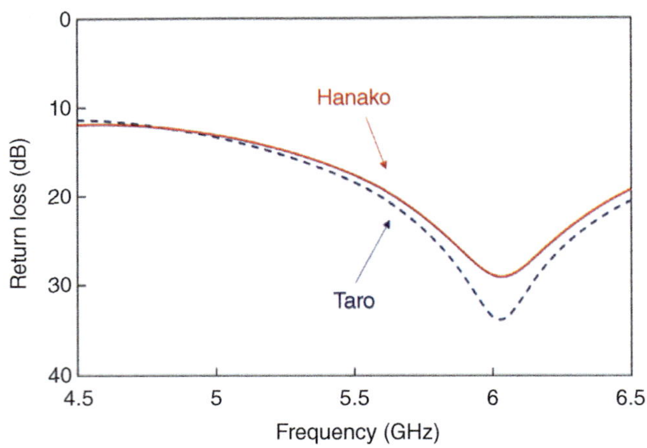

Figure 7.14 Return loss results of the on-body antennas within the 4.5–6.5 GHz band for the Taro and Hanako models.

7.3.3 S_{21} Results

S_{21} results as a function of the on-body antenna movement distance in horizontal direction from the initial position at various points along the vertical axis for the Taro and Hanako model case scenarios are displayed, respectively, in Figures 7.15 and 7.16. The fluctuation of S_{21} results along the vertical axis indicates that the movements of internal organs affected the signal attenuation characteristics for the in-body propagation scenario. It can be observed that the deviation range of attenuation is roughly 30 dB at maximum for both model scenarios. The results highlight the important insight on the variations of signal attenuations caused by the organ movements.

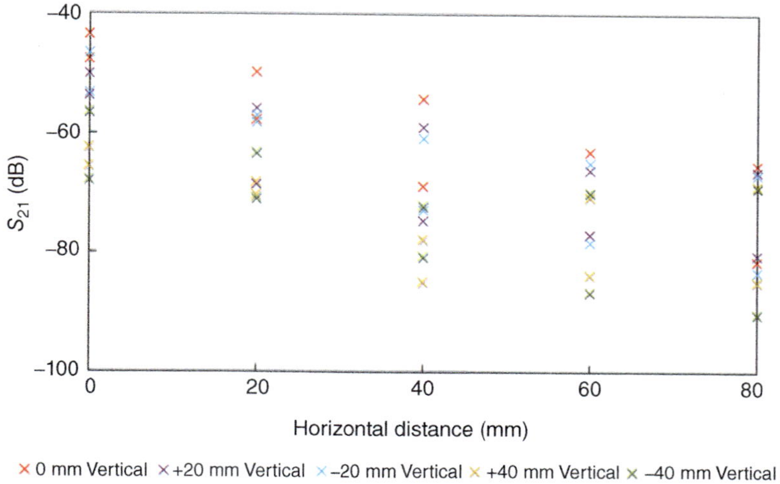

Figure 7.15 S_{21} results as a function of horizontal movement distance of the on-body antenna from its initial position at different locations on vertical axis for the Taro model scenario. (*Source*: Leelatien, P., Ito, K., Saito, K., et al., 2018. © IEEE.)

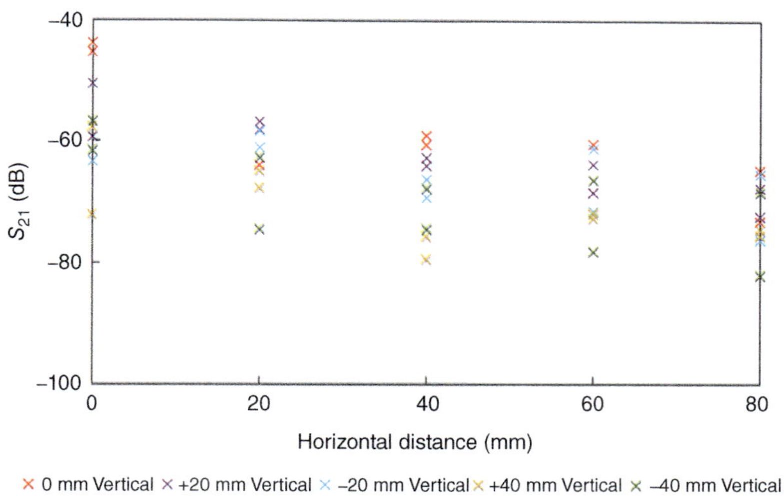

Figure 7.16 S_{21} results as a function of horizontal movement distance of the on-body antenna from its initial position at different locations on vertical axis for the Hanako model scenario.

7.3.4 Path Loss Results

The PL data for both model scenarios were consequently processed from the obtained S_{21} data, as $PL_{dB} = -|S_{21}|$ in decibels. Thereafter, the PL model as a function of the propagation distance was derived using the technique of least-squares fitting. The fitted line for the PL model was applied using Equation (7.1). The PL data is then presented in Figure 7.17 as a function of the logarithmic propagation distances and its linear fitted curve. Table 7.4 shows the corresponding PL parameters calculated for the reference implant depth, d_0. n is the PL exponent indicating the rate of attenuation in the communication environment. S is the shadowing factor that shows the PL variations from the average PL. It is a normally distributed statistical variable with a zero-mean and standard deviation, σ_{dB}.

Overall, the PL is lower in the Hanako model case compared to the PL in the Taro model case. This could be because the female body normally has more low-loss tissues such as fat (its conductivity is 0.21 S m^{-1} at 4.5 GHz), while the male body normally has more high-loss tissues such as muscle (its conductivity is 3.51 S m^{-1} at 4.5 GHz).

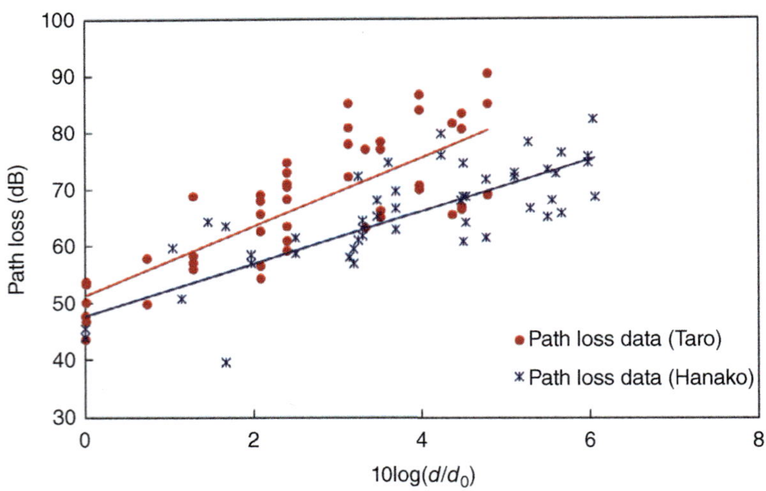

Figure 7.17 Path loss results of Taro and Hanako models vs the logarithmic in- and on-body antenna separation distances. (*Source*: Modified from Leelatien, P., Ito, K., Saito, K., et al., 2018.)

Table 7.4 Path loss parameters for the Taro and Hanako model case scenarios

	d_0 (mm)	PL_0 (dB)	n	σ (dB)
Taro	31.5	51.3	6.1	7.1
Hanako	24	47.7	4.6	6.1

Figures 7.18 and 7.19 show that the normal distribution employed in Equation (7.1) is valid. It is observed that the deviation of the PL is roughly within a range of 7 and 5 dB for the Taro and Hanako cases, respectively. These

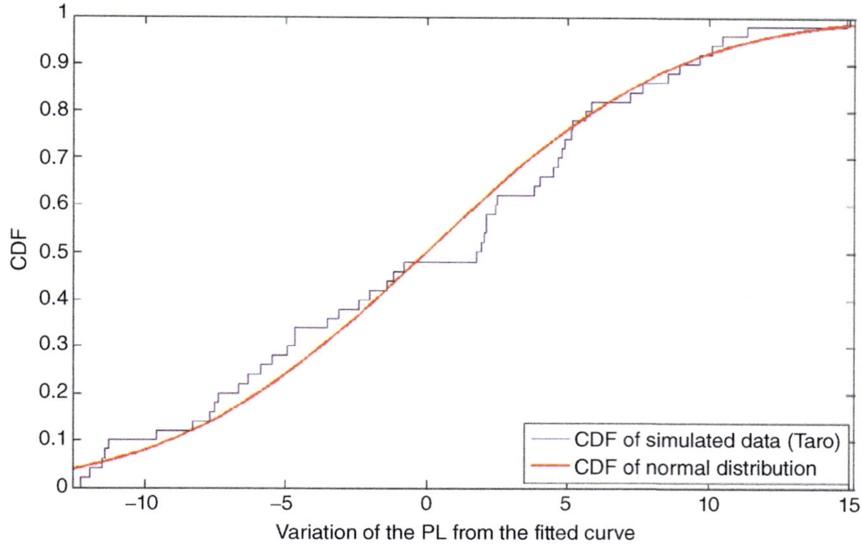

Figure 7.18 CDF of the scattering data for the Taro model case fitted to the normal distribution for the Taro model scenario.

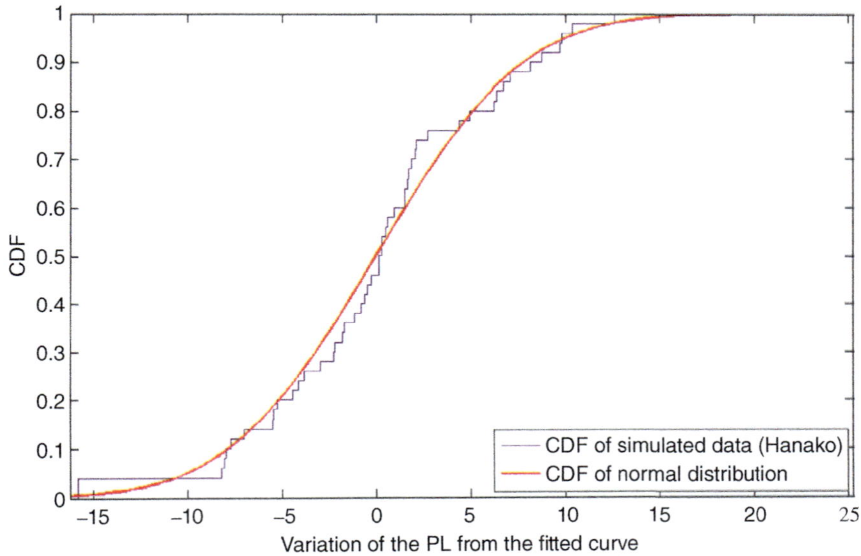

Figure 7.19 CDF of the scattering data for the Hanako model case fitted to the normal distribution.

deviations are caused by the differences of dielectric properties of organs and tissues located along the path of the propagation. It is noticed that the shadowing factor of the Hanako model case is less than that of the Taro model case. This could be attributed to the fact that the body of the Hanako model is smaller; thus, the area around the liver is more compact compared to the Taro model case.

$$PL_{dB}(d) = PL_{0,dB} + 10n\log_{10}\left(\frac{d}{d_0}\right) + S_{dB} \tag{7.1}$$

7.4 The Influence of Antenna Misalignment

In this part, Taro and Hanako digital models were used in our investigation on the effect of antenna misalignment on channel characteristics for liver-implanted wireless communication. The frequency band from 4.5 to 6.5 GHz was considered here. The simulations here were carried out using CST Microwave Studio software.

7.4.1 Simulation Setup

Similar to the earlier parts, we utilized the same UWB antenna manufactured by Queen Mary University of London as in- and on-body antennas and both digital human models of male (Taro) and female (Hanako) [59] in the study. However, different from the configurations in the previous investigation, the antennas were set in the opposite orientations to assess the effect of antenna misalignment, as seen in Figures 7.20 and 7.21 for the Taro model case (the antennas were also applied the same configuration for the Hanako model case), i.e.

1) horizontal-oriented in-body antenna and vertical-oriented on-body antenna
2) vertical-oriented in-body antenna and horizontal-oriented on-body antenna

Consequently, we adopted the same approach as we used previously to both model cases and collected numerical S-parameter results at different gaps between the in- and on-body antennas. Consequently, the PL was calculated by processing the simulated S_{21} data as $PL = -|S_{21}|$ in decibels.

7.4.2 Study Results and Analysis

The PL results of the antennas in alignment scenario collected previously and those of the antenna misalignment scenario for the Taro and Hanako model scenarios are compared and displayed in Figures 7.22 and 7.23, respectively. Figures 7.24 and 7.25 show the probability density function (PDF) for the Taro

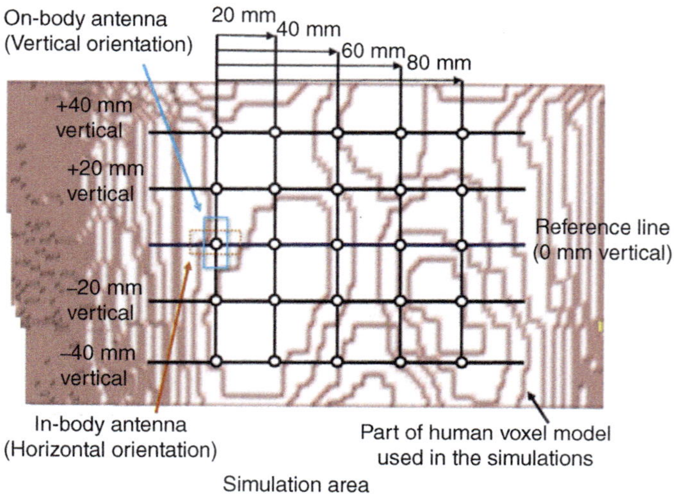

Figure 7.20 Part of Taro model displaying simulation area and all on-body antenna locations for the vertical-oriented on-body antenna and the horizontal-oriented in-body antenna scenario. (*Source*: Leelatien, P., Ito, K., Saito, K., et al., 2018. © IEEE.)

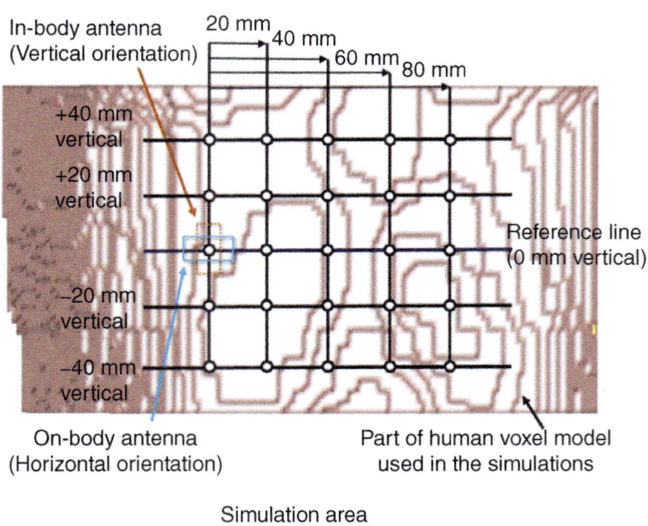

Figure 7.21 Part of Taro model displaying simulation area and all on-body antenna locations for the horizontal-oriented on-body antenna and the vertical-oriented in-body antenna scenario. (*Source*: Leelatien, P., Ito, K., Saito, K., et al., 2018. © IEEE.)

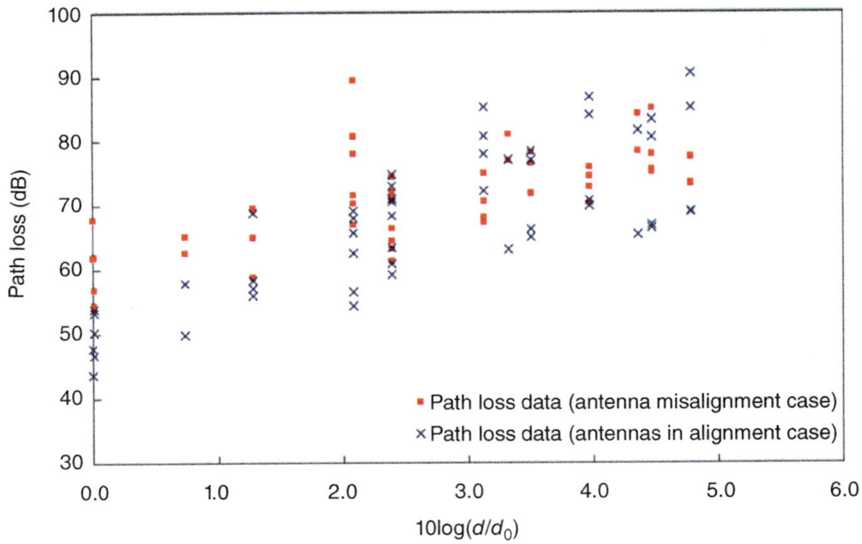

Figure 7.22 Path loss data of the simulated channel versus the logarithmic in- and on-body antenna separation distance comparing between the antenna misalignment case and the antennas in alignment case for the Taro model case.

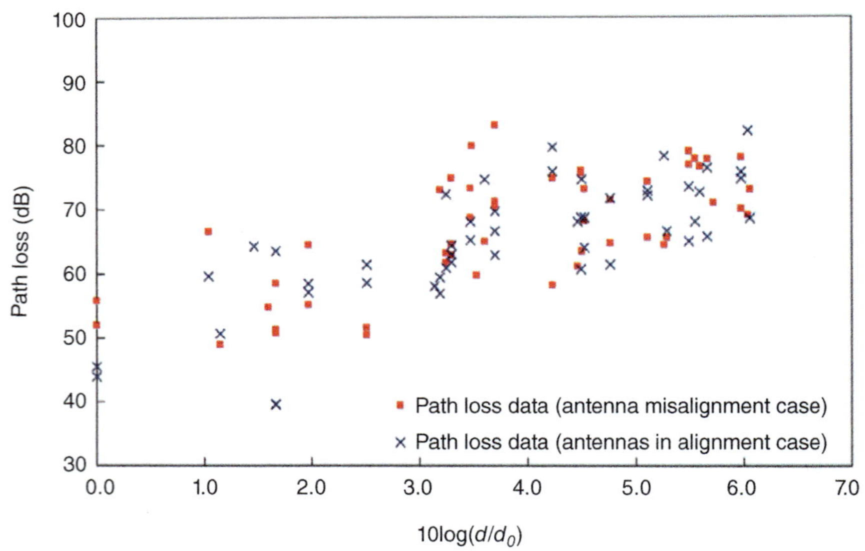

Figure 7.23 Path loss data of the simulated channel versus the logarithmic in- and on-body antenna separation distance comparing between the antenna misalignment case and the antennas in alignment case for the Hanako model case.

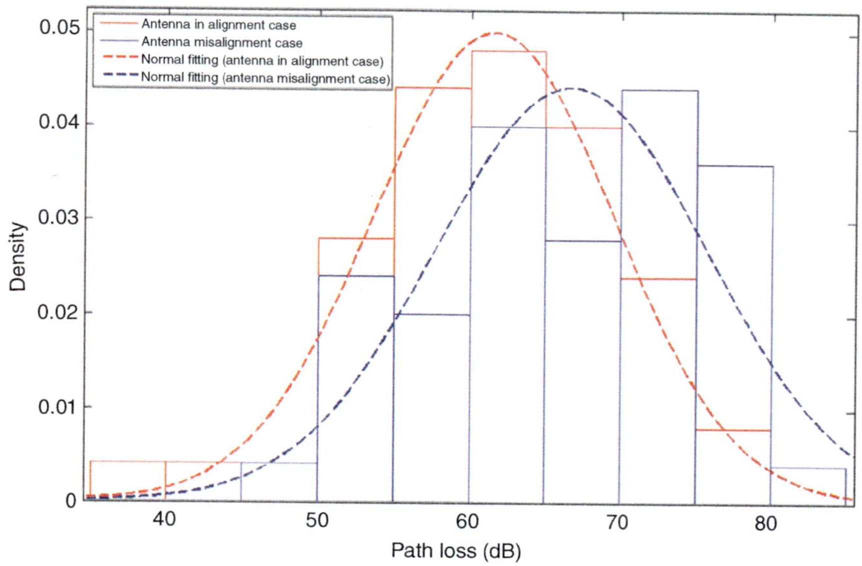

Figure 7.24 PDF of the path loss data for the Taro model case comparing between antennas in alignment scenario and antenna misalignment scenario.

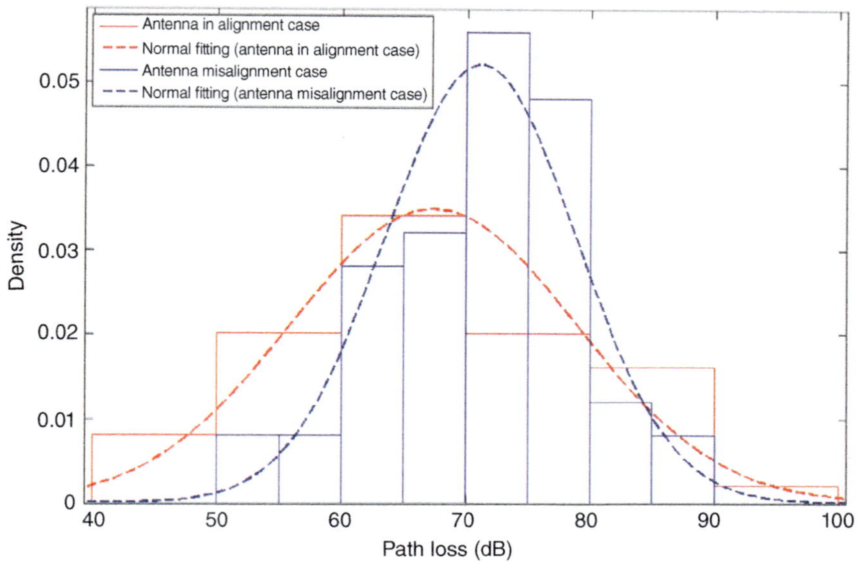

Figure 7.25 PDF of the path loss data for the Hanako model case comparing between antennas in alignment scenario and antenna misalignment scenario.

and Hanako cases correspondingly. It is observed that in antenna misalignment case, the mean PL is higher than the mean PL in the case of antenna in alignment for both model case scenarios by roughly 5 dB. Furthermore, it is noticeable that most PL data in the case of antenna misalignments are between 63 and 80 dB in the Taro case and between 53 and 78 dB in the Hanako case, which are slightly higher than the overall PL data in the case of antennas in alignment.

7.5 Channel Characteristics for the In- to Off-Body Scenario

Our studies so far were for the IN2ON communication scenario. However, in practice, an on-body device may not need to be attached to the skin surface directly, but it may also be placed on clothes, for instance. Therefore, the communication scenario will become an IN2OFF communication scenario as there would be some gaps between an on-body device and skin surface [62]. Subsequently, this would contribute to an increase in signal attenuations.

7.5.1 Simulation Setup

The on-body antenna was located at the off-body distance (d_{off}) = 2 and 5 mm separated from the skin surface in this IN2OFF communication scenario. On the other hand, the in-body antenna was fixed at the liver surface at the same location as of the setup in the previous sections, as illustrated in Figures 7.26 and 7.27 for both Taro and Hanako model cases, respectively. Similarly, the on-body antenna was relocated by 20 mm in the horizontal direction along

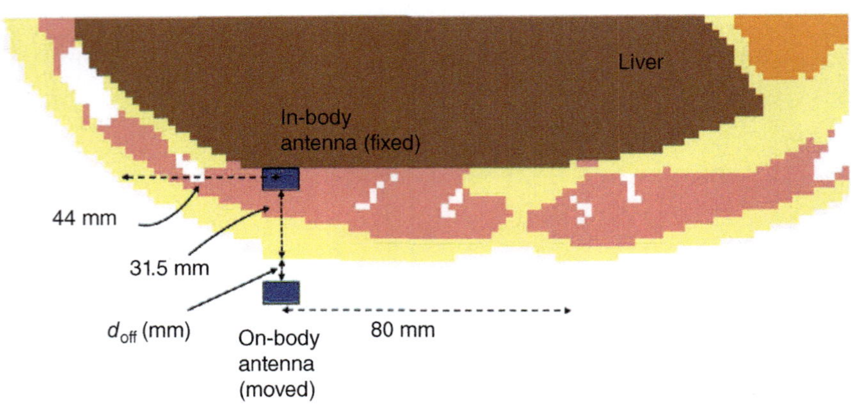

Figure 7.26 Cross-sectional view of the Taro model sliced at a height of 1170 mm (as illustrated in Figure 7.11), showing the on- and in-body antenna positions in the IN2OFF simulation setup where two scenarios of d_{off} (distance from the skin surface) = 2 and 5 mm were configured.

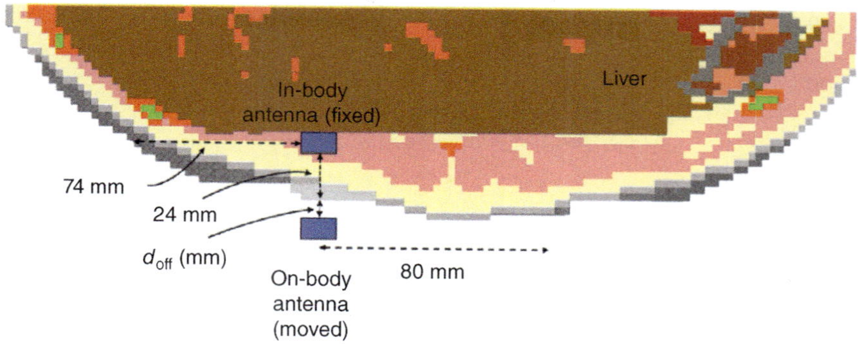

Figure 7.27 Cross-sectional view of the Hanako model sliced at a height of 1170 mm (as illustrated in Figure 7.12), showing the on- and in-body antenna positions in the IN2OFF simulation setup where two scenarios of d_{off} (distance from the skin surface) = 2 and 5 mm were configured.

the reference line up to the 80-mm distance and also above and below the reference line in the vertical direction up to the 40-mm distance, as displayed in Figures 7.11 (Taro case) and 7.12 (Hanako case). Thereafter, *S*-parameter data were collected at different positions of the on-body antenna.

7.5.2 Return Loss Results

Figures 7.28 and 7.29 present the return loss of the on-body antenna for this off-body scenario. It is noticed that the on-body antenna performed well in the 4.5–6.5 GHz band for both model cases. The diversity of return loss could be because of the body curvature.

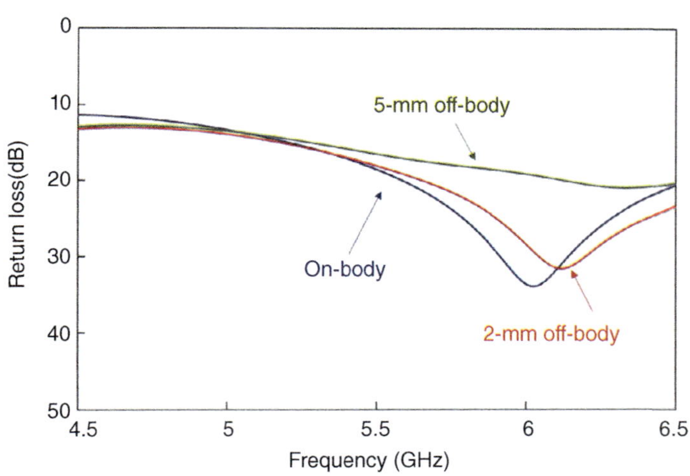

Figure 7.28 Return loss curves of the on-body antennas at the various distances from the body surface within the 4.5–6.5 GHz frequency range for the Taro model case.

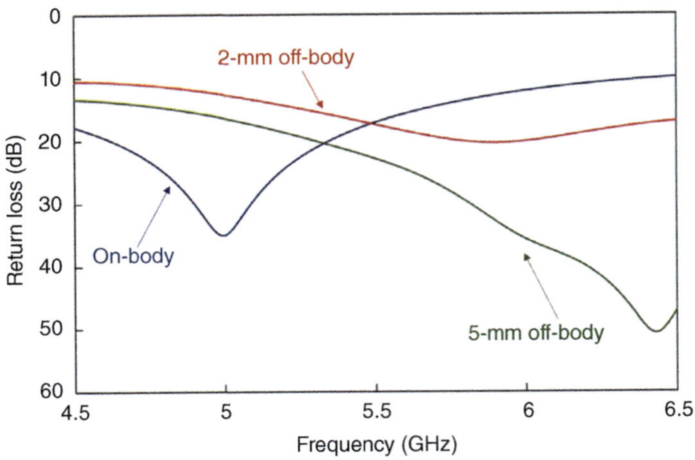

Figure 7.29 Return loss results of the on-body antennas at the various distances from the body surface within the 4.5–6.5 GHz frequency range for the Hanako model case.

7.5.3 Path Loss Results for the In- to Off-Body Scenario

Using Equation (7.1), the PL data for this IN2OFF communication scenario as a function of logarithmic propagation distance and the linear fitted lines for both Taro and Hanako model cases were obtained and displayed in Figures 7.30 and

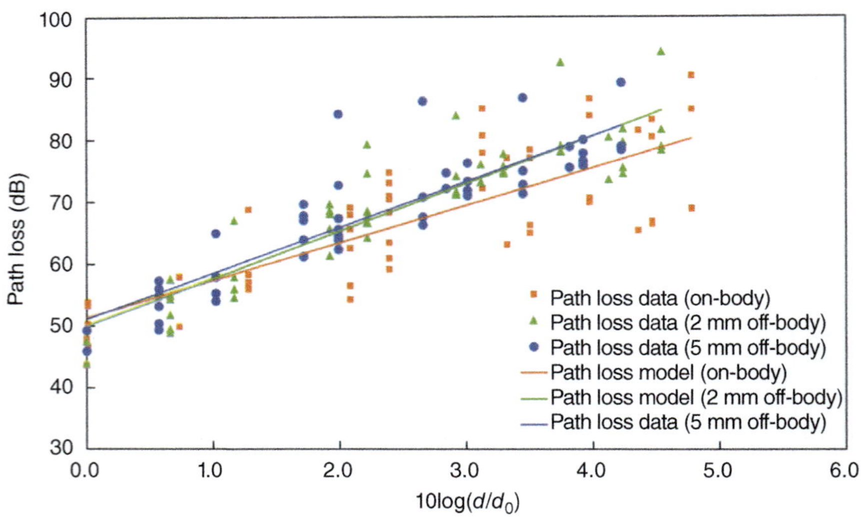

Figure 7.30 Path loss of the simulated channel as a function of the logarithmic propagation distances comparing between the IN2ON and the IN2OFF case scenarios for the Taro model case.

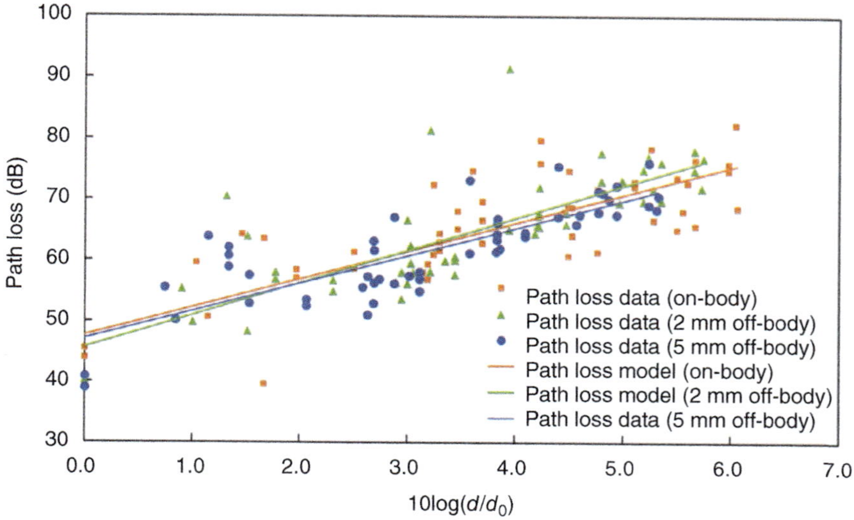

Figure 7.31 Path loss of the simulated channel as a function of the logarithmic propagation distances comparing between the IN2ON and the IN2OFF case scenarios for the Hanako model case.

7.31, respectively, together with the PL data of the IN2ON communication scenario presented earlier. The PL parameters at 2- and 5-mm off-body distances of both model scenarios are shown in Tables 7.5 and 7.6. The similarity between the PL data for IN2OFF communication scenarios at both 2- and 5-mm distances and the PL data for the IN2ON communication scenario are observed. This suggests that the in-body propagation is mainly accountable for the total PL for the IN2OFF channel.

Table 7.5 Path loss parameters for the Taro model case in the IN2OFF scenarios.

	d_0 (mm)	PL_0 (dB)	n	σ (dB)
2-mm off-body	33.5	49.9	7.7	5
5-mm off-body	36.5	51.1	7.4	5

Table 7.6 Path loss parameters for the Hanako model case in the IN2OFF scenarios

	d_0 (mm)	PL_0 (dB)	n	σ (dB)
2-mm off-body	26	45.7	5.3	6.4
5-mm off-body	29	47.2	4.5	4.6

7.6 System Performance Evaluation

A performance of communication system for body area scenario is affected by the operating channel. Moreover, the propagation channels of body area communication are different from the channels of indoor and outdoor communication scenarios since for body area communications, its signal propagates inside, on, or near human body. The difference in the propagation medium presents new topics including channel modeling and evaluation of system performance. The previous sections have addressed in-body channels in terms of signal attenuation and PL. This section will evaluate the system performance for two typical usage scenarios: IN2ON and IN2OFF communication scenarios.

7.6.1 Link Budget Evaluation and Analysis

A link budget evaluation considers all gains and losses from the transmitter via the propagation medium to the receiver in a communication system. It takes into account the propagation attenuation of signal, the gains of antennas, and feedline, for instance. Not only the PL data we obtained previously, the transmitting signal power and the characteristics of noise are also required for link budget analysis.

The emission mask for UWB was stated by the Federal Communications Commission [65] to ensure that UWB signal can operate with other existing radio signals. Then, the allowed transmitting power is limited by the emission mask, i.e. for the UWB ranging from 3.1 to 10.6 GHz, the maximum allowed emission power density, $P_M(f)$, is -41.3 dBm MHz^{-1}. Consequently, for the considered frequency band in this study, from 4.5 to 6.5 GHz, the maximum allowed transmitting power, P_{Max}, is calculated as follows:

$$\begin{aligned} P_{Max}(\text{dBm}) &= 10\log_{10}\int_{4.5\times10^3}^{6.5\times10^3} P_M(f)\text{d}f \\ &= -41.3 + 10\log_{10}(6.5\times10^3 - 4.5\times10^3) \\ &= -8.29\ \text{dBm} \end{aligned} \tag{7.2}$$

With this maximum allowed transmitting power, the system safety margin can be calculated accordingly.

Firstly, we calculate the noise characteristics with an assumption that the noise at the receiver end is additive white Gaussian noise (AWGN) only. Basically, it is thermal noise which is expressed by

$$N_0 = k[T_a + (N_F - 1)T_0] \tag{7.3}$$

where k is the Boltzmann constant equal to 1.38×10^{-23} J K^{-1}, T_a is the temperature at the receiving antenna, N_F is the noise figure of the receiver, and T_0 is

Table 7.7 Parameters for UWB link budget analysis in the considered system scenario.

Frequency (GHz)	4.5–6.5
Transmitting power P_t (dBm)	−8.29
Transmitting antenna gain G_t (dBi)	−24 (Taro), −19 (Hanako)
Receiving antenna gain G_r (dBi)	0 (Taro), 0 (Hanako)
Environment temperature (K)	300
Transmitter losses L_t (dB)	0
Miscellaneous losses L_M (dB)	0
Receiver losses L_r (dB)	0
Front-end noise figure (dB)	6
Boltzmann constant k (J K^{-1})	1.38×10^{-23}
Noise power (dBm)	−104.8
Bit error rate (BER)	10^{-3}
Modulation	Pulse-position modulation (PPM)
Demodulation	Noncoherent energy detection
Channel	Additive white Gaussian noise (AWGN)
$[E_b/N_0]_{spec}$ (dB)	8

the environment temperature, equals to 300 K. Here, the receiver is located on the human body; hence, it is practical to say that T_a and T_0 are 300 K. Therefore, Equation (7.3) becomes

$$N_0 = kT_0N_F \tag{7.4}$$

Then, the receiving power at the receiver end is expressed as the following formula:

$$P_{r,dBW} = P_{t,dBW} + G_{t,dB} - L_{t,dB} - PL_{dB} - L_{M,dB} + G_{r,dB} - L_{r,dB} \tag{7.5}$$

which includes all the losses and gains at both sides of the transmission in the system and also miscellaneous losses such as fading margin and polarization mismatch. The explanation of each parameter is in Table 7.7.

Next, at a given data rate, f_b, the energy per bit to noise power spectral density ($\frac{E_b}{N_0}$), a measure of signal-to-noise ratio, is calculated. In data transmission, the $\frac{E_b}{N_0}$ is an important parameter indicating the best performance that can possibly be accomplished for a communication link at a given transmitting power and a targeted bit error rate (BER). The $\frac{E_b}{N_0}$ is expressed in decibels:

$$\frac{E_b}{N_0} = \frac{P_r}{f_b N_0} \tag{7.6}$$

$$\left[\frac{E_\mathrm{b}}{N_0}\right]_\mathrm{dB} = P_\mathrm{r,dBW} - 10\log_{10} f_\mathrm{b} - N_\mathrm{0,dB} \tag{7.7}$$

Subsequently, the term $\frac{E_\mathrm{b}}{N_0}$ can be rewritten in the term of the communication distance d based on the PL equation (Equation 7.1) as

$$\begin{aligned}\left[\frac{E_\mathrm{b}}{N_0}\right]_\mathrm{dB} &= P_\mathrm{r,dBW} - 10\log_{10} f_\mathrm{b} - N_\mathrm{0,dB} \\ &= P_\mathrm{t,dBW} - \mathrm{PL}_\mathrm{dB} + G - L - 10\log_{10} f_\mathrm{b} - N_\mathrm{0,dB} \\ &= P_\mathrm{t,dBW} - \mathrm{PL}_\mathrm{0,dB} - 10n\log_{10}\left[\frac{d}{d_0}\right] - S_\mathrm{dB} + G - L - 10\log_{10} f_\mathrm{b} - N_\mathrm{0,dB}\end{aligned} \tag{7.8}$$

where $P_\mathrm{t,dBW}$ is the transmitting power, G is the inclusion of all gains in the system, L is the inclusion of all losses in the system, f_b is the data rate, and N_0 is the AWGN.

Lastly, the safety margin of the system M_system can be defined as

$$M_\mathrm{system} = \frac{\frac{E_\mathrm{b}}{N_0}}{\left[\frac{E_\mathrm{b}}{N_0}\right]_\mathrm{r}} \tag{7.9}$$

$\left[\frac{E_\mathrm{b}}{N_0}\right]_\mathrm{r}$ denotes the required $\frac{E_\mathrm{b}}{N_0}$ for the desired communication system. Considering Equation (7.9), if $M_\mathrm{system} \geq 0$, it means that the considered wireless communication is possible.

The performance of the communication system will be assessed using link budget analysis. The acceptable BER was selected to be 10^{-3} for our considered system in this example case. Accordingly, the specification of the signal-to-noise ratio (SNR) or $\frac{E_\mathrm{b}}{N_0}$ of 8 dB is required [54]. Thereafter, with the parameters given in Table 7.7, the possible communication distance can be estimated using Equation (7.9) at the given BER.

7.6.1.1 In- to On-Body Scenario

Based on the maximum allowed transmitting power and PL parameters derived previously, link budget was evaluated with respect to the transmission data rate, the communication distance, and the safety margin of the system for both Taro and Hanako cases for the IN2ON scenario. Figure 7.32 shows that the safety margin of the system depends on both the distance and the data rate. It is observed that at the 1-Mbps data rate, the communication can be achieved approximately up to 90-mm distance for the Taro case and more than 100-mm distance for the Hanako case. At the data rate of 10 Mbps, the communication distances are possible up to the 55-mm distance for the Taro case and the 90-mm distance for the Hanako case.

7.6.1.2 In- to Off-Body Scenario

Using the same approach as the IN2ON scenario, link budget was analyzed for the IN2OFF scenario for both Taro and Hanako cases. Here, the safety margin of the system is also dependent on the communication distance and the data rate as seen in Figures 7.33 and 7.34. For the Taro case, given that the data rate is 1 Mbps, it can be noticed that with the on-body antenna set at 2- and 5-mm distance from the body surface, it is possible to achieve the communication distances up to approximately 80 and 90 mm, respectively. Then, given that the data rate is 10 Mbps, with the on-body antenna set at 2- and 5-mm off-body surface, it is viable to achieve the communication distances up to 60 and 70 mm, respectively for the Taro case. Consequently, the link budget characteristics observed in the Hanako case are similar to that of Taro case. Given the 1-Mbps data rate, it is possible to accomplish the communication distances farther than 100-mm distance for both 2- and 5-mm off-body surface scenario. Then, given the 10-Mbps data rate, it is feasible to accomplish the communication distances up to approximately 70 and 100 mm for the 2- and 5-mm off-body surface scenario, respectively.

7.7 Electromagnetic Compatibility Evaluations

This section demonstrates the investigation of an energy absorption in a human body and an analysis of the system performance for an organ-monitoring application based on the specific absorption rate (SAR). Initially, based on

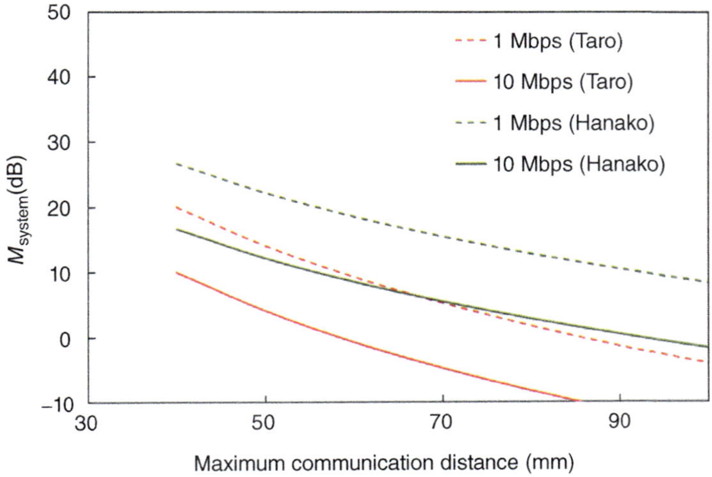

Figure 7.32 The safety margin of the system M_{system} as a function of the communication distance for the in- to on-body scenario of Taro and Hanako model cases at data rate = 1 and 10 Mbps.

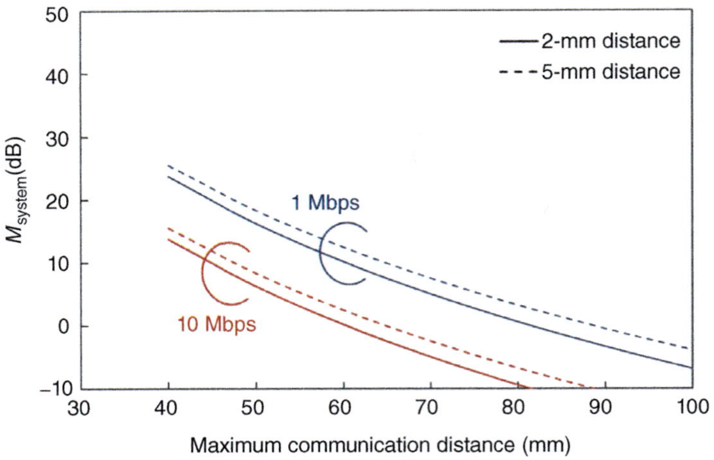

Figure 7.33 The safety margin of the system M_{system} as a function of the communication distance for the in- to off-body scenario with the on-body antenna set at 2- and 5-mm off skin surface of Taro model case at data rate = 1 and 10 Mbps.

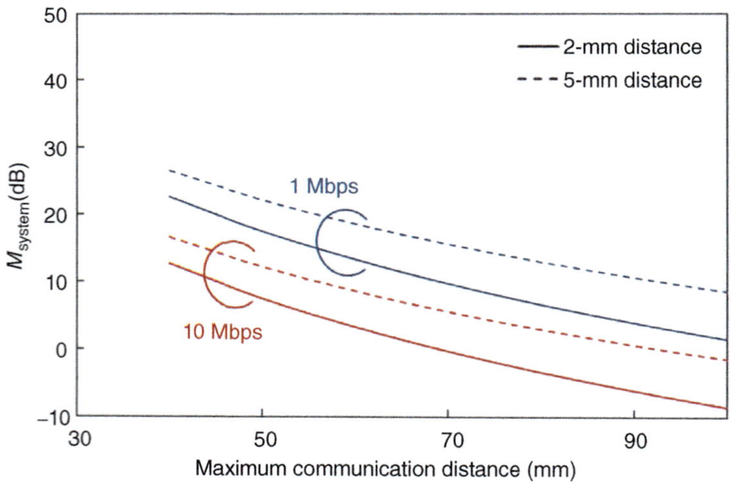

Figure 7.34 The safety margin of the system M_{system} as a function of the communication distance for the in- to off-body scenario with the on-body antenna set at 2- and 5-mm off skin surface of Hanako model case at data rate = 1 and 10 Mbps.

link budget evaluation using the derived PL data in the previous section, the required transmitting power will be calculated given the desired data rate at the specific BER. The corresponding SAR will then be calculated. Finally, taking into account the human safety, the possibility of the communication for liver implant at UWB range is presented.

7.7.1 Analysis

This section evaluates the system performance based on the acceptable BER, which was 10^{-3} for our considered system in this example case scenario. Consequently, the required $\frac{E_b}{N_0}$ or $[\frac{E_b}{N_0}]_r$ is 8 dB [54].

Firstly, the receiving power, $P_{r,dBW}$, is derived as

$$P_{r,dBW} = \left[\frac{E_b}{N_0}\right]_{dB} + 10\log_{10} f_b + N_{0,dB} \tag{7.10}$$

where f_b denotes the data rate, and $N_{0,dB}$ is the noise PSD.

Then, under the parameters given in Table 7.7 and the PL at the communication distance d between the on- and the in-body antenna, the required transmitting power at the distance d can be written as

$$P_{t,dBW} = P_{r,dBW} - G_{t,dB} + L_{t,dB} + PL(d)_{dB} + L_{M,dB} - G_{r,dB} + L_{r,dB} \tag{7.11}$$

This equation shows that the required transmitting power varies according to a distance d at a targeted BER. Hence, SAR also varies according to the distance d. Subsequently, under the transmitting power calculated using Equation (7.11), the values of SAR were computed using CST Microwave Studio software.

7.7.2 SAR Results

As a guideline for the assessment of human safety, the 10-g-averaged spatial peak SAR is used. According to the FCC regulations, the maximum allowed transmitting power for the considered frequency band in this example case scenario is limited to roughly −38 dBW. The examples of the transmitting power required for accomplishing the BER of 10^{-3} versus the propagation distance from the in-body device located on the surface of the liver to the on-body device located on the skin surface at the data rates of 1 and 10 Mbps for the Taro and Hanako model scenarios were calculated at 4.5 GHz and are presented in Figures 7.35 and 7.36. The required transmitting powers clearly depend on the data rate and the communication distance.

Then, SARs were calculated within the 4.5–6.5 GHz band at the given data rates of 1 and 10 Mbps considering the worst-case scenario with the constraint of the transmitting power and the propagation distances. For the Taro model case, the possible communication was up to 55- and 80-mm distances at the

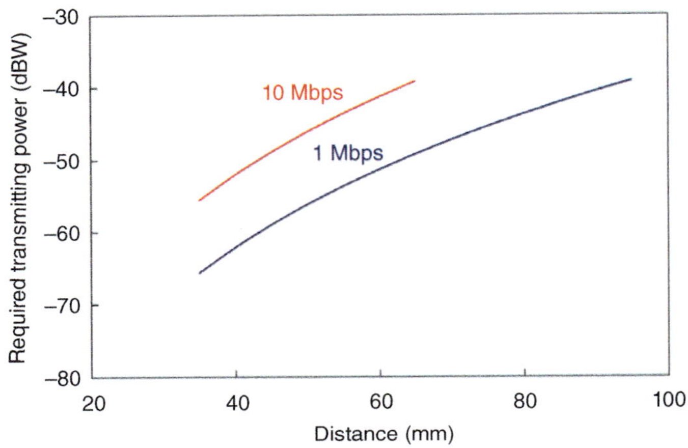

Figure 7.35 Example of required transmitting power versus communication distance or achieving a BER of 10^{-3} for the Taro model scenario at 4.5 GHz.

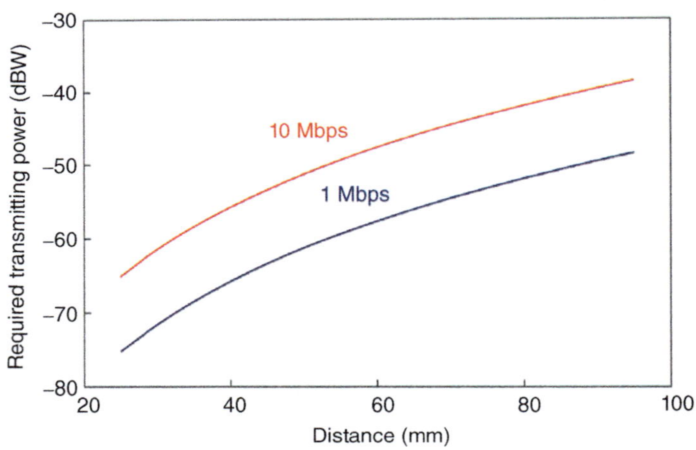

Figure 7.36 Example of required transmitting power versus communication distance or achieving a BER of 10^{-3} for the Hanako model scenario at 4.5 GHz.

data rates of 10 and 1 Mbps, respectively. Consequently, at these maximum communication distances, the required transmitting powers were calculated and used for the calculations of SAR.

Likewise, for the Hanako model case, it was viable to achieve communication distances more than 95 mm at both the 1- and 10-Mbps data rates. Nevertheless, our PL results were valid roughly up to the 95-mm distance. Hence, based on the required transmitting power at the distance of 95 mm, the SARs were calculated.

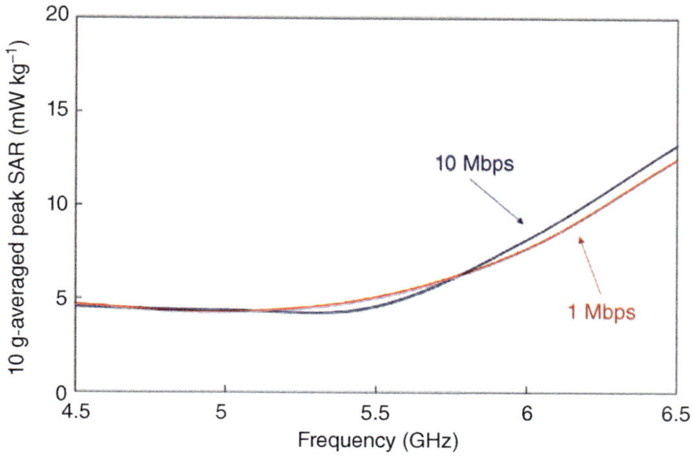

Figure 7.37 10-g-averaged peak SAR under the required transmitting power to meet the desired BER of 10^{-3} for the Taro model case at the given data rate of 1 and 10 Mbps for various frequencies.

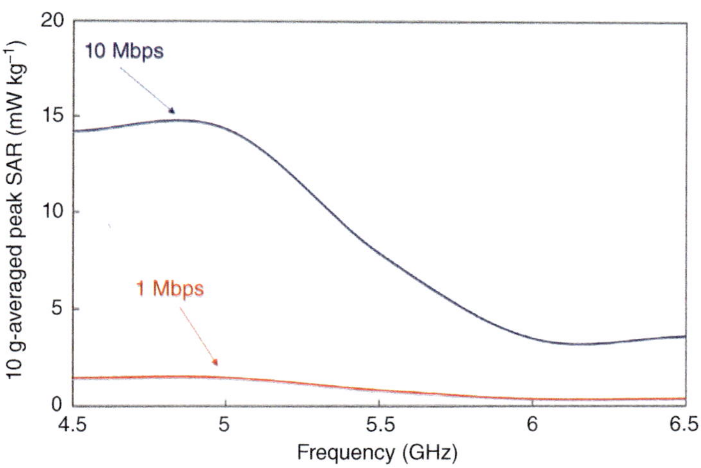

Figure 7.38 10-g-averaged peak SAR under the required transmitting power to meet the desired BER of 10^{-3} for the Hanako model case at the given data rate of 1 and 10 Mbps for various frequencies.

Considering the worst-case scenario described previously, the simulated 10-g-averaged peak SARs according to the required transmitting power at the data rates of 1 and 10 Mbps for both Taro and Hanako model cases were calculated as illustrated in Figures 7.37 and 7.38. For the Taro model case, the SAR results at both the data rates were similar because the transmitting powers were considered at roughly the limit of the allowed transmitting power. For the Hanako model case, the SAR results for both 1- and 10-Mbps data rates were different because they were calculated using the transmitting powers required for the communication distance of 95 mm, which were different for the 1- and 10-Mbps data rates. Moreover, the first approximation of the SAR considering the wideband transmission within the 4.5–6.5 GHz frequency range was obtained by the summation of the SAR values at different frequencies within the considered frequency range. The summation of SAR values for the Taro case were 34.9 mW kg^{-1} and 34 mW kg^{-1} at the data rates of 1 and 10 Mbps, respectively. Similarly, for the Hanako case, the cumulative SAR values were 4.3 and 43.3 mW kg^{-1} at the data rates of 1 and 10 Mbps, respectively. The results showed that, overall, the 10-g-averaged peak SAR for both Taro and Hanako model cases never surpassed the safety limit of 2 W kg^{-1}.

7.8 Conclusions

This investigation addresses to clarify the channel characteristics of the liver-implanted wireless communications at UWB range. Firstly, in Section 7.2, to check the viability of the implementation of the liver-implanted wireless communication links at UWB range, the study was done by means of measurements and simulations using simplified multilayer human-equivalent phantoms. Frequency-dependent attenuation results collected from the experimental measurements and simulations using simplified multilayer phantoms within the frequency band from 4.5 to 6.5 GHz were showed and discussed. The results indicated that the attenuation characteristics of the UWB signal in this communication scenario highly depended on the propagation distance and the frequency. It should be pointed out that multilayer phantoms without skin layer in this work may contribute to an underestimated attenuation result. Nevertheless, the results showed that deploying simplified multilayer phantoms can provide acceptable estimation of the channel characteristics. In addition, multilayer human phantom model can be used to represent a part of the human internal structure which can be a good option for an investigation of wireless communications for in-body scenario at an initial stage since the phantom model can be manufactured easily and also it is not as time consuming as simulations using human voxel models.

Thereafter, Section 7.3 investigated the characteristics of liver-implanted channel at the 4.5–6.5 GHz of UWB range with the consideration of organ movements caused by respiration along with human individuality. In this section, two different numerical human models of male (Taro) and female (Hanako) were deployed. The variations of signal attenuation caused by respiration-induced organ movement were presented in both the model cases. The results illustrated that organ movements can lead to the changes in signal attenuation. Additionally, the maximum variations of attenuation were within the 30-dB range, considering the movements of the upper abdominal organs during normal respirations up to 40 mm. The results indicated that the impact of organ movement should not be neglected when designing the in-body wireless communication system.

Then, PL data and PL model for standard in-body communication channels: the IN2ON and the IN2OFF channels for the two model cases were derived. It is observed that PL data were between 45 and 90 dB for the Taro case and between 40 and 80 dB for the Hanako case for up to an approximate distance of 95 mm. The shadowing factor indicated the effect of lossy environment to the in-body signal propagation. The differences in channel characteristics between the two models suggested that the propagation characteristics of channel are subject specific and, therefore, should be investigated in future researches.

Moreover, the effect of antenna misalignment on the channel characteristics was examined in Section 7.4. The results illustrated that the average PL due to antenna misalignment was higher than the average PL when the antennas were aligned for both Taro and Hanako models. Consequently, Section 7.5 compared the PLs of the IN2OFF scenarios with the PLs of the IN2ON scenario, and it was found that the PLs of the IN2OFF scenarios were similar to the PLs of the IN2ON scenario. These results suggested that the overall PL for the IN2OFF channel is mainly attributed to the propagation inside human body.

The channel performances of the liver-implanted communication system for the IN2ON and the IN2OFF scenarios in terms of link budget were evaluated numerically for both the male and female digital model cases in Section 7.6. It was found that the communication system in the example case scenarios always had a system margin more than 0 dB for the communication distance up to 60 mm even at a high data rate of 10 Mbps. The results suggested that it is possible to accomplish a reliable wireless communication using the UWB channel for the desired application in the considered case scenarios.

Furthermore, Section 7.7 discussed the viability of liver-implanted communications at UWB range considering the safety standard based on the FCC regulations of UWB transmission power and ICNIRP guidelines. The required transmitting powers for achieving the desired BER of 10^{-3} at the data rate of 1 and 10 Mbps were calculated by the method of link budget based on the previously obtained PL data. Thereafter, the 10-g-averaged peak SARs were calculated based on the required transmitting powers for the worst-case scenarios. The results presented the possibility of the implementation of liver-implanted wireless telemetry using UWB technology at the high data rate as 10 Mbps while still obeying the safety standards.

Regarding the future work, there are remaining issues to be explored before actual implementations: (i) more practical in-body antenna, i.e. a more compact and lighter antenna will be specifically developed and investigated for the liver-implanted communication. (ii) The use of circularly polarized antenna for the considered scenario will be studied to ease the problem of antenna misalignment. (iii) Experimental studies using animals will be performed to gain more understanding of the channel under the more realistic propagation environment. (iv) Discussions with medical staff will be held for more precise use-case scenarios such as the monitoring time frame. (v) More accurate methods for SAR evaluation for wideband transmission should be studied. (vi) To enhance the system performance, various techniques such as modulation techniques and MIMO technology will be investigated.

References

1 Gao, Y., Zheng, Y., Diao, S. et al. (2011). Low-power ultrawideband wireless telemetry transceiver for medical sensor applications. *IEEE Transactions on Biomedical Engineering* 58 (3): 768–772.

2 Astaras, A., Arvanitidou, M., Chouvarda, I. et al. (2008). An integrated biomedical telemetry system for sleep monitoring employing a portable body area network of sensors (SENSATION). Proceedings of the 30th Annual International Conference of the IEEE Engineering in Medicine and Biology Society, EMBS'08 Personalized Healthcare through Technology, 5254–5257.

3 Ferguson, J.E. and Redish, A.D. (2011). Wireless communication with implanted medical devices using the conductive properties of the body. *Expert Review of Medical Devices* 8 (4): 427–433.

4 Alemdar, H. and Ersoy, C. (2010). Wireless sensor networks for healthcare: a survey. *Computer Networks* 54 (15): 2688–2710.

5 Huang, F.J., Lee, C.M., Chang, C.L. et al. (2011). Rectenna application of miniaturized implantable antenna design for triple-band biotelemetry communication. *IEEE Transactions on Antennas and Propagation* 59 (7): 2646–2653.

6 Panescu, D. (2008). Emerging technologies: wireless communication systems for implantable medical devices. *IEEE Engineering in Medicine and Biology Magazine* 27 (2): 96–101.

7 Hannan, M.A., Abbas, S.M., Samad, S.A., and Hussain, A. (2012). Modulation techniques for biomedical implanted devices and their challenges. *Sensors* 12 (1): 297–319.

8 Lin, L., Wong, K.J., Tan, S.L., and Phee, S.J. (2008). In-vivo wireless capsule for health monitoring. Proceedings of the International Symposium on Consumer Electronics, ISCE, 1–4.

9 Stankovic, J.A., Cao, Q., Doan, T. et al. (2005). Wireless sensor networks for in-home healthcare. High Confidence Medical Device Software and Systems (HCMDSS) Workshop.

10 Karacolak, T., Cooper, R., and Topsakal, E. (2009). Electrical properties of rat skin and design of implantable antennas for medical wireless telemetry. *IEEE Transactions on Antennas and Propagation* 57 (9): 2806–2812.
11 Asgarian, F. and Sodagar, A.M. (2011). Wireless telemetry for implantable biomedical microsystems. In: *Biomedical Engineering, Trends in Electronics, Communications and Software*. Rijeka, Croatia: InTech. ISBN: 978-953-307-475-7.
12 Yin, M., Borton, D.A., Aceros, J. et al. (2013). A 100-channel hermetically sealed implantable device for chronic wireless neurosensing applications. *IEEE Transactions on Biomedical Circuits and Systems* 7 (2): 115–128.
13 Bechsgaard, T., Honge, J.L., Nygaard, H., and Jensen, M.O. (2015). In vivo wireless monitoring system of cardiovascular force data. *Cardiovascular Engineering and Technology* 6 (1): 2–7.
14 Wang, G., Liu, W., Sivaprakasam, M. et al. (2006). A dual band wireless power and data telemetry for retinal prosthesis. Annual International Conference of the IEEE Engineering in Medicine and Biology – Proceedings, 4392–4395.
15 Chi, Y.J. and Chen, F.C. (2014). On-body adhesive-bandage-like antenna for wireless medical telemetry service. *IEEE Transactions on Antennas and Propagation* 62 (5): 2472–2480.
16 Merli, F., Bolomey, L., Zürcher, J.F. et al. (2011). Design, realization and measurements of a miniature antenna for implantable wireless communication systems. *IEEE Transactions on Antennas and Propagation* 59 (10): 3544–3555.
17 Rahmat-Samii, Y. and Kim, J. (2006). Implanted antennas in medical wireless communications. *Synthesis Lectures on Antennas* 1 (1): 1–82.
18 Chow, E.Y., Chlebowski, A.L., Chakraborty, S. et al. (2010). Fully wireless implantable cardiovascular pressure monitor integrated with a medical stent. *IEEE Transactions on Biomedical Engineering* 57 (6): 1487–1496.
19 Chow, E.Y., Morris, M.M., and Irazoqui, P.P. (2013). Implantable RF medical devices: the benefits of high-speed communication and much greater communication distances in biomedical applications. *IEEE Microwave Magazine* 14 (4): 64–73.
20 Kiourti, A., Psathas, K.A., and Nikita, K.S. (2014). Implantable and ingestible medical devices with wireless telemetry functionalities: a review of current status and challenges. *Bioelectromagnetics* 35 (1): 1–15.
21 Ericson, M., Wilson, M., Coté, G. et al. (2004). Implantable sensor for blood flow monitoring after transplant surgery. *Minimally Invasive Therapy & Allied Technologies* 13 (2): 87–94.
22 Kellar, C.A. (2015). Solid organ transplantation overview and detection criteria. *The American Journal of Managed Care* 21 (Suppl. 1): S4–S11.
23 Grinyó, J.M. (2013). Why is organ transplantation clinically important. *Cold Spring Harbor Perspectives in Medicine* 3 (6): a014985.

24 Kim, I.H., Kisseleva, T., and Brenner, D.A. (2015). Aging and liver disease. *Current Opinion in Gastroenterology* 31 (3): 184–191.

25 Jadlowiec, C.C. and Taner, T. (2016). Liver transplantation: current status and challenges. *World Journal of Gastroenterology* 22 (18): 4438–4445.

26 Black, C.K., Termanini, K.M., Aguirre, O. et al. (2018). Solid organ transplantation in the 21st century. *Annals of Translational Medicine* 6 (20): 409.

27 Akl, T.J., Wilson, M.A., Ericson, M.N. et al. (2014). Wireless monitoring of liver hemodynamics in vivo. *PLoS ONE* 9 (7): e102396.

28 Ghildiyal, A., Amara, K., Molin, R.D. et al. (2010). UWB for in-body medical implants: a viable option. 2010 IEEE International Conference on Ultra-Wideband, ICUWB2010 Proceedings (September), vol. 2, 1–4.

29 Chavez-Santiago, R., Sayrafian-Pour, K., Khaleghi, A. et al. (2013). Propagation models for IEEE 802.15.6 standardization of implant communication in body area networks. *IEEE Communications Magazine* 51 (8): 80–87.

30 Das, R. and Yoo, H. (2017). A multiband antenna associating wireless monitoring and nonleaky wireless power transfer system for biomedical implants. *IEEE Transactions on Microwave Theory and Techniques* 65 (7): 2485–2495.

31 Lopez-Linares Roman, K., Vermeeren, G., Thielens, A. et al. (2014). Characterization of path loss and absorption for a wireless radio frequency link between an in-body endoscopy capsule and a receiver outside the body. *EURASIP Journal on Wireless Communications and Networking* 1: 21.

32 Liao, Y., Leeson, M.S., and Higgins, M.D. (2015). An in-body communication link based on 400 MHz MICS band wireless body area networks. 2015 IEEE 20th International Workshop on Computer Aided Modelling and Design of Communication Links and Networks, CAMAD 2015, 152–155.

33 De Santis, V. and Feliziani, M. (2011). Intra-body channel characterization of medical implant devices. Proceedings of EMC Europe 2011 York – 10th International Symposium on Electromagnetic Compatibility (September), 816–819.

34 Yazdandoost, K.Y. and Kohno, R. (2007). Wireless communications for body implanted medical device. 2007 Asia-Pacific Microwave Conference Proceedings (December), 1–4.

35 Smith, D.B., Miniutti, D., and Hanlen, L.W. (2011). Characterization of the body-area propagation channel for monitoring a subject sleeping. *IEEE Transactions on Antennas and Propagation* 59 (11): 4388–4392.

36 Chandra, R. and Johansson, A.J. (2015). Antennas and propagation for in-mouth tongue-controlled devices in wireless body area networks. *IEEE Antennas and Wireless Propagation Letters* 14: 1518–1521.

37 Kurup, D., Joseph, W., Vermeeren, G., and Martens, L. (2011). In-body path loss model for homogeneous human tissues. *IEEE Transactions on Electromagnetic Compatibility* 54 (3): 556–564.

38 Abidi, B., Jilbab, A., and Mohamed, E.H. (2019). Wireless body area network for health monitoring. *Journal of Medical Engineering and Technology*: 1–9.

39 Shimly, S.M., Movassaghi, S., and Smith, D.B. (2016). Cooperative communications for sleep monitoring in wireless body area networks. *Electronics Letters* 52 (8): 594–596.

40 Shen, Q., Liu, J., Yu, H. et al. (2013). Adaptive cognitive enhanced platform for WBAN. 2013 IEEE/CIC International Conference on Communications in China, ICCC 2013, 739–744.

41 Bala, R., Singh, R., Marwaha, A., and Marwaha, S. (2016). Wearable graphene based curved patch antenna for medical telemetry applications. *Applied Computational Electromagnetics Society Journal* 31 (5): 543–550.

42 Andreu, C., Garcia-Pardo, C., Castelló-Palacios, S. et al. (2018). Frequency dependence of UWB in-body radio channel characteristics. *IEEE Microwave and Wireless Components Letters* 28 (4): 359–361.

43 Garcia-Pardo, C., Chávez-Santiago, R., Cardona, N., and Balasingham, I. (2015). Experimental UWB frequency analysis for implant communications. 2015 37th Annual International Conference of the IEEE Engineering in Medicine and Biology Society (EMBC), Milan, Italy (25–29 August 2015), 5457–5460.

44 Thotahewa, K.M., Redoute, J.M., and Yuce, M.R. (2013). Electromagnetic and thermal effects of IR-UWB wireless implant systems on the human head. 2013 35th Annual International Conference of the IEEE Engineering in Medicine and Biology Society (EMBC), IEEE, 5179–5182.

45 Aziz, N.A., Mohamad, N.R., Abu, M., and Othman, A. (2016). Design of ultrawideband (UWB) implantable antenna for biomedical telemetry. *ARPN Journal of Engineering and Applied Sciences* 11 (5): 3249–3252.

46 Dissanayake, T., Yuce, M.R., and Ho, C. (2009). Design and evaluation of a compact antenna for implant-to-air UWB communication. *IEEE Antennas and Wireless Propagation Letters* 8: 153–156.

47 Khaleghi, A., Chávez-Santiago, R., and Balasingham, I. (2010). Ultra-wideband pulse-based data communications for medical implants. *IET Communications* 4 (15): 1889–1897.

48 Yuce, M.R. and Dissanayake, T. (2012). Easy-to-swallow wireless telemetry. *IEEE Microwave Magazine* 13 (6): 90–101.

49 Pan, G. and Wang, L. (2012). Swallowable wireless capsule endoscopy: progress and technical challenges. *Gastroenterology Research and Practice* 2012, 9pp. doi: https://doi.org/10.1155/2012/841691.

50 Staderini, E.M. (2002). UWB radars in medicine. *IEEE Aerospace and Electronic Systems Magazine* 17 (1): 13–18.

51 Ghildiyal, A., Godara, B., Amara, K. et al. (2010). UWB for low power, short range, in-body medical implants. 2010 IEEE International Conference on Wireless Information Technology and Systems, Honolulu, USA (28 August–3 September 2010), 1–4.

52 Miralles, E., Andreu, C., Cabedo-Fabres, M. et al. (2017). UWB on-body slotted patch antennas for in-body communications. 2017 11th European Conference on Antennas and Propagation (EUCAP), Paris, France (19–24 March 2017), 167–171.

53 Floor, P.A., Chávez-Santiago, R., Brovoll, S. et al. (2015). In-body to on-body Ultrawideband propagation model derived from measurements in living animals. *IEEE Journal of Biomedical and Health Informatics* 19 (3): 938–948.

54 Wang, J. and Wang, Q. (2012). *Body Area Communications: Channel Modeling, Communication Systems, and EMC*. Wiley.

55 Khaleghi, A., Chávez-Santiago, R., and Balasingham, I. (2011). Ultra-wideband statistical propagation channel model for implant sensors in the human chest. *IET Microwaves, Antennas & Propagation* 5 (15): 1805–1812.

56 Bahrami, H., Mirbozorgi, S.A., Rusch, L.A., and Gosselin, B. (2015). Biological channel modeling and implantable uwb antenna design for neural recording systems. *IEEE Transactions on Biomedical Engineering* 62 (1): 88–98.

57 Morimoto, Y., Anzai, D., and Wang, J. (2015). Antenna development, link budget analysis and specific absorption rate evaluation in ultra-wideband implant communications. *IET Microwaves, Antennas & Propagation* 9 (14): 1574–1580.

58 Leelatien, P., Ito, K., Saito, K. et al. (2018). Channel characteristics and wireless telemetry performance of transplanted organ monitoring system using ultrawideband communication. *IEEE Journal of Electromagnetics, RF and Microwaves in Medicine and Biology* 2 (2): 94–101.

59 Sharma, M., Parini, C.G., and Alomainy, A. (2014). Time domain analysis of a miniature tapered-slot UWB antenna. 2014 International Workshop on Antenna Technology: "Small Antennas, Novel EM Structures and Materials, and Applications" (iWAT), Sydney, Australia (4–6 March 2014), 318–321.

60 Felício, J.M., Fernandes, C.A., and Costa, J.R. (2016). Comparing liquid homogeneous and multilayer phantoms for human body implantable antennas. 2016 IEEE International Symposium on Antennas and Propagation (APSURSI), Fajardo, Puerto Rico (26 June–1 July 2016), 1049–1050.

61 Gabriel, S., Lau, R.W., and Gabriel, C. (1996). The dielectric properties of biological tissues: II. Measurements in the frequency range 10 Hz to 20 GHz. *Physics in Medicine and Biology* 41 (11): 2251–2269.

62 Leelatien, P., Ito, K., Saito, K. et al. (2019). Numerical channel characterizations for liver-implanted communications considering different human subjects. *IEICE Transactions on Communications* 102 (4): 876–883.

63 Nagaoka, T., Watanabe, S., Sakurai, K. et al. (2003). Development of realistic high-resolution whole-body voxel models of Japanese adult males and females of average height and weight, and application of models to radio-frequency electromagnetic-field dosimetry. *Physics in Medicine and Biology* 49: 1–15.

64 Bussels, B., Goethalsa, L., Feronb, M. et al. (2003). Respiration-induced movement of the upper abdominal organs: a pitfall for the three-dimensional conformal radiation treatment of pancreatic cancer. *Radiotherapy and Oncology* 68 (1): 69–74.

65 Federal Communications Commission (2002). In the matter of revision of part 15 of the commission's rules regarding ultra-wideband transmission systems. First Report and Order, ET Docket 98-153.

8

High-Efficiency Multicoil Wireless Power and Data Transfer for Biomedical Implants and Neuroprosthetics

Manjunath Machnoor and Gianluca Lazzi

Department of Electrical and Computer Engineering, University of Southern California, Los Angeles, CA, USA

8.1 Introduction

With the advances in low-power integrated circuits and millimeter-size microelectrode arrays, prosthetic devices have become a promising solution for improving the daily life of patients with disabilities. Some of these technologies are currently in clinical trials [1, 2], while several devices are commercially available [3]. Commercial devices are successfully implanted in patients for several applications, such as a retinal prosthetic for artificial vision, spinal cord stimulator for pain management, and deep brain stimulation for Parkinson's disease [4–6]. The power requirement by the implanted electronics depends on the application (e.g. neural stimulator, neural activity recorder, actuator, and sensors), which can range from tens of microwatts to hundreds of milliwatts. Some applications include implanted rechargeable battery, while few implants are powered continuously using wired or wireless power link. To eliminate the transcutaneous wires between the external power source and the implanted device, and to achieve a long lifetime of the implanted device, most commercial devices use wireless power transfer (WPT) to the implanted electronics. Similarly, the data signals are transmitted over the wireless link to configure the implanted electronics in different operating modes. For a few devices, neural signals and sensor data are transmitted from the implant to the external unit: Figure 8.1 shows the relative position of three commercially available neuroprosthetic devices. WPT has become a critical enabling component since implants must often be charged from devices outside the human body. WPT also removes the need for implantable batteries or cabling requirements, making biomedical implants more practical [8, 9]. Besides biomedical implants [10–14], WPT has found application in the fields of electric vehicles battery charging [15–18] and communication [19, 20], to name a few, with more applications rapidly emerging, thanks to the appeal of

Antenna and Sensor Technologies in Modern Medical Applications,
First Edition. Edited by Yahya Rahmat-Samii and Erdem Topsakal.

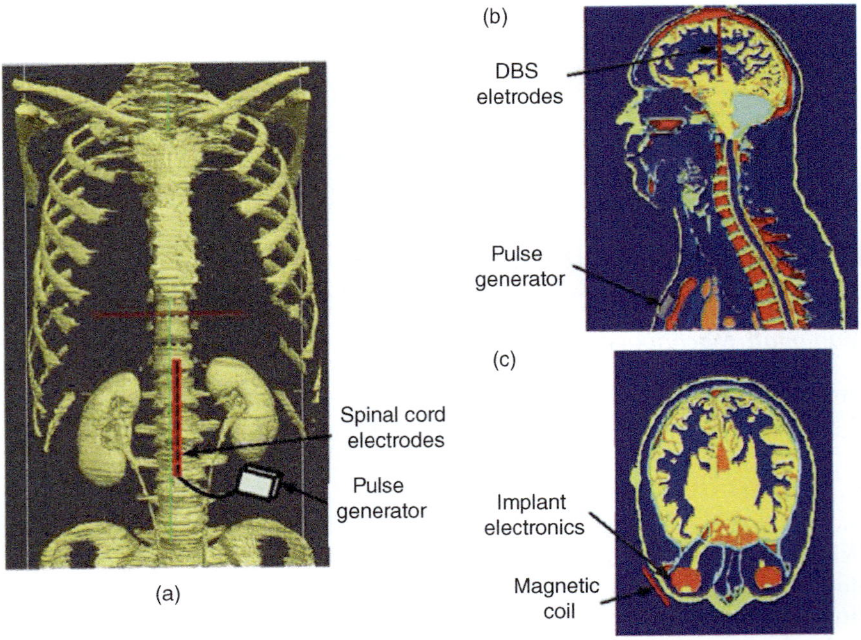

Figure 8.1 (a) Block diagram of a spinal cord stimulator with pulse generator and implanted electrodes, (b) position of deep brain stimulator electrode in the thalamus and pulse generator, and (c) retinal prosthetic implant with external magnetic coil for wireless power and data transfer [7]. (*Source*: Modified from RamRakhyani A. K. and Lazzi, G., 2014.)

charging wirelessly and conveniently. Despite well-established wireless power and data transfer technology, significant research is devoted to improving the power transfer efficiency (PTE) (above 40–70%) and supported data rate for the power and data telemetry.

WPT is commonly implemented using two inductively coupled coils/antennas [8]. In WPT systems, a capacitor is generally used to reduce the reactive power stored in the system by compensating for the inductive coil reactance [21, 22]. The reactance does not contribute to power transfer, and therefore, reducing it leads to a better power factor of the system [16]. Improved coupling and load tolerance is often achieved using more than two inductive coils/antennas [10–13, 23], and impedance matching of the load [14, 24–28] is employed extensively. Load matching can be achieved using additional passive/active components [14, 24–28] or using three- or four-coil systems [10–13, 29, 30]. The ultimate goal of the WPT system is to achieve the required power transfer to a given load with maximum efficiency [31, 32].

WPT systems for biomedical implants have additional constraints: they must comply with electromagnetic safety standards (such as that of complying with the maximum allowable specific absorption rate (SAR) [33]); they must be biocompatible; and they have often specific longevity requirements [34–37]. Both the two-coil [14, 24, 38] and three-coil [11] designs have been successfully employed in biomedical applications: the advantages of using a three- over a two-coil system are generally better misalignment insensitivity, coupling enhancement, lower induced fields in the body, and better bandwidth [10, 11, 17, 39, 40].

The size of the WPT system for biomedical implants is a critical design variable, as the available area is often very limited [41–43]. In addition, it has been demonstrated that a larger size increases the risk of tissue inflammation, cell damage [44, 45], and discomfort to the patient. These challenges associated with the design of WPT systems for biomedical implants are the primary motivation of this chapter.

Summarizing, the overall design goals of WPT for biomedical implants and, therefore, the goals considered in this chapter are small size (inductance) of the coil implanted in the body, low loss in the receiver (RX), and high efficiency and power delivery. There are several popular designs of WPT systems for biomedical implants available in the literature [10, 11, 13]. To effectively achieve the stated goals in a three-coil WPT system, circuit-theory-based design strategies are reviewed in this chapter. The performance of the designs in [10, 11], which have two coils implanted in the body, will be compared with the systems devised through the design strategies outlined here. The chapter is divided into two main sections. Section 8.2 describes the use of multicoil systems in efficient power delivery to the implanted RX. The section mainly deals with the new design techniques to achieve better performance over conventional designs of multicoil system. Section 8.3 describes inductive data transfer. The section describes how a simple update to the proposed technique enhances performance parameters at the data transmission frequency which can help in better data signal delivery.

8.2 Multicoil System to Achieve Efficient Power Transfer

In this section, the design of the conventional two- and three-coil WPT systems is presented, along with the advantages of using multicoil (and three-coil in particular) systems. A convenient circuit design technique to enhance the performance of the three-coil system compared to the conventional design of a three-coil system, and originally presented in [46], is introduced. The system discussed here is advantageous when small implanted RX coils are required. Performance enhancement observed in the load tolerance and the current consumption of the proposed system are shown through simulation results.

8.2.1 Two-Coil WPT Systems

A conventional two-coil (2*Coil*) WPT system consists of two inductively coupled coils, one connected to the transmitter (TX) and another to the RX. The power delivery from the TX coil to the RX coil occurs due to the magnetic coupling between the two coils. The coupling coefficient K_{12} of the two coils indicates the ratio of the magnetic field density in the load ($2Coil_2$) and transmit ($2Coil_1$) coils; a schematic view of the system with a power source at the TX, load at the RX, and compensating capacitors (in the resonance condition, expressed by Equation (8.1)) is shown in Figure 8.2. The theory of a 2*Coil* WPT system can be conveniently explained using matrix theory and reflected impedance theory [10–13]. The reflected impedance theorem uses Kirchhoff's voltage law (KVL) and Kirchhoff's current law (KCL). The KVL equations for the 2*Coil* system can be written in matrix form known as impedance matrix, as shown in Equation (8.2). The determinant of the impedance matrix Z, when expressed in canonical form, can be used to obtain the reflected impedance from $2Coil_2$ to $2Coil_1$, as shown in Equation (8.5). Compared with the explanation offered in [10–13], the various impedances of the system can be derived from the determinant of the matrix, and the system performance is analyzed using the matrix theory. Following the approach in [10–13], we can write (8.1–8.6), where R_1 is the parasitic resistance of $2Coil_1$, R_2 is the parasitic resistance of $2Coil_2$, R_{ref} is the reflected impedance from $2Coil_2$ to $2Coil_1$, $L_{12} = K_{12}\sqrt{(L_1L_2)}$ is the mutual inductance between the coils, and I_1 and I_2 are the currents flowing through $2Coil_1$ and $2Coil_2$, respectively.

The performance parameters of the design considered here are the power delivered to the load (PDL) and the PTE η, which is defined as the ratio of PDL to input power under resonance condition. The reflected impedance

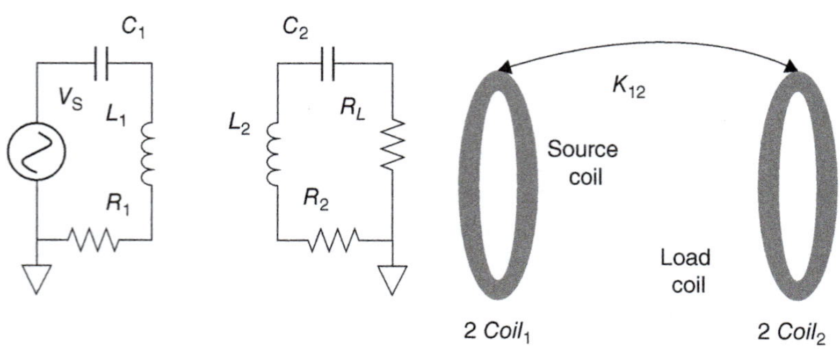

Figure 8.2 Schematic of a traditional two-coil WPT system. (*Source:* Machnoor, M., Rodríguez, E. S. G., Kosta, P., et al., 2018. © IEEE.)

parameters are used to define PTE and PDL. For the 2*Coil* system, η is given by Equation (8.6) [10–13]

$$j\omega L_1 = \frac{1}{j\omega C_1}, \; j\omega L_2 = \frac{1}{j\omega C_2} \tag{8.1}$$

$$V = Z \times I \tag{8.2}$$

$$\begin{pmatrix} V_s \\ 0 \end{pmatrix} = \begin{pmatrix} R_1 & j\omega L_{12} \\ j\omega L_{12} & R_2 + R_L \end{pmatrix} \begin{pmatrix} I_1 \\ I_2 \end{pmatrix} \tag{8.3}$$

$$\text{determinant}(Z\ \text{Matrix}) = Z_1 Z_2 \tag{8.4}$$

$$Z_1 = R_1 + R_{\text{ref}}, \quad Z_2 = R_2 + R_L$$

$$R_{\text{ref}} = \frac{\omega^2 L_{12}^2}{R_2 + R_L} \tag{8.5}$$

$$\eta = \frac{|i_2|^2 R_L}{V_s |i_1|} = \frac{i_2^2\, R_L}{V_s\ i_1\ \text{PF}} \tag{8.6}$$

The definition of the efficiency in (8.6) ignores the imaginary power at the TX as it does not result in power delivery. Cramer's rule can be applied to solve the impedance matrix equation (see (8.3)) to find the values of i_1 and i_2. Substituting the values of currents in (8.6) and rearranging, we can express the efficiency in terms of reflected impedances:

$$i_1 = V_s \frac{(R_2 + R_L)}{R_s(R_L + R_2) + \omega^2 L_{12}^2} = \frac{V_s(R_2 + R_L)}{\text{Determinant}(Z)}$$

$$i_2 = V_s \frac{-j\omega L_{12}}{R_s(R_L + R_2) + \omega^2 L_{12}^2} = \frac{-j\omega L_{12} V_s}{\text{Determinant}(Z)}$$

$$\eta_{2Coil} = \frac{|i_2|^2 R_L}{V_s |i_1|} = \frac{\omega^2 L_{12}^2}{\text{Determinant}(Z)} \times \frac{R_L}{R_L + R_2} = \frac{\omega^2 L_{12}^2}{R_s(R_L + R_2) + \omega^2 L_{12}^2} \times \frac{R_L}{R_L + R_2}$$

$$\eta_{2Coil} = \frac{\frac{\omega^2 L_{12}^2}{(R_L + R_2)}}{R_s + \frac{\omega^2 L_{12}^2}{(R_L + R_2)}} \times \frac{R_L}{R_L + R_2} = \frac{R_{\text{ref}}}{R_{\text{ref}} + R_1} \frac{R_L}{R_L + R_2} \tag{8.7}$$

The total efficiency of 2*Coil* can therefore be expressed as a product of two terms: PTE of $2Coil_1(\eta_{2Coil1})$ and PTE of $2Coil_2(\eta_{2Coil2})$, as given by Equation (8.8) [10–13]. This expression helps us locate the part of the system where maximum losses occur. The term η_{2Coil1} is the efficiency of the TX, and η_{2Coil2} is the efficiency of the RX for the 2*Coil* system considered here.

$$\eta_{2Coil} = \eta_{2Coil1} \times \eta_{2Coil2} \tag{8.8}$$

Let the input power to the 2*Coil* system be given by P_{in}. Then, the definition of PDL connected to the receiver can be expressed in the form of Equation (8.9):

$$\mathrm{PDL}_{2Coil} = P_{in} \times \eta_{2Coil} \tag{8.9}$$

Expressing (8.9) in terms of R_{ref}, one obtains

$$\mathrm{PDL}_{2Coil} = \frac{V_s^2 R_{ref}}{(R_1 + R_{ref})^2} \times \frac{R_L}{R_L + R_2} \tag{8.10}$$

The PDL can also be calculated by measuring the gain (V_{out}/V_{in}) of the system from two-port network parameters [10, 13]. This is very convenient when vector network analyzer is used for system performance analysis, as the exact value of the V_s is not known [10]. Given that the quality factor of the coils in Figure 8.2 can be written as $Q_1 = \omega L_1/R_1$ and $Q_2 = \omega L_2/(R_2 + R_L)$, rewriting ωL_{12}, R_s, and R_2 in terms of Q_1, Q_2, and K_{12} in η_{2Coil}, Equation (8.7) can be rewritten in a form similar to [10–13]

$$\eta_{2Coil} = \frac{K_{12}^2 Q_1 Q_2}{1 + K_{12}^2 Q_1 Q_2} \times \frac{R_L}{R_2 + R_L} \tag{8.11}$$

From the above considerations, the following observations about the two-coil system can be made with specific consideration to biomedical applications. First, if $R_L \gg R_2$, η_{2Coil2} is close to unity, and no power is dissipated in the RX coil of the system: this ensures that the power loss in the RX coils implanted in the body is negligible. This condition also reduces PDL. The load resistance R_L value depends on the battery specifications (if the RX is charging the battery). When a rechargeable battery of 1 or 2 V is being charged at several hundreds of micro- to milliamperes range, it results in a load resistance in the range of kiloohms. If the RX coil is used to drive an ASIC chip, the ranges of voltages and currents still hold true. R_2 is the parasitic resistance of the implanted coil, which is in the range of few ohms.

Further, since R_{ref} is inversely proportional to R_L (see Equation (8.5)), a higher value of R_L (which ensures higher η_{2Coil2}) reduces η_{2Coil1}: this results in poor η_{2Coil} and increased power loss in the $2Coil_1$, an aspect that can be addressed using the three-coil system and is discussed in Section 8.2.2. Finally, the coupling coefficient K_{12} is a function of the physical dimensions of $2Coil_2$ and $2Coil_1$. In biomedical WPT systems, to deliver power to load of kiloohms without dissipating much power into the RX coil, we need coupling coefficient in the range of 0.01. This dependence of the coupling coefficient on the diameter of the RX requires us to implant a coil of diameter of few tens of millimeters [10].

The efficiency of the system is high when the TX coil is held close to the RX coil as the coupling coefficient becomes high ($K_{12} \sim 0.1$). Similarly, the PTE of the system reduces as the RX coil is moved away from the TX coil. It is desirable to know where the efficiency is lost as the RX coil is moved away from the TX. The reduced efficiency implies that the input power is not delivered to the load

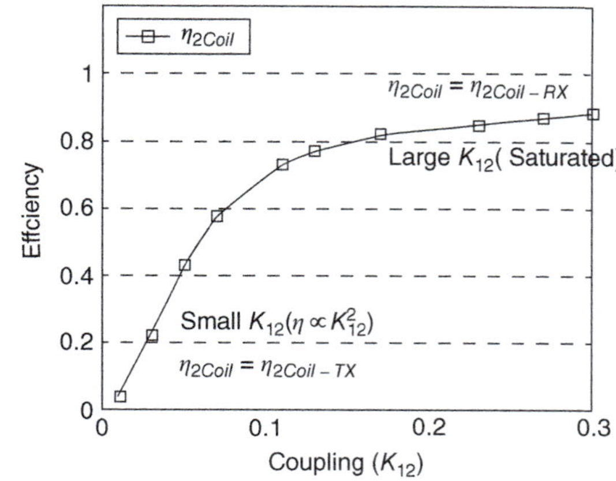

Figure 8.3 Efficiency (η_{2Coil}) versus K_{12} for the two-coil system with $L_1 = L_2 = 2$ μH, $R_1 = R_2 = 1\ \Omega$, $R_L = 100\ \Omega$, and $f = 5$ MHz. (*Source:* Machnoor, M., Rodríguez, E. S. G., Kosta, P., et al., 2018. © IEEE.)

but is dissipated as a heat in the parasitic resistance of a coil. Figure 8.3 shows the plot of η_{2Coil} as a function of K_{12} for a typical embodiment of a two-coil WPT system characterized by $L_1 = L_2 = 2$ μH, $R_1 = R_2 = 1\ \Omega$, $R_L = 100\ \Omega$, and $f = 5$ MHz. The PTE(η) versus K_{12} plot for a typical WPT has a similar trend. Noting that $2Coil_1$ is the TX and $2Coil_2$ is the RX, we can write that $\eta_{2Coil1} = \eta_{2CoilTX}$ and $\eta_{2Coil2} = \eta_{2CoilRX}$. In the design of a *2Coil* system, $\eta_{2CoilRX}$ is constant and does not vary with the distance between the coils, and it is $\eta_{2CoilTX}$ which varies with the distance between the coils. From Figure 8.3, it can be concluded that the RX efficiency (implanted coil $2Coil_2$) can be thought of as the saturation efficiency at high K_{12} (which is found for small distances between coils). The efficiency of the system at low K_{12} is limited by $\eta_{2CoilTX}$, which has square dependence on K_{12} for low K_{12} values.

There are two types of resonances that can be applied to the RX coil. The secondary side of the two-coil system can be connected either in series or parallel resonance. The efficiency of a secondary coil for a parallel and series resonance is given in [47]:

$$\eta_{2Coil2\text{–Parallel}} = \frac{R_L}{R_2 + R_L + \frac{R_2 R_L^2}{\omega^2 L_2^2}}$$

$$\eta_{2Coil2\text{–Series}} = \frac{R_L}{R_2 + R_L}$$

The two resonance conditions can be compared for a case of small RX coil and low frequency. As L_2 becomes small, which is typical for a biomedical implant, for a given ω and R_L, $\eta_{2Coil2-\text{Parallel}}$ is severely limited [47]. Parallel resonance secondary has better reflected impedance compared with the series connected RX, but its RX efficiency is limited. For example, for the *2Coil* system design considered in this chapter, $L_2 = 1$ μH, $R_2 = 0.5\ \Omega$, $f = 5$ MHz, results in $\eta_{2Coil2-\text{Parallel}} = 0.56$, whereas $\eta_{2Coil2-\text{Series}} = 0.99$. For this reason, in this chapter, the series resonance configuration of the secondary for the two-coil system is considered, and its overall efficiency is improved using the three-coil system.

8.2.2 Conventional Three-Coil WPT System

A three-coil (3*Coil*) WPT system consists of three inductively coupled coils; one coil is connected to the TX, and two coils are used at the RX end [11]. The coupling coefficients (K_{12} and K_{23}) and the physical layout and schematic are shown in Figure 8.4. The additional coil used at the RX, termed secondary coil ($3Coil_2$), is responsible for enhancing the PTE of the system under high R_L conditions. The operation of the 3*Coil* WPT system can be also understood using the matrix theory and reflected impedance theory [10–13]. The KVL equations for the resonant (see (8.12)) 3*Coil* system, written in matrix form, lead to the Z matrix whose determinant can be used to obtain the two reflected impedances R_{ref1} and R_{ref2} of the 3*Coil* system, which are given in (8.13) [17]

$$j\omega L_1 = \frac{1}{j\omega C_1},\ j\omega L_2 = \frac{1}{j\omega C_2},\ j\omega L_3 = \frac{1}{j\omega C_3} \tag{8.12}$$

$$\begin{pmatrix} V_s \\ 0 \\ 0 \end{pmatrix} = \begin{pmatrix} R_1 & j\omega L_{12} & 0 \\ j\omega L_{12} & R_2 & j\omega L_{23} \\ 0 & j\omega L_{23} & R_3 + R_L \end{pmatrix} \begin{pmatrix} I_1 \\ I_2 \\ I_3 \end{pmatrix}$$

$$\text{Determinant}(Z) = Z_1 \times Z_2 \times Z_3$$

$$Z_1 = R_{\text{ref1}} + R_1$$

$$Z_2 = R_{\text{ref2}} + R_2$$

$$Z_3 = R_3 + R_L$$

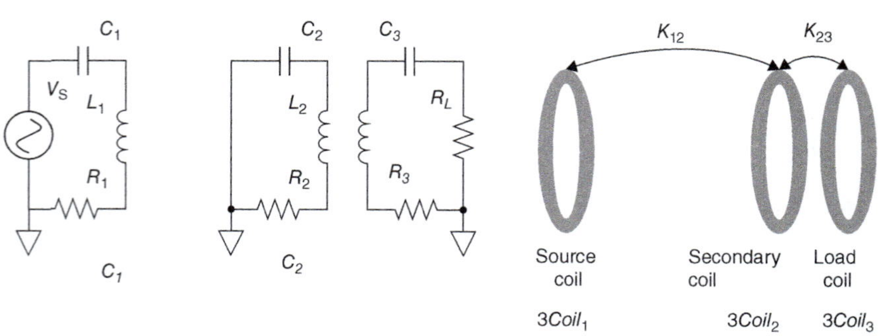

Figure 8.4 Schematic of a conventional three-coil WPT system (3*Coil*) [10–13]. (*Source:* Machnoor, M., Rodríguez, E. S. G., Kosta, P., et al., 2018. © IEEE.)

$$\text{Determinant}(Z) = R_1R_2(R_3 + R_L) + \omega^2L_{12}^2(R_3 + R_L) + \omega^2L_{23}^2R_1$$

$$R_{ref1} = \frac{\omega^2L_{12}^2}{R_2 + \frac{\omega^2L_{23}^2}{R_3+R_L}}, \quad R_{ref2} = \frac{\omega^2L_{23}^2}{R_3 + R_L} \tag{8.13}$$

where R_1 is the parasitic resistance of $3Coil_1$, R_2 is the parasitic resistance of $3Coil_2$, R_3 is the parasitic resistance of $3Coil_3$, R_{ref1} is the reflected impedance from $3Coil_2$ to $3Coil_1$, and R_{ref2} is the reflected impedance from $3Coil_3$ to $3Coil_2$. The mutual inductances between the coils $L_{12} = K_{12}\sqrt{(L_1L_2)}$ and $L_{23} = K_{23}\sqrt{(L_2L_3)}$ are the result of the coupling K_{12}, K_{23} between the coils, while i_1, i_2, and i_3 are the currents flowing through $3Coil_1$, $3Coil_2$, and $3Coil_3$, respectively. Following a similar analysis to that of the $2Coil$ system, the equation for the PTE can be written in terms of reflected impedances R_{ref1} and R_{ref2} as follows:

$$i_1 = \frac{V_s(R_2(R_3 + R_L) + \omega^2L_{23}^2)}{\text{Determinant}(Z)}, i_3 = \frac{-(\omega^2L_{12}L_{23})\,V_s}{\text{Determinant}(Z)}$$

$$\eta_{3Coil} = \frac{|i_3|^2R_L}{V_s|i_1|} = \frac{(\omega^2L_{12}L_{23})^2}{\text{Determinant}(Z)} \times \frac{R_L}{(R_2(R_3 + R_L) + \omega^2L_{23}^2)}$$

$$\eta_{3Coil} = \frac{\frac{\omega^2L_{12}^2}{R_2+\frac{\omega^2L_{23}^2}{R_3+R_L}}}{R_1 + \frac{\omega^2L_{12}^2}{R_2+\frac{\omega^2L_{23}^2}{R_3+R_L}}} \times \frac{\frac{\omega^2L_{23}^2}{R_3+R_L}}{R_2 + \frac{\omega^2L_{23}^2}{R_3+R_L}} \times \frac{R_L}{R_L + R_3}$$

$$\eta_{3Coil} = \frac{R_{ref1}}{R_{ref1} + R_1} \times \frac{R_{ref2}}{R_{ref2} + R_2} \times \frac{R_L}{R_L + R_3} \tag{8.14}$$

The total efficiency of $3Coil$ can therefore be expressed as a product of three terms: PTE of $3Coil_1$ (η_{3Coil1}), PTE of $3Coil_2$ (η_{3Coil2}), and PTE of $3Coil_3$ (η_{3Coil3}), as given by Equation (8.15). This expression helps us to locate the part of the system where maximum losses occur. The term η_{3Coil1} is the efficiency of the TX, and the term $\eta_{3Coil2} \times \eta_{3Coil3}$ is the efficiency of the RX for the $3Coil$ system considered here.

$$\eta_{3Coil} = \eta_{3Coil1} \times \eta_{3Coil2} \times \eta_{3Coil3} \tag{8.15}$$

Let the input power to the $3Coil$ system be given by P_{in}. The definition of PDL connected to the receiver can be expressed in the following form:

$$\text{PDL}_{3Coil} = P_{in} \times \eta_{3Coil}$$

The PDL can also be expressed in terms of reflected impedances, as in (8.16):

$$\text{PDL}_{3Coil} = \frac{V_s^2R_{ref1}}{(R_1 + R_{ref1})^2} \times \frac{R_{ref2}}{R_{ref2} + R_2} \times \frac{R_L}{R_L + R_2} \tag{8.16}$$

From the above considerations, the following observations about the three-coil system can be made with specific consideration to biomedical applications. First, if $R_L \gg R_3$, η_{3Coil3} is close to 1, and no power is dissipated in the $3Coil_3$ of the system. However, this does not guarantee that the power loss in the RX coils implanted in the body is minimized. Nonetheless, this condition does not imply sufficiently high PDL. Further, R_{ref2} is directly proportional to L_2 and L_3. High inductance (obtained through high copper wire length of $3Coil_2$ + $3Coil_2$) results in high R_{ref2} and high η_{3Coil2}. Large $R_{ref2}(>R_2)$ and $R_L(>R_3)$ are sufficient conditions to reduce the power dissipation in the implanted coils of $3Coil$. It is also to be noted that the main functionality of $3Coil_2$ is to invert and scale the contribution of the load coil ($3Coil_3$) on the reflected impedance at $3Coil_1$. Comparing R_{ref} (see (8.5)) of the $2Coil$ system with R_{ref1} (see (8.13)) of the $3Coil$ system, the abovementioned functionality of the $3Coil_2$ can be confirmed (i.e. $R_L \rightarrow (\omega^2 L_{23}^2/(R_L + R_3))$). This is referred to as the impedance-matching capability of the $3Coil$ system. Lastly, the general plot of η_{3Coil} as a function of K_{12} has the same trend as shown in Figure 8.3. Noting that $3Coil_1$ is the TX and $3Coil_2$ and $3Coil_3$ form the RX, we can write $\eta_{3Coil1} = \eta_{3CoilTX}$ and $\eta_{3Coil2} \times \eta_{3Coil3} = \eta_{3CoilRX}$.

8.2.3 Performance of the Two- and Three-Coil Systems as a Function of RX Coil Size

There is no established standard for the design of WPT systems for biomedical implants, but the general designs in the literature include a TX coil larger than the implanted RX coil [10–13, 33, 48]. It is desirable to reduce the size (size can refer to weight, diameter, number of turns, etc.) of the implanted coil to make it suitable for implantation. However, the performance of the RX system in the conventional two- and three-coil systems (discussed above) degrades as the size (inductance determines reflected impedance, see (8.5, 8.13)) of the RX coil reduces.

The design of the three-coil ($3Coil$) WPT system involves placing the additional secondary coil closer to the coil with low Q [49]. Since the TX is outside the human body and is larger, it is possible to design the Q of TX greater than the Q of the RX coil. Thus, in biomedical applications [11] of the $3Coil$ system, two coils are located at the RX side and one coil is at the TX. The additional coil can also be placed at the TX side [10]; such a system will be discussed in later sections. As the size of the two RX coils reduces (either in terms of diameter or the number of turns), L_2, L_3, and their mutual inductance L_{23} reduce. This results in reduced R_{ref2}; as a result, η_{3Coil2} (see (8.14, 8.15)) decreases, and losses in the implanted coil increase. Furthermore, R_{ref1}, which is inversely proportional to R_{ref2}, either increases or saturates, depending on the value of R_{ref2}. The efficiency of the system η_{3Coil} will be limited by η_{3Coil2}: since R_{ref2} decreases and R_{ref1} either increases or saturates, PDL_{3Coil}(see (8.16)) also decreases as the size reduces. Thus, as the size of the RX coils in the 3*Coil* decreases, PTE and PDL of the entire system decrease, and losses in the implanted coils increase. This provides a challenge to design a system with good PTE and PDL.

Similarly, by referring to (8.5, 8.7), PTE and R_{ref} of the 2*Coil* system reduce as the size of $2Coil_2$ reduces. It can also be concluded that in the 2*Coil* and 3*Coil* systems with small RX coils (low L_2 and L_3), performance degradation can be linked to a reduction in reflected impedance. Thus, this chapter proposes a technique to maximize reflected impedance for a 3*Coil* system to achieve good PTE and PDL performance for a small RX three-coil system.

The effects of frequency of operation on the human body are explained in [10]. The choice of 700 kHz in [10] and 13 MHz in [11] is made considering the Q-factor of the coils used, following an optimization process. In this chapter, we chose the frequency of 5 MHz as the copper wire of AWG 20 exhibited $Q = 150$ for $L = 5\ \mu\text{H}$. We have also considered a load resistance $R_{\text{L}} = 1\ \text{k}\Omega$. In this chapter, and unlike [10], no further optimization of coils was undertaken to choose a frequency with higher Q as high Q is not necessary to obtain higher PTE with the approach presented here. Biomedical implants are generally designed to efficiently deliver power of the order of 100 mW (50–300 mW) to the RX [11].

8.2.4 Description of the Proposed Three-Coil System

In this subsection, we introduce a three-coil system which can be used to either increase the efficiency or reduce the size of the implanted coils (inductance). The proposed system makes the R_{ref2} independent of the inductances of the implanted coils. That is, it overcomes the disadvantages observed in the conventional two- and three-coil systems mentioned in Section 8.2.3. The proposed system uses different resonance conditions compared to conventional systems.

The resonant condition for the conventional three-coil system [10–13] is provided in (8.12). In this chapter, we propose a different resonant condition which can be applied to multicoil systems (three-coil, four-coil, etc.): while the layout of the proposed three-coil system ($3Coil_{\text{p}}$) remains the same as Figure 8.4, the resonance condition is changed to (8.17) instead of (8.12). This results in a new schematic equivalent of the $3Coil_{\text{p}}$ system shown in Figure 8.5. Generally, dot convention is used between the coupled coils to indicate the relative phase of voltages and currents. In Figure 8.5, the dot convention is used at the RX coils to indicate the relative phases of the induced voltages.

The performance and functionality of the proposed three-coil system is explained using the matrix theory and reflected impedance theory. The impedance matrix equation for the modified resonant scheme is provided in (8.18): compared with the Z matrix of the conventional 3*Coil* in Equation (8.13), the Z matrix of $3Coil_{\text{p}}$ (see (8.18)) includes the impedance of the capacitor C_{m} used for creating a resonance condition at the RX coils. From the determinant

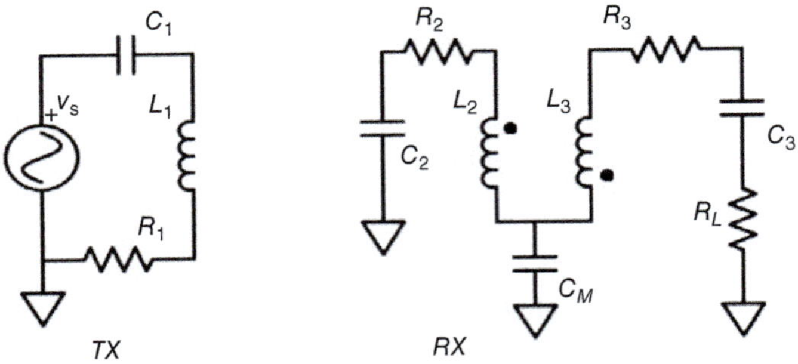

Figure 8.5 Schematic of the proposed efficient and compact three-coil system (3*Coil*$_p$). To maximize R_{ref2} of the small RX size 3*Coil* system, two techniques are adopted: $L_2 = L_3$ and $1/\omega C_2 = 1/\omega C_3 = 0$ along with the appropriate RX system's relative coil polarity required to increase R_{ref2p}.

of the resonant Z matrix (impedance matrix) when expressed in the canonical form, we can obtain the two reflected impedances R_{ref1p} and R_{ref2p} for the proposed three-coil system $3Coil_p$ (see (8.22)). The main advantage of this system is that it increases the effective mutual impedance between the $3Coil_{2p}$ and $3Coil_{3p}$; the equivalent L_{23p} of the system increases, as shown in (8.20).

Since we have noted in Section 8.2.3 that, as the size of the RX in the three-coil system reduces, R_{ref2} reduces, adopting this new resonant condition helps us maximize R_{ref2} of the small RX in the three-coil system. By increasing R_{ref2p}, the PTE and PDL can be increased, and the losses in the implanted coil can be reduced. Both the three-coil systems under consideration (3*Coil* and $3Coil_p$) have the same set of variables to describe the operation; in order to differentiate the variables of the two systems, the proposed three-coil system uses subscript p for all the variables (for example, R_{ref2} is for the 3*Coil* system, and R_{ref2p} is for the $3Coil_p$ system).

$$j\omega L_1 = \frac{1}{j\omega C_1},\quad j\omega L_2 = \frac{1}{j\omega C_2} + \frac{1}{j\omega C_m},\quad j\omega L_3 = \frac{1}{j\omega C_3} + \frac{1}{j\omega C_m} \tag{8.17}$$

$$V = Z \times I \tag{8.18}$$

$$\begin{pmatrix} V_s \\ 0 \\ 0 \end{pmatrix} = \begin{pmatrix} R_1 & j\omega L_{12} & 0 \\ j\omega L_{12} & R_2 & j\omega L_{23} - \frac{1}{j\omega C_m} \\ 0 & j\omega L_{23} - \frac{1}{j\omega C_m} & R_3 + R_L \end{pmatrix} \begin{pmatrix} I_1 \\ I_2 \\ I_3 \end{pmatrix} \tag{8.19}$$

$$j\omega L_{23} \rightarrow j\omega L_{23} - \frac{1}{j\omega C_m} \tag{8.20}$$

$$\text{determinant}(Z) = Z_1 \times Z_2 \times Z_3 \tag{8.21}$$

$$Z_1 = R_1 + R_{ref1p}$$

$$Z_2 = R_2 + R_{\text{ref2p}}$$

$$Z_3 = R_3 + R_{\text{L}}$$

$$\text{Determinant}(Z) = R_1R_2(R_3 + R_{\text{L}}) + \omega^2L_{12}^2(R_3 + R_{\text{L}}) + \left(\omega L_{23} + \frac{1}{\omega C_{\text{m}}}\right)^2 R_1$$

$$R_{\text{ref1p}} = \frac{\omega^2L_{12}^2}{R_2 + \frac{\left(\omega L_{23}+\frac{1}{\omega C_{\text{m}}}\right)^2}{R_3+R_{\text{L}}}}, R_{\text{ref2p}} = \frac{\left(\omega L_{23} + \frac{1}{\omega C_{\text{m}}}\right)^2}{R_3 + R_{\text{L}}} \tag{8.22}$$

In (8.19), R_1 is the parasitic resistance of $3Coil_{1\text{p}}$, R_2 is the parasitic resistance of $3Coil_{2\text{p}}$, and R_3 is the parasitic resistance of $3Coil_{3\text{p}}$. R_{ref1p} is the reflected impedance from $3Coil_{2\text{p}}$ to $3Coil_{1\text{p}}$, and R_{ref2p} is the reflected impedance from $3Coil_{3\text{p}}$ to $3Coil_{2\text{p}}$. R_{L} is, instead, the load resistance. The notation p is adapted for the proposed system; $\eta_{3Coil1\text{p}}$, $\eta_{3Coil2\text{p}}$, and $\eta_{3Coil3\text{p}}$ are the efficiency of $3Coil_{1\text{p}}$, $3Coil_{2\text{p}}$, and $3Coil_{3\text{p}}$, respectively. Following the analysis of the η_{3Coil} system, PTE and PDL for the $\eta_{3Coil\text{p}}$ system can be defined as in (8.14–8.16) with an updated definition of R_{ref2p}. That is, PTE and PDL can be written in terms of reflected impedances R_{ref1p} and R_{ref2p} as follows:

$$i_1 = \frac{V_{\text{s}}\left(R_2(R_3 + R_{\text{L}}) + \left(\omega L_{23} + \frac{1}{\omega C_{\text{m}}}\right)^2\right)}{\text{Determinant}(Z)}, i_3 = \frac{(j\omega L_{12})\left(j\omega L_{23} - \frac{1}{j\omega C_{\text{m}}}\right)V_{\text{s}}}{\text{Determinant}(Z)}$$

$$\eta_{3Coil\text{p}} = \frac{|i_3|^2R_{\text{L}}}{V_{\text{s}}|i_1|} = \frac{(\omega L_{12})^2\left(\omega L_{23} + \frac{1}{\omega C_{\text{m}}}\right)^2}{\text{Determinant}(Z)} \times \frac{R_{\text{L}}}{\left(R_2(R_3 + R_{\text{L}}) + \left(\omega L_{23} + \frac{1}{\omega C_{\text{m}}}\right)^2\right)}$$

$$\eta_{3Coil\text{p}} = \frac{\frac{\omega^2L_{12}^2}{R_2+\frac{\left(\omega L_{23}+\frac{1}{\omega C_{\text{m}}}\right)^2}{R_3+R_{\text{L}}}}}{R_1 + \frac{\omega^2L_{12}^2}{R_2+\frac{\left(\omega L_{23}+\frac{1}{\omega C_{\text{m}}}\right)^2}{R_3+R_{\text{L}}}}} \times \frac{\frac{\left(\omega L_{23}+\frac{1}{\omega C_{\text{m}}}\right)^2}{R_3+R_{\text{L}}}}{R_2 + \frac{\left(\omega L_{23}+\frac{1}{\omega C_{\text{m}}}\right)^2}{R_3+R_{\text{L}}}} \times \frac{R_{\text{L}}}{R_{\text{L}} + R_3}$$

$$\eta_{3Coil\text{p}} = \frac{R_{\text{ref1p}}}{R_{\text{ref1p}} + R_1} \times \frac{R_{\text{ref2p}}}{R_{\text{ref2p}} + R_2} \times \frac{R_{\text{L}}}{R_{\text{L}} + R_3}$$

Similar to conventional three-coil system, if $R_{\text{L}} \gg R_3$ is maintained in the proposed three-coil system, $\eta_{3Coil3\text{p}}$ is close to 1, and no power is dissipated in the load coil of the system. However, this does not guarantee that power loss in the secondary ($3Coil_{2\text{p}}$) coil implanted in the body is minimized. Also, it is worth noting that R_{ref1p} and R_{ref2p} of the $3Coil_{\text{p}}$ system in (8.22) are different from those in (8.13). ωC_{m}, which helps increase R_{ref2p}, results in the decrease of R_{ref1p}.

A decrease of R_{ref1p} will result in the reduction of $\eta_{3Coil1p}$. That is, mutual capacitor at the RX reduces the efficiency of $3Coil_{1p}$, which is used at the TX. This calls for the efficient design of transmit coil. This issue is addressed in Section 8.2.7.

In the conventional three-coil (3*Coil*) system, only the mutual impedance between the two RX coils dominates the R_{ref2}, PTE, and PDL (see (8.13)). In the proposed three-coil ($3Coil_{\text{p}}$) system, all the impedances of the RX contribute to R_{ref2p} (see (8.23)), PTE, and PDL. This effectively enhances the reflected impedance for a given RX system, enabling a smaller and more compact design.

$$R_{\text{ref2p}} = \frac{(\omega L_{23})^2 + \left(\frac{1}{\omega C_{\text{m}}}\right)^2 + \omega^2 L_2 L_{23} + \omega^2 L_3 L_{23}}{R_3 + R_{\text{L}}} \tag{8.23}$$

As can be noted from (8.23), L_2, L_3, C_{m}, and L_{m} contribute (if $1/C_{\text{m}} = \omega^2 L_2 = \omega^2 L_3$) to R_{ref2p} of the $3Coil_{\text{p}}$ system. This leads to the effective utilization of all the impedance sources implanted in the body.

It should be noted that the relative polarity of the proposed three-coil ($3Coil_{\text{p}}$) system (that is, the order of connected ends of the inductors) now becomes more important compared with the conventional 3*Coil* system. If the coils are reversed (as indicated by the adjusted dot locations in Figure 8.6b), then R_{ref2p} reduces like in (8.24) instead of increasing like in (8.22). Therefore, coil polarity should be configured as shown in Figure 8.6a for maximum reflected impedance. The circuit representation under two different polarity connection is shown in Figure 8.6

$$R_{\text{ref2p}} = \frac{\left(\omega L_{23} - \frac{1}{\omega C_{\text{m}}}\right)^2}{R_3 + R_{\text{L}}} \tag{8.24}$$

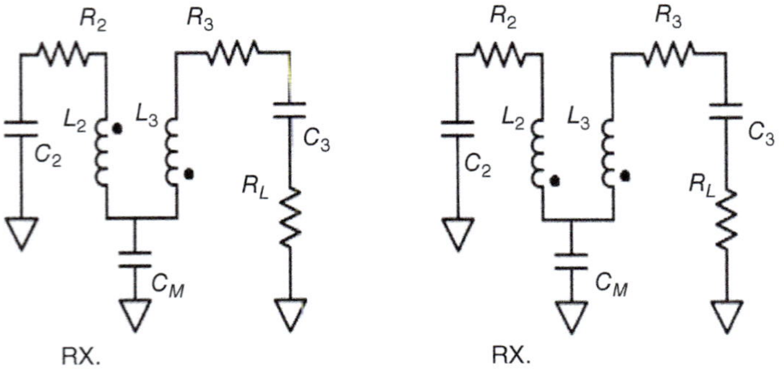

Figure 8.6 (a) Dot convention that results in increase of R_{ref2}. (b) Dot convention that results in decrease of R_{ref2}.

In this chapter, two additional circuit techniques are adopted to maximize R_{ref2p} for the given values of L_2 and L_3. The first technique is related to splitting the given length of wire as L_2 and L_3 equally, to achieve efficient usage of cable length implanted in the body (covered in Section 8.2.5). The second circuit technique leads to $1/\omega C_2 = 1/\omega C_3 = 0$ for the circuit shown in Figure 8.6a; this also results in higher R_{ref2p} covered in Section 8.2.6.

As mentioned before, the proposed circuit technique and resonance condition can be used for any type of multicoil (three- or four-coil) systems. If the additional coil is used at the TX side, we have $\omega L_{12} \rightarrow j\omega L_{12} \pm \frac{1}{j\omega C_1}$, where C_1 is the common capacitor used between the two TX coils as shown in Figure 8.7. The exact value of the $\pm$ sign depends on the relative polarity between the coils. The PTE and PDE for the schematic shown in Figure 8.7 are given by the following equations:

$$\text{PTE} = \frac{\dfrac{\left(\omega M_{12} \pm \frac{1}{\omega C_1}\right)^2}{R_2 + \frac{\omega^2 M_{23}^2}{R_3 + R_L}}}{\dfrac{\left(\omega M_{12} \pm \frac{1}{\omega C_1}\right)^2}{R_2 + \frac{\omega^2 M_{23}^2}{R_3 + R_L}} + R_1} \times \frac{\left(\frac{\omega^2 M_{23}^2}{R_3 + R_L}\right)}{R_2 + \frac{\omega^2 M_{23}^2}{R_3 + R_L}} \times \frac{R_L}{R_3 + R_L}$$

$$\text{PDL} = V_{\text{in}}^2 \frac{\dfrac{\left(\omega M_{12} \pm \frac{1}{\omega C_1}\right)^2}{R_2 + \frac{\omega^2 M_{23}^2}{R_3 + R_L}}}{\left(\dfrac{\left(\omega M_{12} \pm \frac{1}{\omega C_1}\right)^2}{R_2 + \frac{\omega^2 M_{23}^2}{R_3 + R_L}} + R_1\right)^2} \times \frac{\left(\frac{\omega^2 M_{23}^2}{R_3 + R_L}\right)}{R_2 + \frac{\omega^2 M_{23}^2}{R_3 + R_L}} \times \frac{R_L}{R_3 + R_L}$$

It can be noticed that, depending on the polarity employed, the PDL of the system in Figure 8.7 can be enhanced without compromising the PTE (if

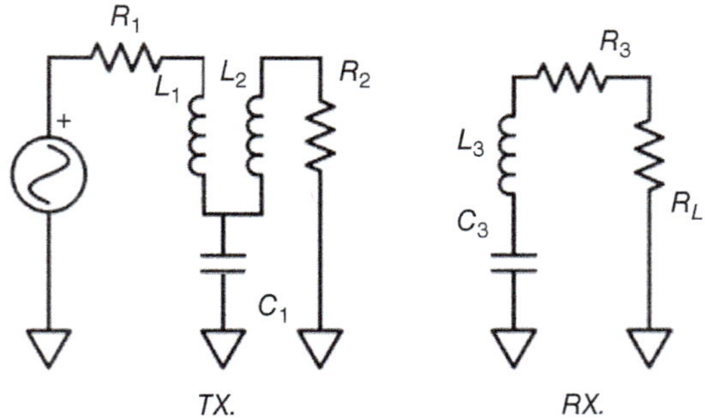

Figure 8.7 Schematic of a three-coil system with an additional coil and the mutual capacitor at the TX. The driver coil (L_1) is connected to the TX coil (L_2) using the mutual capacitance (C_1). The choice of relative voltage polarity of L_1 and L_2 (dot convention not shown here) will determine the PTE and PDL. (*Source:* Machnoor, M., Rodríguez, E. S. G., Kosta, P., et al., 2018. © IEEE.)

$\left(\omega M_{12} - \frac{1}{\omega C_m}\right)^2 / (\omega^2 M_{23}^2/(R_3 + R_L) + R_2) \gg R_1)$, or the PTE of the system can be enhanced. Similarly, a four-coil [13] system with the additional coil at both the TX and the RX sides can use C_1 at the TX side to enhance PDL and C_m at the RX side to enhance the RX efficiency.

8.2.5 Efficient Use of Implanted Wire of the Coil in a Small RX Three-Coil System

8.2.5.1 Circuit Technique Description

We can increase the PTE of the secondary $3Coil_2$ and load coil $3Coil_3$ and reduce the power dissipation in the RX system using higher L_2 and L_3 (8.13–8.15). However, it is always better to use a smaller implant and shorter wire inside the human body. We can consider that the inductance of the coil is approximately proportional to the length of the wire even if the inductance that can be achieved for a coil depends on the process used to make the inductor. The diameters of two coils must be equal to maximize the coupling between the two implanted coils K_{23} of the three-coil system. In this chapter, a diameter of 35 mm has been chosen for the implanted coils to compare with other reported biomedical WPT systems [10, 11, 13]. The proposed technique is independent of the diameter of the coils used. Given a chosen length of coil (fixed maximum inductance, L_{max}), the procedure can be summarized as follows:

$$L_2 + L_3 = L_{max}$$

$$maximize\ R_{ref2} = \frac{\omega^2 L_{23}^2}{R_3 + R_L} = \frac{\omega^2 K_{23}^2 L_2 L_3}{R_3 + R_L}$$

$$\text{i.e.}\ maximize\ L_2 \times L_3, \quad \text{Solution}: L_2 = L_3 = \frac{L_{max}}{2}$$

The maximum reflected impedance from the RX is obtained when the inductances L_2 and L_3 are equal.

8.2.5.2 Testing the Technique: Comparison 1

In this chapter, two tests are performed to present the advantages of the proposed techniques. The implanted coils presented in [10] are considered here in the first test. The efficiency of the implanted coils is enhanced in [10] (increase R_{ref2}) using higher L_2, L_3, and Q_2 at low frequency (700 kHz). An optimization procedure was considered in [10] to find the values of the implanted coil parameters. The equivalent circuit diagram of the two implanted coils in [10] is shown in Figure 8.8a (note that $Q_2 = \frac{\omega L_2}{R_2} = 273$). Reference [10] uses two implanted coils of smaller diameter (and multilayer) but very high secondary coil inductance (L_2) and low load coil inductance (L_3). Since, in this example, only the efficiency

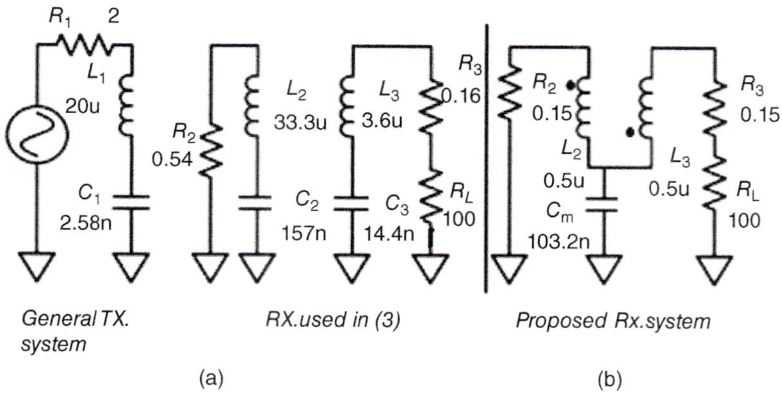

Figure 8.8 (a) Equivalent schematic of the system used in [10] ($K_{23} = 0.62$). (b) Proposed RX system incorporating the equal split inductance ($K_{23p} = 0.84$) along with mutual capacitance and appropriate relative polarity. The two RX systems shown in this figure are compared using the same TX system (left). (*Source:* Machnoor, M., Rodríguez, E. S. G., Kosta, P., et al., 2018. © IEEE.)

of the implanted RX coils ($3Coil_{2p}$ and $3Coil_{3p}$) is compared, the choice of the TX coil does not affect the PTE and PDL comparison. Thus, for comparison purposes, a 20 μH TX is used in Figure 8.8. The efficient use of wires implanted inside the body was not the design requirement in [10]. Hence, the resulting system is characterized by a larger inductance of the implanted coil of 36 μH, with a corresponding longer wire. The RX system of [10] [reproduced here as Figure 8.8a] is compared against the smaller RX system as shown in Figure 8.8b (note that $Q_{2p} = 145$). The TX used in this smaller RX design is the same; Q_2 of this system is smaller by 45%, and the values of L_2 and L_3 are about 10% of the values used in Figure 8.8a. The comparison of the two circuits is carried out at the same frequency, load, and TX conditions. The PTE, PDL, and frequency response of the two systems under comparison are shown in Figures 8.9 and 8.10, respectively. The L_2, L_3, and Q_2 of Figure 8.8b are smaller than that of Figure 8.8a for similar PDL, PTE, and frequency performances. It proves that using $L_2 = L_3$ and mutual coupling capacitor C_m, maximization of R_{ref2} is achieved. This comparison is also summarized in Table 8.1.

8.2.6 Reducing Power Dissipation in the Implanted RX

8.2.6.1 Circuit Technique Description

The term $\eta_{RX-3Coilp}$ has to be maximized to minimize the losses in the RX system. The implant coils (RX section) of the conventional three-coil sys-

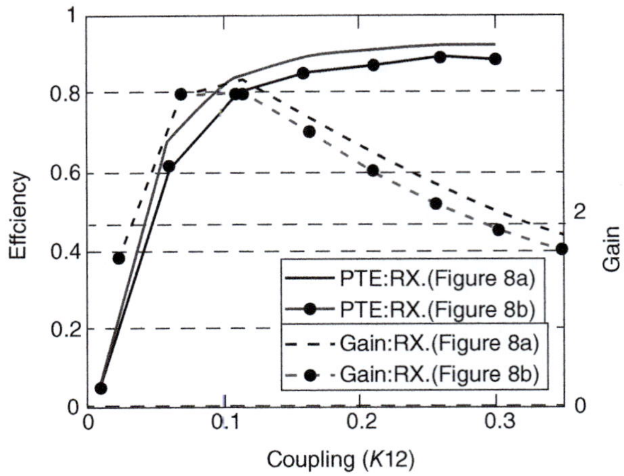

Figure 8.9 Comparison of PTE and gain of two systems in Figure 8.8 (Figure 8.8a representing [10] and Figure 8.8b representing smaller and equal split inductance). (*Source:* Machnoor, M., Rodríguez, E. S. G., Kosta, P., et al., 2018. © IEEE.)

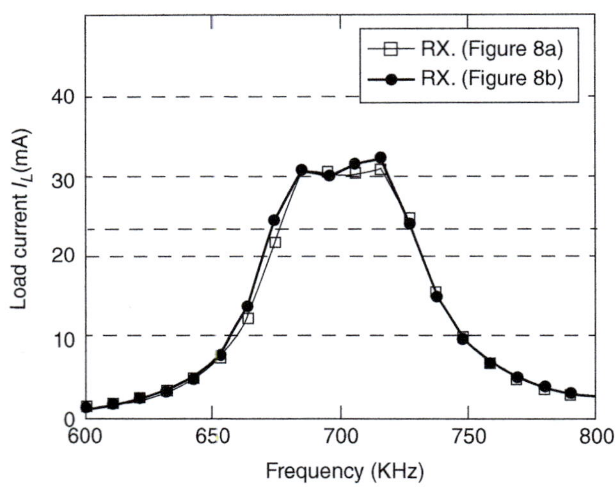

Figure 8.10 Comparison of frequency response of load current of two systems in Figure 8.8 (Figure 8.8a representing [10] and Figure 8.8b representing smaller and equal split inductance). (*Source:* Machnoor, M., Rodríguez, E. S. G., Kosta, P., et al., 2018. © IEEE.)

tems have efficiency given by (8.13–8.15). The $\eta_{RX-3Coil}$ can be rewritten as shown in (8.25). The efficiency of the RX section of the proposed three-coil system $\eta_{RX-3Coilp}$ (8.26) can be maximized by increasing $1/\omega C_m$ and avoiding C_1 and C_2 ($1/\omega C_2 = 1/\omega C_3 = 0$ in (8.17)).

$$\eta_{RX3Coil} = \frac{\left(\frac{\omega^2 L_{23}^2}{R_3+R_L}\right)}{R_2 + \frac{\omega^2 L_{23}^2}{R_3+R_L}} \times \frac{R_L}{R_3 + R_L} \tag{8.25}$$

Table 8.1 Results of two comparison exercises and the advantages of the proposed techniques as compared with the systems in [10, 11].

System	η_{RX}	L_2 (μH), L_3 (μH)	Q_2	Comments
[10] Figure 8.8a (Rx. Only)	0.91	33, 3	273	Testing technique: It is desirable to have less L_2, L_3, and Q_2 for a given receiver efficiency. Thus, to obtain 0.91 receiver efficiency, the L_2, L_3, and Q_2 requirements of the proposed system are less and more practical to attain
Proposed (Figure 8.8b)	0.91	0.5, 0.5	145	
[11] Figure 8.11a	0.75	0.4, 0.4	179	Testing technique: It is desirable to obtain more efficiency for a given set of coils L_2, L_3. In this test, the use of mutual capacitor C_m increases the receiver efficiency
Proposed (Figure 8.11b)	0.96	0.4, 0.4	179	

$$\eta_{RX3Coil} = \frac{\frac{\left(\omega L_{23}+\frac{1}{\omega C_m}\right)^2}{R_3+R_L}}{R_2 + \frac{\left(\omega L_{23}+\frac{1}{\omega C_m}\right)^2}{R_3+R_L}} \times \frac{R_L}{R_3 + R_L} \tag{8.26}$$

8.2.6.2 Testing the Technique: Comparison 2

In this subsection, the second test is carried out to prove the advantages of the proposed design techniques. The implanted coils from [11] are used as a reference for this test. In [11] (given as L_3 and L_4 for a three-coil system in Table 8.1), a conventional three-coil system is considered for the design. Higher frequency (13.56 MHz), Q_2 and low L_2 and L_3 are used in [11] to enhance the efficiency of the implanted coils (to increase R_{ref2}). The equivalent circuit diagram of the system in [11] is shown in Figure 8.11a. The approach considers two implanted coils of equal inductance (L_2) and (L_3), and the obtained RX efficiency is 0.75. The goal of the second test is to increase this implanted RX efficiency and demonstrate the functionality of mutual capacitance (C_m) in the proposed system. It is to be noted that neither the reduction of power dissipation of the coils implanted in the body nor the efficient usage of coils implanted in the body was the design requirement in [11]. As a result, K_{23}= 0.19 is chosen to reduce R_{ref2}. This design choice may increase η_{3Coil1}, although this may come at the expense of higher power dissipation in the body; the resulting system in [11], albeit an efficient one, has 25% of the constant loss in the coils implanted in the body. The RX system of Figure 8.11a is compared against the RX system shown in Figure 8.11b. The coils used in this design are the same; the only difference is that a resonant scheme with $1/\omega C_2 = 1/\omega C_3$= 0 (see (8.17)) is used

Table 8.2 Material properties of various tissue and implant components at 3.156 MHz from [33].

Tissue name	Conductivity (S/m)	Relative permittivity	Mass density (kg/m^3)
Sinus	0	1	1
Cornea	0.790	847	1076
Fat	0.026	20.7	920
Mucous membrane	0.296	612	1102
Muscle	0.570	494	1040
Brain white matter	0.120	279	1043
Gland	0.673	476	1028
Blood vessel	0.333	142	1102
Socket	7.66×10^6	0	8570
Cable (gold)	4.56×10^7	0	19,320
Array (gold)	4.56×10^7	0	19,320
Foam	0	3	1000
External coil enclosure	0	3	1070
Glasses frame	0	8	1550
PCB (FR4)	0	4.4	1850
PCB coils	5.98×10^7	0	8940
Implant coil (gold)	4.56×10^7	0	19,320
Implant coil insulation	0	3.5	2330
Cable insulation	0	3.5	2330
Cerebellum	0.234	797	1045
Bone cortical	0.032	80.6	1908
Cartilage	0.307	531	1100
Tendon	0.396	126	1142
Skin dry	0.067	730	1010
Brain grey matter	0.199	554	1039
Lens	0.452	563	1100
Eye sclera	0.729	691	1170
Blood	0.989	1020	1060
Cerebrospinal fluid	2	109	1007
Vitreous humor	1.5	73.4	1009
Bone marrow	0.0057	30.4	1029
Bone cancellous	0.103	144	1178

Source: Kosta, P., Paknahad, J., Rodríguez, E. S. G. et al. Electromagnetic safety assessment of a cortical implant for vision restoration. IEEE Journal of Electromagnetics, RF and Microwaves in Medicine and Biology 2 (1): 56–63. © 2018 IEEE.

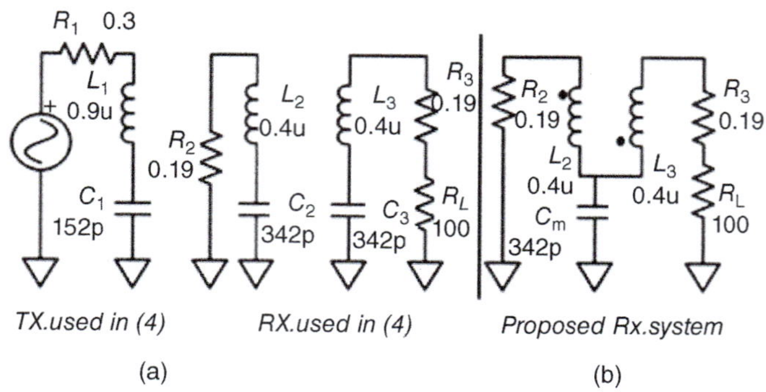

Figure 8.11 (a) Equivalent circuit diagram of the system used in [11]. The system is tested for its losses in the RX implanted in the body. (b) Schematic of the proposed RX system. The two RX systems shown in this figure are compared using the same TX system (left). (*Source:* Machnoor, M., Rodríguez, E. S. G., Kosta, P., et al., 2018. © IEEE.)

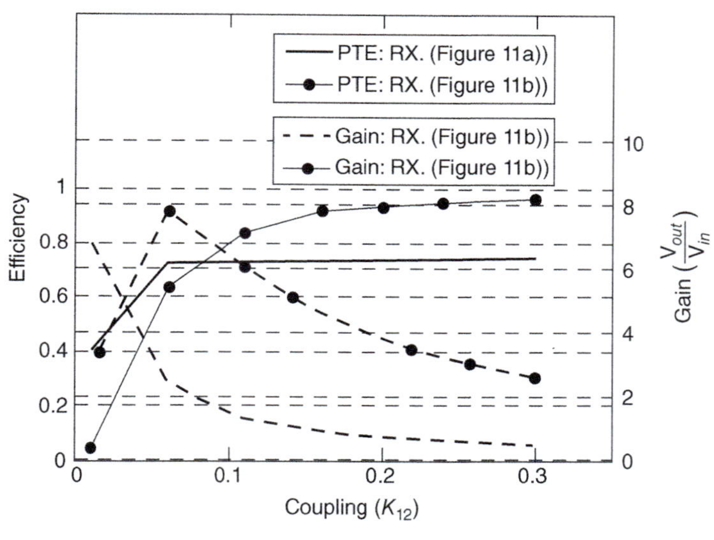

Figure 8.12 Comparison of PTE and gain of systems using two different RX configurations in Figure 8.11 (Figure 8.11a representing [11] and Figure 8.11b representing *Cm*-enhanced system). (*Source:* Machnoor, M., Rodríguez, E. S. G., Kosta, P., et al., 2018. © IEEE.)

to minimize the losses of the implanted system. Both the circuits are compared at the same frequency and load and TX conditions. The PTE and PDL (gain) of the two systems are shown in Figure 8.12. The plots of PTE (see Figure 8.11) of the two systems (Figure 8.11a representing [11] and Figure 8.11b representing $1/\omega C_2 = 1/\omega C_3 = 0$) under consideration indicate that the RX efficiency of the system (see Figure 8.11b) with mutual capacitance is 0.95, while the RX efficiency of the system without mutual capacitance is 0.75. The TX efficiency of the RX-enhanced system is reduced (see Figure 8.12) but can be increased by increasing the mutual impedance with the TX. The plots of PDL (gain) of the two systems under consideration indicate the advantages of the system (see Figure 8.11b) with mutual capacitance at the RX at higher K_{12}. This comparison is also summarized in Table 8.1.

8.2.7 Design Procedure and the Advantages of the Proposed Three-Coil System Over the Conventional Three-Coil System Design

8.2.7.1 Design Procedure

This chapter discusses two circuit concepts to increase the system performance in the proposed three-coil system $3Coil_p$ compared to the conventional design. The use of two equal coils at the RX and common capacitor enhances the reflected impedance of the RX and enables an efficient WPT for small RXs. This results in the efficient use of wires in the body and reduces the power dissipation of the coils in the RX.

The efficiency of the three-coil system can be enhanced by reducing I_1, I_2 for a given I_3 [49]. That is, both I_1/I_3 and I_2/I_3 should be minimized. The terms I_1/I_3 and I_2/I_3 now refer to the efficiency of the TX and RX, respectively. The conventional and the proposed three-coil systems have the following ratios:

$$\frac{I_1}{I_3} = \frac{(R_2(R_3 + R_L) + (\omega M_{23})^2)}{\omega M_{12}(\omega M_{23})}, \quad \frac{I_2}{I_3} = \frac{R_3 + R_L}{j\omega M_{23}} \tag{8.27}$$

$$\frac{I_{1p}}{I_{3p}} = \frac{\left(R_2(R_3 + R_L) + \left(\omega M_{23} + \frac{1}{\omega C_m}\right)^2\right)}{\omega M_{12}\left(\omega M_{23} + \frac{1}{\omega C_m}\right)}, \quad \frac{I_{2p}}{I_{3p}} = \frac{R_3 + R_L}{j\omega M_{23} + \frac{1}{j\omega C_m}} \tag{8.28}$$

The smaller RX system designed with R_2 $(R_L + R_3)$=$2\omega^2 M_{23}^2$ leads to fixed I_1/I_3 if M_{23} is doubled. That is, if the mentioned condition is satisfied, doubling ωM_{23} will not affect the efficiency of the TX. This approximate doubling of ωM_{23} is achieved through the added conductive pathway linking the two RX coils (with the addition of mutual capacitance, C_m). To demonstrate the operation and advantages of the proposed system, an RX system with limited size (smaller M_{23}) is designed, and then, using the proposed technique, the efficiency of the RX is enhanced without compromising the TX efficiency. As an example, we have considered R_L = 1 kΩ, $R_2 = R_3 = 0.5\ \Omega$, $R_1 = 1\ \Omega$, $L_1 = 5\ \mu H$, $L_2 = L_3 = 1\ \mu H$, and $f = 5$ MHz. This accounts for all the conditions proposed in this chapter, that is $L_2 = L_3$, $R_L \gg R_3$, and $R_2(R_L + R_3) = 2\omega^2 M_{23}^2$. The condition $R_2(R_L + R_3) = 2\omega^2 M_{23}^2$ leads to the smaller RX system with poor efficiency, which will be enhanced (doubled) using the proposed system with $1/\omega C_2$= $1/\omega C_3$ = 0 condition. The system [schematic of the proposed RX system shown in Figure 8.13b and the conventional system shown in

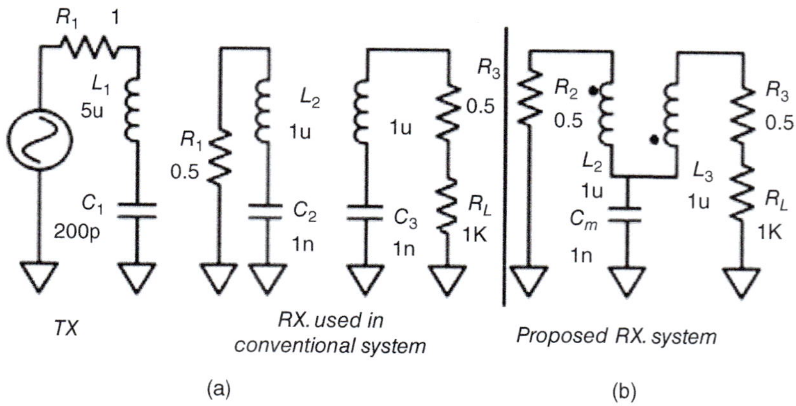

Figure 8.13 (a) Schematic of the implemented conventional three-coil system. (b) Schematic of the implemented proposed three-coil system. The two RX systems shown in this figure are compared using the same TX system (left). (*Source:* Machnoor, M., Rodríguez, E. S. G., Kosta, P., et al., 2018. © IEEE.)

Figure 8.13a] is implemented experimentally, and the results are provided in the measurements section. The simulation results showing the design approach of reducing I_2/I_3 by keeping I_1/I_3 almost fixed are shown in Figure 8.14 (it proves that we can increase the RX performance without affecting the TX efficiency).

8.2.7.2 Tolerance to Load Changes

One of the main advantages of the conventional three-coil system over the two-coil system (parallel secondary) is that its PTE is less sensitive to the variation of load. The efficiency of the RX in the proposed three-coil system is less sensitive to load variations compared with the conventional three-coil system. It is to be noted that while the conventional system achieves insensitivity by reducing R_2 [10] (or higher Q_2), the proposed system improves the insensitivity by increasing mutual coupling. The RX efficiency of the conventional and the proposed three-coil systems for the designed parameters is shown in Figure 8.15. Following the same analysis, it can be noted that $\eta_{\mathrm{RX}-3Coilp}$ is less sensitive to load compared with $\eta_{\mathrm{RX}-3Coil}$:

$$\frac{\partial(\eta_{\mathrm{RX}3Coil})}{\partial R_{\mathrm{L}}} = -\frac{\omega^2 M_{23}^2 R_2}{(\omega^2 M_{23}^2 + R_2 R_{\mathrm{L}})^2} \tag{8.29}$$

$$\frac{\partial(\eta_{\mathrm{RX}3Coilp})}{\partial R_{\mathrm{L}}} = -\frac{\left(\omega M_{23} + \frac{1}{\omega C_{\mathrm{m}}}\right)^2 R_2}{\left(\left(\omega M_{23} + \frac{1}{\omega C_{\mathrm{m}}}\right)^2 + R_2 R_{\mathrm{L}}\right)^2} \tag{8.30}$$

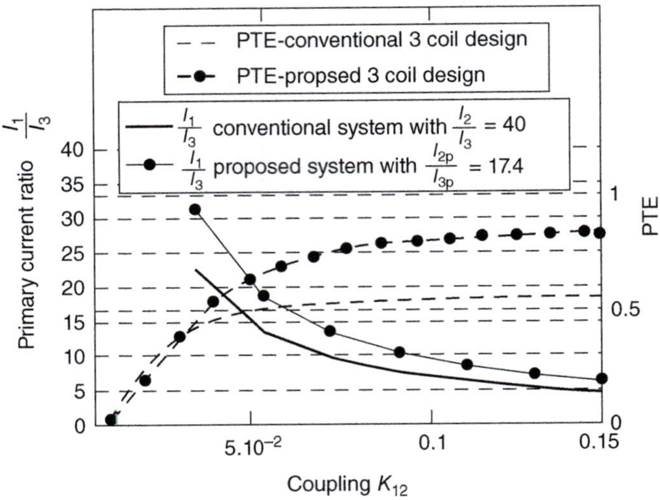

Figure 8.14 I_{2p}/I_{3p} is lesser than I_2/I_3 of the conventional system. It proves that we can increase the RX performance without affecting the TX efficiency. At lower K_{12}, PTE is limited by the TX efficiency, which is the same for both the systems. (*Source:* Machnoor, M., Rodríguez, E. S. G., Kosta, P., et al., 2018. © IEEE.)

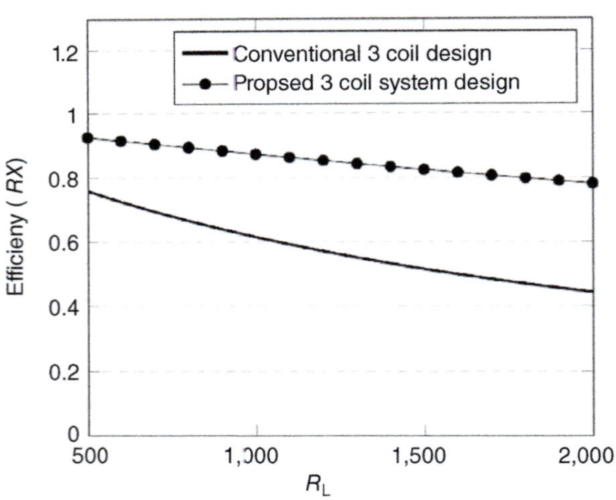

Figure 8.15 Comparison of load sensitivity of the efficiency of implanted systems designed using the conventional and the proposed design techniques. (*Source:* Machnoor, M., Rodríguez, E. S. G., Kosta, P., et al., 2018. © IEEE.)

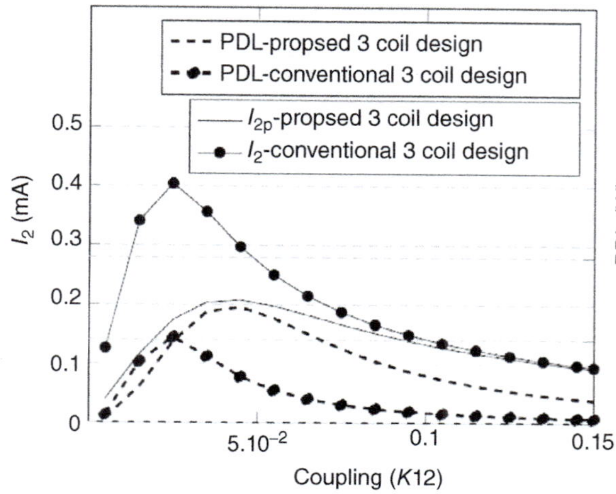

Figure 8.16 Comparison of PDL ($Vin = 1$) and secondary coil currents of the proposed and conventional designs of the three-coil system. It can be noticed that, for a given PDL, the required value of I_{2p} is less than I_2 for all K_{12}. (*Source:* Machnoor, M., Rodríguez, E. S. G., Kosta, P., et al., 2018. © IEEE.)

8.2.7.3 Advantage 2: Reducing Currents in the Secondary Coil

The currents through the intermediate secondary coil of the three-coil system should be reduced for a given load to decrease the losses in the system [49]. The proposed and the conventional systems, for the given design parameters, are evaluated for the secondary coil current for different couplings with the TX coil. The proposed system reduces the current through the secondary coil by enhancing the mutual impedance between the implanted coils, as shown in Figure 8.16. The magnetic field is proportional to the current flowing through the coil, and usually, for a single antenna, electric field is proportional to the magnetic field. In the measurements section, it will be shown that the proposed system achieves the same power delivery of the traditional three-coil system while achieving higher efficiency.

Load Current I_3 and $I_{3\text{p}}$ The simulated PDL ($I_3^2 R_\text{L}$, $I_{3\text{p}}^2 R_\text{L}$, for $V_\text{in} = 1$) and current in $Coil_2$ and $Coil_{2\text{p}}$ for the conventional three-coil (see Figure 8.13a) system and the proposed three-coil see Figure 8.13b) system for a different K_{12} value are shown in Figure 8.16. To analyze the effect of mutual capacitance on the RX currents (I_3, I_2 and $I_{3\text{p}}$, $I_{2\text{p}}$) for the systems under consideration, we solve the matrix in (8.19) for $I_{2\text{p}}$ (similarly for I_2) and rewrite (8.27, 8.28) as (8.31) (where $R_{3t} = R_3 + R_\text{L}$). Thus, it can be noticed in Figure 8.16 that at high K_{12} (the terms with ωM_{12} dominate in I_2 (and I_{2p}) and consequently, I_2 becomes equal to I_{2p}), for a given I_2 value (or I_{2p}), the proposed three-coil system has higher load current (I_{3p}) compared with the conventional three-coil system (I_3)

$$I_2 = \frac{j\omega M_{12} R_{3t}}{R_1 R_2 R_{3t} + \omega^2 M_{23}^2 R_1 + \omega^2 M_{12}^2 R_{3t}}$$

$$I_{2p} = \frac{j\omega M_{12} R_{3t}}{R_1 R_2 R_{3t} + \left(\omega M_{23} + \frac{1}{\omega C_m}\right)^2 R_1 + \omega^2 M_{12}^2 R_{3t}}$$

$$I_3 = \frac{I_2 (j\omega M_{23})}{R_{3t}}, \quad I_{3p} = \frac{I_{2p}\left(j\omega M_{23} + \frac{1}{j\omega C_m}\right)}{R_{3t}} \tag{8.31}$$

Conversely, for a given load current (fixed $I_3 = I_{3p}$) or PDL, the required value of I_{2p} is less than the required value of I_2(at lower K_{12}, the terms with ωM_{23} and $\omega M_{23}+1/\omega C_m$ dominate in I_2 and I_{2p}, respectively, and $I_{2p}/I_2 = (\omega M_{23}/\omega M_{23} + 1/\omega C_m)$. This can be attributed to the increased mutual impedance between the *Coil2p* and *Coil3p* for the proposed three-coil system.

The maxima of the PDL in Figure 8.16 occurs when $R_{ref1} = R_1$ for 3*Coil* and $R_{ref1p} = R_1$ for 3$Coil_p$ systems as given by the MPT theorem. The PDL maxima for the 3$Coil_p$ is higher than the PDL maxima of 3*Coil* and also occurs at slightly higher K_{12}. It is because C_m, which increases R_{ref2}, decreases R_{ref1} slightly. It is to be noted that this relation is also the consequence of the choice of relative coil polarity.

8.2.7.4 K_{12} and C_m for Optimization of System Performance: Layout Design Advantages

In the conventional three-coil (3*Coil*) system, the mutual coupling between the two RX coils K_{23} is used to optimize the reflected impedance R_{ref2} to obtain the desired system performance [10–13]. The maximization of K_{23} increases the RX efficiency but decreases TX efficiency and vice versa. This dependence of system performance on K_{23} puts a constraint on the coil geometry in the conventional three-coil system. The system in [10] uses a larger (multilayer) secondary coil compared with load coil to achieve K_{23} of 0.6. In the system in [11], additional spacing is used between the two RX coils to achieve a lower K_{23} value of 0.22. These geometries are difficult to implement for a real compact implant RX. In this proposed three-coil (3$Coil_p$) system, the adopted architectural update leads to new reflected impedance of the secondary R_{ref2p} (see (8.22)), which depends not only on K_{23} but also on mutual capacitance (C_m) and appropriate relative polarity. Now, C_m have the same effect on the system as K_{23}. This puts less constraints on the K_{23} requirements, and we can optimize the layout of the implanted coils to meet additional requirements like smaller size (inductance) or any other variables, like SAR [33, 48] requirements.

In this chapter, to demonstrate the advantage of the proposed technique, an RX coil with small inductance is considered. The mutual capacitance between the two implanted coils is used to enhance the efficiency of the RX coils. The PTE comparison of the conventional three-coil system and the proposed three-coil system will be verified in the measurements Section 8.2.6.

8.2.7.5 Effects of Tissue and Tissue Parameters on the Power Delivery

The proposed WPT system could be used in a cortical implant for vision restoration [33]. In the model of the human head, there is 4-mm-thick fat and 3.75-mm-thick dry skin in between the RX coil and the air interface. To analyze the effects of the human tissue on the proposed system performance, fat and dry skin layers are used in the CST simulation as shown in Figure 8.17. The material density, electrical conductivity, and relative permittivity of the materials are presented in [32, shown next page]. K_{12}, and PTE of the system are not affected by the tissue, and as a result, the PDL of the system also remains unchanged, as shown in Figure 8.17. The PDL of the proposed system for a separation of 20 mm between the TX and the RX at 5 MHz is 18 mW (gain = 4.25, PDL = $(V_{in} \times \text{Gain})^2/R_L = (1 \times 4.25)^2/1000$). This is verified using measurements in the next section.

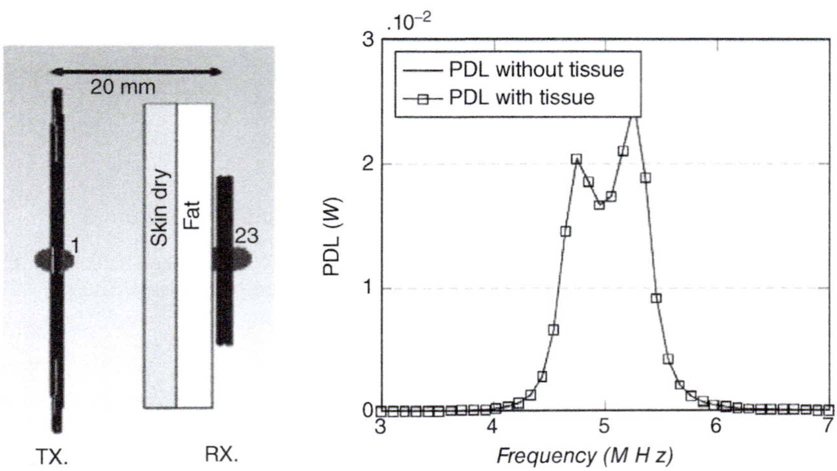

Figure 8.17 Study of the effect of tissue material on the system performance. Left: the proposed three-coil WPT system with skin dry (3.75-mm thick) and fat (4-mm thick) tissue in between the TX and the RX. Right: plot of PDL versus frequency for the system with and without the tissue. It can be noted that tissue has no effect on the PDL. Refer to Table 8.2 for details about the material properties. (*Source:* Machnoor, M., Rodríguez, E. S. G., Kosta, P., et al., 2018. © IEEE.)

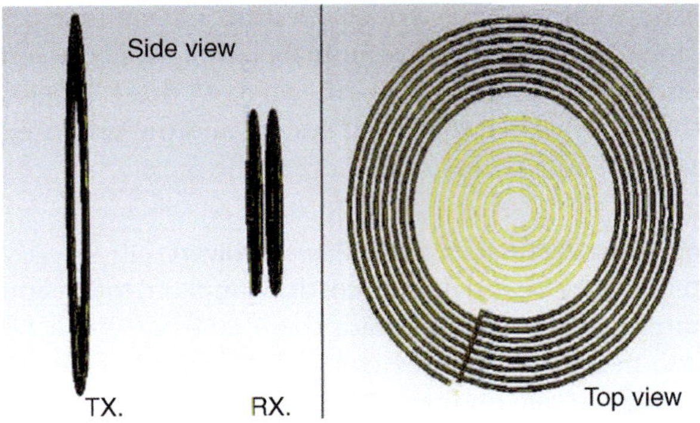

Figure 8.18 Layout of the side view and top view of the three-coil system in CST Design STUDIO. In the top view, $3Coil_1$ highlighted for differentiation. The diameters of the transmit and receive coils are 70 and 35 mm, respectively. (*Source:* Machnoor, M., Rodríguez, E. S. G., Kosta, P., et al., 2018. © IEEE.)

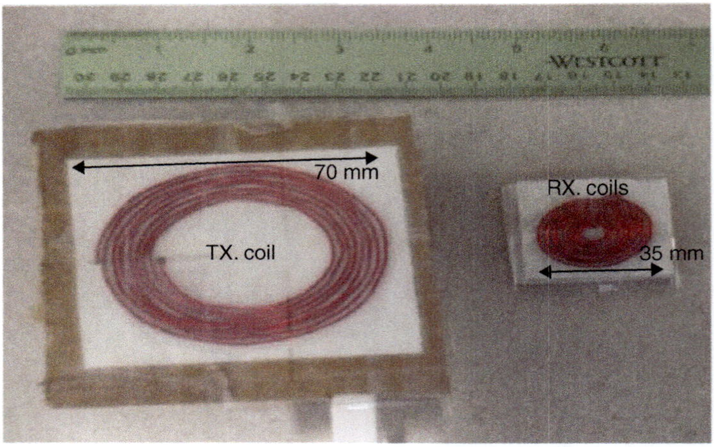

Figure 8.19 Photograph of the measurement setup showing TX coil (left) and RX coil (right). The diameters of the transmit and receive coils are 70 and 35 mm, respectively. (*Source:* Machnoor, M., Rodríguez, E. S. G., Kosta, P., et al., 2018. © IEEE.)

8.2.8 Experiments: Measurements and Results

The proposed three-coil system $3Coil_p$ is compared against a conventional three-coil system 3*Coil* and two-coil system 2*Coil*. The measurement results are compared against simulation. The side view and top view of the layout of the considered three-coil system are shown in Figure 8.18, while the measurement setup is shown in Figure 8.19. It is to be recalled that the layout of 3*Coil* and $3Coil_p$ is the same, but the resonance condition is different. Two-coil system 2*Coil* is formed by removing the $3Coil_3$ of the 3*Coil* system.

Table 8.3 Properties of the coils used.

Coil	Coil diameter (mm)	Number of turns	L (μH)	Q	AWG
TX	70	8	5	150	20
Sec.	35	8	1	70	20
Load	35	8	1	70	20

Table 8.4 Circuit parameters of the three systems under test.

System	L_1 (μH)	L_2 (μH)	L_3 (μH)	R_L (kΩ)	f (MHz)
2*Coil*	5	1		1	5
3*Coil*	5	1	1	1	5
3$Coil_p$	5	1	1	1	5

The physical and electrical parameters of the coils used in the experiments are shown in Tables 8.3 and 8.4, respectively. In the 3$Coil_p$ and 3*Coil* systems, $L_2 = L_3$ is maintained. Furthermore, in the 3$Coil_p$ systems, $1/\omega C_2 = 1/\omega C_3 = 0$ is maintained in the implementation. Finally, in the 3$Coil_p$ system, a smaller RX system is designed with $R_2(R_L + R_3) = 2\omega^2 M_{23}^2$, so that I_1/I_3 remains unchanged if M_{23} is doubled using the proposed design technique. The measurements are performed using a VNA; S-parameters from VNA are converted to Z-parameters. The performance parameters of interest (PTE [see (32)] and PDL) are expressed using Z-parameters [10–13]. Since it is difficult to measure the exact source voltage (V_s) for VNA measurements, measurement is made independent of V_s by measuring the gain instead. PDL is related to the voltage gain by (8.33)

$$\eta = \frac{|Z_{21}|^2}{R_L |Z_{11}| \cos(\text{Phase}(Z_{11}))}, \quad \text{Gain} = \frac{|Z_{21}|}{|Z_{11}|} \tag{8.32}$$

$$\text{PDL} = \frac{|V_2|^2}{2R_L} = \frac{|Z_{21}|^2 V_1^2}{2R_L |Z_{11}|^2} = \frac{\text{Gain}^2 V_1^2}{2R_L} \tag{8.33}$$

The PTE comparison (see Figure 8.20) shows that for a small RX system with large R_L, $\eta_{3Coilp} > \eta_{3Coil} > \eta_{2Coil}$ for all the distances. Also, η_{3Coilp} at large distances (small K_{12}) does not fall below 3*Coil*. The PTE of the 3*Coil* at 20 cm separation is 0.4, whereas the PTE of the 3$Coil_p$ at 20 cm is 0.8. It can be concluded that, in the considered case, the 3$Coil_p$ has double the PTE of 3*Coil*. The

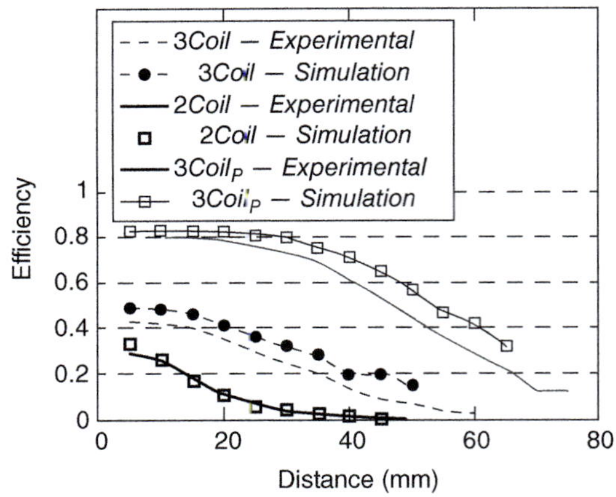

Figure 8.20 Experimental and simulation results of PTE of three systems under comparison. (*Source:* Machnoor, M., Rodríguez, E. S. G., Kosta, P., et al., 2018. © IEEE.)

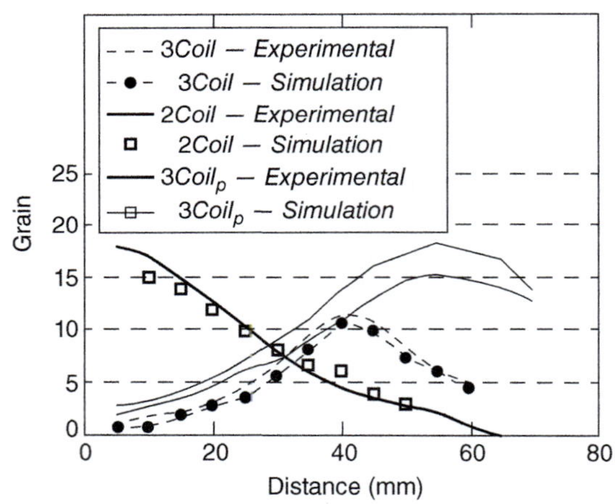

Figure 8.21 Experimental and simulation results of gain of three systems under comparison. (*Source:* Machnoor, M., Rodríguez, E. S. G., Kosta, P., et al., 2018. © IEEE.)

gain performance (see Figure 8.21) of the three-coil system is better than the two-coil system at larger distances for higher loads and smaller coils. The common capacitor circuit ($3Coil_p$) performs better than the conventional three-coil ($3Coil$) system, both in terms of efficiency and gain for all the distances between the TX and the RX.

8.3 Justifying the Advantages of Using Multicoil WPT Systems for Data Transfer

In biomedical implants and neural prosthesis, data transmission is a crucial part of maintaining the consistent performance of the system. Data transmission can be used to transmit the recorded data to the external system [1–3, 7]. Several techniques are presented in the literature to achieve wireless power and data transmission [7, 50–52]. Since the inductive power and data is the focus of this chapter, we briefly mention several techniques adopted in the literature. The simplest technique is to use a separate coil for power and data transmission [53]. The use of separate coils can lead to reduced communication quality [54] as well as reduced Q of the power transmission coil due to proximity effect, if the dimensions of the two coils are comparable. Dual-band performance is achieved by frequency splitting [54–56] and SPRC (series and parallel resonator circuits) [57–59] circuits in the literature. While the SPRC systems need more complex RXs, frequency splitting is a high coupling phenomenon [60] reserved for electric vehicles. The RX electronics implanted in the body need to be reliable, low power, and simple to avoid any failure. Hence, amplitude modulation (AM) and frequency modulation (FM) are popular modulation techniques for biomedical applications [50]. Other modulation and coding techniques, for example amplitude shift keying (ASK) [61], frequency shift keying (FSK) [62], cyclic ON–OFF keying (COOK) [63], load shift keying schemes [64], and others [65–68], are also studied to explore their advantages. The use of separate frequencies for power and data transmission is usually adopted as a higher quality factor is often needed to achieve high-power transmission efficiency. It is to be noted that dual-band systems designed with a goal of comparable PTE at the two bands experience a reduction in maximum efficiency [58]. This is not acceptable as the power transmission must be conducted at high-efficiency levels for better battery performance. Thus, in this work, three-coil systems are used to improve PF and gain at an assumed data delivery frequency.

In this work, we have discussed PTE, PDL (gain), and PF as performance parameters. Improvement in any of these parameters enhances the power delivery capability of a system. Improvement in PF ensures appropriate matching and reduced reflection; improvement in PTE reduces resistive losses, and gain improvement enables higher power delivery for a given voltage source. A higher Q requirement of the coil reduces the bandwidth available for data transmission and necessitates allotment of the separate band for the data transfer. Also, to achieve the desired power delivery, sometimes in a multicoil system, the coupling between the driver and TX coil is varied, and in an LCC system, LCC parameters are varied [16]. The variation in the coupling parameters or the values of the matching network also varies the bandwidth of the PTE, gain, and PF, influencing the frequency characteristics available for the data transmission. Thus, to avoid the influence of power delivery properties on data transmission, dual bands are adopted in the literature [69]. It is to be noted that, even though separate bands are used for power and data transmission, in several wireless data and power transmission works, no additional circuit element is added to enhance the system performance at data transmission frequency [10, 70]. This may severely limit the range of data communication systems where simple RX architectures are used.

The performance of the inductive link-based communication system depends on the Q-factors of the coils, magnetic coupling between them, and the carrier frequency. The goal of the antennas is to provide favorable frequency characteristics for power and data transmission. The data transfer frequency is usually chosen to be different from the power delivery frequency in high Q systems (dual band [7]). In this section, the advantage of using a multicoil topology for wireless power and data transmission compared to a standard two-coil system is described.

The goal is to provide better frequency characteristics at the data transfer frequency without affecting the performance at power transmission resonance frequency. The gain and power factor of the data transmission frequency in a three-coil system is enhanced compared to the two-coil system. Further, the designer must be able to choose the data transmission frequency independent of the gain performance requirements at the power transmission frequency. This is important because the same system can be tuned to deliver different power to the RX for a fixed data transmission band.

The schematic and the performance parameters of an example two-coil system are shown in Figure 8.22. The system is designed for a power transmission resonance frequency of 5.030 MHz. The salient feature of this system is that the frequency response of PTE, PDL, gain, and PF achieves maximum at the resonance frequency. There are no other maxima in the frequency response of these performance parameters. The advantage of such a simple system is that the TX coil is operating at its maximum efficiency possible. The system does not have sufficient degrees of freedom to achieve secondary resonances at any arbitrary data delivery frequencies. The additional degree of freedom can come from the use of multicoil systems.

The three-coil systems can help achieve better PF and gain performance at a chosen data transmission frequency without compromising the efficiency at the power transmission frequency. Also, this can be achieved in a three-coil system by changing only one capacitor marked as C_m in the schematics shown in Figures 8.23 and 8.24. The tuning of C_m allows changing an example data transmission frequency marked as B (3.9 MHz) in Figure 8.23 to C (4.56 MHz) in Figure 8.24. The power transmission gain, PTE, and PF of the system are maintained at a fixed value for both the circuits in Figures 8.23 and 8.24. This means that we can design a system whose data frequency resonance can be tuned independently of the performance parameters at the power transfer frequency.

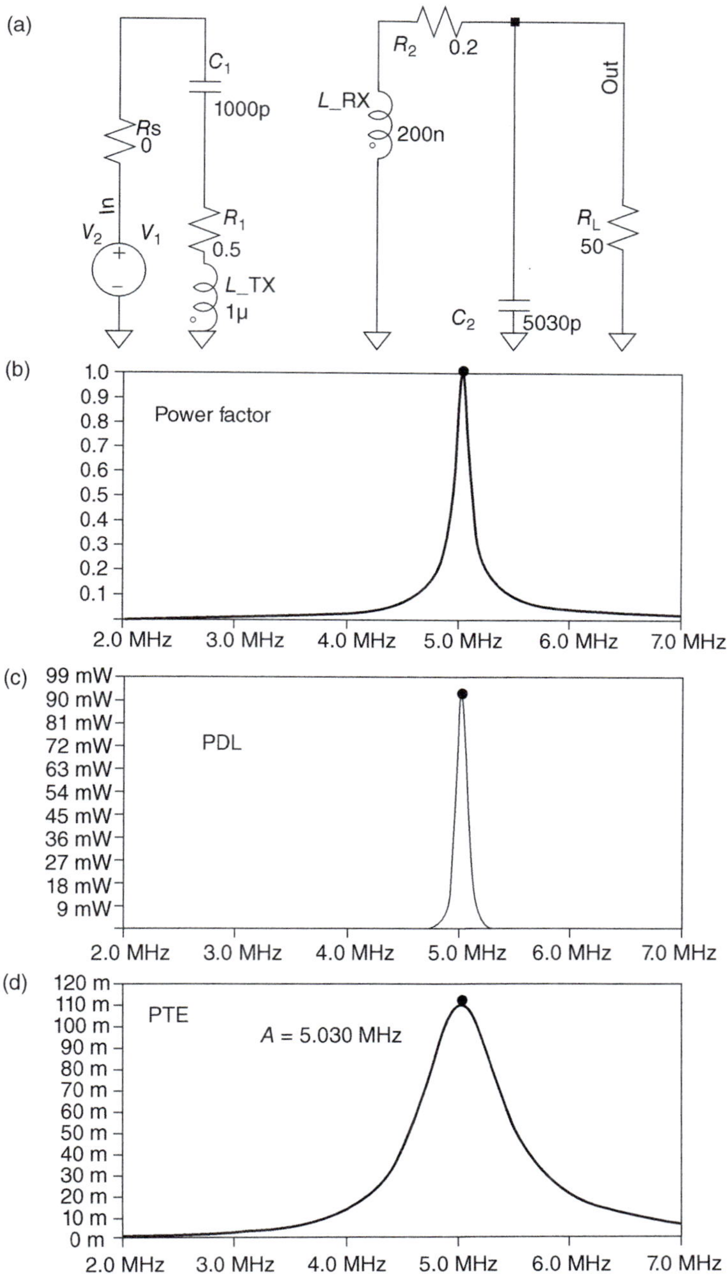

Figure 8.22 (a) The schematic of the two-coil system under study. The coupling coefficient (K_{12}) between the transmitter coil (L_{TX}) and the receiver coil (L_{RX}) is 0.02. (b) The unity power factor observed at the resonance frequency of 5.030 MHz. (c) The PDL (gain) achieves peak at the resonance frequency. (d) The PTE achieves peak at the resonance frequency.

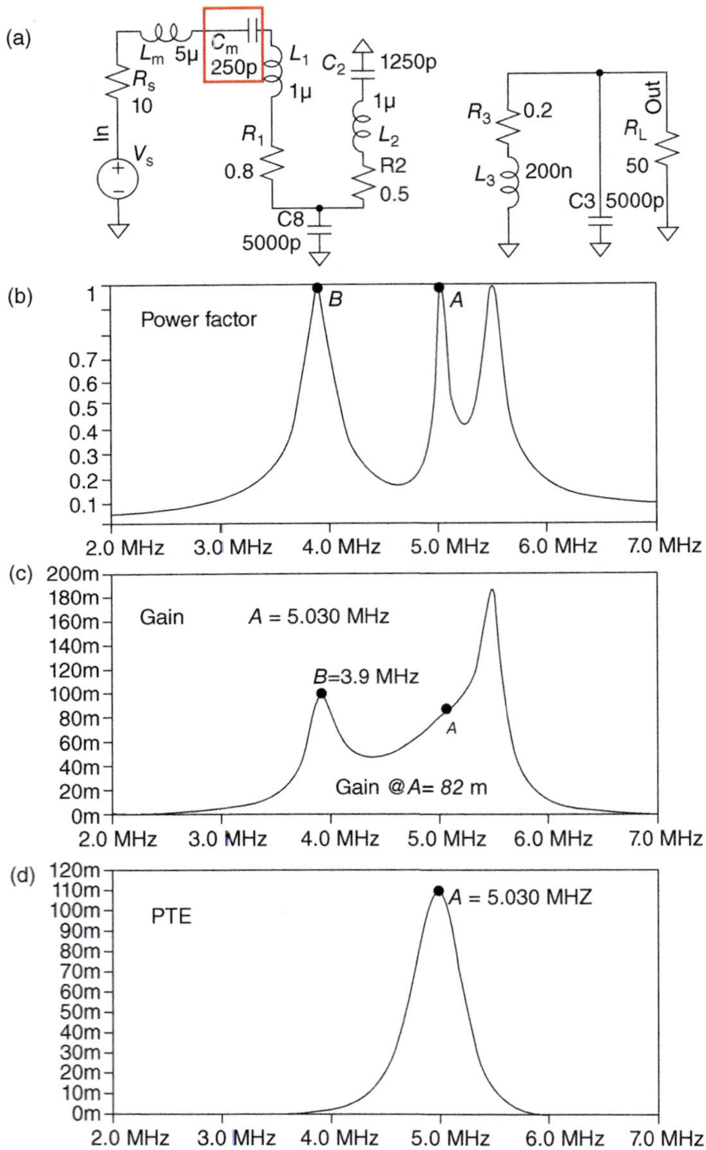

Figure 8.23 (a) The schematic of the three-coil system under study. Note that the value of C_m is 250 *pF*. The coupling coefficient (K_{12}) between the driver coil (L_1) and the transmitter coil (L_2) is 0.5. The coupling coefficient (K_{23}) between the transmitter coil (L_2) and the receiver coil (L_3) is 0.02. (b) The unity power factor observed at the power transfer resonance frequency 5.030 MHz (A) and an example data transmission frequency 3.9 MHz (B). (c) The PDL (gain) achieves a maxima at B, and the gain at A is 82 m. (d) The PTE achieves peak at power transfer resonance frequency (A).

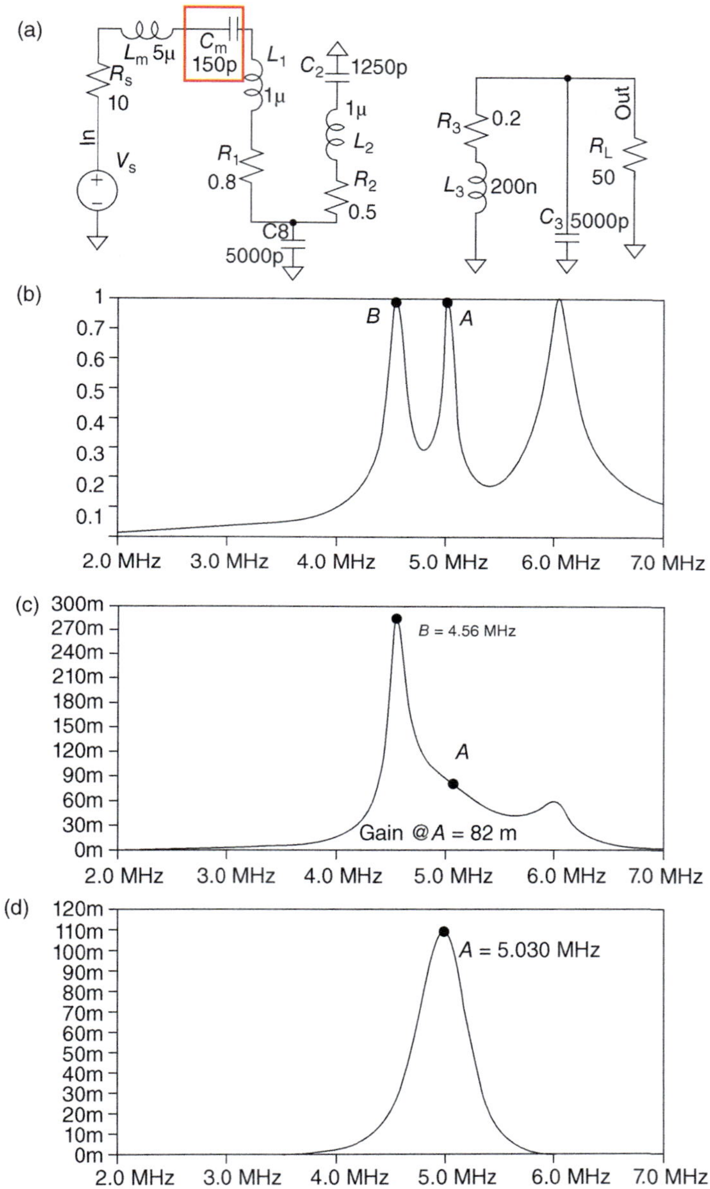

Figure 8.24 (a) The schematic of the three-coil system under study. Note that the value of C_m is now 150 pF to change the example data transfer frequency from 3.9 to 4.56 MHz. The coupling coefficient (K_{12}) between the driver coil (L_1) and the transmitter coil (L_2) is 0.5. The coupling coefficient (K_{23}) between the transmitter coil (L_2) and the receiver coil (L_3) is 0.02. (b) The unity power factor observed at the power transfer resonance frequency 5.030 MHz (A) and an example data transmission frequency 4.56 MHz (C). (c) The PDL (gain) achieves a maxima at C and maintains the gain of 82 m at A. (d) The PTE achieves peak at power transfer resonance frequency (A).

8.4 Conclusion

Multicoil WPT systems, in general, provide several advantages over conventional two-coil systems. The use of additional coils, in general, leads to higher coupling, higher efficiency, insensitivity to load, and misalignments. The use of multicoil systems also enables us to provide better PF and gain characteristics at the data transfer frequency.

In this chapter, a modified three-coil system configuration is proposed that introduces additional degrees of freedom in the design process. The appropriate relative voltage polarity between coils and the mutual capacitance can now be used in addition to K_{23} in the conventional three-coil systems to control the reflected impedance and hence the system performance. In this design, these additional variables are used to improve the systems with low RX inductance and RX efficiency. Two techniques are considered: 1) equal split of two RX coils in the three-coil WPT system ($L_2 = L_3$)) and 2) $1/\omega C_2 = 1/\omega C_3 = 0$. The combined effect of these concepts leads to a system with high R_{ref2p}. Experiments verify the assertions, with results demonstrating the proposed three-coil system with twice the efficiency of a conventional system for small RX coils. The proposed system design results in a PTE and gain of 0.45 and 15 at 60 mm separation between the TX and the RX at a resonance frequency of 5 MHz and $R_L = 1\ \text{k}\Omega$.

In comparison, under the same operating conditions, the conventional three- and two-coil system result in a PTE of less than 0.1 and again of less than 5. The proposed system also achieves RX designs with better insensitivity to load variation while also reducing the fields induced in the body due to secondary coil current. Finally, we show that, at the considered frequency, the system performance is robust to the presence of human tissue. The inductive WPT technique has been successfully applied to transmit power to the commercial retina prosthesis [3, 33].

Commonly Used Symbols

η	symbol for efficiency
η_{Coil-n}	efficiency of coil n
LCC	inductor capacitor (used as a matching circuit in [16])
L_n	self-inductance of coil n
R_n	parasitic resistance of coil n
R_L	load resistor
C_m	mutual capacitor; it is used in between two coils
C_k	$k = 1, 2, 3$ is the capacitor used in each coil for resonance purposes
K_{mn}	mutual coupling symbol between coils m and n
Q_m	quality factor of coil m

L_{12}	mutual inductance between coils m and n
M_{12}	mutual inductance between coils m and n
ω	angular frequency, $\omega = 2\pi f$
I_k	$k = 1, 2, 3$ the current flowing in the coil k of a conventional system
I_{kp}	$k = 1, 2, 3$ the current flowing in the coil k of the proposed system
PDL	power delivered to the load
Z_{mn}	Z parameters between ports m and n

References

1 Song, D., Robinson, B.S., Hampson, R.E. et al. (2018). Sparse large-scale nonlinear dynamical modeling of human hippocampus for memory prostheses. *IEEE Transactions on Neural Systems and Rehabilitation Engineering* 26 (2): 272–280.

2 Lee, B., Kramer, D., Armenta Salas, M. et al. (2018). Engineering artificial somatosensation through cortical stimulation in humans. *Frontiers in Systems Neuroscience* 12: 24. https://doi.org/10.3389/fnsys.2018.00024.

3 Roksana, S., Arathy, K., Michael, B. et al. (2019). Thermal and distance image filtering improve independent mobility in Argus II retinal implant. *Journal of Vision* 19: 23. https://doi.org/10.1167/19.15.23.

4 Taccola, G., Sayenko, D., Gad, P. et al. (2018). And yet it moves: recovery of volitional control after spinal cord injury. *Progress in Neurobiology* 160: 64–81.

5 Gross, R.E., Krack, P., Rodriguez-Oroz, M.C. et al. (2006). Electrophysiological mapping for the implantation of deep brain stimulators for Parkinson's disease and tremor. *Movement Disorders* 21: S259–S283.

6 Humayun, M. and de Juan, E. (1998). Artificial vision. *Eye* 12: 605–607.

7 Ramrakhyani, A.K. and Lazzi, G. (2015). *Wireless Applications: Dual Band Power and Data Telemetry*. New York: Springer.

8 Bashirullah, R. (2010). Wireless implants. *IEEE Microwave Magazine* 11 (7): S14–S23.

9 Chen, G., Stang, J., Haynes, M. et al. (2018). Realtime three-dimensional microwave monitoring of interstitial thermal therapy. *IEEE Transactions on Biomedical Engineering* 65 (3): 528–538.

10 Ram Rakhyani, A.K., Mirabbasi, S., and Chiao, M. (2011). Design and optimization of resonance-based efficient wireless power delivery systems for biomedical implants. *IEEE Transactions on Biomedical Circuits and Systems* 5 (1): 48–63.

11 Kiani, M., Jow, U.-M., and Ghovanloo, M. (2011). Design and optimization of a 3-coil inductive link for efficient wireless power transmission. *IEEE Transactions on Biomedical Circuits and Systems* 5 (6): 579–591.

12 Kiani, M. and Ghovanloo, M. (2012). The circuit theory behind coupled-mode magnetic resonance-based wireless power transmission. *Transactions on Circuits and Systems I: Regular Papers* 59 (9): 2065–2074.
13 RamRakhyani, A.K. and Lazzi, G. (2013). On the design of efficient multi-coil telemetry system for biomedical implants. *IEEE Transactions on Biomedical Circuits and Systems* 7 (1): 11–23.
14 Knecht, O., Bosshard, R., and Kolar, J.W. (2015). High-efficiency transcutaneous energy transfer for implantable mechanical heart support systems. *IEEE Transactions on Power Electronics* 30 (11): 6221–6236.
15 Musavi, F. and Eberle, W. (2014). Overview of wireless power transfer technologies for electric vehicle battery charging. *IET Power Electronics* 7 (1): 60–66.
16 Li, S., Li, W., Deng, J. et al. (2015). A double-sided LCC compensation network and its tuning method for wireless power transfer. *IEEE Transactions on Vehicular Technology* 64 (6): 2261–2273.
17 Zhang, J., Yuan, X., Wang, C., and He, Y. (2017). Comparative analysis of two-coil and three-coil structures for wireless power transfer. *IEEE Transactions on Power Electronics* 32 (1): 341–352.
18 Moon, S., Kim, B.-C., Cho, S.-Y. et al. (2014). Analysis and design of a wireless power transfer system with an intermediate coil for high efficiency. *IEEE Transactions on Industrial Electronics* 61 (11): 5861–5870.
19 Bi, S., Ho, C.K., and Zhang, R. (2015). Wireless powered communication: opportunities and challenges. *IEEE Communications Magazine* 53 (4): 117–125.
20 Huang, K. and Zhou, X. (2015). Cutting the last wires for mobile communications by microwave power transfer. *IEEE Communications Magazine* 53 (6): 86–93.
21 Ko, W.H., Liang, S.P., and Fung, C.D.F. (1977). Design of radio-frequency powered coils for implant instruments. *Medical & Biological Engineering & Computing* 15 (6): 634–640.
22 Wu, K., Choudhury, D., and Matsumoto, H. (2013). Wireless power transmission, technology, and applications [scanning the issue]. *Proceedings of the IEEE* 101 (6): 1271–1275.
23 Kurs, A., Karalis, A., Moffatt, R. et al. (2007). Wireless power transfer via strongly coupled magnetic resonances. *Science* 317 (5834): 83–86.
24 Kiani, M., Lee, B., Yeon, P., and Ghovanloo, M. (2015). A Q-modulation technique for efficient inductive power transmission. *IEEE J. Solid-State Circuits* 50 (12): 2839–2848.
25 Zhong, W.X. and Hui, S.Y.R. (2015). Maximum energy efficiency tracking for wireless power transfer systems. *IEEE Transactions on Power Electronics* 30 (7): 4025–4034.

26 Zhang, W. and Mi, C.C. (2016). Compensation topologies of high-power wireless power transfer systems. *IEEE Transactions on Vehicular Technology* 65 (6): 4768–4778.
27 Tan, X. and Ruan, X. (2016). Equivalence relations of resonant tanks: a new perspective for selection and design of resonant converters. *IEEE Transactions on Industrial Electronics* 63 (4): 2111–2123.
28 Xue, R.-F., Cheng, K.-W., and Je, M. (2013). High-efficiency wireless power transfer for biomedical implants by optimal resonant load transformation. *Transactions on Circuits and Systems I: Regular Papers* 60 (4): 867–874.
29 Chen, C.-J., Chu, T.-H., Lin, C.-L., and Jou, Z.-C. (2010). A study of loosely coupled coils for wireless power transfer. *IEEE Transactions on Circuits and Systems II: Express Briefs* 57 (7): 536–540.
30 Qusba, A., RamRakhyani, A.K., So, J.-H. et al. (2014). On the design of microfluidic implant coil for flexible telemetry system. *IEEE Sensors Journal* 14 (4): 1074–1080.
31 Rodríguez, E.S.G., RamRakhyani, A.K., Schurig, D., and Lazzi, G. (2016). Compact low-frequency metamaterial design for wireless power transfer efficiency enhancement. *IEEE Transactions on Microwave Theory and Techniques* 64 (5): 1644–1654.
32 RodrÃguez, E.S.G., Machnoor, M., and Lazzi, G. (2017). On the generation of nondiffracting beams in extremely subwavelength applications. *IEEE Transactions on Antennas and Propagation* 65 (10): 5228–5237.
33 Kosta, P., Paknahad, J., Rodríguez, E.S.G. et al. (2018). Electromagnetic safety assessment of a cortical implant for vision restoration. *IEEE Journal of Electromagnetics, RF and Microwaves in Medicine and Biology* 2 (1): 56–63.
34 IEEE Standard for Safety Levels With Respect to Human Exposure to Radio Frequency Electromagnetic Fields, 3 KHz to 300 GHz, IEEE Standard C95.1-2005 (Revision of IEEE Std C95.1-1991) (April 2006), 1–238.
35 Gabriel, S., Lau, R.W., and Gabriel, C. (1996). The dielectric properties of biological tissues: II. Measurements in the frequency range 10 Hz to 20 GHz. *Physics in Medicine and Biology* 41 (11): 2251.
36 Hui, S.Y.R., Zhong, W., and Lee, C.K. (2014). A critical review of recent progress in mid-range wireless power transfer. *IEEE Transactions on Power Electronics* 29 (9): 4500–4511.
37 Chen, X.L. et al. (2014). Human exposure to close-range resonant wireless power transfer systems as a function of design parameters. *IEEE Transactions on Electromagnetic Compatibility* 56 (5): 1027–1034.
38 Van Paemel, M. (2011). High-efficiency transmission for medical implants. *IEEE Solid-State Circuits Magazine* 3 (1): 47–59.
39 RamRakhyani, A.K. and Lazzi, G. (2012). Multi-coil telemetry system for compensation of coil misalignment effects in implantable systems. *IEEE Antennas and Wireless Propagation Letters* 11: 1675–1678.

40 Zhong, W.X., Zhang, C., Liu, X., and Hui, S.Y.R. (2015). A methodology for making a three-coil wireless power transfer system more energy efficient than a two-coil counterpart for extended transfer distance. *IEEE Transactions on Power Electronics* 30 (2): 933–942.

41 Sodagar, A.M., Wise, K.D., and Najafi, K. (2009). A wireless implantable microsystem for multichannel neural recording. *IEEE Transactions on Microwave Theory and Techniques* 57 (10): 2565–2573.

42 Harrison, R.R. et al. (2007). A low-power integrated circuit for a wireless 100- electrode neural recording system. *IEEE J. Solid-State Circuits* 42 (1): 123–133.

43 Lee, S.B., Lee, H.-M., Kiani, M. et al. (2010). An inductively powered scalable 32-channel wireless neural recording system-on-a-chip for neuroscience applications. *IEEE Transactions on Biomedical Circuits and Systems* 4 (6): 360–371.

44 Karumbaiah, L. et al. (2013). Relationship between intracortical electrode design and chronic recording function. *Biomaterials* 34 (33): 8061–8074.

45 McConnell, G., Rees, H., Levey, A. et al. (2009). Implanted neural electrodes cause chronic, local inflammation that is correlated with local neurodegeneration. *Journal of Neural Engineering* 6: 056003.

46 Machnoor, M., Rodríguez, E.S.G., Kosta, P. et al. (2018). Analysis and design of a 3-coil wireless power transmission system for biomedical applications. *IEEE Transactions on Antennas and Propagation*: 1–1.

47 Liu, X., Ng, W.M., Lee, C.K., and Hui, S.Y. (2008). Optimal operation of contactless transformers with resonance in secondary circuits. Proceedings of the 23rd Annual IEEE Applied Power Electronics Conference and Exposition, Austin, TX, USA (February 2008), 645–650.

48 Ahn, D. and Hong, S. (2013). A study on magnetic field repeater in wireless power transfer. *IEEE Transactions on Industrial Electronics* 60 (1): 360–371.

49 RamRakhyani, A.K. and Lazzi, G. (2014). Multi-coil approach to reduce electromagnetic energy absorption for wirelessly powered implants. *Healthcare Technology Letters* 1 (1): 21–25.

50 Kim, H., Hirayama, H., Kim, S. et al. (2017). Review of near-field wireless power and communication for biomedical applications. *IEEE Access* 5: 21264–21285.

51 Lee, B. and Ghovanloo, M. (2019). An overview of data telemetry in inductively powered implantable biomedical devices. *IEEE Communications Magazine* 57 (2): 74–80.

52 Hirai, J., Kim, T.-W., and Kawamura, A. (1999). Practical study on wireless transmission of power and information for autonomous decentralized manufacturing system. *IEEE Transactions on Industrial Electronics* 46 (2): 349–359.

53 Jung, L.H., Byrnes-Preston, P., Hessler, R. et al. (2007). A dual band wireless power and FSK data telemetry for biomedical implants. Proceedings of the

29th Annual International Conference of the IEEE Engineering in Medicine and Biology Society, Lyon, France (August 2007), 6596–6599.
54 Kim, J., Wei, G., Kim, M. et al. (2018). A splitting frequencies-based wireless power and information simultaneous transfer method. *IEEE Transactions on Circuits and Systems I: Regular Papers* 65 (12): 4434–4445.
55 Jiang, J., Song, K., Wei, G. et al. (2015). Capacity and bandwidth analysis of symmetric two-coil resonant magnetic communication using frequency divarication. *IEEE Antennas and Wireless Propagation Letters* 14: 370–373.
56 Hu, H. and Georgakopoulos, S.V. (2017). Multiband and broadband wireless power transfer systems using the conformal strongly coupled magnetic resonance method. *IEEE Transactions on Industrial Electronics* 64 (5): 3595–3607.
57 Kung, M. and Lin, K. (2014). Investigation of dual-band coil module for nearfield wireless power transfer systems. Proceedings of the IEEE Wireless Power Transfer Conference, Jeju, South Korea (May 2014), 265–268.
58 Kim, J., Wei, G., Kim, M. et al. (2019). A wireless power and information simultaneous transfer technology based on 2fsk modulation using the dual bands of series–parallel combined resonant circuit. *IEEE Transactions on Power Electronics* 34 (3): 2956–2965.
59 Kim, J., Wei, G., Kim, M. et al. (2018). A comprehensive study on composite resonant circuit-based wireless power transfer systems. *IEEE Transactions on Industrial Electronics* 65 (6): 4670–4680.
60 Zhang, Y. and Zhao, Z. (2014). Frequency splitting analysis of two-coil resonant wireless power transfer. *IEEE Antennas and Wireless Propagation Letters* 13: 400–402.
61 Wang, Y., Ye, D., Lyu, L. et al. (2018). A 13.56 MHz wireless power and data transfer receiver achieving 75.4% effective-power-conversion efficiency with 0.1% ask modulation depth and 9.2mw output power. Proceedings of the 2018 IEEE International Solid – State Circuits Conference – (ISSCC), San Francisco, CA, USA (February 2018), 142–144.
62 Hoeher, P.A. (2019). FSK-based simultaneous wireless information and power transfer in inductively coupled resonant circuits exploiting frequency splitting. *IEEE Access* 7: 40183–40194.
63 Ha, S., Kim, C., Park, J. et al. (2016). Energy recycling telemetry IC with simultaneous 11.5 mw power and 6.78 mb/s backward data delivery over a single 13.56 MHz inductive link. *IEEE Journal of Solid-State Circuits* 51 (11): 2664–2678.
64 Tang, Z., Smith, B., Schild, J.H., and Peckham, P.H. (1995). Data transmission from an implantable biotelemeter by load-shift keying using circuit configuration modulator. *IEEE Transactions on Biomedical Engineering* 42 (5): 524–528.

65 Kiani, M. and Ghovanloo, M. (2015). A 13.56-mbps pulse delay modulation based transceiver for simultaneous near-field data and power transmission. *IEEE Transactions on Biomedical Circuits and Systems* 9 (1): 1–11.
66 Meng, M. and Kiani, M. (2019). Gastric seed: Toward distributed ultrasonically interrogated millimeter-sized implants for large-scale gastric electrical wave recording. *IEEE Transactions on Circuits and Systems II: Express Briefs* 66 (5): 783–787.
67 Kiani, M. and Ghovanloo, M. (2013). A 20-mb/s pulse harmonic modulation transceiver for wideband near-field data transmission. *IEEE Transactions on Circuits and Systems II: Express Briefs* 60 (7): 382–386.
68 Jia, Y., Mirbozorgi, S.A., Zhang, P. et al. (2019). A dual-band wireless power transmission system for evaluating mm-sized implants. *IEEE Transactions on Biomedical Circuits and Systems*: 1–1.
69 Kung, M. and Lin, K. (2015). Enhanced analysis and design method of dual band coil module for near-field wireless power transfer systems. *IEEE Transactions on Microwave Theory and Techniques* 63 (3): 821–832.
70 Sample, A.P., Meyer, D.T., and Smith, J.R. (2011). Analysis, experimental results, and range adaptation of magnetically coupled resonators for wireless power transfer. *IEEE Transactions on Industrial Electronics* 58 (2): 544–554.

9

Wireless Drug Delivery Devices

Yang Hao[1], Ahsan Noor Khan[1], Alexey Ermakov[2] and Gleb Sukhorukov[3]

[1] *School of Electronic Engineering and Computer Science, Queen Mary University of London, London, UK*
[2] *I.M. Sechenov First Moscow State Medical University, Moscow, Russia*
[3] *School of Engineering and Materials Science, Queen Mary University of London, London, UK*

9.1 Introduction

The burgeoning research interests in advanced therapeutic modalities have paved the way to cure wide range of chronic ailments by employing wirelessly controlled drug delivery devices [1]. The major motive of drug delivery devices is to overcome the limitations of systemic administration methods, such as injection, oral, and topical, that are unable to impair the harmful side effects on healthy body tissues [2]. Moreover, these methods are not adept to provide high drug concentration at the tumor location and thus require multiple administrations for treatment. The recurrent intake of drug and pharmaceutical compounds can ensue inconvenience to patients and hence affect the required pharmacokinetics due to imperfections in administration location particularly by aging patients. In addition, the intricate location of tumor and its composition can degrade drug efficacy.

Drug delivery devices pose a possible alternative to overcome the limitations of systemic administration as they can provide patients or physicians the control on release mechanism and drug regimen. Several methods can be adapted for drug delivery to the desired organs, cells, and tissues through implantable devices [3, 4]. The precise medicine technology can benefit patients who are suffering from chronic diseases by improving the therapeutic index that can lead to uniform spatial distribution of drugs around tumors [5]. Recent advances in micro-electro-mechanical systems (MEMS) and microfabrication technologies have provided the platform to manufacture compact drug delivery devices that can release drug with controlled pharmacokinetics and efficacy [1, 6, 7]. The cancer tumors require high drug concentration and controlled

Antenna and Sensor Technologies in Modern Medical Applications,
First Edition. Edited by Yahya Rahmat-Samii and Erdem Topsakal.

pharmacokinetics for early recovery, and thus, drug delivery devices have been adapted as the most prevalent technology in current medical practice [8].

9.2 Active and Passive Drug Delivery Devices

Drug delivery devices are categorized into passive and active systems. In a passive system, drug is released from the device due to the availability of specific environment conditions at the targeted disease-infected site or body's natural response to the physiochemical characteristics of drug [9]. There are several passive actuating mechanisms for drug delivery, such as shape memory alloys [10], temperature [11, 12], hydrogels [13, 14], pH [15, 16], and photoresponsive materials [17, 18]. In an active system, drug is expelled from the device after remote actuation or triggering [19, 20]. The active systems are more commercialized, as passive systems for drug delivery result in small actuation force and complex system packaging [2].

9.3 Capsule-Mediated Active Drug Delivery Process

Capsule-shaped devices have been widely used in medical practice for wireless endoscopy [21, 22] and drug absorption rate studies [23]. However, in general, wirelessly controlled capsule devices have only been considered to treat pathologies of the digestive tract and thus unable to provide therapeutic benefits. Due to recent progressions in pharmaceutical research to combine diagnosis and therapy for clinical needs, drug delivery capsules have been envisioned as next-generation therapeutic devices [21, 24, 25].

A typical active capsule device consists of an antenna, onboard electronics, drug-carrying reservoirs, and battery for supplying power in the device [2, 26]. An implant's battery increases the overall size of a device, and for this reason, miniaturization techniques are required for implantable applications. The concept of a drug delivery process using an ingestible capsule is illustrated in Figure 9.1. The capsule-shaped device is swallowed by the patient and then traverses through the body until it reaches the close vicinity of a targeted tumor. The external interrogator triggers the release mechanism through the wireless signal to initiate the drug delivery process. Several release patterns of drugs are discussed in the literature, such as zero-order release, environment responsive release, differential release, and targeted release [27].

The on-body antennas are used to establish bidirectional wireless communication link with the capsule for data, power transfer, and drug dosage monitoring [28].

Drug delivery process from a device is strongly pertinent to a number of key design parameters, such as device materials, packaging of components, and

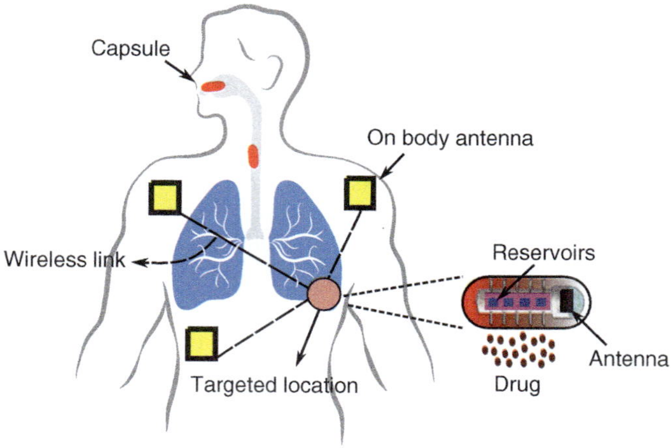

Figure 9.1 Targeted drug delivery concept using ingestible capsule device [26]. (*Source*: Hao, Y., Khan, A. N., Giddens, H., et al., 2019.)

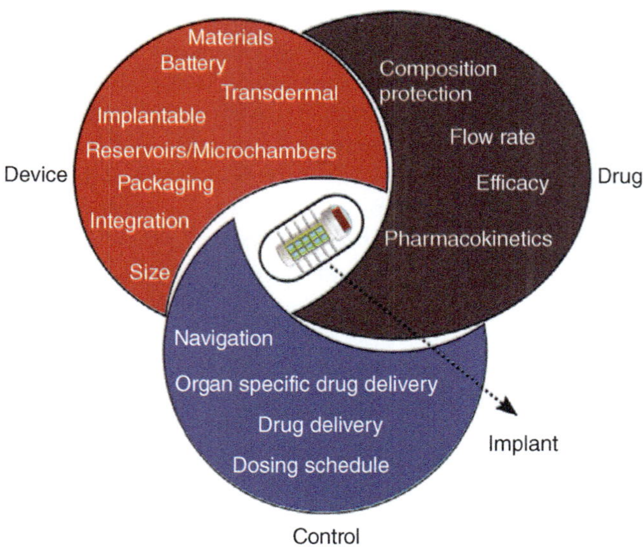

Figure 9.2 Features of a traditional drug delivery device.

drug flow rate and control circuitry for dose scheduling, as shown in Figure 9.2. The recent innovations in biomedical engineering and material science are addressing the challenges in therapeutics delivery. Some of the device features are elucidated in detail in the next part of this chapter.

9.4 Transdermal and Implantable Devices

Drug delivery devices encompass a wide assortment of systems that are distinguishable in terms of their biocompatibility, mechanical stability, materials, and administration methods. Various kinds of flexible materials have been explored for the development of transdermal drug delivery devices that offer sustained drug delivery and stable drug levels with reduced side effects [29–31]. Moreover, transdermal systems pose benefits of convenient therapy interruption by the removal of transdermal drug delivery patch [32]. Current progress in microfabrication technologies has integrated microneedle patches in the transdermal devices that penetrate through the skin with less pain [32, 33]. The smart microneedle systems are evolving in recent past that can release drug after monitoring the physiological conditions using sensors. The microneedles can also be used to increase the permeability of skin for enhanced drug absorption [31].

For implantable drug delivery systems, microchips have been envisioned as a promising platform for storing drugs in tiny reservoirs that are fabricated through micromachined technology [34]. The microchip-based drug delivery devices are implanted around the tumor-infected tissues through surgery and pose the advantage of releasing drugs in single or mixed formulations. Moreover, microchips protect stored drug formulations from external environment and thus offer long-term drug stability. Microchips miniaturize the overall device and thus can offer convenience to patients at the implant location. Microchip-based implantable drug delivery devices are categorized into active and passive devices. Active chips are based on silicon and mainly considered for controlled and pulsatile drug release systems, whereas passive chips employ resorbable polymeric microchip for predetermined drug release systems [35].

9.5 Micro- and Nanoscale Devices

The rapid advancements in fabrication and packaging technologies have facilitated drug delivery devices with compact design and integrated systems, leveraging micro- and nanoscale drug delivery mechanisms for in vivo treatment of diseases (Figure 9.3). The nanorobots or motors have emerged to improve therapeutic treatment as they can cargo drugs to the targeted tumor site with less discomfort to the patients [36–38]. The nanodrug delivery devices offer the advantage of accessing the intricate parts of the body tissues for drug delivery, increasing uptake of drugs as compared to systemic administration. Moreover, the nanostructures can utilize chemical or external energy to produce mechanical motions for traversing through the body and delivering drug effectively without excessive degradation before reaching the targeted tumor [39].

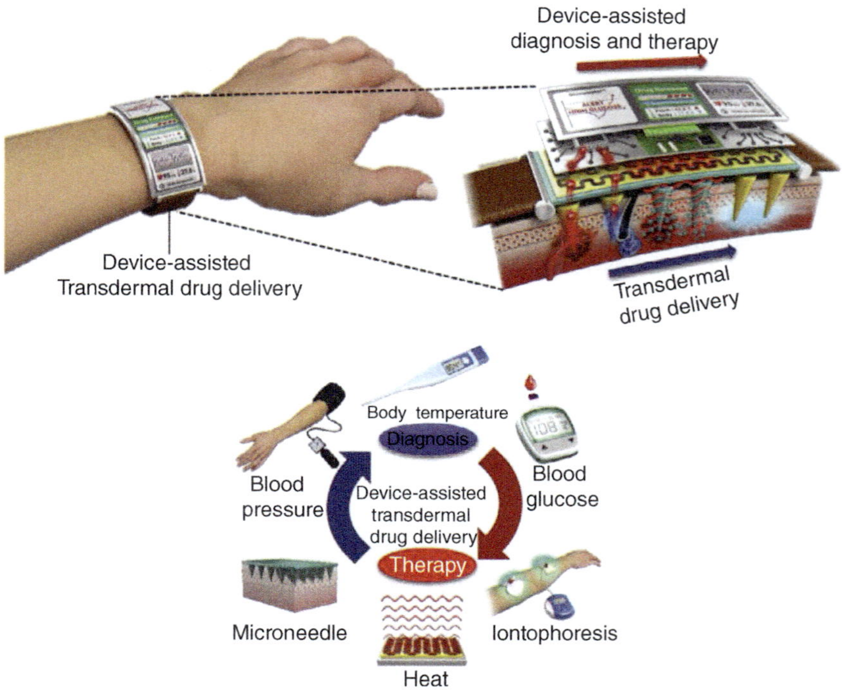

Figure 9.3 Schematic illustration of a device-assisted transdermal drug delivery. (*Source*: Lee, H., Song, C., Baik, S., et al., 2018. © Elsevier.)

9.6 Packaging and Integration of Components

As a drug delivery device encompasses several components, the microfabrication and compact system integration technologies are required to miniaturize the overall size, particularly for implantable applications. Moreover, the implantable drug delivery device should be compatible with the characteristics of the surrounding tissues [40]. The protective packaging methods and biocompatible materials are thus essential to implant drug delivery device with minimum toxicity. In the literature, insulating materials, such as aluminum oxide, polyethyleneglycol, polytetrafluoroethylene, and silicon nitride, are mostly used for packaging and interconnecting power source with other components in the drug delivery module [35]. The packaging should also provide compatibility among several components of the device while minimizing drug contamination.

The packaging can vary according to transdermal and implantable applications. For instance, transdermal drug delivery devices based on microneedles require minimal packaging as drug is stored in microcontainers and delivered through the attached microneedles. However, implantable devices with controlled release mechanism require MEMS and integrated circuit (IC) technology for the packaging of integrating components [6].

9.7 Materials for Drug Delivery Devices

A broad assortment of biocompatible materials has been explored to devise various kinds of diagnostic and therapeutic devices [41]. The selection of appropriate materials can be beneficial for seamless integration and packaging of components within compact space. In recent past, biocompatible materials comprising flexible nature have emerged for the encapsulation of carriers for drug delivery inside the body. The encapsulation protects stored therapeutics from light, humidity, and temperature that can alter the composition and formulation before releasing from the device [42]. Moreover, the carrier materials should be compatible with drug composition to avoid any degradation in its purity, stability, and efficacy.

In the literature, several materials, such as hydrogels [43], titania (TiO_2) nanotube [44], polymers [45], liposome [46], photoresponsive [18], and nanomaterials [47–49], have been used for drug delivery applications. The passive drug release mechanisms are mostly dependent on hydrogels [13, 50] and photoresponsive [18] materials.

Magnetically activated membranes have shown their potential for programmable drug delivery systems that can control therapeutic levels within desired range [51]. The biodegradable nonporous silicon membranes and metal-based nanoshells have also been used for controlled release drug delivery systems owing to their rapid kinetics capability [7, 52]. Nanoparticles-mediated drug delivery has emerged as the most prevalent modality for antitumor therapy [46, 53]. Variety of antibodies and vaccines have been delivered using nanoparticles for therapy and diagnosis [46]. Particularly, nanoparticles have been employed for drug delivery in brain due to their ability to pass the blood–brain barrier [54].

9.8 Organ-Specific Drug Delivery Devices

The routes of drug administration should be convenient when patients are particularly prescribed with high dosing frequency. The transdermal, pulmonary, and oral routes have been considered as a paramount strategy to deliver drugs in the human body [4]. Targeted drug delivery techniques can enhance therapeutics concentration at the specific organs and tissues [3] to treat wide spectrum of afflictions. This approach can reduce harmful side effects on the healthy organs as drug is mostly diffused around disease-infected organ compartments. However, drug carriers must bypass various cells, molecules, and membranes to reach in the close vicinity of a desired organ. For this reason, several requirements need to be met by the device to tailor pharmaceutical compounds toward targeted organ or even a part of organ. The chemical or physical characteristics of tissues can also be exploited for organ-specific drug delivery [4]. In the literature, breadth of approaches has been used to deliver drugs in different regions of the gastrointestinal tract, such as mouth, stomach, esophagus, small intestine, and colon [3]. Apart from gastrointestinal tract, MEMS-based devices have shown their potential for drug delivery to organs protected by blood–brain barriers, such as brain and eyes [6].

9.9 Wireless Communication for Drug Delivery Devices

The tendency of implementing wirelessly controlled electronics and sensors is actively underway to provide patient's autonomy on drug administrations. By connecting an implantable device with external controller over a wireless link, patients having debility to administer medication can benefit themselves as drug delivery process can be controlled by remote physicians. Moreover, dosing schedule can be wirelessly programmed according to the physician's prescription that can modify with the periods of time.

In recent past, wireless actuation is the most promising noninvasive strategy for releasing drug compounds in the human body. The specific dose administration can maximize therapeutic benefits for effective dosing regimens with minimum toxicity. In the literature, wireless communication has been actively considered for the actuation of brain implants [55], drug delivery [1], glucose dosage monitoring [56], capsule endoscopy [20], and transdermal medical devices for physiological monitoring [57].

Rapid developments in understanding the interactions of electromagnetic (EM) waves with body tissues have ushered in devising bidirectional communication strategies that can perform data telemetry between an implant and external interrogator [58]. The received data can be beneficial for physicians to delineate the requirements for further optimization of drug delivery procedure and dosing schedules. The bidirectional communication is also advantageous to follow device status before and after releasing drug compounds. In addition, information related to number of reservoirs triggered for delivery, battery voltage status, and implant location can also be transferred wirelessly through the body [59]. Apart from data telemetry, wireless communication has been predominantly considered for power transfer to the implant on the near-field inductive link [60]. Wireless power transfer technique poses the advantage of excluding battery requirements in the implant and thus offers miniaturized device design for patient convenience.

For aforementioned reasons, radio-frequency (RF) system has become an integral part of current drug delivery devices for data telemetry, wireless power transfer, and remote actuation. With the advancements in understanding path loss associated with radio waves propagating through the body, optimum frequency range and power levels of an implant can be tailored further for maximizing the device performance [58]. This book chapter recapitulates wirelessly controlled drug delivery devices and different mechanisms that are essential for drug delivery. Moreover, drug carriers and materials that are now widely used for drug delivery have been explained in detail.

9.9.1 Microchips-Mediated Drug Delivery Devices

With the emergence of microfabrication techniques, microchips have been conceived as a potent technology for controlled drug delivery systems, owing to their capability of storing drugs for long periods of time [61, 62]. Microchips are categorized into solid-state silicon chip and resorbable polymeric chip [35].

Traditional microchip-based drug delivery systems consist of a substrate that contains tiny reservoirs to store drugs in solid, liquid, or a gel form [35]. The microfabrication techniques are capable of etching thousands of tiny reservoirs in a single microchip that also contains power source, electronics, antenna systems, and a microprocessor [1]. In terms of protecting drug composition from external environment, microchips are capable of providing sealing to each reservoir [34]. The sealing is generally formed using metallic material, such as titanium (Ti) and platinum (Pt) [63]. The metallic sealing, also known as membrane, is connected with a microprocessor using wired connection. The microprocessor can be programmed wirelessly to release current into the metallic membrane for its diffusion through electrothermal process that initiates the release of drug from the reservoirs.

Due to the recent trends of empowering patients with self-management of therapeutic treatment, wireless systems have been emerged as a prevalent technology for programming the dosing schedule in an implanted microchip. The complementary metal oxide semiconductor (CMOS)-based system on chip (SoC) technology offers low power consumption and thus has been investigated for implantable drug delivery devices [64]. The 0.35 μm CMOS technology has the capability to etch tiny reservoirs in the chip ($1.77 \times 1.4\,mm^2$) to store 5 nl drug formulations in each reservoir as shown in Figure 9.4a. The final prototype in Figure 9.4b shows the bonding of polydimethylsiloxane (PDMS) reservoirs layer with chip. The tiny reservoirs can be addressed individually through a microcontroller-based processor that is triggered wirelessly over the Medical Implant Communication Service (MICS, 402–405 MHz) band. Once the device is externally triggered, the electrothermal process is

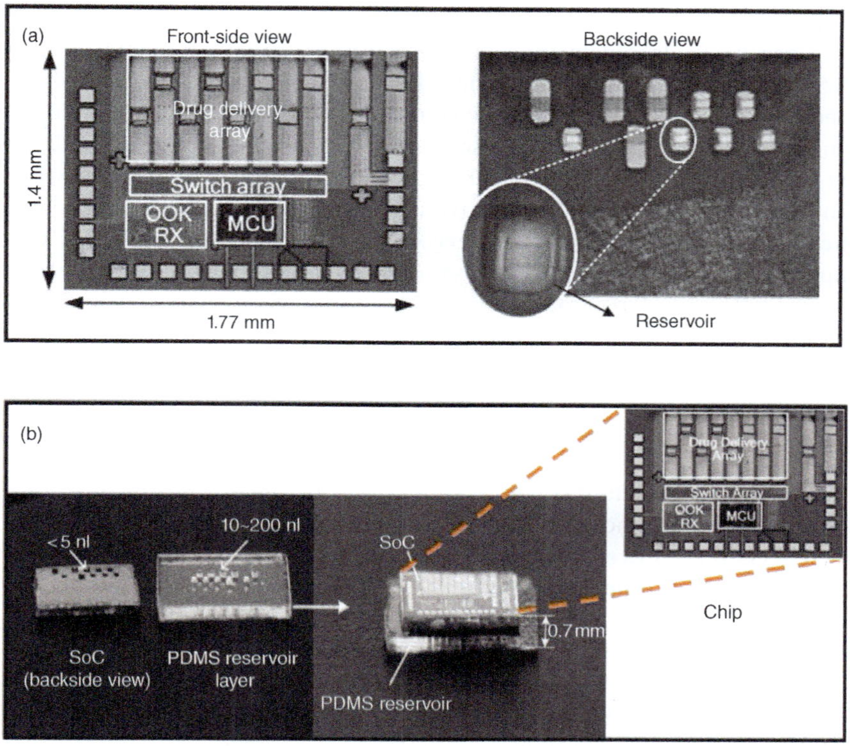

Figure 9.4 (a) Chip micrographs post IC processing. (*Source*: Reprinted with permission from International Solid-State Circuits Conference-Digest of Technical Papers, 2009. © IEEE.) (b) Fabricated drug delivery device. (*Source:* Reprinted with permission from Association for Computing Machinery, 2012. © Association for Computing Machinery.)

activated, which results in melting the reservoir membranes to spout drug outside the chip.

The intraocular drug delivery has always been challenging due to the size constrains of an implant. Battery is considered to be the main contributor in the physical size of an implanted ocular drug delivery system. In [65], a silicon-based microchip ($3\times 3\,mm^2$) is fabricated by anisotropic wet etching process for ocular drug delivery applications. The implant can be powered wirelessly at 7.1 MHz frequency through inductive link between an external transmitter and implanted coil, thus excluding the requirements of a battery. The chip contains a decoder, demultiplexer, microreservoirs, and ferrite rod antenna. The chip has been experimentally tested under the influence of an external RF signal (1-W RF power) that actuates the control circuitry to dissolve gold membranes of reservoirs for delivering drugs.

Clinical tests of an implanted device are useful to evaluate the impact of lossy body tissues on drug delivery rate. The controlled drug delivery techniques leverage physicians to adjust dosing schedules according to the therapeutic needs that can be varied during the course of treatment. For aforementioned benefits, a microchip-based drug delivery device was implanted surgically in the patients [66]. The device can be tracked and programmed over the MICS band for controlled release, thus providing real-time scheduling and tracking. The device contains an array of reservoirs on two silicon microchips. A thin impermeable metallic membrane was used to encase apertures of reservoirs that can be dissolved using electrothermal ablation process. The antenna of an implant transmits drug release acknowledgement and battery voltage status to the external receiver.

9.9.2 Micropumps and Microvalves-Mediated Drug Delivery Devices

Therapeutic treatment involves a wide range of precise dosing methods. By keeping drug concentration within a therapeutic window, the adverse side effects due to overdosing can be reduced. Recently, MEMS technology has opened a set of new possibilities to fabricate compact micropumps and microvalves for controlled drug delivery. A typical micropump-based system consists of drug storage chamber, flow sensor, controller, and outlet valve [67]. The advanced microfabrication technologies are currently developing low-cost micropumps that can be seamlessly integrated with wireless systems to achieve noninvasive control on the pumping process.

On the other hand, microvalves can assist the functionality of implanted pumps by controlling the flow routes of delivered drugs. Moreover, multiple microvalves can be actuated wirelessly at the same time so that the dose quantity can be adjusted according to therapeutic requirements [68]. In the literature, wirelessly actuated microvalves are mostly fabricated using hydrogels [43, 69], ionic polymer metal composite (IPMC) [70], parylene [71, 72], and piezoelectric materials [68]. A piezoelectric microvalve that is activated by an inductor capacitor LC resonant circuit for drug delivery is shown in Figure 9.5a [68]. The device contains a PDMS reservoir to store 88.9 μl fluid (Figure 9.5b). The piezoelectric actuator (PEA) is actuated by an LC resonant multilayer coil that produces a pressure difference under the influence of external magnetic fields (operating at 10 kHz). Pressure difference squeezes the reservoir to release stored fluids when external magnetic fields are activated as shown in Figure 9.5c.

Another application of LC resonant heater for actuating the drug delivery process is presented in [73]. The spiral coil is fabricated from a biocompatible nitinol material that is used to actuate the pump chamber. The coil is excited by RF magnetic fields that are operating at 185 MHz and generates cantilever actuation to pump drug out of the chip ($10 \times 10 \times 2\ mm^3$) (Figure 9.6a). The chip

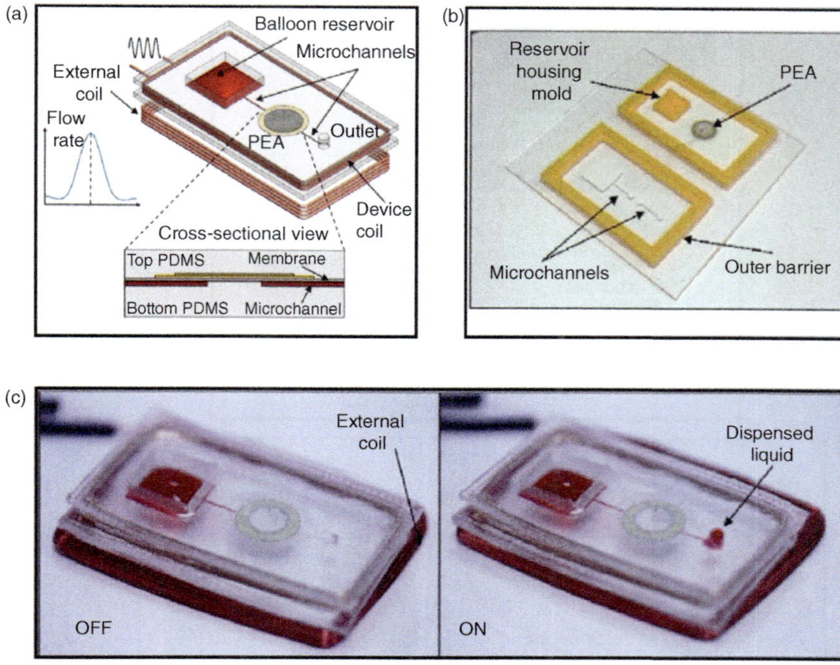

Figure 9.5 (a) Schematic illustration of the working principle of the proposed device. (b) Fabricated prototype of the piezoelectrically actuated microvalve (PEA). (c) Demonstration of active and inactive controls on the release mechanism of the device under the influence of external RF magnetic fields. (*Source:* Reprinted with permission from Nafea, M., Nawabjan, A., and Ali, M. S. M., 2018. © Elsevier.)

was fabricated with biocompatible materials. The polyimide casing (305 μm) is used to package the whole device as shown in Figure 9.6b. The release of 76 μl stored agents from the reservoir is experimentally demonstrated in water after exposing the device with radio waves (1.1 W). The scanning electron image of the device indicates the outlet nozzle that is used to eject drug out of the chip (Figure 9.6c).

A thermopneumatic micropump that is encompassing a frequency-controlled LC heater has been developed for a reliable drug delivery operation (Figure 9.7a) [74]. The LC heater can be frequency controlled to trigger micropump for drug delivery. Maximum heat is generated when the frequency of external magnetic fields is tuned to the resonant frequency of the heater. The micropump ($22 \times 7 \times 4\,mm^3$) consists of three flexible layers, and it was fabricated using MEMS technology as shown in Figure 9.7b. The LC heater is activated when RF signal (0.22 W) operating at 81.5 MHz is applied from an external source. The generated heat is quickly transferred to the pump

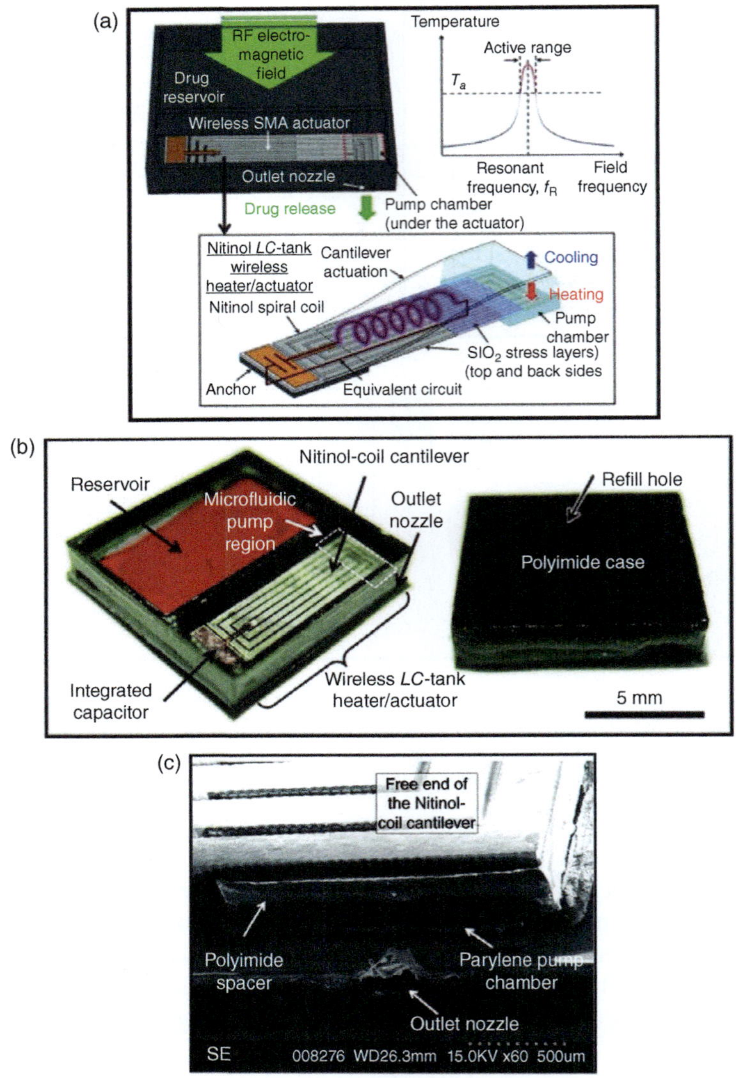

Figure 9.6 (a) Conceptual illustration of Nitinol LC wireless resonant heater integrated in the chip to perform cantilever actuation for drug delivery. (b) Fabricated drug delivery chip without (left) and with (right) polyimide casing. *Source*: Reprinted with permission from Lab Chip, (2015), 15, 1050–1058. Copyright 2015, Royal Society of Chemistry. (c) Scanning electron microscope (SEM) image of the Nitinol actuator coupled with pump chamber. The SEM image also shows the outlet nozzle for ejecting stored agents from the device. (*Source*: Reprinted with permission from Lab Chip, (2015), 15, 1050–1058. Copyright 2015, Royal Society of Chemistry)

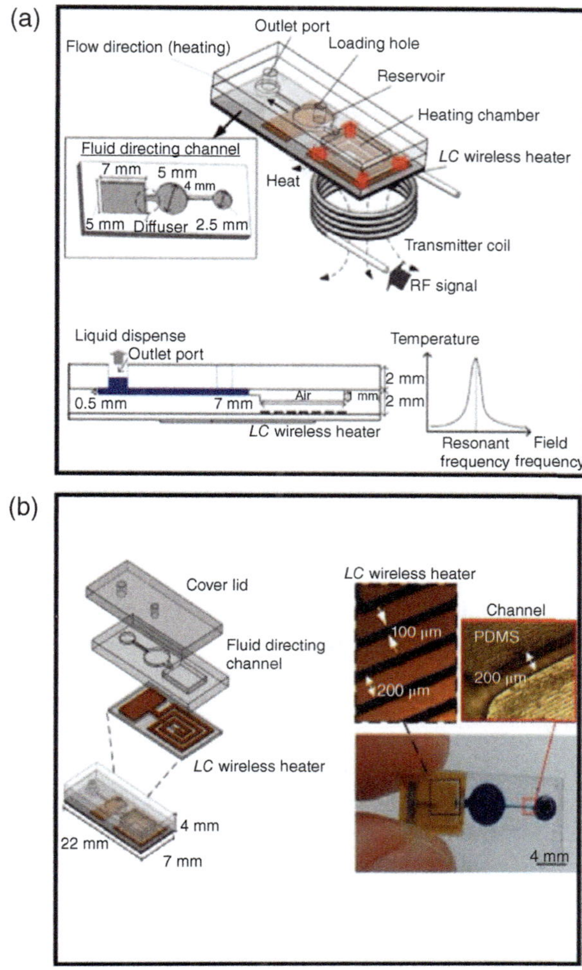

Figure 9.7 (a) Schematic illustration of a thermopneumatic micropump. (b) The fabricated micropump with multiple layers of cover lid, fluid-directing channel, and LC wireless heater. (*Source*: Reprinted with permission from Chee, P.S., Minjal, M. N., Leow, P. L., and Ali, M. S. M., 2015. © Elsevier.)

chamber for the transportation of stored fluid and thus validates its potential for drug delivery applications.

9.9.3 Microrobots-Mediated Drug Delivery

Untethered medical microrobots are revolutionizing therapeutic treatments due to their diverse characteristics, in particular, facilitating disease prognosis and treatment in inaccessible convoluted areas of the human body [75]. Contrary to traditional large-scale mechanical robots, medical applications necessitate robots to be soft, miniaturized, and biocompatible due to their interaction with the human body [76]. The key features of a microrobot, such as small size, low weight, and ability to traverse through the body, have stimulated their applications for drug delivery. The confluence of MEMS and microfabrication technologies has enabled the development of magnetically controlled microrobots that can perform drug delivery tasks at very small scales [77]. Magnetic microrobots can be steered in the human body by an external EM-actuating system. Magnetic robots for drug delivery encompass magnetic bodies along with several other components that are responsible for locomotion, control, and wireless communication through the human body. In general, microrobots utilize thin layers of biocompatible Ti [78] or gold [79] for implantable applications.

In [77], a helical-shaped microrobot that can be controlled wirelessly has demonstrated its potential to traverse through twisted and narrow tubular environments in the human body for delivering drugs. It consists of rotating and fixed magnets that produce torque to navigate microrobot with drilling motion, in response to the external magnetic fields operating in the frequency range of 0–15 Hz. Moreover, the attractive and repulsive forces in between magnets can be controlled with external magnetic manipulator to deliver drugs out of the nozzle.

In [80], a capsule-shaped microrobot with the ability to perform pick-and-drop motion has been demonstrated. The microrobot contains a plunger and cap. The microrobot encapsulates drugs in the container by the pick-and-drop motion. The transportation of microparticles is demonstrated through pick-and-drop motion that holds particles within a confined volume. To transport drugs, the microrobot exhibits corkscrewing motion.

Another wirelessly controlled magnetic robot is demonstrated in [81] for drug delivery in the posterior segment of human eye. The robot is fabricated using electrodeposition method, and magnetic cobalt–nickel (CoNi) alloy is employed as a conformal coating so that it can be wirelessly steered using magnetic fields. An external induction heating system generates magnetic fields to induce heating on the gold-coated CoNi substrate for increasing the surface temperature. Similar kind of work is demonstrated in [82] that utilizes EM actuation mechanism to magnetize the microrobot for its orientation toward the targeted site.

9.9.4 Material-Mediated Drug Delivery

Materials for advanced actively controlled systems have recently attracted wide attention due to the progress in biomedical engineering. Since bulky scaffolds and devices with batteries have several limitations due to the size of their components, the direct influence of external fields to the sensitizer has been widely investigated. In this fashion, the direct exposure of radio waves to nanoparticles has been investigated as a therapeutic approach for noninvasive or minimally invasive thermal ablation [27].

This approach is based on nanoparticles which serve as a sensitizer to RF fields due to their ability to absorb the energy in RF range. To reach a direct therapeutic in this way, nanoparticles have to be concentrated in the specific area (such as tumor). A range of nanoparticles has been shown to exhibit ability to be heated under the influence of RF fields. The initial work in this area was based on conductive gold nanoparticles that enabled local thermal ablation and can be used for local treatment [83, 84]. This noninvasive method called nano-radio-frequency ablation has suggested highly localized therapy of tumor or selective treatment of cancer cells in some cases.

However, the exact peculiarities of heat generation by nanoparticles are not completely clear; some points of view are discussed by Liu et al. [85], which shows that the most probable mechanism is joule heating produced by electrical currents on the surface of conductive nanoparticles [86]. The ohmic nature of the heat generation also has been suggested based on the experimental data on the nanoparticles size dependence of the heating values. Moran et al. have demonstrated inverse dependence of heat generation under the influence of RF fields in suspensions of gold nanoparticles with a size under 50 nm, while at larger sizes, this dependence has not been revealed [86, 87]. Gold nanoparticles with a size lower than 50 nm have been shown to heat twice more efficiently. The possible reason is the higher electrical resistivity of the nanoparticles with a size under 50 nm. In this way, Kruse et al. have demonstrated that the gold nanoparticles with a size of 5 nm exhibit higher efficacy in terms of RF-induced heating in comparison to the gold nanoparticles of larger sizes [87]. It should be noted that the heating of the gold nanoparticles increases linearly with the increase in concentration followed by saturation. The experiment was performed by means of noncontact RF–EM systems.

Groups of San and Tamarov have also shown that the temperature increase linearly is dependent on the nanoparticle's concentration of Pt and Si [88, 89]. However, it seems to be a more complicated process in suspensions of single-walled carbon nanotubes (SWCNTs). A nonlinear temperature increase that is dependent on the concentration of SWCNTs has been demonstrated by Gannon et al. [90]. Nevertheless, the heat-generation process in suspensions of nanoparticles was found to be dependent on a range of factors including the chemical nature of the medium, heat and electrical conductivity, permittivity, and many others, thus emphasizing that RF-induced heat generation has not been in pure ohmic nature [88]. Some reports also demonstrate that the shape of nanoparticles, their presence, and ratio of nonaggregated conductive nanoparticles cannot affect heating process at certain rates [91–93]. These reports suggest that the heat-generation process is basically the consequence of the ions movement on the surrounding medium. These reports also argue that the cell death in the presence of nanoparticles could be induced by cationic cytotoxicity of the nanoparticles rather than increased temperature in the biological medium. It should be noted that the so-called protein corona was found to affect the response of the nanoparticles to RF fields with a higher rates of the heat generation that was attributed to the enhancement of RF energy loss at the gold nanoparticle–protein interface [93]. Nevertheless, to date, many independent experimental studies have confirmed the high therapeutic efficacy of different NPs in the treatment of tumor and cancer cells for both in vitro and in vivo applications. Control samples in these studies have shown low cytotoxicity of the nanoparticles and low side effects [88, 90, 94–96]. Some of the studies have also applied nanoparticles to the sites of interest by antibody agents that are specific to the chosen cells in order to reach the highest efficacy of the therapy.

A variety of agents employed for absorbing RF fields is mostly represented by electrically conductive and magnetic nanoparticles. The initial works on nanoparticle-mediated RF thermal ablation were based on gold nanoparticles and carbon nanotubes [86, 90, 94]. Relatively high concentrations of the nanoparticles ($1\,\mathrm{mg\,ml^{-1}}$) were shown to be necessary to reach heating at a rate of $20\,\mathrm{K\,s^{-1}}$ induced by RF field with a frequency of 13.6 MHz and a power of 600 W. Noninvasive thermal ablation of cancer cells was shown to be induced with the RF field of these parameters for in vitro scenario. Properties of gold nanoparticles can be tuned with a high accuracy by changing their size, shape, and composition in order to obtain desired characteristics such as extinction spectra. For example, gold–silica core–shell structures can be synthesized with different ratio between the silica core and layer of gold that defines the absorption characteristics of the particle.

With respect to in vitro and in vivo experiments, gold nanoparticles can be chemically modified by a number of agents, including antibodies and different peptides/proteins, to provide targeting to cancer cells [95]. In this way, antibodies specific to cancer cells can be chemically attached to the surface of gold nanoparticles, resulting in increased internalization of the nanoparticles in comparison with gold NPs modified with nonspecific antibodies or without chemical modification of the particle surface. There is significant improvement of nanoparticles internalization when specific antibody modification is applied in comparison to modification by nonspecific antibody. Covalent functionalization and noncovalent wrapping have been employed in order to target carbon nanotubes to specific cells [90]. Furthermore, not only conductive nanoparticles have been shown to produce heat under RF fields but heating effect has also been revealed in suspensions of magnetic particles. In this case, magnetic nanoparticles (mostly iron base, for example, magnetite) are used to produce heat as a result of their interaction with the magnetic component of the EM fields in a wide range of frequencies, such as from 0.2 to 30 MHz [97–100]. The heat production in this case was mainly attributed to the relaxation losses (Neel–Brownian); however, it should be noted that at frequencies of about 30 MHz, nonspecific and irrelevant heating of the magnetic NPs has a high contribution to this process.

Later, conductive particles of different compositions have been shown to produce heat under the influence of RF fields. For example, crystalline silicon nanoparticles were heated with a high performance at the corresponding powers of RF fields [88, 89] as well as Pt nanoparticles which exhibit even higher efficacy in comparison with gold nanoparticles [89]. A few promising works based on quantum dots (QDs) demonstrated their application as a sensitizer agent for RF ablation with efficacy close to gold nanoparticles [101]. Furthermore, high quantum yield of QDs could also be useful in cell imaging along with RF sensitization.

More recently, a number of chemical routes allowed synthesis of nanoparticles with different functions that can serve as new agents for RF ablation, for example, hybrid of gold nanoparticles and magnetic compounds such as Fe_3O_4, resulting in contrasting the magnetic resonance imaging (MRI) and fluorescence along with responsiveness toward RF field [96] [102–104].

9.10 Carrier Types for Drug Delivery

A range of researches demonstrated that the RF-sensitive particles can be employed as vehicles/carriers for drug delivery with an RF-triggered release of the cargo. RF field-sensitive porous silicon nanoparticles were shown to be effective nanocarriers for delivery of cargo [105]. In this case, a polymer sensitive to the temperature was absorbed on the surface of the porous particle and served as a shutter that enables the release of the encapsulated cargo from pores in response to the RF-induced heating. In another case, titania nanotubes were employed as drug carriers functionalized by gold nanoparticles that allowed RF-triggered release of the cargo [44]. Magnetic nanoparticles have also demonstrated a great prospect for RF-triggered drug release with repeatable mechanism. A spongelike material (PDMS elastomer) was functionalized with ferromagnetic carbonyl iron microparticles that allowed using it as a microspouter for precise and repeatable drug delivery system with release-on-demand function triggered by RF irradiation [27].

In this case, the magnetic sponge can be deformed in a controlled manner by external magnetic fields as a trigger. The deformations induced in the sponge are reversible and enable release of the cargo. The release was demonstrated by means of methylene blue as a model substance, and it was activated at different strengths of the magnetic fields. The concept of incorporation of RF-sensitive nanoparticles to the structure of drug delivery vehicles has been applied in the development of nanocomposite hydrogels. The properties of hydrogel can be remotely controlled in order to release the drug and to sense the environment that has a great prospect as a theragnostic system. These composite systems can be made using a wide range of the RF sensitizers (such as magnetite NPs, gold NPs, carbon nanotubes, and others) and thermos-responsive hydrogels, which exhibit a strong response in their mechanical properties (including deformation, shrinking, and pore size change) upon heating [51, 106, 107].

In general, described particles (magnetite and gold nanoparticles, SWCNTs, and others) are traditional components of drug delivery nano and microcarriers. These particles are widely applied as functional components in the structure of different drug delivery vehicles in order to provide sensitivity to different types of external fields. The presence of magnetic and conductive nanoparticles in vehicles can be utilized in order to absorb EM energy, resulting in increase of the temperature in medium or thermally triggered opening of the vehicles.

A wide range of nano and microcarriers with colloidal particle shells are based on liposomes [108]. Conductive and magnetic nanoparticles were shown to provide responsiveness of liposome-based nanocomposite vesicle to pulsed electric and magnetic fields, which enables targeting and triggered release of cargo [109–112]. Another broad type of drug delivery carriers is based on hydrogels which, together with great biocompatibility and extensive choice of materials with desired properties, have a tremendous prospective in EM field-mediated drug delivery [113]. Hydrogels offer a range of thermally responsive compositions and enable simple functionalization by colloidal nanoparticles, both magnetic [114] and conductive [115]. Recent advances in the synthesis of hollow nanocomposite alginate microcapsules functionalized with nanoparticles have demonstrated both susceptibility to magnetic field and in vivo opening by laser treatment [116, 117]. Majority of structures synthesized by means of the pickering-emulsion route should be noted as it offers extensive variety of routes for obtaining nano and microshells functionalized by different nanoparticles; for review, please refer [118].

Microcontainers synthesized via layer-by-layer (LbL) assembly of oppositely charged species should be highlighted as it offers great possibility for versatile tailoring of stimuli-responsive materials with demanded properties. The LbL assembly employs the bottom-up approach, which enables to provide control over the structure and physical properties of multilayer shells at nanoscale. LbL technique suggests a sequential adsorption of oppositely charged species on top of a template which can be a planar substrate or a suspension of microparticles. Usually, polyelectrolytes (polymers that become charged in water medium) are applied to create the polymer matrix, which can be functionalized by charged fillers such as nanoparticles. Combination of different materials in highly determined order (at nanoscale range) enables tailoring of the carriers with a wide range of specific properties [119, 120]. Traditionally, microparticles are employed as a template for LbL assembly of polyelectrolytes, which enables fabrication of microcapsules suspension with a highly ordered multilayer shell. The scheme of the process is shown in Figure 9.8. Polyelectrolyte microcapsules were shown to encapsulate both low and high molecular weight molecules [121, 122]. Recent study has

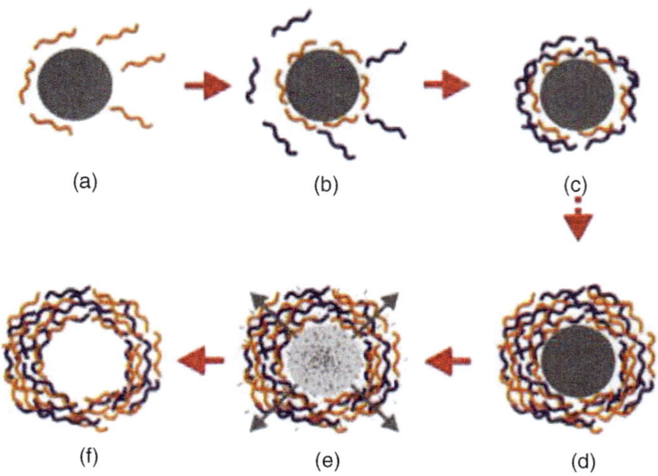

Figure 9.8 Schematic illustration of the microcapsule fabrication via layer-by-layer assembly followed by core decomposition. (*Source*: Reprinted with permission Donath, E., Sukhorukov, G. B., Caruso, F., et al., 1998.)

demonstrated that circulation of large polyelectrolyte microcapsules in blood does not obstruct blood flow [123].

Recently, Kiryukhin and coworkers have reported an approach to synthesize a patterned array of hollow microchambers via LbL assembly; a schematic picture of this process is shown in Figure 9.9. In order to fabricate microchambers, a template with an array of microwells of predetermined sizes and shapes is fabricated. Secondly, the template is suggested to be covered with a polyelectrolyte multilayer film of oppositely charged polyelectrolytes. At this step, the coated microwells are supposed to be filled with a desired cargo. Then, mechanical pulling out or dissolving of the template enables a patterned array of microchambers loaded with cargo. Such an array of microchambers provides a site-specific release of the desired cargo in extremely low and precisely defined quantities and represents an alternative to microelectromechanical systems (like valves and pumps described above), which electronically trigger the release of the cargo from a reservoir. The LbL technique offers a range of possibilities to provide high responsiveness of the microcontainer shells toward external stimuli of different nature [124]. Modification of multilayer shells by nanoparticles or polymers with specific properties is employed with this purpose. Due to electrostatic adsorption during the LbL assembly, charged nanoparticles can be incorporated into the multilayer shell. In this way, polyelectrolyte microcontainers that are made via LbL assembly with shells containing gold NPs, magnetite, carbon-based materials, and many other magnetic and conductive species have been successfully fabricated and shown

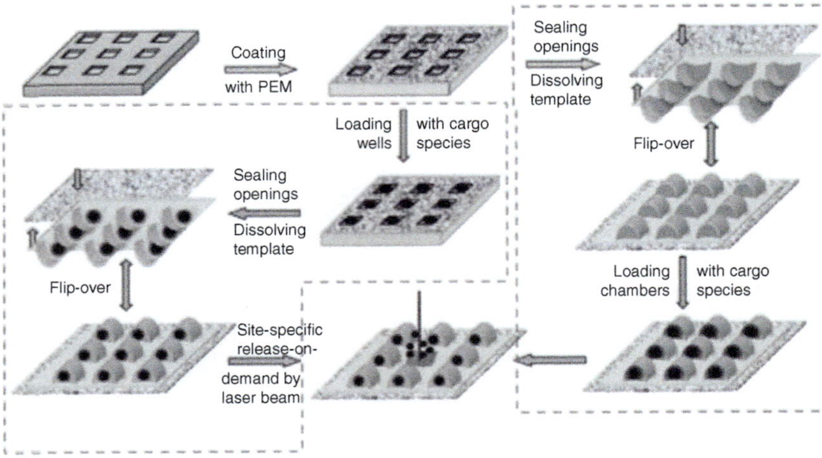

Figure 9.9 Schematic illustration of the microchambers fabrication and their loading with cargo followed by site-specific release. (*Source*: Reprinted with permission from Kiryukhin, M. V., Gorelik, S. R., Man, S. M., et al., 2012. © John Wiley & Sons.)

to be effective functional carriers. Polyelectrolyte microcapsules containing magnetite were widely investigated and shown to be effectively triggered and opened by magnetic fields and employed as an MRI agent [125–127]. Conductive and plasmon resonance nanoparticles, including graphene, carbon nanotubes, and gold and silver nanoparticles, were included in the structure of polyelectrolyte shells by electrostatic adsorption and were shown to provide responsiveness of the capsules toward laser irradiation [128–131]. Discovered recently, carbon dots with highly conductive properties and biocompatibility were also shown to be a great alternative to gold nanoparticles as a functional part of microcontainers [132, 133]. In terms of RF-induced heating, one of the most important factors is the thermal responsiveness of the carriers. The LbL assembly offers a range of tools to tailor high thermal responsiveness of polyelectrolyte multilayer shells [134]. For example, the presence of thermally responsive polymers (such as poly(*N*-isopropylacrylamide) PNIPAM) in the microcapsule structure makes it possible to provide control over the microcapsule permeability by means of thermal treatment [135].

References

1 Khan, A.N., Ermakov, A., Sukhorukov, G., and Hao, Y. (2019). *Applied Physics Reviews* 6: 041301.
2 Ali, M.M. and Takahata, K. (2011). *Journal of Micromechanics and Microengineering* 21: 075005.

3 Pinto, J.F. (2010). *International Journal of Pharmaceutics* 395: 44.
4 Pettit, D.K. and Gombotz, W.R. (1998). *Trends in Biotechnology* 16: 343.
5 Weiser, J.R. and Saltzman, W.M. (2014). *Journal of Controlled Release* 190: 664.
6 Lee, H.J., Choi, N., Yoon, E.-S., and Cho, I.-J. (2018). *Advanced Drug Delivery Reviews* 128: 132.
7 Shawgo, R.S., Grayson, A.C.R., Li, Y., and Cima, M.J. (2002). *Current Opinion in Solid State and Materials Science* 6: 329.
8 Senapati, S., Mahanta, A.K., Kumar, S., and Maiti, P. (2018). *Signal Transduction and Targeted Therapy* 3: 1.
9 Rani, K. and Paliwal, S. (2014). *Scholars Journal of Applied Medical Sciences* 2: 328.
10 Reynaerts, D., Peirs, J., and Brussel, H.V. (1997). *Sensors and Actuators A: Physical* 61: 455. Proceedings of EUROSENSORS X.
11 Fitzpatrick, S.D., Fitzpatrick, L.E., Thakur, A. et al. (2012). *Expert Review of Medical Devices* 9: 339.
12 Bikram, M. and West, J.L. (2008). *Expert Opinion on Drug Delivery* 5: 1077.
13 Atta, S. et al. (2015). *International Journal of Biological Macromolecules* 80: 240.
14 Deen, G.R. and Loh, X.J. (2018). *Gels* 4: 13.
15 Zhu, Y.-J. and Chen, F. (2015). *Chemistry: An Asian Journal* 10: 284.
16 Balamuralidhara, V. et al. (2011). *American Journal of Drug Discovery and Development* 1: 25.
17 Zhou, Y., Ye, H., Chen, Y. et al. (2018). *Biomacromolecules* 19: 1840.
18 Cho, H.J., Chung, M., and Shim, M.S. (2015). *Journal of Industrial and Engineering Chemistry* 31: 15.
19 Wang, Y. and Kohane, D.S. (2017). *Nature Reviews Materials* 2: 17020.
20 Munoz, F., Alici, G., and Li, W. (2014). *Advanced Drug Delivery Reviews* 71: 77.
21 Woods, S.P. and Constandinou, T.G. (2013). *IEEE Transactions on Biomedical Engineering* 60: 945.
22 Suzan Miah, M., Khan, A.N., Icheln, C. et al. (2019). *IEEE Transactions on Antennas and Propagation* 67: 2687.
23 Wilding, I., Hirst, P., and Connor, A. (2000). *Pharmaceutical Science & Technology Today* 3: 385.
24 Jiang, H., Yu, W., Oscai, M., and Ziaie, B. (2018). *IEEE Transactions on Biomedical Engineering* 65: 2808.
25 Pi, X. et al. (2010). *Sensors and Actuators A: Physical* 159: 227.
26 Hao, Y., Khan, A.N., Giddens, H., and Sukhorukov, G. (2019). Characterization of microchamber arrays for targeted drug delivery. Proceedings of the IEEE International Symposium on Antennas and Propagation and USNC-URSI Radio Science Meeting (2019), 1–2.

27 Shademani, A., Zhang, H., Jackson, J.K., and Chiao, M. (2017). *Advanced Functional Materials* 27: 1604558.

28 Huang, H. et al. (2014). *IEEE Journal of Translational Engineering in Health and Medicine* 2: 1.

29 Lee, H. et al. (2017). *Science Advances* 3: e1601314.

30 Lee, H. et al. (2018). *Advanced Drug Delivery Reviews* 127: 35.

31 Prausnitz, M.R. and Langer, R. (2008). *Nature Biotechnology* 26: 1261.

32 Rosen, Y., Gurman, P., and Elman, N. (2017). *Drug Delivery: An Integrated Clinical and Engineering Approach*. Boca Raton, FL: CRC Press.

33 He, X. et al. (2019). *Dose-Response* 17: 1559325819878585.

34 Eltorai, A.E., Fox, H., McGurrin, E., and Guang, S. (2016). *BioMed Research International* 2016.

35 Sutradhar, K.B. and Sumi, C.D. (2016). *Drug Delivery* 23: 1.

36 Saadeh, Y. and Vyas, D. (2014). *American Journal of Robotic Surgery* 1: 4.

37 Luo, M., Feng, Y., Wang, T., and Guan, J. (2018). *Advanced Functional Materials* 28: 1706100.

38 Li, J., de Avila, B.E.-F., Gao, W. et al. (2017). *Science Robotics* 2: eaam6431.

39 Wang, S., Liu, K., Wang, F. et al. (2019). *Chemistry: An Asian Journal* 14: 2336.

40 Wong, C., Moon, K.-S., and Li, Y. (2010). *Nano-Bio-Electronic, Photonic and MEMS Packaging*. New York: Springer.

41 Lim, H.-R. et al. (2019). *Advanced Materials* 32: 1901924.

42 Mitragotri, S. and Lahann, J. (2012). *Advanced Materials* 24: 3717.

43 Rahimi, S. and Takahata, K. (2011). A wireless implantable drug delivery device with hydrogel microvalves controlled by field-frequency tuning. Proceedings of the IEEE 24th International Conference on Micro Electro Mechanical Systems (IEEE, 2011), 1019–1022.

44 Bariana, M., Aw, M.S., Moore, E. et al. (2014). *Nanomedicine* 9: 1263.

45 Lahann, J. (2011). *Small* 7: 1149.

46 Tiwari, G. et al. (2012). *International Journal of Pharmaceutical Investigation* 2: 2.

47 Hubbell, J.A. and Chilkoti, A. (2012). *Science* 337: 303.

48 Mukherjee, B. et al. (2014). Current status and future scope for nanomaterials in drug delivery. In: *Application of Nanotechnology in Drug Delivery* (ed. A.D. Sezer). Rijeka: IntechOpen, chap. 16.

49 Vasilev, K., Chen, H., and Murray, P. (2012). *Journal of Nanomaterials* 2012.

50 Deen, G.R. and Loh, X.J. (2018). *Gels* 4: 13.

51 Hoare, T. et al. (2009). *Nano Letters* 9: 3651.

52 Meng, E. and Sheybani, R. (2014). *Therapeutic Delivery* 5: 1167.

53 Li, C. et al. (2019). *Acta Pharmaceutica Sinica B* 9: 1145.

54 Suri, S.S., Fenniri, H., and Singh, B. (2007). *Journal of Occupational Medicine and Toxicology* 2: 16.

55 Ando, H. et al. (2016). *IEEE Transactions on Biomedical Circuits and Systems* 10: 1068.
56 Christiansen, M. et al. (2017). *Journal of Diabetes Science and Technology* 11: 567.
57 Dias, D., Paulo, J., and Silva, J.P. (2018). *Sensors* 18: 2414.
58 Ramesh, M.V., Mohan, K.S., and Nadarajan, D. (2014). An in-body wireless communication system for targeted drug delivery: Design and simulation. Proceedings of the International Symposium on Technology Management and Emerging Technologies (IEEE, 2014), 56–61.
59 Walton, A.J., et al. (2006). Miniaturised drug delivery system with wireless power transfer and communication. The Institution of Engineering and Technology Seminar on MEMS Sensors and Actuators 2006, London, 2006, 155–162. doi: https://doi.org/10.1049/ic:20060457.
60 Tang, T. et al. (2008). *IET Nanobiotechnology* 2: 72.
61 Lee, S.H. et al. (2012). *AAPS PharmSciTech* 13: 211.
62 Maloney, J.M. et al. (2005). *Journal of Controlled Release* 109: 244. Proceedings of the Twelfth International Symposium on Recent Advances in Drug Delivery Systems.
63 Yang, Y.-J., et al. (2009). A release-on-demand wireless CMOS drug delivery SoC based on electrothermal activation technique. Proceedings of the IEEE International Solid-State Circuits Conference-Digest of Technical Papers (IEEE, 2009), 288–289.
64 Huang, Y.-J. et al. (2012). *Journal on Emerging Technologies in Computing Systems* 8: 12:1.
65 Smith, S. et al. (2007). *IET Nanobiotechnology* 1: 80.
66 Farra, R. et al. (2012). *Science Translational Medicine* 4: 122ra21.
67 Nisar, A., Afzulpurkar, N., Mahaisavariya, B., and Tuantranont, A. (2008). *Sensors and Actuators B: Chemical* 130: 917.
68 Nafea, M., Nawabjan, A., and Ali, M.S.M. (2018). *Sensors and Actuators A: Physical* 279: 191.
69 Yi, Y., et al. (2015). Electromagnetically powered electrolytic pump and thermo-responsive valve for drug delivery. Proceedings of the 10th IEEE International Conference on Nano/Micro Engineered and Molecular Systems (IEEE, 2015), 5–8.
70 Cheong, H.R., Nguyen, N.-T., Khaw, M.K. et al. (2018). *Lab on a Chip* 18: 3207.
71 Li, P.-Y., Givrad, T.K., Holschneider, D.P. et al. (2009). *Journal of Microelectromechanical Systems* 18: 1184.
72 Li, P.-Y. et al. (2010). *Lab on a Chip* 10: 101.
73 Fong, J., Xiao, Z., and Takahata, K. (2015). *Lab on a Chip* 15: 1050.
74 Chee, P.S., Minjal, M.N., Leow, P.L., and Ali, M.S.M. (2015). *Sensors and Actuators A: Physical* 233: 1.
75 Sitti, M. et al. (2015). *Proceedings of the IEEE* 103: 205.

76 Li, J., de Ávila, B.E.-F., Gao, W. et al. (2017). *Science robotics* 2.
77 Koppisetti, V. and Sahiti, B. (2011). *International Journal of Drug Development and Research* 3: 260.
78 Dogangil, G., et al. (2008). Toward targeted retinal drug delivery with wireless magnetic microrobots. Proceedings of the IEEE/RSJ International Conference on Intelligent Robots and Systems (IEEE, 2008), 1921–1926.
79 Fusco, S. et al. (2014). *Expert Opinion on Drug Delivery* 11: 1815.
80 Lee, S. et al. (2018). *Advanced Healthcare Materials* 7: 1700985.
81 Sivaraman, K.M., et al. (2013). Functional polypyrrole coatings for wirelessly controlled magnetic microrobots. Proceedings of the IEEE Point-of-Care Healthcare Technologies (PHT) (IEEE, 2013), 22–25.
82 Jeong, J., Jang, D., and Chung, S.K. (2018). Target drug delivery technology (Carrying, releasing, penetrating) using acoustic bubbles embedded in an electromagnetically driven microrobot. Proceedings of the Micro Electro Mechanical Systems (MEMS) (IEEE, 2018), 59–61.
83 Szymanski-Exner, A. et al. (2003). *Journal of Pharmaceutical Sciences* 92: 289.
84 Goldberg, S. (2001). *European Journal of Ultrasound* 13: 129.
85 Liu, X. et al. (2015). *Applied Physics Reviews* 2: 011103.
86 Moran, C.H. et al. (2009). *Nano Research* 2: 400.
87 Kruse, D.E. et al. (2011). *IEEE Transactions on Biomedical Engineering* 58: 2002.
88 Tamarov, K.P. et al. (2014). *Scientific Reports* 4: 7034.
89 San, B.H., Moh, S.H., and Kim, K.K. (2013). *International Journal of Hyperthermia* 29: 99.
90 Gannon, C.J. et al. (2007). *Cancer: Interdisciplinary International Journal of the American Cancer Society* 110: 2654.
91 Hanson, G.W., Monreal, R.C., and Apell, S.P. (2011). *Journal of Applied Physics* 109: 124306.
92 Mackeyev, Y., Mark, C., Kumar, N., and Serda, R.E. (2017). *Acta Biomaterialia* 53: 619.
93 Mironava, T., Arachchilage, V.T., Myers, K.J., and Suchalkin, S. (2017). *Langmuir* 33: 13114.
94 Cardinal, J. et al. (2008). *Surgery* 144: 125.
95 Cherukuri, P., Glazer, E.S., and Curley, S.A. (2010). *Advanced Drug Delivery Reviews* 62: 339.
96 Park, S.-I. et al. (2018). *Colloids and Surfaces A: Physicochemical and Engineering Aspects* 538: 304.
97 Samanta, B. et al. (2008). *Journal of Materials Chemistry* 18: 1204.
98 Prigo, E.A. et al. (2015). *Applied Physics Reviews* 2: 041302.
99 Hervault, A. and Thanh, N.T.K. (2014). *Nanoscale* 6: 11553.
100 Cervadoro, A. et al. (2013). *PLoS One* 8: e57332.
101 Glazer, E.S. and Curley, S.A. (2011). *Therapeutic Delivery* 2: 1325.

102 Warsi, M.F. and Chechik, V. (2011). *Physical Chemistry Chemical Physics* 13: 9812.

103 Glazer, E.S., Massey, K.L., Zhu, C., and Curley, S.A. (2010). *Surgery* 148: 319.

104 Jose, A., Surendran, M., Fazal, S. et al. (2018). *Colloids and Surfaces B: Biointerfaces* 165: 371.

105 Tamarov, K. et al. (2016). *Journal of Controlled Release* 241: 220.

106 Satarkar, N.S. et al. (2010). *Journal of Applied Polymer Science* 117: 1813.

107 He, Z., Satarkar, N., Xie, T. et al. (2011). *Advanced Materials* 23: 3192.

108 Lee, Y. and Thompson, D. (2017). *WIREs Nanomedicine and Nanobiotechnology* 9: e1450.

109 Gulyaev, Y.V. et al. (2015). *Journal of Communications Technology and Electronics* 60: 1097.

110 Khomutov, G.B. et al. (2017). *Colloids and Surfaces A: Physicochemical and Engineering Aspects* 532: 26. 30th European Colloid and Interface Society Meeting, Rome 2016.

111 Rasch, M.R., Yu, Y., Bosoy, C. et al. (2012). *Langmuir* 28: 12971.

112 Hardiansyah, A. et al. (2017). *Nanoscale Research Letters* 12: 355.

113 Li, J. and Mooney, D.J. (2016). *Nature Reviews Materials* 1: 16071.

114 Zhao, W., Odelius, K., Edlund, U. et al. (2015). *Biomacromolecules* 16: 2522.

115 Li, T. et al. (2016). *The AAPS Journal* 18: 146.

116 Lengert, E. et al. (2018). *Nanoscale* 10: 17249.

117 Lengert, E. et al. (2019). *Materials Science and Engineering C: Materials for Biological Applications* 98: 1114.

118 Thompson, K.L., Williams, M., and Armes, S.P. (2015). *Journal of Colloid and Interface Science* 447: 217.

119 Sukhorukov, G.B. et al. (1998). *Polymers for Advanced Technologies* 9: 759.

120 Donath, E., Sukhorukov, G.B., Caruso, F. et al. (1998). *Angewandte Chemie International Edition* 37: 2201.

121 De Temmerman, M.-L., Demeester, J., De Vos, F., and De Smedt, S.C. (2011). *Biomacromolecules* 12: 1283.

122 Ermakov, A.V. et al. (2019). *Macromolecular Rapid Communications* 40: 1800200.

123 Sindeeva, O.A. et al. (2019). *ACS Biomaterials Science & Engineering*.

124 Antipina, M.N., Kiryukhin, M.V., and Sukhorukov, G.B. (2012). *Stimuli-Responsive Polymer Composite Multilayer Microcapsules and Microchamber Arrays*, 851–890. John Wiley & Sons, Ltd, chap. 36.

125 German, S.V. et al. (2016). *Physical Chemistry Chemical Physics* 18: 32238.

126 Voronin, D.V. et al. (2017). *ACS Applied Materials and Interfaces* 9: 6885.

127 Grigoriev, D., Gorin, D., Sukhorukov, G.B. et al. (2007). *Langmuir* 23: 12388.

128 Gorin, D.A. et al. (2008). *Physical Chemistry Chemical Physics* 10: 6899.

129 Bukreeva, T., Parakhonsky, B., Skirtach, A. et al. (2006). *Crystallography Reports* 51: 863.

130 Yashchenok, A.M. et al. (2010). *Advanced Functional Materials* 20: 3136.

131 Ermakov, A. et al. (2019). *Macromolecular Rapid Communications* 40: 1700868.

132 Sindeeva, O.A. et al. (2018). *Soft Matter* 14: 9012.

133 Ermakov, A.V. et al. (2019). *Journal of Applied Polymer Science* 136: 47718.

134 Gao, C., Leporatti, S., Moya, S. et al. (2003). *Chemistry A European Journal* 9: 915.

135 Prevot, M., Djugnat, C., Mhwald, H., and Sukhorukov, G.B. (2006). *ChemPhysChem* 7: 2497.

10

Minimally Invasive Microwave Ablation Antennas

Hung Luyen[1], Yahya Mohtashami[2], James F. Sawicki[3], Susan C. Hagness[1] and Nader Behdad[1]

[1] *Department of Electrical and Computer Engineering, University of Wisconsin, Madison, WI, USA*
[2] *Department of Electrical and Computer Engineering, University of California, Santa Barbara, CA, USA*
[3] *Direct Imaging Center of Excellence, Boston Scientific Corporation, Marlborough, MA, USA*

10.1 Introduction

10.1.1 Overview of Microwave Ablation Therapy

Microwave-induced heating of tumors has emerged as an effective treatment strategy for a variety of clinical applications in oncology. There are two target temperature regimes for microwave thermal therapies, as illustrated in Figure 10.1. Moderate hyperthermia, defined here as elevating the temperature of cancer cells up to 45°C for an extended period of time, typically 60–90 minutes, results in increased blood flow, heat shock, and the induction of apoptosis [1]. Since thermal sensitization renders the tumor more susceptible to chemotherapy and radiation therapy [2], microwave-induced hyperthermia has been used as an adjunct to standard of care treatments for superficial tumors within a couple of centimeters of the skin surface as well as deep-seated tumors [3–6]. The modest target temperature rise makes it feasible to perform microwave hyperthermia noninvasively using external waveguide applicators or phased-array systems designed to focus the microwave energy at the tumor site and selectively heat the tumor and its margins while maintaining normal physiological temperatures in the surrounding healthy tissue.

Extreme hyperthermia involves elevating the temperature of cancer cells above 50–60°C. In this so-called ablation regime, the absorption of microwave energy results in protein denaturation and coagulation necrosis [7]. The rapid and irreversible thermal damage is vividly seen through color changes of the ablated tissue [8, 9], as illustrated in Figure 10.2. Microwave ablation (MWA) is minimally invasive, requiring the use of an interstitial antenna inserted

Antenna and Sensor Technologies in Modern Medical Applications,
First Edition. Edited by Yahya Rahmat-Samii and Erdem Topsakal.

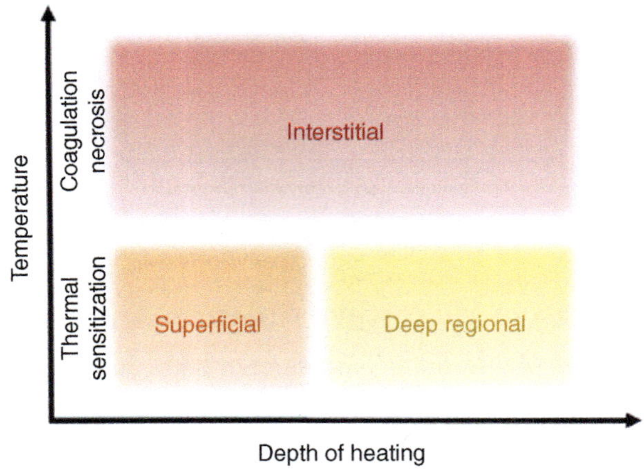

Figure 10.1 Microwave thermal therapies that include (i) lower temperature superficial and deep regional microwave hyperthermia techniques, which weaken the tumor via thermal sensitization and render it more susceptible to chemo- and radiation therapy and (ii) higher temperature interstitial microwave ablation techniques, which induce direct cell death via coagulation necrosis.

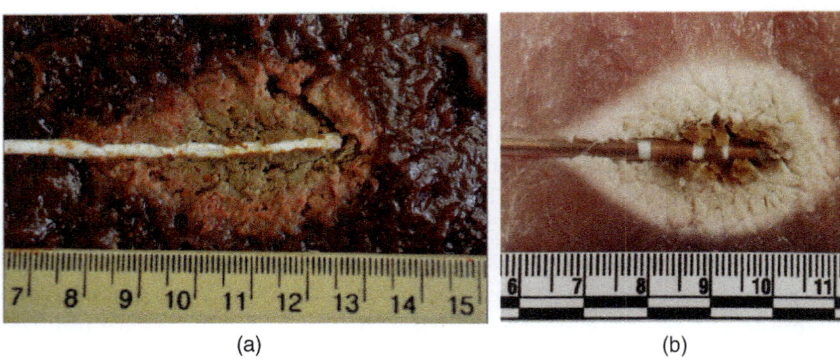

Figure 10.2 Photographs of representative bisected coagulation zones in ex vivo (a) bovine liver [8] (*Source*: Luyen, H., Hagness, S. C., and Behdad, N., 2015. © IEEE.) and (b) porcine muscle [9] vividly illustrate the physiological changes that occur during ablation. (*Source*: Luyen, H., Hagness, S. C., and Behdad, N., 2017. © IEEE.)

directly into the tumor. Tissue temperatures in the immediate vicinity of the antenna can reach well over 100°C.

To date, MWA has been most widely investigated in treating unresectable malignant hepatic tumors [10]. It also shows promise for treating a variety of other cancers, including kidney, lung, bone, breast, prostate, and pancreas [11–16]. Interest in MWA is fueled in part by concerns about the risks and limited effectiveness of conventional treatments. Consider breast cancer treatment, for example, where surgical resection is commonly combined with radiation, chemotherapy, and/or endocrine therapy to achieve long-term survival [17]. All of these treatment options carry risks of short-term side effects and chronic morbidities as well as some life-threatening toxicities. MWA offers the potential for quicker recovery and poses fewer risks.

There are a number of significant advantages of MWA over other types of thermal ablation technologies, including radio-frequency ablation (RFA), high-intensity focused ultrasound (HIFU), and laser ablation [10]. For example, microwave propagation is not impeded by dessicated tissue, and the rapid rate of heating overcomes heat-sink effects of nearby vessels [10]. Furthermore, MWA achieves higher temperatures, larger ablation volumes (as needed), and shorter ablation times, i.e. ~5 minutes compared to ~15 minutes for RFA, ~30 minutes for laser, and ~60 minutes for HIFU [13]. Consequently, MWA devices are rising in popularity among interventional oncologists [18].

10.1.2 Historical Development and Current Landscape of Research on MWA Antennas

The idea of delivering electromagnetic (EM) radiation into the human body for medical purposes dates back to the early twentieth century [19]. One of the first works in this area is described in a US patent issued to W. M. Hahnemann in 1939 in which some of the important challenges of efficiently delivering the energy of short-wavelength EM waves into the body were identified, and techniques for circumventing them were proposed [19]. The use of cavity magnetron as a high-power microwave source, which was arguably the most critical component of allies' radar technology during World War II, was extended to the medical field shortly after the war. One of the first medical devices that used the cavity magnetron was Raytheon's Microtherm introduced in the 1940s for the purpose of heating human tissue [20]. However, most of the research conducted in this area prior to the 1960s focused on therapeutic applications of microwave that involved delivering EM energy to the body using external applicators [20–22]. One of the first devices developed for delivering EM energy into a body cavity was conceived as early as 1960 by G. Seifert [23]. This device resembles many interstitial antennas developed in later decades for microwave hyperthermia and ablation applications. In the same decade, R. W. P. King and K. Iizuka developed the theory of dipole antennas radiating in dissipative media [24–26]. Among its other applications, this theory is highly relevant to the design of interstitial antennas radiating inside biological tissues. These studies were followed on by additional theoretical studies in the 1970s and 1980s investigating other aspects of the operation of dipole antennas immersed in dissipative or conductive environments [27–31].

The development of antennas for delivering EM energy into the body, either through body cavities or interstitially, continued in the 1970s. Early examples of such antennas included simple coaxial probes with extended center conductors [32–34] and coaxial-fed monopole or dipole antennas [35–38]. Experimental techniques were often used to characterize and optimize the performances of such simple antennas [39, 40]. One of the early examples of a more sophisticated interstitial antenna is a coax-fed helical coil developed for microwave hyperthermia [41], which was shown to be superior to a conventional interstitial dipole antenna in producing more localized heating patterns [42]. With the development and widespread use of numerical EM simulation and optimization techniques, numerous other more sophisticated interstitial antennas were developed starting in the late 1980s and the early 1990s. Such techniques allowed for optimizing the antenna performance metrics important to MWA and hyperthermia applications. These include the impedance matching, specific absorption rate (SAR) pattern, heating profile, and insensitivity of the antenna response to the insertion depth. Examples of these early studies included the development of multisection monopoles [43, 44] and end-fire applicators for microwave hyperthermia [45]. These techniques also allowed for conveniently comparing the performances of various interstitial antennas together [44, 46].

As the use of MWA as a means of treating cancer began to gain more traction, several challenges in designing interstitial antennas had to be addressed. In particular, the temperature levels required for MWA are significantly higher than those needed for hyperthermia. Therefore, interstitial antennas used for MWA must produce localized heating patterns without long tails and with minimal heating of the healthy tissue surrounding the antenna shaft along its insertion path. As a result, many simple monopole or dipole antennas that had been widely used for microwave hyperthermia would not be suitable for MWA as they tend to produce elongated heating patterns. Moreover, the input impedances of such antennas are often highly dependent on the insertion depth of the antenna into the tissue as well as the dielectric properties of the tissue surrounding the active tip of the antenna, which changes drastically during ablation process. This impedance variability complicates the task of delivering high-power microwaves to the tissue to be ablated and maintaining this power transfer during the ablation process. One of the early antenna designs that addressed these challenges was a coax-fed insulated dipole with a coaxial balun that was capable of producing localized heating patterns [47]. In this design, the coaxial balun was used to choke the RF currents flowing on the outer surface of the outer conductor of the feeding coaxial cable. This is important since these currents run along the healthy tissue surrounding the shaft of the antenna along its insertion path and can cause unwanted heating and damage to the healthy tissue. Suppressing these currents and insulating the antenna from the lossy tissue surrounding it allowed for achieving a localized heating pattern and reduced the impedance variations of the antenna as a function of the insertion depth and the changing dielectric properties of the environment. Figure 10.3a illustrates the topology

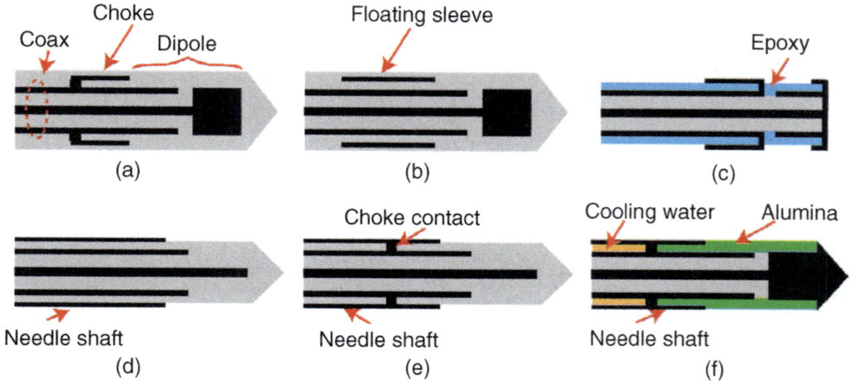

Figure 10.3_1 Topology of various MWA antenna designs. (a) Choke dipole [47]. (*Source*: Modified from Hurter, W., Reinbold, F., and Lorenz, W.J., 1991.) (b) Floating-sleeve dipole [48]. (*Source*: Modified from Yang, D., Bertram, J. M., Converse, M.C., et al., 2006.) (c) Cap-choke antenna [49]. (*Source*: Modified from Lin, J.C. and Wang, Yu-Jin, 1996.) (d) Triaxial antenna [50]. (*Source*: Modified from Brace, C. L., Laeseke, P. F., van der Weide, D. W., et al., 2005.) (e) Dipole with a sliding choke [51]. (*Source*: Modified from Longo, I., Gentili, G. B., Cerretelli, M., et al., 2003.) (f) Closed-tip antenna with a coaxial choke [52]. (*Source*: Modified from Cavagnaro, M., Amabile, C., Bernardi, P., et al., 2011.)

of the coax-fed choked dipole antenna reported in [47]. The coaxial balun in this design was implemented using a third conductor, referred to as a coaxial sleeve, that encompassed the outer conductor of the feeding coaxial cable. The coaxial sleeve and the outer conductor of the coaxial cable formed a quarter-wavelength transmission line, which was short-circuited at the proximal end, to present a high input impedance at the distal end to choke the undesired currents flowing on the outer conducting surface of the coaxial cable. Other innovative designs that used coaxial baluns to perform a similar task were reported in the 1990s and the 2000s. Notable examples among these include the cap-choke antenna [49, 58], a coax-fed dipole with a miniaturized sleeve choke [51] and its variants [52, 59], the coaxial-dipole antenna [60], the floating-sleeve dipole (FSD) antenna [48], the expanded wire tip antenna [61], and the triaxial antenna [50]. These antennas are all coax-fed monopoles or dipoles (symmetric or asymmetric) and use different variations of a coaxial balun to achieve localized heating patterns and good impedance matching during the ablation process. Figure 10.3b and c shows examples of two other ways to implement coaxial baluns using different terminations and/or lengths for the coaxial sleeve, such as an open-ended half-wavelength sleeve (e.g. used in [48]) or a sleeve short-circuited at the distal end instead of at the proximal end (e.g. used in [49]). The use of a coaxial balun, however, increases the overall diameter of the interstitial antenna, which is undesired for a minimally invasive therapy. Therefore, a great deal of effort in the past two decades has

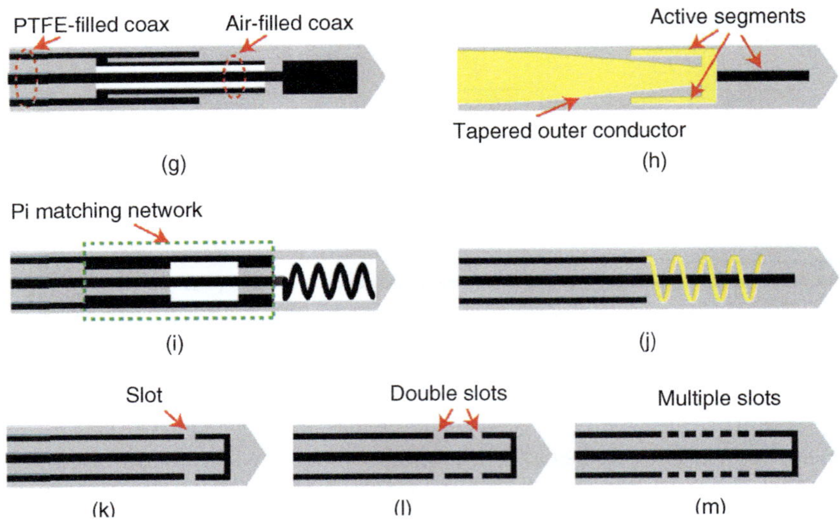

Figure 10.3_2 (g) Reduced-diameter, balun-equipped dipole [9]. (*Source*: Luyen, H., Hagness, S. C., and Behdad, N., 2017.) (h) Coax-fed antenna with a tapered-slot balun [53]. (*Source*: Modified from Luyen, H., Hagness, S. C., and Behdad, N., 2018.) (i) Balun-free helical monopole with a pi-matching network [8]. (*Source*: Luyen, H., Hagness, S. C., and Behdad, N., 2015.) (j) Balun-free helical dipole [54]. (*Source*: Mohtashami, Y., Behdad, N., and Hagness, S.C., 2020.) (k) Single-slot [55] (*Source*: Modified from Hamada, L., Saito, K., Yoshimura, H., et al., 2000.) (l) double-slot [56] (*Source*: Modified from Saito, K., Yoshimura, H., Ito, K., et al., 2004.) and (m) multiple-slot antennas [57]. (*Source*: Modified from Wang, T., Zhao, G., and Qiu, B., 2015.) Black represents metal, gray represents dielectric, and white represents air.

been put in reducing the invasiveness of interstitial antennas compared to conventional coax-fed, balun-equipped designs.

Various solutions have been proposed in recent years for minimizing the invasiveness of coax-fed MWA antennas, which can be classified into two general groups. The first group represents solutions that target innovative implementations of coaxial baluns. On the other hand, the second group involves novel antenna designs that provide localized heating profiles without the need of any coaxial baluns, referred to as balun-free antennas. A prominent solution belonging to the first group associates with taking advantages of a metallic biopsy needle used for guiding the antenna to an ablation site and doubling its function as a coaxial balun. The needle shaft was used to make a floating sleeve for a triaxial antenna [50], as shown in Figure 10.3d, or a sliding choke for an asymmetric dipole [51], as shown in Figure 10.3e, or a fixed choke for a closed-tip antenna [52], as shown in Figure 10.3f. Another solution for reduced-diameter coaxial balun implementations was presented in [9], which proposed using an impedance-matched transition between a dielectric-filled feed line and an air-filled coax section. Because air has smaller permittivity than polytetrafluoroethylene (PTFE), the air-filled coax has a smaller diameter outer conductor compared to the PTFE-filled coax for the same characteristic impedance and inner conductor size. Therefore, this smaller diameter air-filled coax can be leveraged to implement the coaxial balun and active part of the antenna, as shown in Figure 10.3g, to achieve diameter reduction compared to a similar antenna topology implemented on the PTFE-filled coax. Aside from tweaking coaxial-sleeve baluns, a different approach was presented in [53] that relies on using a less-invasive balun topology for MWA antenna designs. The balun in this design was realized by tapering the outer conductor of the coaxial cable to provide a smooth transition from a coaxial line to a parallel-wire line that can be used to feed a dipole antenna, as illustrated in Figure 10.3h.

Alternatively, several novel balun-free MWA antenna designs have been proposed for achieving localized SAR patterns. Notable designs include a half-wavelength helical monopole antenna [8], a low-impedance helical dipole antenna [54], and a family of slot antennas [55–57, 62–66]. The balun-free operation of a helical monopole antenna reported in [8] was achieved by operating the antenna at its second resonant frequency where the electrical current is minimum at the base of the helix. This creates a natural choke point for the current that tends to get excited on the outer conducting surface of the coax, resulting in a highly localized SAR pattern at this frequency. Due to the maximum voltage and minimum current at the base of the helix, the helical monopole had a high input impedance and needed to be impedance matched to a standard 50 Ω coaxial feed line via an internal impedance matching network, as shown in Figure 10.3i. Interestingly, it was shown that not only a high impedance but also a low impedance at the feed point can be utilized to choke undesired outer-surface currents in coax-fed antennas, as demonstrated in the asymmetric dipole antenna design reported in [54]. Figure 10.3j shows the topology of this antenna, which consists of a three-quarter-wavelength helical arm connected to the outer conductor and a quarter-wavelength straight arm connected to the inner conductor of the coax. The current flowing in the inner surface of the coax's outer conductor to the junction (feed point of the dipole arms) sees a lower impedance path via the helix and higher impedance path via the outer surface of the coaxial cable. This results in a small fraction of current flowing back to the outer conducting surface of the coaxial cable, creating a localized SAR pattern. Besides the balun-free helical monopole and dipole designs, numerous publications reported different variations of slot antennas. Figure 10.3k–m illustrates the general topologies of single-, double-, and multislot antennas examined in various publications in the literature [55–57, 62–66]. In these designs, the inner and outer conductors of the coax are typically short-circuited at the distal end, and one or multiple annular slots are cut in the outer conductor. In [55], a single dielectric-loaded annular slot was proposed for improved control of the longitudinal heating pattern of the coax-fed antenna. It has been reported that using an additional slot provides much more localized SAR patterns and more spherical ablation zones [56, 67, 68], leading to the widespread of studies on double-slot antennas [63, 64, 69–72]. Multislot antennas which consist of more than three periodic slots were also investigated and optimized for achieving nearly spherical ablation zones [57, 65, 66].

In addition to linear dipole/monopole and slot antennas designed for general use in MWA, other interstitial antenna topologies have also been examined to address more specific applications. A helical slit cut in the outer conductor of a feeding coax was reported in [73] as part of a multiantenna hyperthermia array. A coax-fed spiral antenna, featuring an expanded aperture lateral to the coax's axis, was proposed for achieving large heating zones for cardiac ablation [74, 75]. Flexible implementations of the single-slot antenna, which can be guided through a catheter, have been examined for treatment of bile duct carcinoma [76]. Other exotic types of single-element interstitial antennas have also been developed recently. Examples include antennas capable of producing directional heating patterns [77, 78], non-coax-fed MWA antennas with symmetric or asymmetric heating patterns [79], and a baseball-bat-shaped interstitial antenna capable of producing large ablation zones with low input power levels [80]. Several review articles comparing the performances of different antennas [81–84] and comparing the performance of MWA in different tissues [85] or at different frequencies [86–89] have also been reported over the years, and the interested reader is encouraged to review them.

10.1.3 Impact of Frequency on MWA Performance

Most MWA devices are designed to operate in the 915-MHz or 2.45-GHz industrial, scientific, and medical (ISM) bands. At these frequencies, the penetration depth of microwaves in tissue is on the order of the desired lesion radius, making them a reasonable choice. A theoretical and experimental study comparing ablation performance at 915 MHz and 2.45 GHz reported greater power deposition and larger diameter ablation zones for the higher frequency [89]. Operation at higher frequencies (e.g. >2.45 GHz) reduces the microwave penetration depth and increases undesired heating in the feeding cable due to ohmic losses. However, the long active radiators employed by lower frequency antennas tend to produce aspherical ablation zones that may not both ablate tumors with sufficient safety margin and preserve as much healthy tissue as possible [88, 89]. Higher frequency MWA devices would comprise shorter radiators that would allow more design flexibility.

A few studies have examined MWA at frequencies up to the 24.125-GHz ISM band. A 9.2-GHz MWA system was used in clinical trials for treating endometrial bleeding [90]. 14.5-GHz applicators have also been developed to both measure and ablate tumors [91] and have been studied in ex vivo human liver [92]. Several other studies directly compared the performance of MWA at multiple frequencies [86–88, 93, 94]. One demonstrated that MWA performed at 10 GHz yields ablation volumes comparable to those attained at 1.9 GHz in ex vivo bovine liver when input power and heating duration are the same. This suggests that the growth of ablated tissue is a function of not only direct microwave heating but also of thermal conduction [86]. A second paper utilized computer simulations and compared the performance of 2.45 and 24.125 GHz antennas, showing that the lower frequency MWA yielded a less-compact and more elliptical heating pattern [93]. A third comparison of MWA in the 0.9–18-GHz range showed that, at low power, the 18-GHz system induced the highest tissue temperatures near the microwave applicator [94]. Higher frequency operation also produced the highest differentiation between cancerous and fatty tissues. Another study compared the ablation performance at multiple discrete frequencies in the 1.9–26-GHz range using the same antenna type, input power level, and duration [87]. Simulation results for ex vivo and in vivo settings as well as experimental results for ex vivo ablation with porcine muscle demonstrated relatively consistent maximum lateral dimensions for the ablation zones acquired across the frequency range. A follow-up study conducted later investigated ablation performance over the frequency range of 1.9–18 GHz in the presence of perfusion [88], concluding that higher frequency MWA produces comparable ablation zone sizes as those achieved at lower frequencies even in strongly perfused tissue. These highlighted studies suggest promising performance characteristics of higher frequency MWA. The use of higher microwave frequencies for tissue ablation would enable shorter and potentially less-invasive applicators.

10.1.4 Focus of this Chapter

The chapter is intended to provide a quick review on recent advances in minimally invasive MWA antenna designs and emphasize the authors' collective works in this area. A major fraction of the chapter was compiled from our previous publications on MWA, which highlight two main aspects: (i) investigation of higher frequency microwaves for tissue ablation and (ii) novel MWA antenna designs with reduced-diameter topology for general and specific usage scenarios. Section 10.2 summarizes the key details and main findings of our two studies (presented in [87, 88]) investigating MWA performance at multiple discrete frequencies from 1.9 to 18 GHz. Section 10.3 discusses methods for reducing diameters of balun-equipped coax-fed antennas, starting with a comprehensive literature review and then shifting focus to our two proposed antenna designs, which were previously reported in [9, 53], with more details. Section 10.4 is dedicated to balun-free coax-fed antenna designs which represent a different group of solutions for minimizing invasiveness of MWA antennas. We first review notable studies from other researchers and subsequently dive deeper into the designs of the half-wavelength helical monopole [8] and asymmetric helical dipole [54]. Finally, our effort in developing flexible antennas as well as directional-heating antennas, aimed for increasing the flexibility and customization of MWA treatment, is documented in Section 10.5.

10.2 Toward Length Reduction for Ablation Antennas: Demonstration of Higher Frequency Microwave Ablation

This section highlights our investigation of using higher frequency microwaves for tissue ablation, which is motivated by the aspect of reduced antenna lengths as the operating frequency increases. An MWA applicator with a shorter length is clearly more flexible in various clinical scenarios whether the tumor is deep seated or near the surface of the tissue. A shorter applicator is also more amenable for implementation with flexible embodiments, further reducing the invasiveness of MWA treatment for scenarios where the antenna can be routed through a natural ductal pathway to reach the ablation site. The content presented in this section is derived in part from an article published in the *International Journal of Hyperthermia* in 2017 [87] as well as an article recently published in *IEEE Transactions on Biomedical Engineering* in 2018 [88].

10.2.1 Electromagnetic Evaluation of Microwave Ablation Antennas Operating in the 1.9–18-GHz Range

In this section, a study of the frequency dependence of achievable ablation zones is presented. Performance at discrete frequencies between 1.9 and 18 GHz, a range chosen to include the ISM bands at 2.45 and 5.8 GHz, is demonstrated. SAR patterns and ablation zones at these discrete frequencies are shown for a series of FSD antennas operating in a tissue model.

Figure 10.4a and b shows two cross sections of the coaxial FSD antenna used in this analysis, which was originally introduced by Yang et al. [48] for MWA at 2.45 GHz. Five design frequencies were chosen: from 1.9 and 18 GHz, spaced by 4 GHz (or 4.1 GHz in the case of the spacing between the two lowest frequencies). Antenna design parameters were optimized to achieve good impedance matching for efficient power delivery and a compact SAR pattern wherein minimal radiation occurs behind the floating sleeve.

EM simulations of MWA performance were conducted using CST Microwave Studio. The simulation domain consisted of a block of porcine liver tissue into which the antenna was inserted. The wideband dielectric properties for the liver used in the simulation model were taken from [95]

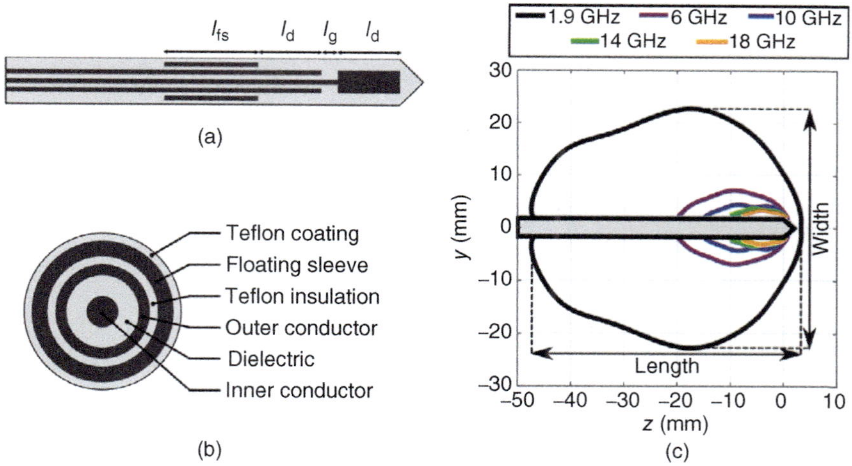

Figure 10.4 (a) Longitudinal cross section and (b) transverse cross section of floating-sleeve dipole (FSD) antennas used in computational and experimental studies of MWA. The length dimensions are customized for seven different frequencies between 1.9 and 18 GHz. (c) Simulated constant power absorption contours bounding the volume in which 75% of power radiated by the FSD antenna (shown in cross-sectional view) is absorbed, as a function of frequency. Measurement axes for the 1.9 GHz contour are shown.

assuming room-temperature tissue. The dimensions of the tissue region within the computational domain were chosen so that the microwaves were highly attenuated before reaching the tissue boundary. First, an analysis is presented of the simulated power deposition patterns for the 1.9-, 6.0-, 10-, 14-, and 18-GHz antennas. A typical analysis of SAR patterns normalizes the SAR distribution to the peak calculated value, but since peak SAR can vary substantially across antenna designs and operating frequencies, such normalized patterns are difficult to compare. This analysis instead utilizes a SAR isosurface for each antenna that encloses the volume of tissue in which 75% of the power radiated by the antenna is absorbed, shown in Figure 10.4c. Figure 10.5 shows the dimensions of these surfaces along and perpendicular to the antenna's axis as well as the volume of tissue enclosed by the surface. As the microwave frequency increases from 1.9 to 18 GHz, the linear dimensions of the SAR isosurfaces shrink by a factor of more than 5, and their volumes fall by a factor of about 350. This represents a substantial decrease in absorption volume across the frequency range of 1.9–18 GHz.

10.2.2 Performance of Higher Frequency Microwave Ablation in the Presence of Perfusion

Blood perfusion acts as a heat sink during hyperthermal therapy, carrying thermal energy away from the treatment site and hindering the production

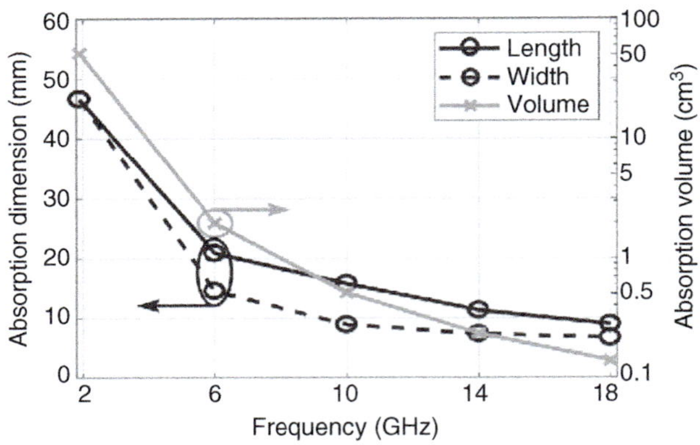

Figure 10.5 Linear dimensions of and volumes enclosed by constant power absorption surfaces enclosing 75% of absorbed power as a function of frequency.

of thermal lesions. This heat-sink effect is particularly pronounced in heavily perfused organs such as the liver, which has a per-mass flow rate that is at least twice as large as that in other commonly ablated organs such as the lung and the prostate [96]. In this section, the performance of MWA across a wide band of frequencies in both perfused and nonperfused ex vivo porcine liver is discussed. The thermal lesions produced in ex vivo porcine liver were measured, and their linear dimensions, volumes, and sphericity ratios were compared. The results illustrate the effects of both perfusion and operating frequency on the dimensions of the thermal lesions.

Unique antennas were designed for each of the five operating frequencies: 1.9, 6.0, 10, 14, and 18 GHz. The antennas were driven by a signal generator and microwave power amplifier, shown in Figure 10.6a. The available power at the antenna was limited to 25 W at the highest operating frequency, so this power was applied in all experiments. Ablations had a five-minute duration. The FSD antennas of the type used in these experiments have been shown to maintain good impedance matching during the ablation process [86]. The reflected power for each antenna was consistently in the range of 1–3 W over the course of each ablation.

Porcine livers were chosen to satisfy the size constraint of the perfusion chamber as well as the quantity of organs needed to reach the targeted number of trials. Eleven days of experiments over a four-month period were required to complete the study, totaling 40 livers and 134 individual ablation sites. Thirty-four experiments were discarded due to antenna failure or thermal lesion overlap with excessively large vessels. In the final dataset, there were data from 10 experiments at each of five frequencies, with and without active perfusion, for a total of 100 ablation experiments. Natural perfusion of the liver organ was approximated in the laboratory using a perfusion chamber,

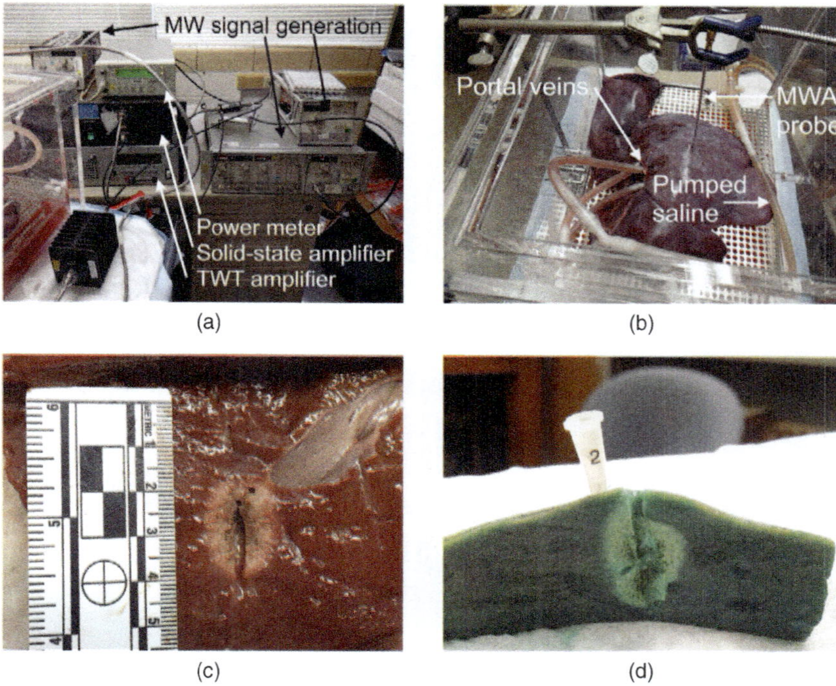

Figure 10.6 Experimental setup and verification of perfusion. (a) Microwave generation equipment. (b) Perfusion chamber with porcine liver. (c) Ablation zone of nonperfused liver. (d) Ablation zone of liver perfused with saline and green India ink to demonstrate complete perfusion. (*Source*: Sawicki, J. F., Luyen, H. Mohtashami, Y. et al., 2018. © IEEE.)

a peristaltic pump, Tygon® tubing, and a ($9\,\mathrm{g\,L^{-1}}$) saline perfusate pumped at 1 liter per minute. Figure 10.6b shows the perfusion chamber. Complete perfusion was demonstrated by adding green India ink to the saline perfusate and observing the staining in liver bisections. Sample ablation zones in perfused and nonperfused livers can be seen in Figure 10.6c and d.

The tissue was bisected along the antenna insertion track and then the lateral and longitudinal diameters (denoted as d_a and d_b, respectively) of the thermal lesions upon gross inspection at the completion of each ablation experiment. Figure 10.7 shows representative ablation zones for each frequency and perfusion state. The boundary between the red unaffected tissue and light brown coagulated tissue was considered the boundary of the thermal lesion. Ablation zone volumes for experiments were estimated as $\frac{4}{3}\pi\left(\frac{d_a}{2}\right)^2\left(\frac{d_b}{2}\right)$ and are shown in Figure 10.8. Error bars representing one standard deviation from the mean are included. Experiments yielded a relatively constant mean volume of ablated

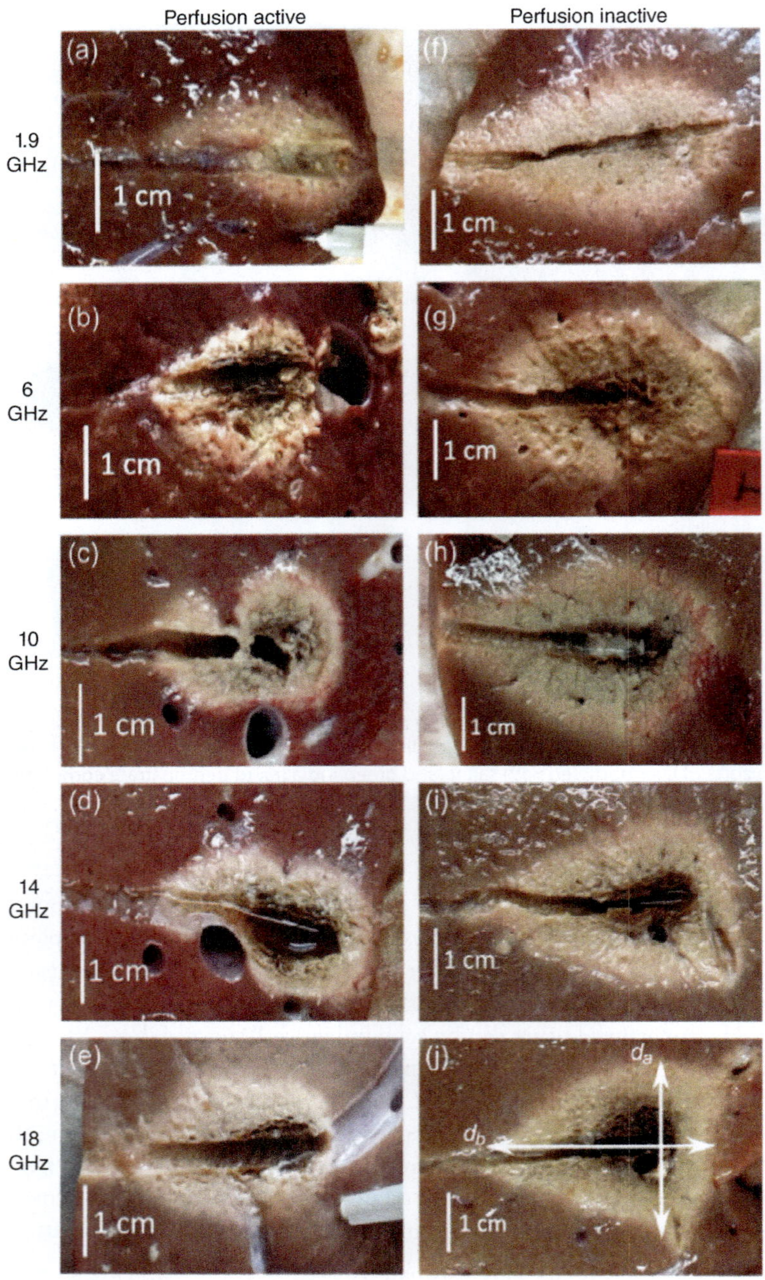

Figure 10.7 Representative images of ablated porcine liver tissue. 25 W of power was applied to the antenna input for five minutes. The frequency of applied microwave power is shown in the leftmost column, and column headers denote the perfusion state. (*Source*: Sawicki, J. F., Luyen, H. Mohtashami, Y., et al., 2018. © IEEE.)

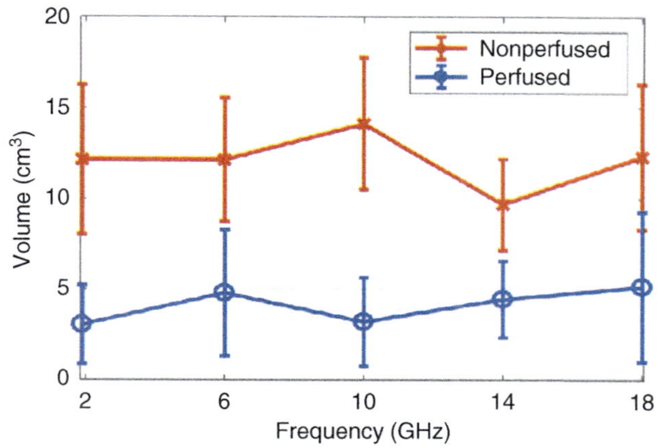

Figure 10.8 Volume of the thermal lesion in ablation experiments as a function of frequency. The variability bars span one standard deviation from the mean (denoted by symbols).

tissue across all frequencies, and the high rate of perfusion clearly reduced the size of achievable thermal lesions.

A comparison between the volumes of microwave power absorption in Figure 10.5 and the volumes of ablated tissue in Figure 10.8 shows that SAR pattern dimensions alone do not predict the size of ablation zones. The volume comprising 75% of the microwave power deposition shrinks by two orders of magnitude as frequency increases from 1.9 to 18 GHz, while experimental results show relatively constant ablation volumes throughout the frequency range. This is consistent with the results reported in [86, 87], which suggested that heat diffusion plays a major role in MWA thermal lesion production, especially at frequencies higher than the 915 MHz and 2.45 GHz typically employed in MWA.

Perfusion was shown to reduce the volume of thermal lesions by a factor of 2–3 compared to nonperfused tissue; however, its impact did not differ appreciably with frequency. Despite the increased reliance on thermal diffusion at higher frequencies, thermal lesion volumes were comparable from 1.9 to 18 GHz. Thus, higher frequency ablation is not impeded more by perfusion than lower frequency ablation, even in highly perfused tissues like the liver. This key result further supports the viability of higher frequency MWA designs.

10.3 Reduced-Diameter, Balun-Equipped Microwave Ablation Antenna Designs

Most coax-fed MWA antennas utilize coaxial baluns, implemented by encompassing the coaxial cable with a hollow conductor, to choke unwanted currents flowing on the outer conducting surface of the cable to minimize detrimental heating of healthy tissue along the feed line. These coaxial balun implementations have been demonstrated to be effective in providing localized heating patterns and making the input impedance of the antenna independent of the insertion depth [47–49, 58]. The only undesirable effect of a coaxial balun of this type is that it increases the overall diameter of the antenna beyond that of the feed cable and makes the antenna more invasive. Simply scaling down the diameter of the antenna using smaller diameter coaxial cables comes with the trade-off of increased ohmic losses and lower average power-handling capabilities. Therefore, solutions that reduce the overall diameter in the geometry of MWA antennas are generally preferable.

Several studies addressed this problem by exploiting a metallic biopsy needle, typically used for guiding the antenna to an ablation site, and turning it into a coaxial balun [50–52]. This helps eliminate an extra layer of conductor that would otherwise be needed in a conventionally implemented coaxial balun and therefore, reduce the antenna's overall diameter. The triaxial antenna reported in [50] used a metallic biopsy needle as a sleeve to adjust the insertion depth of a monopole antenna to enhance impedance matching and improve energy deposition. In [51], the biopsy needle served as a sliding metallic sleeve to create an adjustable choke for an asymmetric dipole antenna. The choke had a short-circuited end realized by soldering a copper collar to the outer conductor of the feed cable at a fixed position to make an electrical contact with the biopsy needle. Cavagnaro et al. [52] proposed another idea for integrating the metallic needle as the choke and protected shaft of the MWA antenna with some differences compared to the design reported in [51]. Specifically, the needle in the new design is fixed with the antenna structure instead of being retractable, which aimed to eliminate potentially unpredictable movements of the antenna caused by retraction movement of the biopsy needle. Additionally, the channel formed between the needle shaft's inner surface and coaxial cable's outer surface in the region behind the short-circuit contact of the choke was utilized for circulating cooling water to prevent the needle shaft from overheating during treatment with high-power levels. Furthermore, alumina with high permittivity was used instead of PTFE to surround the active region of the antenna to reduce the antenna's length. The combination of a shaft-cooling mechanism and antenna length miniaturization was effective in helping the antenna produce large, close-to-spherical ablation zones with longitudinal and later diameters of up to 7.0 and 5.2 cm, respectively, in 15-minute ablations using 60 W power.

Two other approaches for reducing invasiveness of coax-fed, balun-equipped MWA antennas were presented in our previously published studies [9, 53], which will be discussed further in this section. Section 10.3.1 presents the first approach which relies on using an impedance-matched transition between a dielectric-filled (e.g. PTFE-filled) coax and an air-filled coax to implement conventional coaxial baluns [9]. Section 10.3.2 discusses the second approach based on using a different balun topology that is less invasive than a coaxial sleeve. A coaxial line with a tapered outer conductor, which has been used as a wideband balun design to transform an unbalanced coaxial line to a balanced parallel-wire line [97, 98], is a viable candidate for such balun implementation. Two possible implementations of the tapered slot baluns and corresponding dipole antennas were reported in [53], including a single-slot tapered balun connecting to a two-segment dipole and a double-slot tapered balun connecting to a three-segment dipole. The latter implementation using the double-slot tapered balun was found to provide a slightly better impedance match for the antenna and more symmetric heating patterns compared to the other implementation. Therefore, key details of the coax-fed, three-segment dipole antenna using the double-slot tapered balun will be summarized in Section 10.3.2 to illustrate the proposed design concept.

10.3.1 Antennas with Conventional Coaxial Baluns Implemented on Air-Filled Coax Sections

The technique presented in this section is applicable for balun-equipped antennas constructed from coaxial cables using insulating materials with noticeably higher permittivities than air. As PTFE is widely used in low-loss, small-diameter, and commercially available coaxial cables, we illustrate this technique for PTFE-filled coaxial cables. The idea is to introduce an impedance-matched air-filled coax section at the end of the PTFE-filled coax feed, which is shown in Figure 10.9a. Because air has a lower permittivity than PTFE ($\varepsilon_{r,\,air} = 1$ compared with $\varepsilon_{r,\,PTFE} = 2.1$), the air-filled coax has a smaller outer conductor than the PTEF-filled coax for the same characteristic impedance and inner-conductor diameter. The ratio between the outer

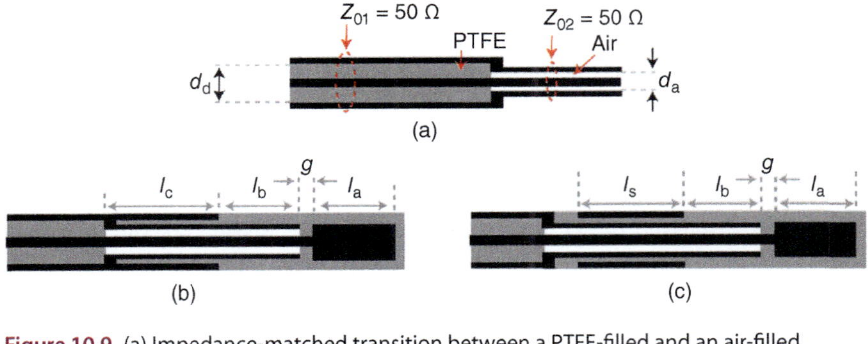

Figure 10.9 (a) Impedance-matched transition between a PTFE-filled and an air-filled coaxial cable. Topology of (b) a modified choke dipole and (c) a modified floating-sleeve dipole implemented on the air-filled coax sections. Black represents metal, gray represents PTFE, and white represents air.

conductors' inner diameters of the air-filled and PTFE-filled coax sections can be easily derived and expressed as $\frac{d_a}{d_d} = \sqrt{\frac{\varepsilon_{r,air}}{\varepsilon_{r,PTFE}}} = \sqrt{\frac{1}{2.1}} = 0.69$. Therefore, the active part of the antenna and coaxial balun can be implemented on the air-filled coax section without exceeding the overall diameter of the PTFE-filled feed line. To demonstrate the effectiveness of this technique, we built prototypes of a choke dipole (CD) and FSD based on the coax transition and compared their performance with conventionally implemented CD and FSD prototypes.

Figure 10.9b and c shows the topology of the modified CD and FSD, respectively, each of which has a dipole and coaxial balun implemented on the air-filled coax of the coaxial transition. Each dipole has two arms with lengths l_a and l_b and a feed gap with a length g. The short-circuited choke for the modified CD and the floating sleeve for the FSD have lengths of l_c and l_s, respectively. The outer diameters of the coaxial baluns of the modified CD and FSD are the same as those of the PTFE-filled feed lines. Clearly, if these baluns are to be implemented directly on the PTFE-filled coaxial cables as in conventional implementations, the overall diameters of the antennas will be larger than those of the feed lines.

Four antenna prototypes were designed and compared against each other: a modified CD, a modified FSD, a conventional CD, and a conventional FSD. Each antenna is fed by a 50-Ω UT-085C semirigid coaxial cable with the outer diameters of 0.511, 1.676, and 2.197 mm for the inner conductor, PTFE insulation layer, and outer conductor, respectively. A brass tube with inner and outer diameters of 1.05 and 1.50 mm was used for the outer conductor of the air-filled coax of the modified CD and FSD antennas. Hollow tubes with inner/outer diameters of 1.68/2.20 mm and 2.5/3.2 mm were used to create the coaxial baluns for the modified and conventional designs, respectively. The antennas were enclosed in Teflon catheters with overall diameters of 2.5 mm for the modified CD and FSD, which are 1 mm (30%) smaller than the 3.5-mm-diameter Teflon catheters used for the conventional counterparts.

We simulated the four antennas in CST Microwave Studio and tuned their feature dimensions for operation at 7 GHz in porcine muscle tissue, which has a relative permittivity of 41.9 and effective conductivity of 7.2 S m^{-1} at 7 GHz. One benefit of this chosen frequency over lower frequencies such as 2.45 GHz or 915 MHz is that the main radiating section of the MWA probe can be made shorter, as discussed in Section 10.2. Moreover, the feeding coaxial cable has a lower ohmic loss at this frequency compared to relatively higher frequencies such as 18 GHz. Fabricated prototypes of these antennas were used to perform ex vivo ablation experiments in pork loin samples. Figure 10.10 shows simulation and measurement results for the input reflection coefficients of the four antennas. The measured and simulated $|S_{11}|$ values of each antenna agree well with each other and demonstrate good impedance matching at the intended

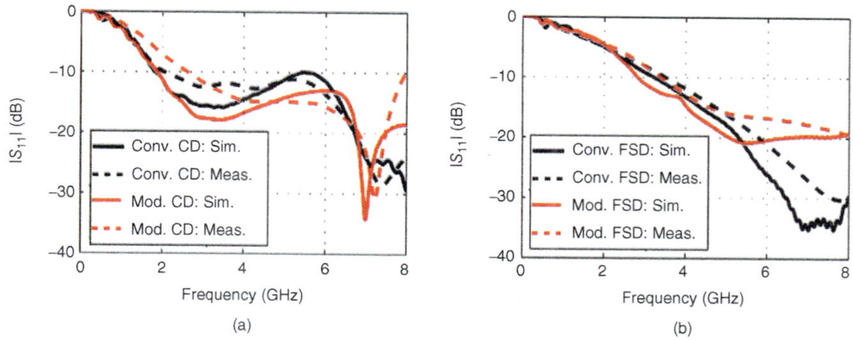

Figure 10.10 Simulation and measurement results for the input reflection coefficient of the (a) conventional and modified CD and (b) conventional and modified FSD antennas.

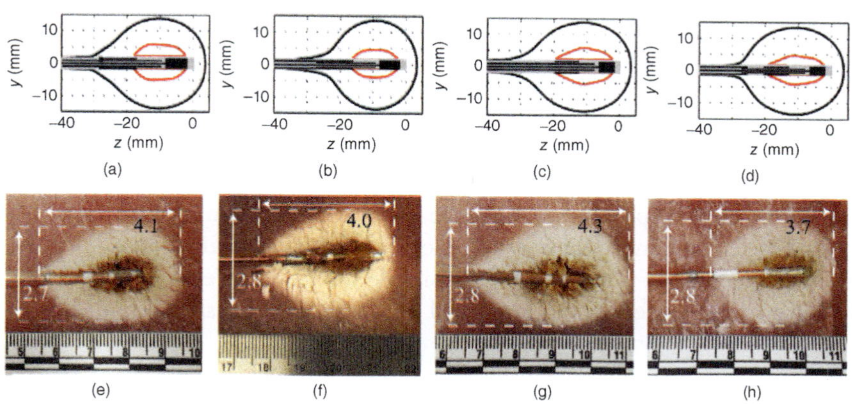

Figure 10.11 (a–d) Simulated 60°C contours (black) and −10 dB normalized SAR contours (red) at 7 GHz of the (a) conventional CD, (b) modified CD, (c) conventional FSD, and (d) modified FSD antennas. (e,f) Photographs of ablation zones generated by the fabricated (a) conventional CD, (b) modified CD, (c) conventional FSD, and (d) modified FSD antennas using an input power of 30 W at 7 GHz for five minutes. The measured values for the maximum long-axis diameters and maximum short-axis diameters of the ablation zones are displayed in centimeters. (*Source*: Luyen, H., Hagness, S. C., and Behdad, N., 2017. © IEEE.)

operating frequency of 7 GHz. The measured $|S_{11}|$ values at 7 GHz were −24 dB for the conventional CD, −23 dB for the modified CD, −27 dB for the conventional FSD, and −18 dB for the modified FSD. Additionally, the measured input reflection coefficients for the antennas were unchanged when their insertion depths were varied, indicating the effectiveness of the baluns in suppressing the outer-surface currents of the feed lines.

Figure 10.11a–d shows the simulated and −10 dB normalized SAR contours at 7 GHz of the four antennas. These contours are well confined to the active dipole arms and baluns of the antennas. The simulated 60°C contours, used to predict boundaries of ablation zones produced by the antennas after five-minute ablation with an input power level of 30 W, are also shown in black curves in Figure 10.11a–d. The simulation results predicted that all antennas generate compact ablation zones with the same maximum lateral dimensions of 2.7 cm and comparable maximum longitudinal dimensions ranging from 3.5 to 4.0 cm. Figure 10.11e–h shows photographs of ablation zones created by the fabricated antenna prototypes using 30 W input power after five minutes of ablation in ex vivo pork loin samples. Each ablation zone consisted of a coagulated zone (white) surrounding a small region of charred tissue (dark brown/black) in the center. The charred regions of the ablation zones are commensurate with the regions encompassed by the simulated −10 dB SAR contours of the antennas, where strongest energy deposition occurs. The longitudinal and lateral diameters of the ablation zones were measured and are reported in Figure 10.11e–h. The ablation zone dimensions were $4.1 \times 2.7\ cm^2$ for the conventional CD, $4.0 \times 2.8\ cm^2$ for the modified CD, $4.3 \times 2.8\ cm^2$ for the conventional FSD, and $3.7 \times 2.8\ cm^2$ for the modified FSD. These maximum longitudinal and lateral dimensions are close to the predicted values for all four antennas. The results demonstrated that the modified antennas delivered similar ablation performance as the conventional prototypes while having 30% smaller diameters. Furthermore, the coaxial transition is not expected to reduce the average power-handling capability of the antenna, which is mainly limited by the maximum temperature level in the PTFE region. Therefore, the proposed technique is an effective yet simple solution for reducing the overall diameters of coax-fed, balun-equipped antennas without sacrificing ablation performance.

10.3.2 Coax-Fed Antenna with a Tapered Slot Balun

Figure 10.12a shows the topology of a coax-fed antenna equipped with a tapered slot balun. The outer conductor is gradually tapered into two parallel strips, leaving two opposite slots for placing two active segments of the antenna. The two active segments are connected to the conductive ring at the distal end of the tapered outer conductor and form one arm of a dipole. The other dipole arm is formed by an extended section of the inner conductor of the coax. The tapered outer conductor creates a smooth transition from a coaxial interface to a parallel-line interface, minimizing returning currents flowing on the outer surface of the outer conductor. The topology of the tapered outer conductor and two active segments connected to its distal end is further illustrated in Figure 10.12b where these parts are unrolled and placed on a flat surface. The slots in the outer conductor required for forming the tapered balun and dipole arms can be etched with high precision using laser fabrication technology. Figure 10.12c shows photographs of an outer conductor machined with such fabrication technology.

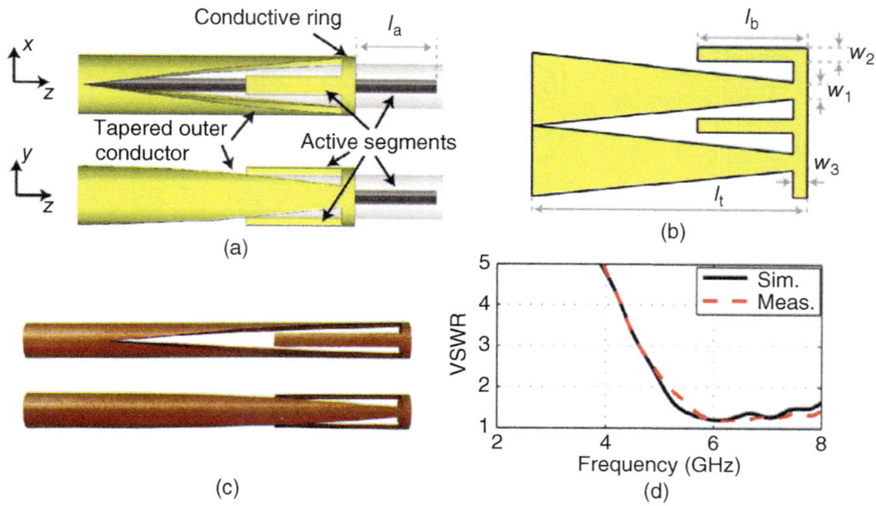

Figure 10.12 (a) Topology of the interstitial antenna design with a double-slot tapered balun and three active segments viewed in the x–z and y–z planes. (b) Drawing of the tapered outer conductor and the two active segments connecting to it when they are unrolled and placed on a flat surface. (c) Photographs of the fabricated outer conductor for the double-slot tapered balun. (d) Simulated and measured input VSWR of the antenna equipped with the tapered slot balun. Dimensions of the antenna are as follows: $l_a = 7$ mm, $l_b = 8$ mm, $l_t = 18$ mm, $w_1 = w_3 = 0.5$ mm, and $w_2 = 0.7$ mm.

A prototype of the coax-fed ablation antenna equipped with the tapered slot balun was designed for operation at 6 GHz in ex vivo bovine liver tissue. Frequency-dependent dielectric properties of liver tissue were modeled with the one-pole Cole Cole model presented in [95]. The antenna was constructed out of a 50-Ω UT-085C semirigid coaxial cable with an outer diameter of 2.2 mm and enclosed in a Teflon catheter with an outer diameter of 2.6 mm. Feature dimensions of this antenna, which are labeled in Figure 10.12a and b, were tuned in full-wave EM simulations in CST Microwave Studio to provide a localized SAR pattern and good impedance match at the intended operating frequency. The final values for these dimensions are shown in the caption of Figure 10.12. Figure 10.12d shows the simulated and measured voltage standing wave ratios (VSWRs) of the antenna prototype. The simulation and measurement results agree well with each other, and both show low VSWR values of less than 1.2 at the operating frequency of 6 GHz. Figure 10.13 shows the simulated and normalized SAR patterns of the proposed antenna at 6 GHz in the x–z and y–z planes. The SAR patterns in these two cut planes are slightly different due to the fact that the tapered outer conductor and two active segments connecting to it are not rotationally symmetric. Nevertheless, the SAR patterns are localized surrounding the active region of the antenna as

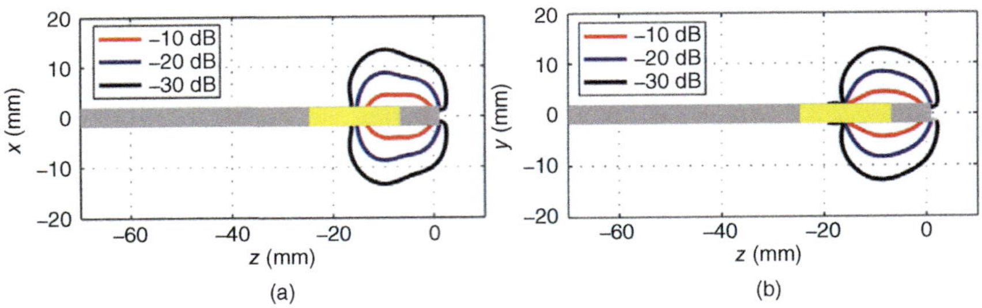

Figure 10.13 Simulated and normalized SAR patterns in the (a) x–z-plane and (b) y–z-plane.

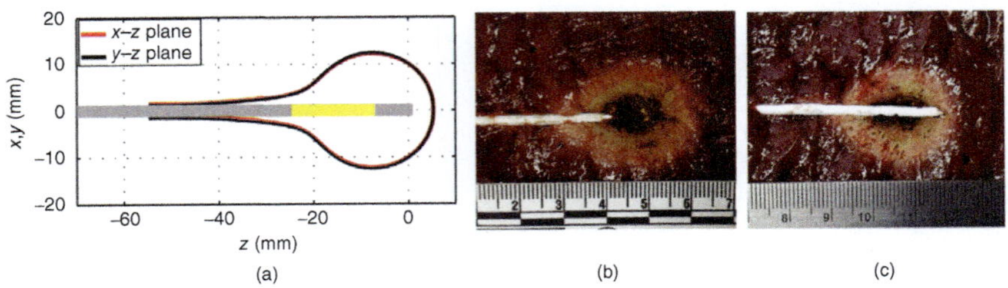

Figure 10.14 (a) Simulated 60°C contours in the x–z and y–z planes. (b,c) Photographs of ablation zones produced by the fabricated antenna in five-minute ablation experiments with 20 W input power in the (b) x–z-plane and (c) y–z-plane. (*Source*: Modified from Luyen, H., Hagness, S. C., and Behdad, N., 2018. © IEEE.)

normalized SAR values fall to −30 dB near the proximal ends of the two active arms connected to the tapered outer conductor.

Subsequently, we conducted thermal simulations using CST Multiphysics Suite to predict ablation performance of the antenna. The thermal simulations treated the absorbed EM energy in liver tissue, which was computed in previous EM simulations and scaled for an input power of 20 W, as the heat source. Thermal conductivity and specific heat capacity of liver tissue were modeled as temperature dependent. Specifically, the thermal conductivity of liver tissue followed the measurement data reported in [99] for temperature from 20 to 90°C and remained constant for temperature levels above 90°C (an assumption made due to the lack of such data in the literature). The specific heat capacity of liver was modeled using the method presented in [100], which takes into account water evaporation as a function of tissue temperature from 20°C to over 100°C. Figure 10.14a shows the predicted ablation zones bounded by the simulated 60°C contours in liver tissues in the *x*–*z* and *y*–*z* planes after five minutes of ablation. The ablation zones in both cut planes are symmetric with respect to the antenna axis and have identical longitudinal dimensions. The maximum lateral dimensions in the *y*–*z* plane (2.3 cm) are just about 0.1 cm larger than that in the *x*–*y* plane (2.2 cm).

Figure 10.14b and c shows photographs of the ablation zones produced by the fabricated antenna in ex vivo liver after five-minute experiments with 20 W input power. The ablation zone dimensions, defined by the maximum longitudinal and lateral dimensions, are $3.2 \times 2.5\ \text{cm}^2$ in the x–z plane and $3.0 \times 2.4\ \text{cm}^2$ for the y–z plane. It should be noted that the ablation zones in these two cut planes were acquired in two separate ablation experiments, and therefore, the impact of variation in tissue samples on achievable ablation zone dimensions is unavoidable. Nevertheless, the ablation zone sizes observed in the two cut planes are close enough and are commensurate with the values predicted in the thermal simulations. Additionally, the aspect ratios of the ablation zones, defined by the ratio of the maximum longitudinal dimension and the maximum lateral dimension, are less than 1.3 in both cases, indicating compact shapes close to that of a sphere (with aspect ratio of 1).

10.4 Balun-Free Microwave Ablation Antenna Designs

In the previous section, we discussed several methods for reducing the invasiveness of MWA antennas by targeting the coaxial balun implementations, which are responsible for the added thickness on top of the feed line in conventional coax-fed, balun-equipped antennas. Clearly, a different approach to achieve diameter reduction is to design antennas that are capable of providing localized heating patterns without the need of baluns. Several balun-free antennas capable of producing localized SAR patterns have been presented in the literature. Prominent examples include double-slot antennas [56, 63, 64], multislot antennas [57, 65, 66], a high input-impedance helical monopole with integrated matching network [8], and a low-impedance helical dipole [54].

Much attention has been paid in investigating and optimizing different variations of slot antennas [55–57, 62–66]. A coax-fed antenna having a single dielectric-loaded annular slot was studied in [55], but this antenna provided relatively elongated SAR patterns compared to balun-equipped antennas. Saito et al. [56] later compared the performance of single- and double-slot antennas and reported that the addition of an extra slot helped the double-slot antennas achieve a much more localized SAR pattern, which was also less dependent on the antenna's insertion depth. The ability to produce localized SAR patterns of double-slot antennas was explained by the destructive interference of two slots placed a half wavelength apart [63]. A few other studies also compared the performance of single- and double-slot antennas and confirmed the better performance for the double-slot antennas in creating wider ablation zones [67, 68, 101]. The significant improvement of going from a single-slot configuration to a double-slot design has motivated some researchers to examine MWA designs with even higher numbers of slots in attempts to extract more performance enhancement. These studies [57, 65, 66] treated the design of coax-fed antennas consisting of periodic annular slots as an optimization problem where parameters such as the total number, widths, and relative positions of slots were derived at the end of the optimization process. In [65], an optimization procedure was conducted to determine the position and number of periodic slots for minimizing the input reflection coefficient of the antenna. Another numerical study [57] conducted by Wang et al. used a genetic algorithm (GA) optimization procedure with the goal of minimizing the overtreatment of a targeted tumor with a predefined size and shape. Bidirectionally coupled EM and thermal simulations, which accounted for temperature-dependent dielectric and thermal properties of liver tissue, were conducted to solve the transient temperature changes in the tissue. The computed spatial temperature distributions at the end of each ablation were used to evaluate the overtreatment ratio as the goal function for optimization. The periodicity of the slots was fixed at 1 mm, while the slot length and number of slots were variables in this optimization. Reported simulation results showed that an antenna configuration with 10 uniformly distributed, 0.064-mm wide, annular slots provided the ablation zone with the closest shape and size to those of a targeted spherical tumor [57]. However, this study did not consider the antenna's input reflection coefficient nor report how the impedance matching was impacted with the changes of the antenna's design features. Ge et al. [66] later performed a similar optimization for a multislot MWA to determine the number, width, and spacing of periodic slots for achieving spherical ablation zones. It was found out that the optimized antenna configuration providing closest-to-spherical heating profiles had a poor impedance match at the intended operating frequency. However, the impedance mismatch problem was easily resolved by employing an internal pi-matching network, similar to the one presented in [8]. Reported ablation zones that were experimentally achieved from experiments with ex vivo porcine livers had nearly spherical shapes with aspect ratios up to 0.95, validating the effectiveness of the proposed optimization.

This section focuses on the two other balun-free antenna designs, which are the helical monopole antenna reported in [8] and the asymmetric helical dipole reported in [54]. Key details regarding the operating principles, simulation results, and experimental characterization of these two antenna designs will be discussed.

10.4.1 High-Input Impedance Helical Monopole with an Integrated Impedance-Matching Section

Figure 10.15 illustrates the topology and operating principle of a balun-free, high-impedance helical monopole antenna. As seen in Figure 10.15a, the monopole antenna is a helix connected to the inner conductor of the coaxial feed line. While the helical shape is particularly chosen here to reduce the longitudinal dimension of the antenna, the design concept is not limited to any

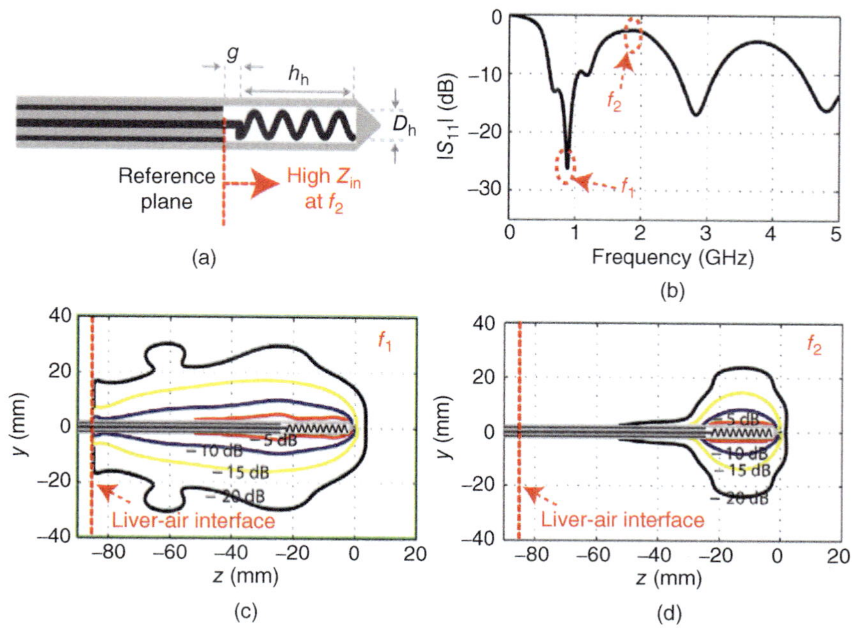

Figure 10.15 (a) Topology of a balun-free helical monopole. (b) Simulated input reflection coefficient seen at the reference plane placed at the base of the helix; the first resonant frequency, $f_1 = 0.9$ GHz, and the second resonant frequency, $f_2 = 1.9$ GHz, are marked. Normalized SAR patterns of the antenna, which are inserted 85 mm deep into liver tissue, at (c) f_1 and (d) f_2.

specific geometry of the monopole. The proposed design relies on operating the helical monopole at its second resonant frequency where the helix is approximately half a wavelength. At this frequency, the electrical current at the feed point of the helix is minimum, creating a natural choke point for currents that tend to flow on the outer surface of the coaxial line. As a result, the antenna provides a localized SAR pattern without using any balun. However, the inherently localized SAR pattern comes with a side effect of a high input impedance at the feed point of the helical monopole, due to the maximum voltage and minimum current at this point. Figure 10.15b shows the simulated input reflection coefficient S_{11}, seen at the feed point of the helix, as a function of frequency. Observe that two frequency points are marked on the plot, labeled as f_1 and f_2, which denote the first and second resonant frequencies of the helical monopole, respectively. At f_1, where the electrical length of the helix is approximately a quarter of the wavelength, the monopole is well matched to 50 Ω as $|S_{11}| < -25$ dB. In contrast, the impedance matching at f_2 is poor, which is exhibited by a high $|S_{11}|$ value (∼−3 dB), due to the high input impedance of the helical monopole. Figure 10.15c and d shows the simulated and normalized SAR patterns produced by the helical monopole at the two resonant frequencies. The SAR pattern at f_1 is not localized and has elongated tails for the −10, −15, and −20 dB contours along the shaft of the feed cable. This would cause excessive heating to healthy tissue along the cable shaft and, therefore, is undesirable for ablation purpose. If the antenna is to use for tissue ablation at $f_{1,}$ a coaxial balun is needed to suppress the unwanted outer-surface currents of the feed line, which is exactly the case for conventional balun-equipped MWA antennas. On the other hand, the SAR pattern at f_2 is highly localized due to the inherent current choking effect mentioned previously. To operate the antenna at $f_{2,}$ the impedance mismatch problem needs to be addressed, e.g. by deploying an impedance matching section between the helical monopole and the 50-Ω coaxial feed line.

Figure 10.16 shows two possible implementations for the integrated impedance matching section used for the balun-free helical monopole. The first implementation is a simple quarter-wavelength transformer as shown in Figure 10.16a. To match the high-impedance antenna (with input impedance Z_{in}) to the feed line ($Z_0 = 50\ \Omega$), the quarter-wavelength section should have a characteristic impedance of $Z_{01} = \sqrt{Z_0 Z_{in}}$. This transformer can be implemented by modifying a section of the 50-Ω coaxial line to achieve a characteristic impedance higher than 50 Ω. Specifically, we can increase the inductance per unit length, $\overline{L} = \frac{\mu}{2\pi} \ln\left(\frac{b}{a_1}\right)$, and decrease the capacitance per unit length, $\overline{C} = \frac{2\pi\varepsilon}{\ln\left(\frac{b}{a_1}\right)}$, of the line. Here a_1 and b are the outer diameter of the inner conductor and inner diameter of the outer conductor of the modified

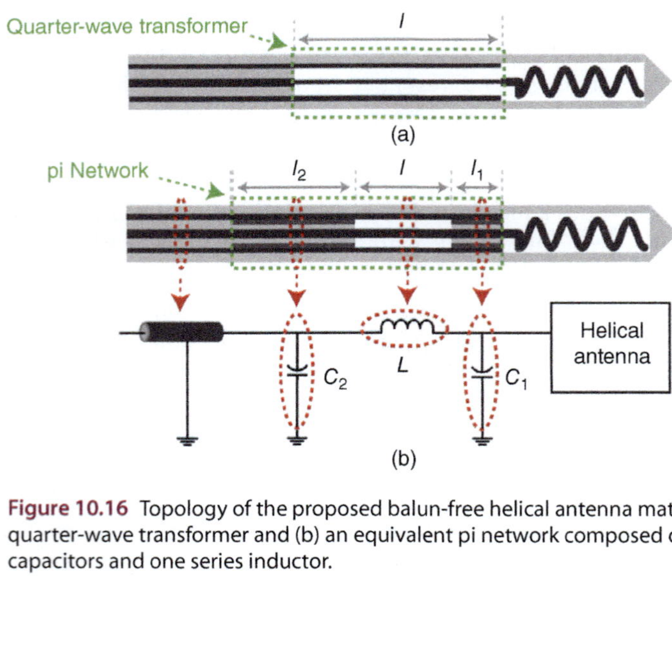

Figure 10.16 Topology of the proposed balun-free helical antenna matched by (a) a quarter-wave transformer and (b) an equivalent pi network composed of two parallel capacitors and one series inductor.

coax section, respectively, and ε and μ are the permittivity and permeability of the insulating layer. By removing the PTFE insulation layer between the inner and outer conductors and making the inner conductor thinner (reducing a_1), we can achieve the desired characteristic impedance of Z_{01}. Simulation results reported in [8] show that the quarter-wave transformer is effective in providing impedance matching for the helical monopole antenna. However, the requirement for making the center conductor of the coax thinner posed some difficulties for the fabrication process. Thus, we chose to proceed with the other impedance-matching method, which is a pi network shown in Figure 10.16b. The capacitors C_1 and C_2 of the pi network were realized using short sections of a low-impedance coaxial line, while the inductor L was realized using a short section of a high-impedance coaxial line. Each low-impedance coax section was implemented by inserting a hollow copper tube in the inner region between the inner and outer conductors of the 50-Ω coax to form a new outer conductor with the reduced inner diameter b_2. This increases the capacitance per unit length and reduces the inductance per unit length of the coaxial line, hence the decreased characteristic impedance. The high-impedance coax section was implemented by simply removing the insulating dielectric layer of the 50-Ω coax to reduce the capacitance per unit length. The design process for the pi-matching network started with choosing values of C_1, C_2, and L to impedance match the helical antenna to the 50-Ω feed line. Then, the length of each capacitive and inductive segment was estimated assuming short transmission line approximation for the reactive elements. Subsequently, these lengths were fine-tuned in full-wave simulations of the impedance-matched helical antenna to yield a low input reflection coefficient at the desired frequency.

We designed and fabricated a prototype of the balun-free helical monopole antenna that is impedance matched to a 50-Ω, 2.2-mm-thick coaxial line by a pi network. Copper tubes with inner diameters of 0.876 mm were used to implement the capacitive segments for the pi network. Dimensions of the helical monopole and pi network are reported in the caption of Figure 10.17. Figure 10.17 shows the simulated and measured input reflection coefficients of the antenna prototype inserted in bovine liver tissue. The measurement and simulation results demonstrated the effectiveness of using the pi network to match the helical monopole to the feed line at the intended operating frequency of 1.9 GHz. Figure 10.18 shows the simulated and normalized SAR patterns for the antenna prototype at 1.9 GHz. The SAR pattern is localized and similar to that produced by the helical monopole without the matching network as shown in Figure 10.15d.

We used the fabricated antenna prototype to conduct two ablation experiments, one with a 5-minute duration and the other one with a 10-minute duration, in ex vivo bovine liver. In both experiments, the power applied at the input of the coaxial feed line was 42 W. Figure 10.19a and b shows photographs of

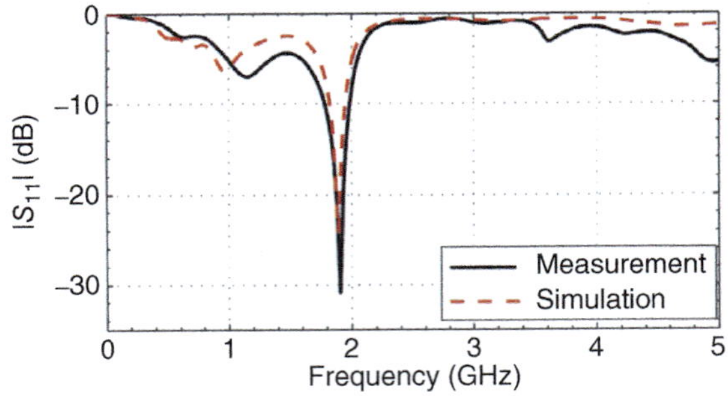

Figure 10.17 Simulation and measurement of $|S_{11}|$ for the balun-free helical antenna, matched by the pi network, operating in bovine liver tissue. The parameters of the helical monopole are as follows: $n = 10$ turns, $h_h = 20$ mm, $D_h = 1.63$ mm, and $g = 2$ mm. The dimensions for the pi-matching network are as follows: $l_1 = 6$ mm, $l_2 = 22$ mm, and $l = 18$ mm.

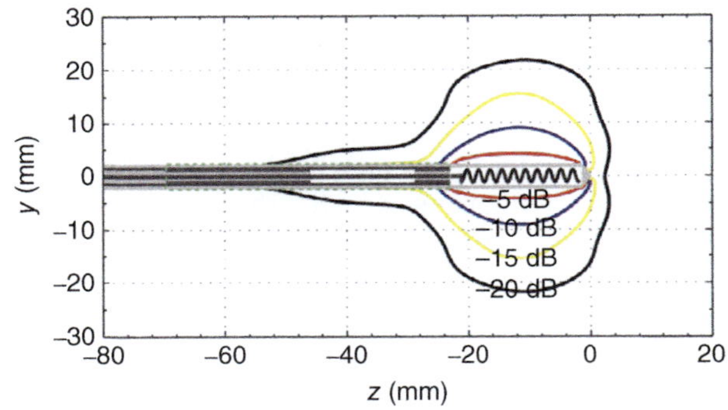

Figure 10.18 Simulated and normalized SAR patterns of the balun-free helical antenna matched by the pi network. The antenna is inserted in the liver tissue with an insertion depth of 85 mm. The boundary of the matching section is highlighted by the dotted green rectangle.

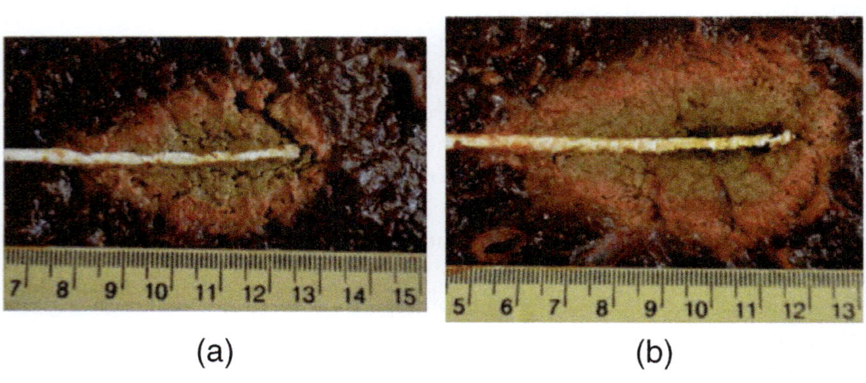

Figure 10.19 Photographs of ablation zones created in ex vivo bovine liver by applying 42 W to the input of the balun-free helical antenna equipped with pi-network matching section for (a) 5 minures and (b) 10 minutes. (*Source*: Luyen, H., Hagness, S. C., and Behdad, N., 2015. © IEEE.)

the ablation zones viewed in the insertion plane of the antenna at the end of the 5- and 10-minute experiments, respectively. The dimensions of the ablation zones were $5.7 \times 3.4\ cm^2$ for the 5-minute ablation and $7.3 \times 3.8\ cm^2$ for the 10-minute ablation. The sizes and shapes of the ablation zones produced by the balun-free helical monopole are similar to those created by a balun-equipped MWA antenna reported in [86] with the same input power and durations. This demonstrates the validity of the balun-free antenna design concept as a promising solution for reducing the overall diameter of the interstitial antenna.

10.4.2 Low-Input Impedance Helical Dipole Design

Figure 10.20a shows the topology of the balun-free, low-input impedance helical dipole antenna. The antenna was designed to use a custom-built semirigid coaxial feed line and operate at 1.9 GHz in egg white. Egg white was chosen as the ablation medium because its transparency helped real-time monitoring of the ablation zone. The proposed antenna is a dipole antenna wherein one arm of the dipole is the extended inner conductor of the coaxial cable and the other arm is a helix which is wrapped around the extended inner conductor and is connected to the coax's outer conductor. In this dipole antenna, the two arms of the dipole are parallel to each other, contrary to the well-known dipole antenna in which the two dipole arms make an angle of 180° between them. Nonetheless, the underlying physics behind the dipole antenna's operating principle does not change. For instance, the currents that flow on these two arms are still relatively sinusoidal and drop to zero at the two ends of the

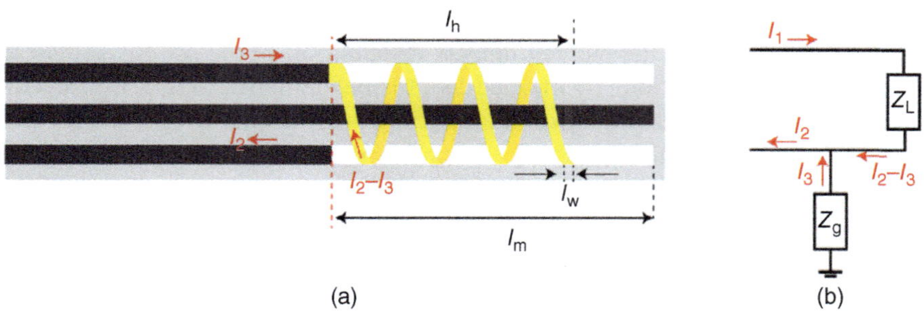

Figure 10.20 Antenna topology and its equivalent circuit model. (a) The diameter of the inner conductor of the coaxial cable is 0.51 mm. The inner and outer diameters of the outer conductor of the coaxial cable are 1.67 and 2.38 mm, respectively. The diameter of the Teflon catheter is 2.8 mm. The feed point of the antenna is shown as a dashed red line. Red arrows show representative current directions. The diagram is not to scale. Yellow and black show copper, gray shows Teflon, and white shows air. Optimized values for l_m (monopole or inner dipole arm length), l_h (longitudinal span of the helix), and N (number of turns in the helix) are 24 mm, 18 mm, and 9.9, respectively, for operation at 1.9 GHz in egg white. (b) Equivalent circuit model of a dipole antenna fed with a coaxial cable [102]. (*Source*: Balanis, C. A., 2005.)

dipole arms. Since the dipole arms are not connected to the coaxial cable in the same way, they create an imbalance [102]. As a result, current I_3 will flow on the outer surface of the outer conductor of the coaxial cable.

Figure 10.20b shows an approximate equivalent circuit model for a dipole antenna connected to a coaxial cable, where Z_L is the dipole's input impedance, and Z_g is the impedance seen by I_3 toward the ground [102]. To reduce I_3, the ratio Z_g/Z_L should be as large as possible. There are two ways to implement this: increasing Z_g, which is the ubiquitous method of using a balun, or decreasing Z_L. In the proposed helical dipole design, shown in Figure 10.20a, the latter approach has been used to eliminate the need for a balun. We have to note that a balanced transmission line or antenna can be represented with a single circuit element Z_L. For the case of an unbalanced element, however, this equivalent circuit model does not represent a complete picture. Nonetheless, it is the authors' belief that this equivalent circuit model still intuitively shows the behavior of a dipole antenna connected to a coaxial cable.

This helical dipole antenna is essentially an off-center-fed dipole where the two arms of the dipole need not necessarily be equal. Assume that the length of the straight arm connected to the coax's inner conductor is chosen to be a constant value of $\lambda_{eff}/4$, where λ_{eff} is the effective wavelength for an insulated monopole antenna created by the extended inner conductor and insulating dielectric layers. Now, let us choose four different values of $\lambda_{eff}/4$, $\lambda_{eff}/2$, $3\lambda_{eff}/4$, and λ_{eff} as the overall length of the helical arm of the dipole. Note that the overall length of the helix is given by $\sqrt{l_h^2 + (\pi ND)^2}$, where N is the number of turns in the helix, D is the mean value of the inner and outer diameters of the outer conductor of the coaxial cable, and l_h is the longitudinal span of the helix (refer to Figure 10.20).

Figure 10.21 shows the current density distribution of the proposed helical dipole design for the four mentioned lengths of the helical arm. The current flowing on the outer conductor's outer surface is substantially reduced for the overall helix lengths of $\sim\lambda_{eff}/4$ and $\sim 3\lambda_{eff}/4$. Specifically, the I_3/I_2 ratio is 0.18 and 0.28 for the overall helix lengths of $\sim\lambda_{eff}/4$ and $\sim 3\lambda_{eff}/4$, respectively, while I_3/I_2 is 0.61 and 0.81 for the overall helix lengths of $\sim\lambda_{eff}/2$ and $\sim\lambda_{eff}$, respectively. The main reason for effective suppression of unwanted current I_3 for the cases where the overall length of the helix is an odd multiple of $\lambda_{eff}/4$ is as follows. When the length of the helix is $\lambda_{eff}/4$, the two arms of the dipole form a half-wavelength dipole. For a half-wavelength dipole, the direction of current becomes maximum at the feed point and goes to zero at the two ends of the arms. The direction of the current, however, does not change as current travels on the arms of the dipole, regardless of the angles the arms make with each other. This is evident from Figure 10.21a, where the current on the arms of the dipole does not experience a reversal of direction. Note, however, that

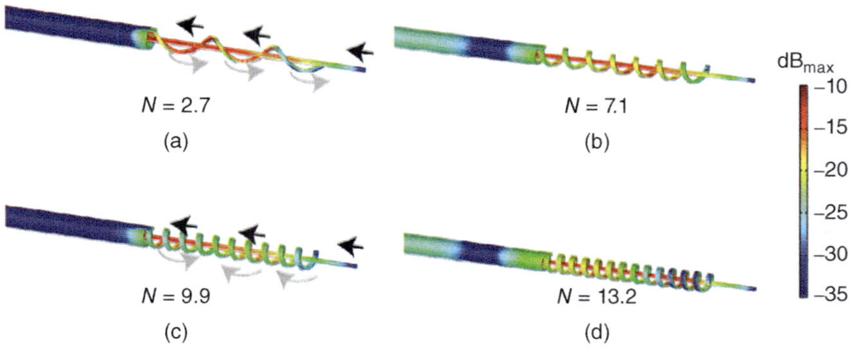

Figure 10.21 Current density distributions of the proposed helical dipole antenna shown in Figure 10.20a for different N values: (a) $N = 2.7$, (b) $N = 7.1$, (c) $N = 9.9$, and (d) $N = 13.2$. Each distribution is normalized to its maximum value (dB max). The N values are chosen such that the overall helix lengths correspond to the first four multiples of $\lambda_{eff}/4$. l_h is fixed at 18 mm. The directions of currents have been schematically added to $N = 2.7$ and $N = 9.9$ for better illustration. Black arrows indicate the current direction on the extended inner conductor, and the gray ones show the direction of current on the helical arm.

because of the special geometry of this dipole, which is similar to a bent dipole, these two currents oppose and almost completely cancel each other. This significantly reduces the input impedance of the antenna, Z_L, which results in effective reduction of unwanted current I_3. However, because the input impedance is very low, the antenna is mismatched. To remedy this, the length of the helical arm is increased to 3 $\lambda_{eff}/4$. The current distribution of this antenna is shown in Figure 10.21c. Since this antenna is one wavelength long, current must drop to zero, half a wavelength from the end of each arm. Therefore, the direction of current on the helical arm reverses $\lambda_{eff}/4$ away from the feed point and becomes aligned with the current that is traveling on the straight arm of the antenna. This partial field cancellation rather than full cancellation of electric fields increases the radiation resistance of the antenna, improving the impedance match. The compromise, however, is that there will be a slightly larger current flowing on the outer surface of the outer conductor. Figure 10.22a shows the simulated and measured $|S_{11}|$ of the antenna prototype with the total helix length of ~3 $\lambda_{eff}/4$. The antenna has a $|S_{11}|$ below −10 dB, and the measurement and simulation results agree reasonably well.

A fabricated prototype of the antenna, shown in Figure 10.22b, was used to perform 40-W ablation experiments in egg white at 1.9 GHz for five minutes. During the ablation process, the $|S_{11}|$ of the antenna was closely monitored. We observed that the $|S_{11}|$ of the fabricated helical dipole antenna remained below −10.0 dB throughout the experiment. Figure 10.23 shows the snapshots of the

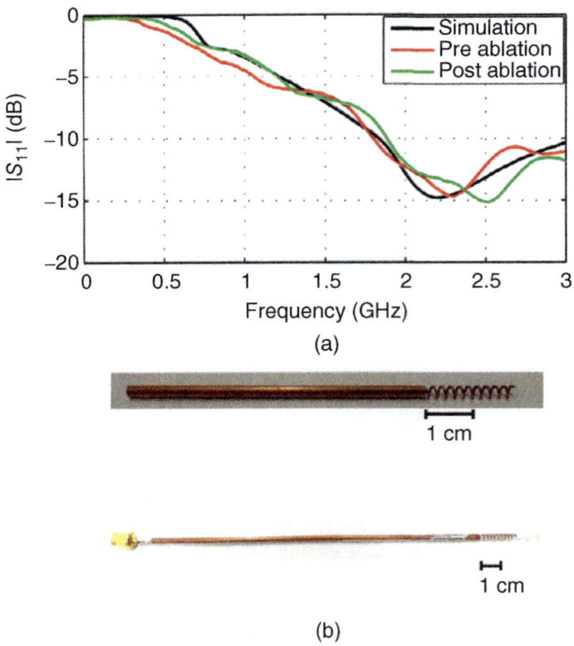

Figure 10.22 (a) $|S_{11}|$ of the optimized helical dipole antenna operating in egg white obtained through simulation and measurement. (b) *Top*: The section of the fabricated prototype showing a section of the outer conductor of the coaxial cable and the helical arm of the dipole antenna. The center conductor of the coaxial cable and the straight arm of the antenna are not shown in this picture. *Bottom*: The fabricated antenna and its feed line. Dimension scales are different for the two photographs.

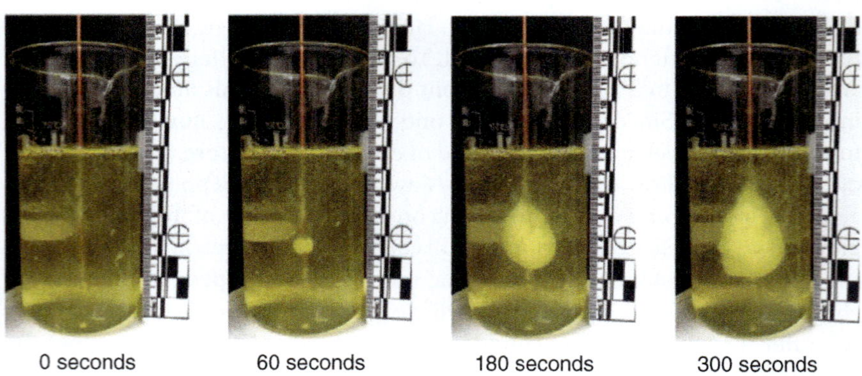

Figure 10.23 Photographs showing the temporal evolution of the ablation zone created by the optimized helical dipole antenna in egg white, in an ablation experiment. The applied power was 40 W. (*Source*: Mohtashami, Y., Behdad, N., and Hagness, S.C., 2020. © IEEE.)

ablation zone generated by the antenna in egg white as ablation progressed. The longitudinal and lateral dimensions of the generated ablation zone, after five minutes, were 3.8 and 3.2 cm, respectively, and no tail was observed along the insertion path of the antenna. This demonstrated the antenna's capability to produce localized heating patterns.

10.5 Toward More Flexibility and Customization in Microwave Ablation Treatment

Most MWA antennas presented in the literature are implemented with semirigid coaxial cables and designed to generate symmetric ablation zones. However, there are clinical scenarios where it is highly desirable to have a flexible antenna that can reach the targeted tumor through catheters or an antenna that is capable of producing directional heating patterns. Consider ablating tumors in lung as an example; the use of rigid MWA probes can increase the risk of pneumothorax due to percutaneous insertion [103, 104]. In this case, it would be much more advantageous to use a flexible applicator that can be routed through a catheter guided through natural ductal pathways to reach the tumor location in lung. On the other hand, MWA antennas having directional heating patterns can see demand in cases where the tumor has an irregular, asymmetric shape, or the central region of the tumor is not easily accessible. For example, a vital organ that should not be ablated may be in the vicinity of the targeted ablation zone, blocking the insertion path to the center of the tumor. In a clinical scenario, this could be hepatic tumors in the vicinity of the bowel or diaphragm, renal tumors in the vicinity of the bowel, or breast tumors adjacent to the chest wall [77]. In such situations, it is helpful to have an antenna that can be placed close to the periphery of the tumor and provide directional heating into the tumor while having negligible radiation on the other side of the antenna shaft where the healthy tissue is. Therefore, designs of MWA antennas that have flexible embodiments or produce asymmetric heating profiles are valuable additions to the mainstream symmetric heating, rigid/semirigid ablation applicator designs, and help extend the flexibility and customization of the MWA treatment. This section is dedicated to discussing our works related to flexible antenna characterization and directional-heating antenna designs for MWA. Section 10.5.1 reports an experimental study examining ablation performance of a flexible antenna which was based on the design of the balun-free helical dipole antenna reported in [54]. Two antenna designs for achieving asymmetric ablation zones were previously reported in [77, 79], and the key details of these studies will be highlighted in Sections 10.5.2 and 10.5.3.

10.5.1 Ex Vivo Performance of a Flexible Microwave Ablation Antenna

In MWA, usually a rigid or semirigid antenna is percutaneously inserted into the tumor. This rigidity, however, may increase the invasiveness of the MWA procedure. One such example is tumors in lung, where close proximity to heart or diaphragm may prevent the use of the rigid antennas. If a flexible antenna is used instead of the rigid antenna, the antenna can be routed through natural ductal pathways to those deep-seated tumors less invasively, decreasing possible contraindications of using a rigid MWA probe. Since the space within a flexible catheter is generally limited, employing a balun for suppression of unwanted currents becomes extremely difficult, if not impossible. While a number of reduced-diameter balun-equipped as well as balun-free antenna designs capable of generating localized ablation zones have been introduced in the literature, most of them have been mostly restricted to implementations with semirigid coaxial cables. Among the balun-free antenna designs introduced thus far, the helical dipole antenna introduced in Section 10.4.2 is a promising candidate for implementation in a flexible embodiment.

Figure 10.24a shows the topology of the flexible helical dipole antenna. The antenna was constructed out of a TGE055D M-Flex flexible coaxial cable. The outer diameters of the inner conductor, dielectric layer, and outer shield (which is a combination of braided wires on top of a wound silver tape) of this cable are 0.287, 0.864, and 1.118 mm, respectively. An added layer of FEP results in an overall diameter of 1.397 mm for the cable. The helical section of the antenna was implemented by a spring made from beryllium copper wire with an overall diameter of 0.2 mm. The antenna assembly was put in a heat shrink tube which was sealed at the far end by epoxy. The heat shrink was then shrunk to make an overall diameter of 1.64 mm for the structure. The antenna was designed for operation in ex vivo porcine liver at 1.9 GHz. Following the same design procedure of the balun-free helical dipole antenna presented in Section 10.4.2, the final dimensions of the helical antenna were acquired and are shown in the caption of Figure 10.24. Figure 10.24b shows the simulated and normalized SAR patterns with −5, −10, −15, and −20 dB contours of the antenna at 1.9 GHz. The

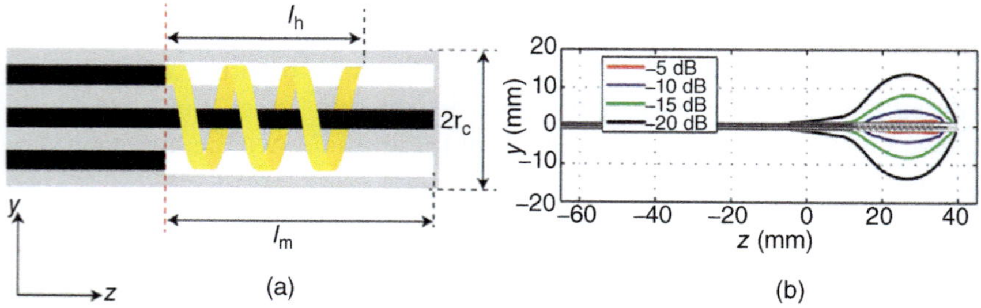

Figure 10.24 (a) Topology of the helical dipole antenna. The inner conductor of the coaxial cable has an overall diameter of 0.287 mm. The overall diameter of the Teflon catheter, $2r_c$, is 1.64 mm. Diagram is not to scale. Optimized values for l_m, l_h (longitudinal span of the helix), and N (number of turns in the helix) are 23 mm, 20 mm and 21, respectively, for operation at 1.9 GHz in the liver. (b) Simulated SAR pattern, normalized to the maximum value, of the antenna at 1.9 GHz, in decibel.

SAR pattern is compact, and little energy absorption is observed along the shaft of the antenna.

The $|S_{11}|$ of the antenna was measured as it passed through a test fixture that had tubes with different radii of curvature, shown in Figure 10.25a. The test fixture had three curved tubes, each having an inner diameter of 2.1 mm, with bend radii of 20, 15, and 10 mm, respectively. The antenna passed through each tube and got immersed in a reference liquid. The reference liquid was a 45 : 55 mixture of methanol and deionized water, mimicking dielectric properties of the porcine liver tissue. Figure 10.25b shows the measured $|S_{11}|$ of the antenna for the case where the antenna was straightly immersed into the reference liquid and for three cases where it was deployed through the curved tubes. The antenna maintained its good impedance match even when it passed through the tube with a tight 10-mm-radius bend.

A fabricated prototype of the antenna was used to perform ablation experiments in perfused porcine livers at 1.9 GHz and at a power level of 10 W. The liver was placed inside a perfusion chamber, as shown in Figure 10.26a. The chamber was filled with perfusate at room temperature (25°C). The perfusate was prepared by solving 36 g of salt in 4 l of water. Salt was used to mimic the salinity of blood. The perfusate was drawn by a pump and then fed into a Y branch, the output of which was fed into two narrower diameter tubes that would go inside the liver through its vessels. The antenna was inserted vertically into relatively thick parts of the liver and left to radiate EM energy for five minutes. The average longitudinal and lateral diameters of the generated ablation zones in perfused porcine liver across five ablation experiments were

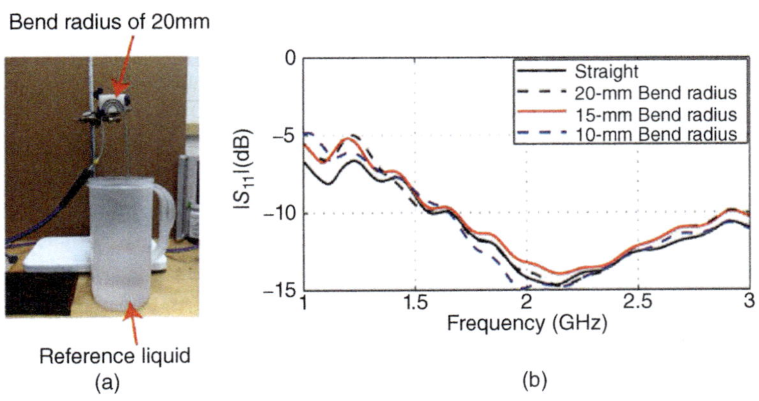

Figure 10.25 (a) The antenna is deployed through the curved tube into the reference liquid. The reference liquid mimics the dielectric properties of the porcine liver. (*Source*: (Not yet published) Mohtashami, Y., Behdad, N., and Hagness, S.C.) (b) Measured $|S_{11}|$ of the flexible antenna in four different deployment scenarios. © IEEE.

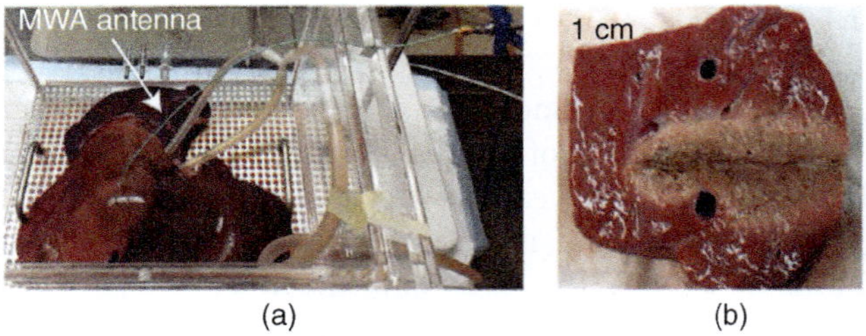

Figure 10.26 The 10-W, CW ablation experiments with the flexible helical dipole antenna in perfused liver. (a) The experimental setup. (b) Representative photograph of the generated ablation zone. (*Source*: (Not yet published) Mohtashami, Y., Behdad, N., and Hagness, S.C. © IEEE.)

4.2 and 2.7 mm, respectively. Figure 10.26b shows an image of one representative ablation zone. Overall, the ablation zones were compact, demonstrating the antenna's capability of generating relatively large ablation zones with low power levels. If the power level were to increase, a cooling mechanism would have been needed to prevent excessive tail heating caused by substantial ohmic losses of the narrow-diameter coaxial cable.

10.5.2 Hybrid Slot/Monopole Antenna with Directional Heating Patterns

Figure 10.27a shows the proposed antenna design for generation of directional heating patterns. The antenna was designed to work at 7 GHz in egg white and fed with a semirigid coaxial cable (UT-085C). The monopole's length, l_m, was chosen to be approximately 0.25 λ_{eff} = 7 mm, where λ_{eff} is the effective wavelength of the EM wave in the surrounding environment. The lower half of the outer conductor of the coaxial cable is extended along the monopole section by a length of l_r. This section acts as a reflector and reduces the magnitude of the electric fields at the back of the reflector, i.e. $y < -r_c$. To further reduce the radiation on the backside of the reflector, a semicylindrical slot, with a length of l_s, is created in the outer conductor of the feeding coaxial cable as shown in Figure 10.27a. This slot is semiannular and only exists in the $y > 0$ region. The role of this slot can be intuitively understood by examining the individual components of the antenna. Figure 10.28 shows the evolution of the near-field electric field distribution as individual radiating components of the proposed hybrid slot/monopole antenna (shown in Figure 10.27a) are added to the design. Figure 10.28a shows the electric field distribution for the case where there is no slot, and the monopole is radiating in the presence of the reflector. The electric field behind the reflector in this case is pointing in the $-y$-direction. Figure 10.28b shows the electric field distribution in the near-field region of the antenna in Figure 10.27a if the length of monopole is set to zero and only the reflector and the slot exist. Upon examination of the fields, we observed

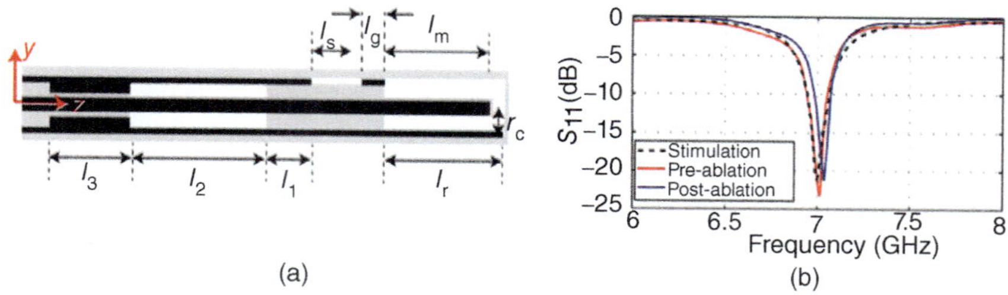

Figure 10.27 (a) The proposed hybrid slot/monopole antenna. The antenna is designed to operate in egg white at 7.0 GHz. Black, gray, and white show copper, Teflon, and air, respectively. r_c is the outer radius of the outer conductor. $l_m = 7$ mm, $l_s = 4$ mm, $l_r = 9$ mm, and $l_g = 1$ mm. The values of the matching network are chosen as $l_1 = 4$ mm, $l_2 = 12$ mm, and $l_3 = 7$ mm. The inner diameter of the copper tube used in the segment denoted as l_3 is 0.78 mm. The whole diameter of the antenna including its catheter is 2.9 mm. (b) The antenna's corresponding simulated and measured S_{11} curves.

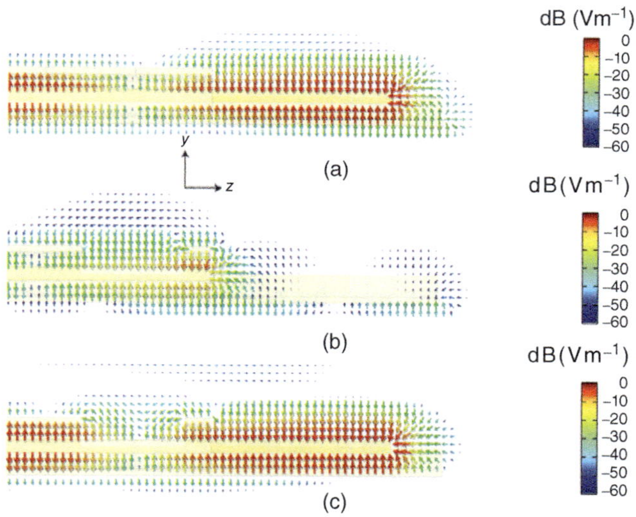

Figure 10.28 Intensity and direction of simulated electric fields for three different structures. The values of the electric field intensity presented in each plot are normalized to that plot's corresponding maximum electric field for the (a) hybrid slot/monopole antenna if the length of the slot is set to zero, (b) hybrid slot/monopole antenna if the length of the monopole is set to zero, and (c) hybrid/slot monopole antenna shown in Figure 10.27a.

that the fields generated by the slot in the back of the reflector toward the tip of the reflector have opposite directions to those of the fields generated by the monopole in Figure 10.28a in the same region. Therefore, it is expected that the combination of the slot and the monopole in the vicinity of the reflector will further reduce the SAR levels at the back of the reflector.

The presence of the reflector behind the monopole antenna and in its close vicinity reduces the feed-point impedance of the antenna. Therefore, an internal π-impedance-matching structure, shown in Figure 10.27a, is used to solve the mismatch problem. The network consists of a high-impedance section with a length of l_2, placed between a low-impedance section with a length of l_3 and a 50-Ω impedance section with a length of l_1. The high-impedance section was constructed by removing the dielectric between the inner and outer conductors, while the low-impedance section was created by decreasing the distance between the inner and outer conductors through inserting a copper tube into the region denoted as l_3. The simulated and measured S_{11} of the antenna are shown in Figure 10.27b and confirm the capability of the proposed matching network in matching the antenna to the 50-Ω coaxial cable. The measured S_{11} shows a dip at 7.05 GHz, which is 0.05 GHz higher than the intended operating frequency of 7.00 GHz. This can be attributed to small uncertainty in the dielectric permittivity of egg white and fabrication tolerances.

A fabricated prototype of the proposed antenna was used to perform ablation experiments in egg white at 7.05 GHz with an input power level of 20 W. The monitored reflected power during the measurements did not go beyond 1 W, indicating that the antenna remained impedance matched throughout the experiments. Figure 10.29 shows different snapshots of an ablation zone as time progressed. The generated ablation zone was highly directional and confined to the region in the vicinity of the antenna. Specifically, no noticeable ablated tail was observed along the insertion path of the antenna. The size of the ablation zone in the x–y plane was $2.0 \times 2.0\,\text{cm}^2$ and in the x–z plane was $2.0 \times 2.0\,\text{cm}^2$. The small ablated region in the back of the reflector can be mainly considered a consequence of the heat diffusion. The fact that this ablated region did not exist at the early stages of the ablation process supports this hypothesis.

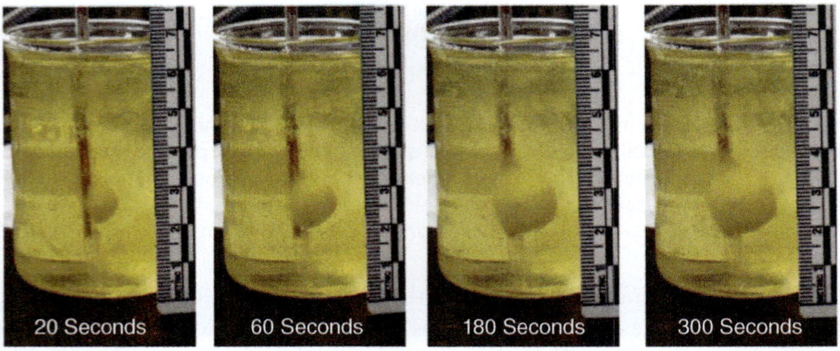

Figure 10.29 Progression of the ablation zone generated by the antenna in egg white. (*Source*: Mohtashami, Y., Hagness, S. C., and Behdad, N., 2017. © IEEE.)

10.5.3 Non-Coaxial-Based Microwave Ablation Antennas with Symmetric and Asymmetric Heating Patterns

A majority of MWA antennas presented to date use coaxial cables as feed lines, which are unbalanced transmission lines and allow for unwanted currents flowing on the outer conducting surfaces of the cables. Therefore, most coax-fed MWA antennas need to utilize some techniques to suppress these outer-surface currents to prevent undesirable heating of healthy tissues along the antenna shafts. Various techniques have been proposed for this purpose, ranging from using coaxial baluns to novel coax-fed antenna designs with balun-free operation, as discussed throughout the chapter. All these techniques are narrowband in nature, meaning they help provide localized SAR patterns for the antennas over a narrow frequency range. A common practice in MWA antenna design is to optimize the antenna to provide localized SAR patterns in a tissue with preablation dielectric properties. As the tissue undergoes significant changes in dielectric properties during ablation process, the frequency range for localized SAR patterns may shift, degrading ablation performance of the antenna. If a balanced transmission line is used to feed the antenna instead of a coaxial cable, localized SAR patterns can be inherently achieved over a wide frequency range.

This section discusses a new class of non-coaxial-based balanced antennas for MWA. Figure 10.30a and b shows two cross-sectional views of a shielded parallel-wire line used to feed a dipole antenna. The feed line consists of two parallel, differentially fed wires covered in Teflon insulation layers and placed inside a metallic tube. The tube is used as a shield to prevent the waves propagated along the line from penetrating into the surrounding healthy tissue. The two parallel wires extend beyond the shield to form two dipole arms which are deployed at certain angles with respect to the axis of symmetry of the feed line. Due to the balanced nature of the feed line and antenna, no currents are excited on the outer surface of the shield, and therefore, the active portions of the antenna are strictly confined to the dipole arms. This allows for exploiting different orientation of the dipole arms to create either symmetric or asymmetric ablation zones. Figure 10.30c and d shows two different embodiments of the dipole arms investigated in this study. In Type I deployment shown in Figure 10.30c, two dipole arms are bent in different directions and make angles of ϕ_1 and ϕ_2 with respect to the vertical y–z-plane. A configuration with $\phi_1 = \phi_2$ generates a symmetric heating pattern, while one with $\phi_1 \neq \phi_2$ creates an asymmetric heating pattern. A higher degree of asymmetry in the heating patterns can be achieved using Type II deployment shown in Figure 10.30d, where both dipole arms are bent in the same direction making angles of θ_1 and θ_2 with respect to the horizontal x–y-plane.

We illustrated the design concept with two antenna prototypes: one generating symmetric heating patterns at 10 GHz in porcine muscle and the other

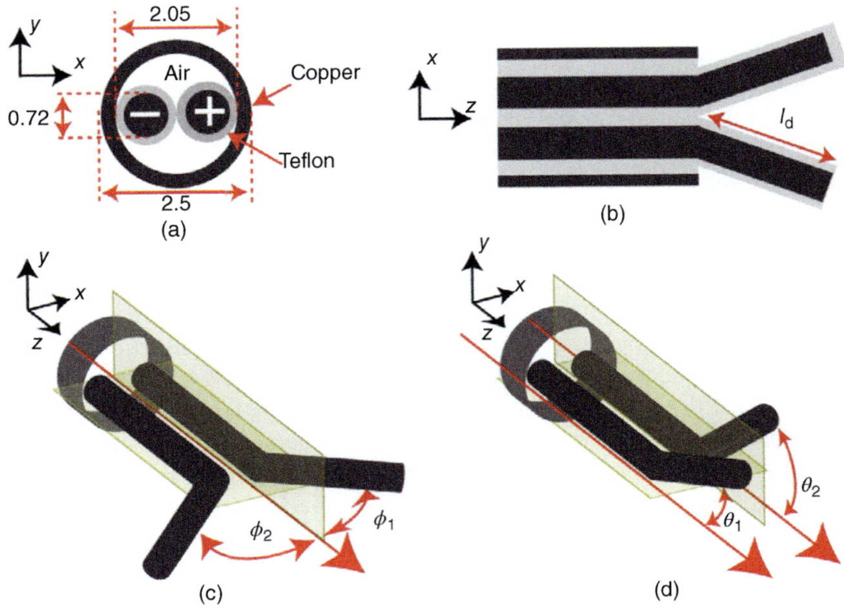

Figure 10.30 Topology of the non-coaxial-based balanced antenna. (a) Cross section of the shielded parallel-wire line feeding the antenna. All dimensions are in millimeters. (b) Side view of the parallel-wire line connecting to a dipole. (c) Type I deployment of the dipole arms: azimuthal control. (d) Type II deployment of the dipole arms: elevation control.

generating asymmetric heating patterns at 6.4 GHz in egg white. Egg white was chosen as the operating medium for the asymmetric-heating antenna prototype because its transparency allows for real-time monitoring of the formulation and expansion of the asymmetric coagulation zone. The choices of different tissue environment and operating frequencies for the two prototypes were intended to demonstrate the frequency scalability and flexibility of the balanced antenna design concept. The parallel wires and dipole arms for the two prototypes were made from 0.72-mm-diameter wires. A hollow copper tube with inner and outer diameters of 2.05 and 2.50 mm, respectively, was used to create a shield for each balanced line. The shielded two-wire transmission line with this implementation has a characteristic impedance of 50 Ω. For comparison, a 50-Ω coaxial cable having an inner conductor with a diameter of 0.72 mm (e.g. the same as one of the two parallel wires) and using a PTFE insulation layer would have an outer conductor with an inner diameter of 2.4 mm (compared to 2.05 mm for the balanced line). Each fabricated antenna prototype used an external coax to two-wire line adapter, which has a similar design to the one reported in [105], to connect the 50-Ω coaxial output of the power amplifier to the input of the parallel-wire transmission line.

The symmetric-heating antenna prototype was initially simulated in CST Microwave Studio by differentially exciting the two wires of the balanced line. We varied the flare angle ($\phi_1 = \phi_2$) from 10° to 35° with an increment of 5° and observed that the impedance matching improved as the flare angle was increased. However, no significant improvement was observed by increasing ϕ_1 beyond 30°, hence the choice of $\phi_1 = \phi_2 = 30°$ for the final design. Simulated VSWR of the balanced antenna (with an ideal differential excitation for the parallel-wire line) exhibited a wide band impedance matching as VSWR < 2 from 6.3 GHz to beyond 13 GHz. Moreover, simulation results also showed that the antenna provides localized SAR patterns across a very wide frequency range. This is illustrated by the simulated −25 dB SAR contours at 7, 10, and 13 GHz in the y–z-plane (shown in Figure 10.31a) and the x–z-plane (shown in Figure 10.31b) provided by the antenna inserted in porcine muscle.

Figure 10.32a shows the measured and simulated VSWRs, seen at the input of the coax-to-balanced-line transition, of the symmetric-heating antenna prototype. The results show a good impedance match for the antenna over a frequency range of 9–11 GHz. Due to the limitation of the specific coax-to-balanced-line transition used in this work, the fabricated prototype did not achieve such wideband operation as the simulated model using ideal differential excitation. The fabricated antenna prototype was used to conduct ex vivo experiments with an input power level of 18 W and duration of 10 minutes. Figure 10.32b and c shows photographs of the ablation zones in the y–z and x–z planes, respectively. The coagulation zones, measured as 3.6×2.4 cm^2 in the y–z-plane and 3.5×2.5 cm^2 in the x–z-plane, were localized with minimal tail heating.

We conducted a numerical study to investigate both the implementations shown in Figure 10.30c (Type I deployment) and Figure 10.30d (Type II deployment) for realizing asymmetric heating patterns. Simulated 60°C contours were

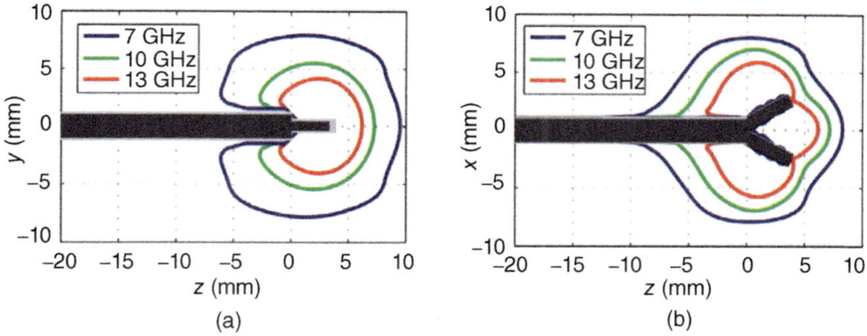

Figure 10.31 Simulated and normalized SAR patterns showing −25 dB contours at 7, 10, and 13 GHz in the (a) y–z-plane and (b) x–z-plane for the case where $\phi_1 = \phi_2 = 30°$ and $l_d = 3.5$ mm.

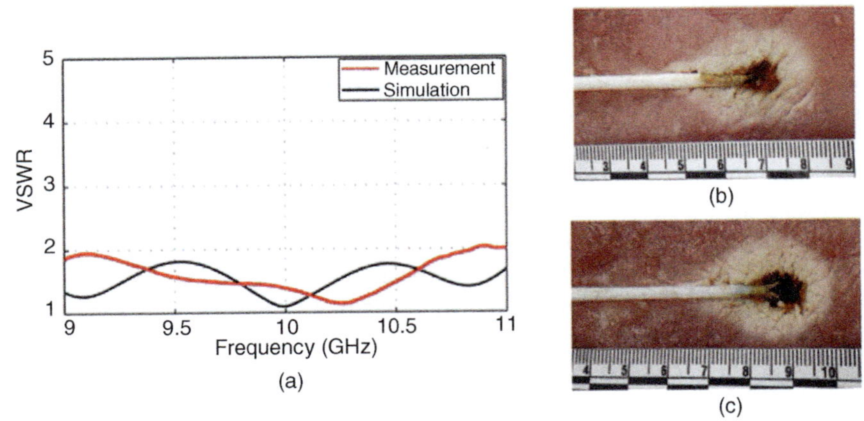

Figure 10.32 (a) Simulated and measured input VSWRs of the symmetric-heating antenna (with $\phi_1 = \phi_2 = 30°$) as seen from the coaxial input of a coax-to-balanced-line transition.

used to define the boundaries of the coagulation zones produced in egg white by the antennas. We defined a directionality ratio as $100 \times \frac{|d_2 - d_1|}{d_2 + d_1}$, where d_1 and d_2 are the lateral distances between the edges of the coagulation zone and the center of the antenna on each side of the feed line (as illustrated in Figure 10.33a and b), to quantify the degree of directionality of each generated ablation zone. Nine Type-I antennas were simulated, each corresponding to a pair of (ϕ_1, ϕ_2) chosen as a combination of $\phi_1 = 0°, 40°, 80°$ and $\phi_2 = 0°, 40°, 80°$. Similarly, nine Type-II antennas were evaluated, corresponding to nine combinations of (θ_1, θ_2) picked from $\theta_1 = 0°, 40°, 80°$ and $\theta_2 = 20°, 40°, 60°$ Figure 10.33a shows the simulated coagulation zones produced by three antenna samples of Type I deployment with ϕ_1 varied between 0°, 40°, and 80° and ϕ_2 fixed at 80°. The maximum directionality for these cases was observed to be 15.8, corresponding to the case with $\phi_1 = 0°$ and $\phi_2 = 80°$. Figure 10.33b shows the simulated ablation zones produced by three antenna samples of Type II deployment with θ_1 varied from 0° to 80° and θ_2 fixed at 60°. The maximum directionality ratio is 33.3 and occurs for the two cases with $(\theta_1 = 80°, \theta_2 = 60°)$ and $(\theta_1 = 80°, \theta_2 = 40°)$. The maximum directionality ratio achievable with the Type II deployment is significantly greater than what can be achieved with the Type I deployment. Therefore, we chose a Type II configuration with $\theta_1 = 80°$ and $\theta_2 = 40°$ as the final design for the asymmetric-heating antenna prototype.

A fabricated prototype of the asymmetric-heating antenna was used to conduct ex vivo ablation experiments in egg white. Figure 10.34a shows the measured and simulated VSWRs of the antenna, which have reasonable agreement and indicate a good impedance match with VSWR lower than 1.3 at the operating frequency of 6.4 GHz. Figure 10.34b and c shows the simulated and experimentally obtained coagulation zones produced by the

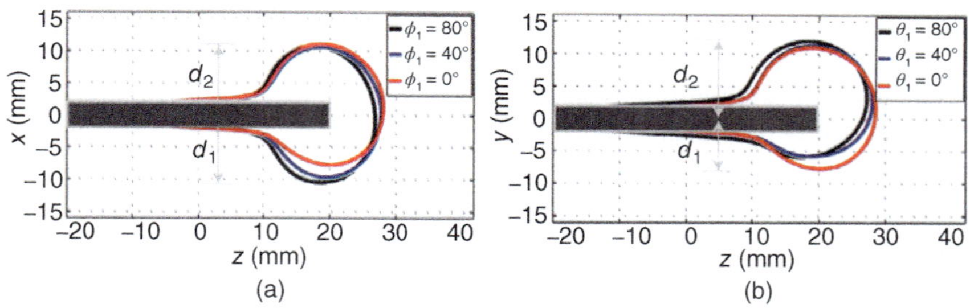

Figure 10.33 (a) Simulated 60°C contours for the balanced antenna with two different deployment mechanisms depicted in Figure 10.30. (a) Type I deployment with variable ϕ_1 and fixed $\phi_2 = 80°$. (b) Type II deployment with variable θ_1 and fixed $\theta_2 = 60°$.

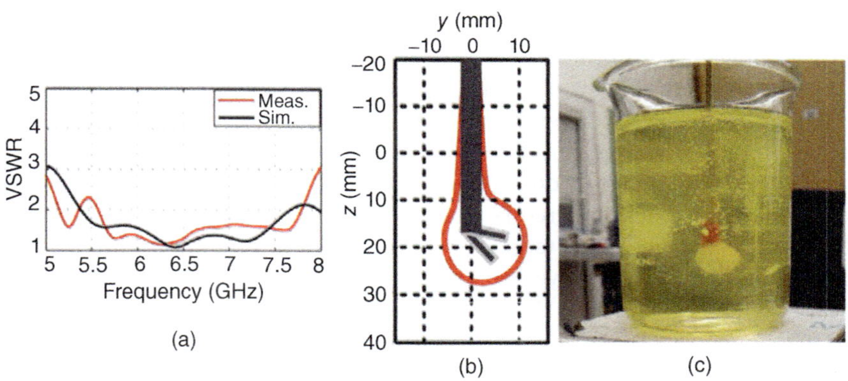

Figure 10.34 (a) Simulated and measured input VSWRs of the asymmetric-heating antenna (with $l_d = 6$ mm, $\theta_2 = 40°$, and $\theta_1 = 80°$) as seen from the coaxial input of a coax-to-balanced-line transition. (b) The simulated 60°C contour of the asymmetric-heating antenna. (c) A photograph of the coagulation zone obtained after five minutes of ablation at a power level of 25 W in egg white.

antenna fed with 25 W power for five minutes. The coagulation zone produced in the experiment was estimated to have dimensions of 20×18 mm^2 in the y–z-plane and 19×20 mm^2 in the x–z-plane as well as a directionality ratio of 40%. This directionality ratio is slightly larger than the predicted value of 33% and confirms the asymmetric-heating feature of the antenna prototype.

10.6 Conclusions

This chapter discussed recent advances in minimally invasive MWA antenna designs with an emphasis on antenna miniaturization to reduce the invasiveness and to increase the flexibility of the treatment. The motivation for reducing interstitial antennas' lengths has resulted in a number of studies investigating the use of higher frequency microwaves for tissue ablation, the main findings of which were briefly summarized in Section 10.1. Section 10.2 highlighted the key details of two studies (reported in [87, 88]) that compared MWA performance at multiple frequencies from 1.9 to 18 GHz for the same input power level and ablation duration. Simulation and measurement results reported in these two studies suggested that higher frequency MWA produces comparable ablation zone sizes as those achieved at lower frequencies in both nonperfused and strongly perfused tissues. This demonstrates the feasibility of using higher microwave frequencies for tissue ablation, which would enable shorter and potentially less-invasive applicators. However, increased ohmic losses at higher frequencies result in more cable heating and may limit the applicability of high-power MWA. Therefore, further investigations are needed to fully explore the performance of high-frequency MWA at higher power levels using actively cooled MWA probes.

A great amount of effort has been put into miniaturization of MWA antennas' diameters to reduce the invasiveness of the treatment. Sections 10.3 and 10.4 summarized various novel MWA antenna designs with reduced-diameter topologies compared to conventional coax-fed, balun-equipped antennas. These innovative designs are classified into two general groups: one group represents solutions that target less-invasive implementations of coaxial baluns, and the other involves novel balun-free antenna designs that provide localized heating patterns. A detailed discussion of the authors' proposed approaches toward diameter reduction was presented. It was demonstrated through numerical simulations and experimental investigations that the proposed antennas could provide good impedance matching and localized heating patterns. The simulation and measurement results also suggest that the ablation zones generated by these reduced-diameter antennas have comparable dimensions as those produced by conventional balun-equipped antennas, at the same input power and ablation duration. The proposed techniques allow for effectively reducing the antenna diameter by about 30% compared to conventional balun-equipped antennas without sacrificing the ablation performance. Given a number of different diameter-reduction techniques presented in the literature to date, comprehensive studies that directly compare these techniques in several aspects such as shapes of ablation zones, power-handling capabilities, and cable heating issues are potential works of interest.

Advances in interstitial antenna designs with shorter radiating lengths and smaller diameters naturally facilitate the development of flexible antennas that can be routed through natural ductal pathways to deep-seated tumors less invasively than a rigid applicator. Among various available antenna designs with reduced-diameter topologies, the balun-free helical dipole presented in Section 10.4.2 is particularly promising for implementation in a flexible embodiment. Preliminary results from ex vivo ablation experiments in porcine liver presented in Section 10.5.1 show that a flexible prototype of this antenna was able to maintain good impedance matching and to produce substantial ablation zones even after being guided through a tube with a tight 10-mm-radius bend. These promising results warrant further research to evaluate the performance of such antennas in various clinical scenarios such as ablating lung tumors or treating bile duct carcinoma.

Section 10.5 also discussed the authors' recent works on designing interstitial antennas capable of generating directional-heating patterns. Two different directional-heating antenna designs were reported: one uses a coaxial feed line, while the other uses a shielded, balanced parallel-wire line to feed a dipole antenna. Ablation experiments of these antennas inserted in egg white showed coagulation zones with relatively high directionality ratios. Future research on novel interstitial applicators that can provide custom shapes of ablation zones or adaptively reconfigure the heating profiles is expected to significantly increase the customization and flexibility of MWA treatment.

References

1 Ahmed, K., Tabuchi, Y., and Kondo, T. (2015). Hyperthermia: an effective strategy to induce apoptosis in cancer cells. *Apoptosis* 20 (11): 1411–1419. https://doi.org/10.1007/s10495-015-1168-3.

2 Kampinga, H.H. (2006). Cell biological effects of hyperthermia alone or combined with radiation or drugs: a short introduction to newcomers in the field. *International Journal of Hyperthermia* 22 (3): 191–196. https://doi.org/10.1080/02656730500532028.

3 Overgaard, J., Gonzalez Gonzalez, D., Hulshof, M.C. et al. (1995). Randomised trial of hyperthermia as adjuvant to radiotherapy for recurrent or metastatic malignant melanoma. *The Lancet* 345 (8949): 540–543. https://doi.org/10.1016/S0140-6736(95)90463-8.

4 van der Zee, J., González, D., van Rhoon, G.C. et al. (2000). Comparison of radiotherapy alone with radiotherapy plus hyperthermia in locally advanced pelvic tumours: a prospective, randomised, multicentre trial. *The Lancet* 355 (9210): 1119–1125. https://doi.org/10.1016/S0140-6736(00)02059-6.

5 Jones, E.L., Oleson, J.R., Prosnitz, L.R. et al. (2005). Randomized trial of hyperthermia and radiation for superficial tumors. *Journal of Clinical Oncology* 23 (13): 3079–3085. https://doi.org/10.1200/JCO.2005.05.520.

6 Cihoric, N., Tsikkinis, A., van Rhoon, G. et al. (2015). Hyperthermia-related clinical trials on cancer treatment within the ClinicalTrials.gov registry. *International Journal of Hyperthermia* 31 (6): 609–614. https://doi.org/10.3109/02656736.2015.1040471.

7 Hildebrandt, B., Wust, P., Ahlers, O. et al. (2002). The cellular and molecular basis of hyperthermia. *Critical Reviews in Oncology/Hematology* 43 (1): 33–56. https://doi.org/10.1016/S1040-8428(01)00179-2.

8 Luyen, H., Hagness, S.C., and Behdad, N. (2015). A balun-free helical antenna for minimally invasive microwave ablation. *IEEE Transactions on Antennas and Propagation* 63 (3): 959–965. https://doi.org/10.1109/TAP.2015.2389223.

9 Luyen, H., Hagness, S.C., and Behdad, N. (2017). Reduced-diameter designs of coax-fed microwave ablation antennas equipped with baluns. *IEEE Antennas and Wireless Propagation Letters* 16: 1385–1388. https://doi.org/10.1109/LAWP.2016.2637874.

10 Martin, R.C.G., Scoggins, C.R., and McMasters, K.M. (2010). Safety and efficacy of microwave ablation of hepatic tumors: a prospective review of a 5-year experience. *Annals of Surgical Oncology* 17 (1): 171–178. https://doi.org/10.1245/s10434-009-0686-z.

11 Simon, C.J., Dupuy, D.E., and Mayo-Smith, W.W. (2005). Microwave ablation: principles and applications. *RadioGraphics* 25 (suppl 1): S69–S83. https://doi.org/10.1148/rg.25si055501.

12 Brace, C.L. (2010). Microwave tissue ablation: biophysics, technology, and applications. *Critical Reviews in Biomedical Engineering* 38 (1): 65–78. https://doi.org/10.1615/CritRevBiomedEng.v38.i1.60.

13 Zhou, W., Zha, X., Liu, X. et al. (2012). US-guided percutaneous microwave coagulation of small breast cancers: a clinical study. *Radiology* 263 (2): 364–373. https://doi.org/10.1148/radiol.12111901.

14 Huston, T.L. and Simmons, R.M. (2005). Ablative therapies for the treatment of malignant diseases of the breast. *American Journal of Surgery* 189 (6): 694–701. https://doi.org/10.1016/j.amjsurg.2005.03.011.

15 Cheng, H.-L.M., Haider, M.A., Dill-Macky, M.J. et al. (2008). MRI and contrast-enhanced ultrasound monitoring of prostate microwave focal thermal therapy: an in vivo canine study. *Journal of Magnetic Resonance Imaging* 28 (1): 136–143. https://doi.org/10.1002/jmri.21415.

16 Carrafiello, G., Ierardi, A.M., Piacentino, F. et al. (2012). Microwave ablation with percutaneous approach for the treatment of pancreatic adenocarcinoma. *Cardiovascular and Interventional Radiology* 35 (2): 439–442. https://doi.org/10.1007/s00270-011-0189-8.

17 Eccles, S.A., Aboagye, E.O., Ali, S. et al. (2013). Critical research gaps and translational priorities for the successful prevention and treatment of breast cancer. *Breast Cancer Research* 15 (5): R92. https://doi.org/10.1186/bcr3493.

18 Medtech Solutions (2018). Interventional oncology devices | MedTech 360 | Market Insights | United States [Online]. https://decisionresourcesgroup.com/report/550881-medtech-interventional-oncology-devices-medtech-360 (accessed 2 January 2020).

19 Max, H.W. (1939). Radiating device. United States Patent Appl. 2161292, 1939 [Online]. http://www.freepatentsonline.com/2161292.html

20 Osborne, S.L. and Frederick, J.N. (1948). Microwave radiations: heating of human and animal tissues by means of high frequency current with wavelength of twelve centimeters (the microtherm). *Journal of the American Medical Association* 137 (12): 1036–1040. https://doi.org/10.1001/jama.1948.82890460002007.

21 Martin, G.M. and Erickson, D.J. (1950). Medical diathermy. *Journal of the American Medical Association* 142 (1): 27–32. https://doi.org/10.1001/jama.1950.72910190003007.

22 Roberts, J.E. and Cook, H.F. (1952). Microwaves in medical and biological research. *British Journal of Applied Physics* 3 (2): 33–40. https://doi.org/10.1088/0508-3443/3/2/301.

23 Gerhard, S. (1966). High frequency therapeutic apparatus. United States Patent Appl. 3230957, 1966 [Online]. http://www.freepatentsonline.com/3230957.html

24 Iizuka, K. and King, R.W.P. (1962). The dipole antenna immersed in a homogeneoous conducting medium. *IRE Transactions on Antennas and Propagation* 10 (4): 384–392. https://doi.org/10.1109/TAP.1962.1137882.

25 King, R.W.P. and Iizuka, K. (1963). The complete electromagnetic field of a half-wave dipole in a dissipative medium. *IEEE Transactions on Antennas and Propagation* 11 (3): 275–285. https://doi.org/10.1109/TAP.1963.1138041.

26 King, R.W.P. (1964). Theory of the terminated insulated antenna in a conducting medium. *IEEE Transactions on Antennas and Propagation* 12 (3): 305–318. https://doi.org/10.1109/TAP.1964.1138215.

27 King, R.W.P., Mishra, S., Kuan, L., and Smith, G. (1975). The insulated monopole: admittance and junction effects. *IEEE Transactions on Antennas and Propagation* 23 (2): 172–177. https://doi.org/10.1109/TAP.1975.1141044.

28 King, R.W.P. (1976). The many faces of the insulated antenna. *Proceedings of the IEEE* 64 (2): 228–238. https://doi.org/10.1109/PROC.1976.10094.

29 Prasad, S. and King, R.W.P. (1982). Experimental study of embedded insulated antennas. *IEEE Transactions on Antennas and Propagation* 30 (5): 1013–1017. https://doi.org/10.1109/TAP.1982.1142896.

30 King, R.W.P., Trembly, B.S., and Strohbehn, J.W. (1983). The electromagnetic field of an insulated antenna in a conducting or dielectric medium. *IEEE Transactions on Microwave Theory and Techniques* 31 (7): 574–583. https://doi.org/10.1109/TMTT.1983.1131547.

31 Casey, J.P. and Bansal, R. (1986). The near field of an insulated dipole in a dissipative dielectric medium (short paper). *IEEE Transactions on Microwave Theory and Techniques* 34 (4): 459–463. https://doi.org/10.1109/TMTT.1986.1133370.

32 Mendecki, J., Friedenthal, E., Botstein, C. et al. (1978). Microwave-induced hyperthermia in cancer treatment: apparatus and preliminary results. *International Journal of Radiation Oncology* 4 (11): 1095–1103. https://doi.org/10.1016/0360-3016(78)90026-3.

33 Taylor, L.S. (1978). Electromagnetic syringe. *IEEE Transactions on Biomedical Engineering* BME-25 (3): 303–304. https://doi.org/10.1109/TBME.1978.326349.

34 Szwarnowski, S., Sheppard, R.J., Grant, E.H., and Bleehen, N.M. (1980). A broad band microwave applicator for heating tumours. *The British Journal of Radiology* 53 (625): 31–33. https://doi.org/10.1259/0007-1285-53-625-31.

35 Mendecki, J., Friedenthal, E., Botstein, C. et al. (1980). Microwave applicators for localized hyperthermia treatment of cancer of the prostate. *International Journal of Radiation Oncology, Biology, Physics* 6 (11): 1583–1588. https://doi.org/10.1016/0360-3016(80)90019-X.

36 Paglione, R.W., Sterzer, F., Mendecki,J. et al. (1980). Microwave applicators for localized hyperthermia treatment of malignant tumors. Presented at the 1980 IEEE MTT-S International Microwave symposium Digest, 1980, 351–354. doi: https://doi.org/10.1109/MWSYM.1980.1124284.

37 Paglione, R.W. (1980). Coaxial applicator for microwave hyperthermia. United States Patent Appl. 4204549, 1980 [Online]. http://www.freepatentsonline.com/4204549.html

38 Taylor, L.S. (1980). Implantable radiators for cancer therapy by microwave hyperthermia. *Proceedings of the IEEE* 68 (1): 142–149. https://doi.org/10.1109/PROC.1980.11594.

39 de Sieyes, D.C., Douple, E.B., Strohbehn, J.W., and Trembly, B.S. (1981). Some aspects of optimization of an invasive microwave antenna for local hyperthermia treatment of cancer. *Medical Physics* 8 (2): 174–183. https://doi.org/10.1118/1.594930.

40 Broschat, S.L., Chou, C., Luk, K.H. et al. (1988). An insulated dipole applicator for intracavitary hyperthermia. *IEEE Transactions on Biomedical Engineering* 35 (3): 173–178. https://doi.org/10.1109/10.1359.

41 Satoh, T., Seilhan, T.M., Stauffer, P.R. et al. (1988). Interstitial helical coil microwave antenna for experimental brain hyperthermia. *Neurosurgery* 23 (5): 564–569. https://doi.org/10.1227/00006123-198811000-00004.

42 Satoh, T., Stauffer, P.R., and Fike, J.R. (1988). Thermal distribution studies of helical coil microwave antennas for interstitial hyperthermia. *International Journal of Radiation Oncology* 15 (5): 1209–1218. https://doi.org/10.1016/0360-3016(88)90206-4.

43 Iskander, M.F. and Tumeh, A.M. (1989). Design optimization of interstitial antennas. *IEEE Transactions on Biomedical Engineering* 36 (2): 238–246. https://doi.org/10.1109/10.16471.

44 Tumeh, A.M. and Iskander, M.F. (1989). Performance comparison of available interstitial antennas for microwave hyperthermia. *IEEE Transactions on Microwave Theory and Techniques* 37 (7): 1126–1133. https://doi.org/10.1109/22.24558.

45 Cerri, G., Leo, R.D., and Primiani, V.M. (1993). 'Thermic end-fire' interstitial applicator for microwave hyperthermia. *IEEE Transactions on Microwave Theory and Techniques* 41 (6): 1135–1142. https://doi.org/10.1109/22.238538.

46 Labonte, S., Blais, A., Legault, S.R. et al. (1996). Monopole antennas for microwave catheter ablation. *IEEE Transactions on Microwave Theory and Techniques* 44 (10): 1832–1840. https://doi.org/10.1109/22.539941.

47 Hurter, W., Reinbold, F., and Lorenz, W.J. (1991). A dipole antenna for interstitial microwave hyperthermia. *IEEE Transactions on Microwave Theory and Techniques* 39 (6): 1048–1054. https://doi.org/10.1109/22.81680.

48 Yang, D., Bertram, J.M., Converse, M.C. et al. (2006). A floating sleeve antenna yields localized hepatic microwave ablation. *IEEE Transactions on Biomedical Engineering* 53 (3): 533–537. https://doi.org/10.1109/TBME.2005.869794.

49 Lin, J.C. and Wang, Y.-J. (1996). The cap-choke catheter antenna for microwave ablation treatment. *IEEE Transactions on Biomedical Engineering* 43 (6): 657–660. https://doi.org/10.1109/10.495286.

50 Brace, C.L., Laeseke, P.F., van der Weide, D.W., and Lee, F.T. (2005). Microwave ablation with a triaxial antenna: results in ex vivo bovine liver. *IEEE Transactions on Microwave Theory and Techniques* 53 (1): 215–220. https://doi.org/10.1109/TMTT.2004.839308.

51 Longo, I., Gentili, G.B., Cerretelli, M., and Tosoratti, N. (2003). A coaxial antenna with miniaturized choke for minimally invasive interstitial heating. *IEEE Transactions on Biomedical Engineering* 50 (1): 82–88. https://doi.org/10.1109/TBME.2002.807320.

52 Cavagnaro, M., Amabile, C., Bernardi, P. et al. (2011). A minimally invasive antenna for microwave ablation therapies: design, performances, and experimental assessment. *IEEE Transactions on Biomedical Engineering* 58 (4): 949–959. https://doi.org/10.1109/TBME.2010.2099657.

53 Luyen, H., Hagness, S.C., and Behdad, N. (2017). A minimally invasive coax-fed microwave ablation antenna with a tapered balun. *IEEE Transactions on Antennas and Propagation* 65 (12): 7280–7287. https://doi.org/10.1109/TAP.2017.2755258.

54 Mohtashami, Y., Behdad, N., and Hagness, S.C. (2020). Toward flexible microwave ablation antennas with a balun-free helical dipole design. *IEEE Transactions on Antennas and Propagation* 68 (7): 5052–5060.

55 Hamada, L., Saito, K., Yoshimura, H., and Ito, K. (2000). Dielectric-loaded coaxial-slot antenna for interstitial microwave hyperthermia: longitudinal control of heating patterns. *International Journal of Hyperthermia* 16 (3): 219–229. https://doi.org/10.1080/026567300285240.

56 Saito, K., Yoshimura, H., Ito, K. et al. (2004). Clinical trials of interstitial microwave hyperthermia by use of coaxial-slot antenna with two slots. *IEEE Transactions on Microwave Theory and Techniques* 52 (8): 1987–1991. https://doi.org/10.1109/TMTT.2004.832005.

57 Wang, T., Zhao, G., and Qiu, B. (2015). Theoretical evaluation of the treatment effectiveness of a novel coaxial multi-slot antenna for conformal microwave ablation of tumors. *International Journal of Heat and Mass Transfer* 90: 81–91. https://doi.org/10.1016/j.ijheatmasstransfer.2015.06.030.

58 Pisa, S., Cavagnaro, M., Bernardi, P., and Lin, J.C. (2001). A 915-MHz antenna for microwave thermal ablation treatment: physical design, computer modeling and experimental measurement. *IEEE Transactions on Biomedical Engineering* 48 (5): 599–601. https://doi.org/10.1109/10.918599.

59 Prakash, P., Converse, M.C., Webster, J.G., and Mahvi, D.M. (2009). An optimal sliding choke antenna for hepatic microwave ablation. *IEEE Transactions on Biomedical Engineering* 56 (10): 2470–2476. https://doi.org/10.1109/TBME.2009.2025264.

60 Saito, K., Hosaka, S., Okabe, S. et al. (2003). A proposition on improvement of a heating pattern of an antenna for microwave coagulation therapy: Introduction of a coaxial-dipole antenna. *Electronics and Communications in Japan (Part I: Communications)* 86 (1): 16–23. https://doi.org/10.1002/ecja.10049.

61 Chiu, H.-M., Mohan, A.S., Weily, A.R. et al. (2003). Analysis of a novel expanded tip wire (ETW) antenna for microwave ablation of cardiac arrhythmias. *IEEE Transactions on Biomedical Engineering* 50 (7): 890–899. https://doi.org/10.1109/TBME.2003.813541.

62 Terakawa, T., Ito, K., Hyodo, M. et al. (1990). Heating patterns of interstitial ring-slot array applicator for microwave hyperthermia. 1990 Proceedings of the Twelfth Annual International Conference of the IEEE Engineering in Medicine and Biology Society, 1990, 1556–1556. doi: https://doi.org/10.1109/IEMBS.1990.691893.

63 Brace, C.L. (2011). Dual-slot antennas for microwave tissue heating: parametric design analysis and experimental validation. *Medical Physics* 38 (7): 4232–4240. https://doi.org/10.1118/1.3601019.

64 Zafar, J., Zafar, T., Zafar, H., and Sharif, F. (2015). Design, development and microwave inter-comparison of dual slot antenna configurations for localized hepatic tumor management. *Australas. Phys. Eng. Sci. Med. Dordr.* 38 (4): 593–601. https://doi.org/10.1007/s13246-015-0384-z.

65 Gas, P. (2017). Optimization of multi-slot coaxial antennas for microwave thermotherapy based on the S11-parameter analysis. *Biocybernetics and Biomedical Engineering* 37 (1): 78–93. https://doi.org/10.1016/j.bbe.2016.10.001.

66 Ge, M., Jiang, H., Huang, X. et al. (2018). A multi-slot coaxial microwave antenna for liver tumor ablation. *Physics in Medicine and Biology* 63 (17): 175011. https://doi.org/10.1088/1361-6560/aad9c5.

67 Rattanadecho, P. and Keangin, P. (2013). Numerical study of heat transfer and blood flow in two-layered porous liver tissue during microwave ablation process using single and double slot antenna. *International Journal of Heat and Mass Transfer* 58 (1): 457–470. https://doi.org/10.1016/j.ijheatmasstransfer.2012.10.043.

68 Keangin, P., Rattanadecho, P., and Wessapan, T. (2011). An analysis of heat transfer in liver tissue during microwave ablation using single and double slot antenna. *International Communications in Heat and Mass Transfer* 38 (6): 757–766. https://doi.org/10.1016/j.icheatmasstransfer.2011.03.027.

69 Chiang, J., Hynes, K.A., Bedoya, M., and Brace, C.L. (2013). A dual-slot microwave antenna for more spherical ablation zones: ex vivo and in vivo validation. *Radiology* 268 (2): 382–389. https://doi.org/10.1148/radiol.13122128.

70 Ibitoye, Z.A., Nwoye, E.O., Aweda, M.A. et al. (2015). Optimization of dual slot antenna using floating metallic sleeve for microwave ablation. *Medical Engineering & Physics* 37 (4): 384–391. https://doi.org/10.1016/j.medengphy.2015.01.015.

71 Ibitoye, A.Z., Nwoye, E.O., Aweda, A.M. et al. (2016). Microwave ablation of ex vivo bovine tissues using a dual slot antenna with a floating metallic sleeve. *International Journal of Hyperthermia* 32 (8): 923–930. https://doi.org/10.1080/02656736.2016.1211323.

72 Jiang, Y., Zhao, J., Li, W. et al. (2017). A coaxial slot antenna with frequency of 433 MHz for microwave ablation therapies: design, simulation, and experimental research. *Medical & Biological Engineering & Computing* 55 (11): 2027–2036. https://doi.org/10.1007/s11517-017-1651-9.

73 Terakawa, T., Ito,K., Kurokawa, S., and Ueno, K. (1988). An improved microwave antenna array for interstitial hyperthermia. The Proceedings of the Annual International Conference of the IEEE Engineering in Medicine and Biology Society, 1988, vol. 3, 1331. doi: https://doi.org/10.1109/IEMBS.1988.95129.

74 Gu, Z., Rappaport, M., Wang, P.J., and VanderBrink, B.A. (2000). Development and experimental verification of the wide-aperture catheter-based microwave cardiac ablation antenna. *IEEE Transactions on Microwave Theory and Techniques* 48 (11): 1892–1900. https://doi.org/10.1109/22.883868.

75 Vanderbrink, B.A., Gu, Z., Rodriguez, V. et al. (2000). Microwave ablation using a spiral antenna design in a porcine thigh muscle preparation: in vivo assessment of temperature profile and lesion geometry. *Journal of Cardiovascular Electrophysiology* 11 (2): 193–198. https://doi.org/10.1111/j.1540-8167.2000.tb00319.x.

76 Saito, K., Itakura, H., Takahashi, M., and Ito, K. (2012). "Microwave heating for treatment of bile duct carcinoma: evaluations on influence of metallic stent. 2012 International Conference on Electromagnetics in Advanced Applications, Cape Town, WP, South Africa, 2012, 156–158. doi: https://doi.org/10.1109/ICEAA.2012.6328612.

77 Mohtashami, Y., Hagness, S.C., and Behdad, N. (2017). A hybrid slot/monopole antenna with directional heating patterns for microwave ablation. *IEEE Transactions on Antennas and Propagation* 65 (8): 3889–3896. https://doi.org/10.1109/TAP.2017.2714020.

78 McWilliams, B.T., Schnell, E.E., Curto, S. et al. (2015). A directional interstitial antenna for microwave tissue ablation: theoretical and experimental investigation. *IEEE Transactions on Biomedical Engineering* 62 (9): 2144–2150. https://doi.org/10.1109/TBME.2015.2413672.

79 Mohtashami, Y., Luyen, H., Hagness, S.C., and Behdad, N. (2018). Non-coaxial-based microwave ablation antennas for creating symmetric and asymmetric coagulation zones. *Journal of Applied Physics* 123 (21): 214903. https://doi.org/10.1063/1.5019267.

80 Hassan, E.G.M.I., Takruri, H., and Zaki, A. (2019). Realization and experimental assessment of baseball-bat microwave antenna for low power cancer ablation. *IEEE Journal of Electromagnetics, RF and Microwaves in Medicine and Biology*: 1–1. https://doi.org/10.1109/JERM.2019.2955709.

81 Bertram, J.M., Yang, D., Converse, M.C. et al. (2006). A review of coaxial-based interstitial antennas for hepatic microwave ablation. *Critical Reviews in Biomedical Engineering* 34 (3): 187–213. https://doi.org/10.1615/CritRevBiomedEng.v34.i3.10.

82 Fallahi, H. and Prakash, P. (2018). Antenna designs for microwave tissue ablation. *Critical Reviews in Biomedical Engineering* 46 (6): 495–521. https://doi.org/10.1615/CritRevBiomedEng.2018028554.

83 Hoffmann, R., Rempp, H., Erhard, L. et al. (2013). Comparison of four microwave ablation devices: an experimental study in ex vivo bovine liver. *Radiology* 268 (1): 89–97. https://doi.org/10.1148/radiol.13121127.

84 Mohtashami, Y., Luyen, H., Sawicki, J.F. et al. (2018). Tools for attacking tumors: performance comparison of triaxial, choke dipole, and balun-free base-fed monopole antennas for microwave ablation. *IEEE Antennas and Propagation Magazine* 60 (6): 52–57. https://doi.org/10.1109/MAP.2018.2870657.

85 Zhou, W., Liang, M., Pan, H. et al. (2013). Comparison of ablation zones among different tissues using 2450-MHz cooled-shaft microwave antenna: results in ex vivo porcine models. *PLoS One* 8 (8): e71873. https://doi.org/10.1371/journal.pone.0071873.

86 Luyen, H., Gao, F., Hagness, S.C., and Behdad, N. (2014). Microwave ablation at 10.0 GHz achieves comparable ablation zones to 1.9 GHz in ex

vivo bovine liver. *IEEE Transactions on Biomedical Engineering* 61 (6): 1702–1710. https://doi.org/10.1109/TBME.2014.2300692.

87 Sawicki, J.F., Shea, J.D., Behdad, N., and Hagness, S.C. (2017). The impact of frequency on the performance of microwave ablation. *International Journal of Hyperthermia* 33 (1): 61–68. https://doi.org/10.1080/02656736.2016.1207254.

88 Sawicki, J.F., Luyen, H., Mohtashami, Y. et al. (2018). The performance of higher-frequency microwave ablation in the presence of perfusion. *IEEE Transactions on Biomedical Engineering*: 1–1. https://doi.org/10.1109/TBME.2018.2836317.

89 Curto, S., Taj-Eldin, M., Fairchild, D., and Prakash, P. (2015). Microwave ablation at 915 MHz vs 2.45 GHz: a theoretical and experimental investigation. *Medical Physics* 42 (11): 6152–6161. https://doi.org/10.1118/1.4931959.

90 Hodgson, D.A., Feldberg, I.B., Sharp, N. et al. (1999). Microwave endometrial ablation: development, clinical trials and outcomes at three years. *BJOG: An International Journal of Obstetrics & Gynaecology* 106 (7): 684–694. https://doi.org/10.1111/j.1471-0528.1999.tb08368.x.

91 Hancock, C.P., Dharmasiri, N., White, M., and Goodman, A.M. (2013). The design and development of an integrated multi-functional microwave antenna structure for biological applications. *IEEE Transactions on Microwave Theory and Techniques* 61 (5): 2230–2241. https://doi.org/10.1109/TMTT.2013.2255620.

92 Jones, R.P., Kitteringham, N.R., Terlizzo, M. et al. (2012). Microwave ablation of ex vivo human liver and colorectal liver metastases with a novel 14.5 GHz generator. *International Journal of Hyperthermia* 28 (1): 43–54. https://doi.org/10.3109/02656736.2011.610428.

93 Komarov, V.V. (2014). Numerical study and optimization of interstitial antennas for microwave ablation therapy. *European Physical Journal Applied Physics* 68 (1): 10901. https://doi.org/10.1051/epjap/2014140175.

94 Yoon, J., Cho, J., Kim, N. et al. (2011). High-frequency microwave ablation method for enhanced cancer treatment with minimized collateral damage. *International Journal of Cancer* 129 (8): 1970–1978. https://doi.org/10.1002/ijc.25845.

95 Lazebnik, M., Converse, M.C., Booske, J.H., and Hagness, S.C. (2006). Ultrawideband temperature-dependent dielectric properties of animal liver tissue in the microwave frequency range. *Physics in Medicine and Biology* 51 (7): 1941–1955. https://doi.org/10.1088/0031-9155/51/7/022.

96 IT'IS Foundation (2011). Tissue Properties Database V1.0. IT'IS Foundation [Online]. https://itis.swiss/virtual-population/tissue-properties/downloads/database-v1-0 (accessed 2 January 2020).

97 Duncan, J.W. and Minerva, V.P. (1960). 100:1 bandwidth balun transformer. *Proceedings of the IRE* 48: 156–164.

98 Choi, J.-G., Yi, S.-H., and Kim, K.-H. (2004). Development of a novel tapered balun for the UWB UHF coupler. Presented at the IEEE Power Modulator Symposium, 2004, 493–496.

99 Guntur, S.R., Lee, K.I., Paeng, D.-G. et al. (2013). Temperature-dependent thermal properties of ex vivo liver undergoing thermal ablation. *Ultrasound in Medicine & Biology* 39 (10): 1771–1784. https://doi.org/10.1016/j.ultrasmedbio.2013.04.014.

100 Yang, D., Converse, M.C., Mahvi, D.M., and Webster, J.G. (2007). Expanding the bioheat equation to include tissue internal water evaporation during heating. *IEEE Transactions on Biomedical Engineering* 54 (8): 1382–1388. https://doi.org/10.1109/TBME.2007.890740.

101 Karampatzakis, A., Kühn, S., Tsanidis, G. et al. (2013). Antenna design and tissue parameters considerations for an improved modelling of microwave ablation in the liver. *Physics in Medicine and Biology* 58 (10): 3191–3206. https://doi.org/10.1088/0031-9155/58/10/3191.

102 Balanis, C.A. (2005). *Antenna Theory: Analysis and Design*, 3e. Hobeken, NJ: Wiley.

103 Bui, J.T., Gaba, R.C., Grace Knuttinen, M. et al. (2011). Microwave lung ablation complicated by bronchocutaneous fistula: case report and literature review. *Seminars in Interventional Radiology* 28 (2): 152–155. https://doi.org/10.1055/s-0031-1280654.

104 Alexander, E.S., Healey, T.T., Martin, D.W., and Dupuy, D.E. (2012). Use of endobronchial valves for the treatment of bronchopleural fistulas after thermal ablation of lung neoplasms. *Journal of Vascular and Interventional Radiology* 23 (9): 1236–1240. https://doi.org/10.1016/j.jvir.2012.06.009.

105 Li, R., Wu, T., Pan, B. et al. (2009). Equivalent-circuit analysis of a broadband printed dipole with adjusted integrated balun and an array for base station applications. *IEEE Transactions on Antennas and Propagation* 57 (7): 2180–2184. https://doi.org/10.1109/TAP.2009.2021967.

11

Inkjet-/3D-/4D-Printed Nanotechnology-Enabled Radar, Sensing, and RFID Modules for Internet of Things, "Smart Skin," and "Zero Power" Medical Applications

Manos M. Tentzeris, Aline Eid, Tong-Hong Lin, Jimmy G.D. Hester, Yepu Cui, Ajibayo Adeyeye, Bijan Tehrani and Syed A. Nauroze

School of Electrical and Computer Engineering, Georgia Institute of Technology, Atlanta, GA, USA

11.1 Introduction

The advent of wearable and Internet of Things (IoT)-connected technologies has enabled and brought to light the potential for a cornucopia of new health-applied wearable devices. Coupled with the exponentially growing capabilities of artificial-intelligence and machine-learning algorithms, these new technological trends hold the promise for the constant gathering, processing, and curating of data to establish longitudinal studies and predictions of chronic or acute health condition and events.

Nevertheless, wide gaps in the capabilities of wearable wireless systems have remained opened and are largely restricting the extent and scope of the application of such far-reaching and valuable devices. The centerpiece critically limiting such hardware implementations is their need for a source of power. Indeed, while a few portable devices, such as a phone or a watch, soon become unreasonably burdensome in their daily maintenance (charging, predominantly), the servicing of a multiplication of sticker-like system whose placement on the body is often critical to guaranteeing their measurement performance—this is, for instance, the case for electrodes-mediated measurement such as electrocardiogram (EKG) and electroencephalogram (EEG) or with electrochemistry-based sensors such as sweat analyzers—would require periodic and careful removal and installation by patients or caregivers. An alternative option could rely on the use of ultra-low-cost disposable flexible devices that are battery powered and could be disposed of once discharged or damaged. This option, however, would induce the production of mountains of small and difficult-to-recycle electrochemical cells at a consequently high cost to the environment.

Antenna and Sensor Technologies in Modern Medical Applications,
First Edition. Edited by Yahya Rahmat-Samii and Erdem Topsakal.

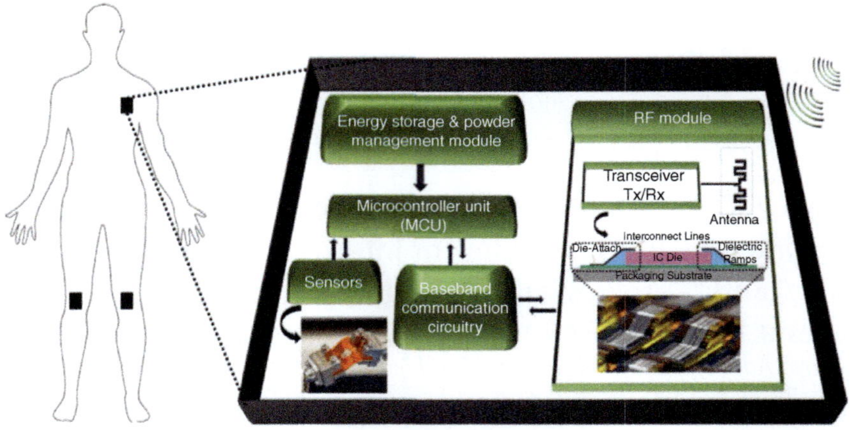

Figure 11.1 A system schematic of a typical wearable IoT wireless sensor module.

The use of additive manufacturing technologies—such as the commonly encountered inkjet-printing technology or the popular forms of 3D printing approaches—enables, through their versatility, a surprising wealth of solutions to the aforementioned limitations of the state-of-the-art health wearables. The innovations presented in this chapter, centered around the peculiar needs of wearable health devices, tackle their requirements from a variety of perspectives as shown in Figure 11.1. In Section 11.2, new strategies enabling the powering of printed wearable systems using both legacy radio-frequency (RF) wireless networks and upcoming 5G millimeter-wave implementations are presented. Next, in Section 11.3, are reported innovations required for the additive integration of mature state-of-the-art RF and millimeter-wave chips into both partially printed flexible boards and compact fully 3D printed millimeter-wave multilayer modules. Wearable systems also require—due to their need for energy autonomy and ultralow power consumption in an on-body setting—the development of new communications and shape-shifting electromagnetic shielding schemes which are described in Section 11.4. Finally, Section 11.5 reports ultra-low-cost printed architectures capable of sensitizing printed devices to a near-infinite variety of gaseous and dissolved or dispersed (through microfluidic means) chemical analytes, before a conclusion is drawn in Section 11.6.

11.2 Batteryless "Green" Powering Schemes for Perpetual Wearables

Our era is witnessing a rapid development in the field of millimeter-wave and IoT technologies with a projected 50 billion IoT devices to be installed by the end of the decade. Those devices, responsible for sensing and communicating, require the use of batteries that need to be continuously recharged or replaced. Since the number of IoT devices will be massive, it is highly desirable to equip them with harvesting capabilities and to manufacture them using low-cost and environmentally friendly processes. Electromagnetic scavenging is one form of energy harvesting relying on collecting the ambient signals and converting them to usable dc power. Among the most popular low-frequency band allocations exploited for energy scavenging are the 900 MHz and 2.4 GHz industrial, scientific, and medical (ISM) bands, where approximately 36 dBm equivalent isotropic radiated power (EIRP) is allowed in transmission. Another powerful source is millimeter-wave energy, present in the 5G bands (above 24 GHz), where the limits of allowable transmitted power by the Federal Communication Commission (FCC) regulations are pushed beyond that of their lower frequency counterparts. Another opportunity at such high-frequency bands is the ability to design scalable antenna-array systems with slim form factors and finely tunable aperture sizes.

The work presented below showcases the freedom accompanied with the design of RF and millimeter-wave energy-harvesting systems, prioritizing specific requirements such as flexibility, compactness, long range, omnidirectionality, and more.

11.2.1 Wearable Rectennas Compatible with Legacy Wireless Networks

As mentioned earlier, the 2.4-GHz RF power is an abundantly available source originating from Wi-Fi routers and access points. An antenna within this frequency band can be made relatively compact compared to the increased challenges in the ultrahigh frequency (UHF) bands. In addition, commercial Schottky diodes are highly available and easy to model at these frequencies with a wide selection depending on the desired RF power sensitivity, breakdown voltage, and diode packaging. For ambient electromagnetic energy, where the received RF power at the input of the rectifier is less than 0 dBm, the diode is required to have a relatively high sensitivity translated through low turn-on power densities. The SMS7630 zero-bias Schottky diode, from Skyworks, falls within this description. It has a low built-in potential that is about 170 mV for 1 mA forward current. The rectenna circuit—rectifier + antenna—presented in Figure 11.2a represents the receiving system responsible of scavenging the RF power and converting it into DC power [1]. It is fabricated on a 180-μm-thick liquid crystal polymer (LCP) substrate (dielectric constant of 3) using an inkjet-printed masking technique followed by etching. The overall size of the 2.4-GHz system is $50 \times 11.5\ mm^2$. In order to test the suitability of this system for wearable applications and the powering of sensors on-body, the rectenna was placed 65 cm away from an RF source, such as the received power at the

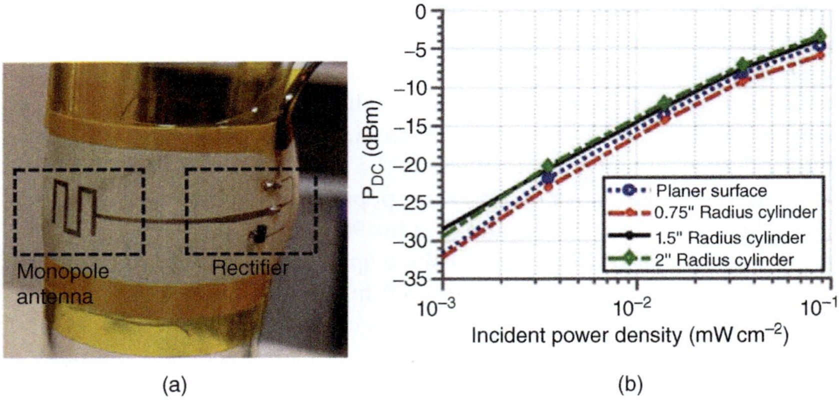

Figure 11.2 (a) Picture of the 2.4-GHz rectenna measurement on the 0.75″ radius cylinder. (b) Measured output DC powers for different cylinders radii.

input of the rectifier ranges between −20 and 0 dBm. Added to the wireless test—that validates the operation of a system in an ambient electromagnetic harvesting environment—the rectenna was placed over cylinders with different radii to test its rectification behavior under bending. Figure 11.2b—displaying the output DC powers versus the incident power densities—demonstrates the robustness and stability of this fabricated compact rectenna under bending down to a 0.75″ radius cylinder, where less than 57% was observed in DC power variations. The output of this rectenna can be used to power microwave on-body sensors or even amplified using dc–dc boost converters to realize self-sufficient health-monitoring devices.

11.2.2 New Opportunities for Power Harvesting from 5G Cellular Networks

11.2.2.1 28-GHz Rotman Lens-Based Energy-Harvesting System

The 5G bands constitute a smart choice when it comes to energy-harvesting applications. As mentioned earlier, those bands are equipped with very high allowable transmitted powers by the FCC (up to 75 dBm) which enable long-range and efficient harvesting capabilities. However, with higher frequencies, more directive antennas are required to counterbalance the increased path loss; these perform best only when perfectly aligned with the source of the RF power. Taking into account the need for a system that enables both high gain and large angular coverage at those 5G bands, the Rotman lens—one form of beam-forming networks—was implemented for the first time for millimeter-wave energy harvesting in Eid et al. [2]. The right side of Figure 11.3 shows the fully flexible rectenna system based on a dual combination: RF + dc. The RF combination occurs through the lens, where the RF power received

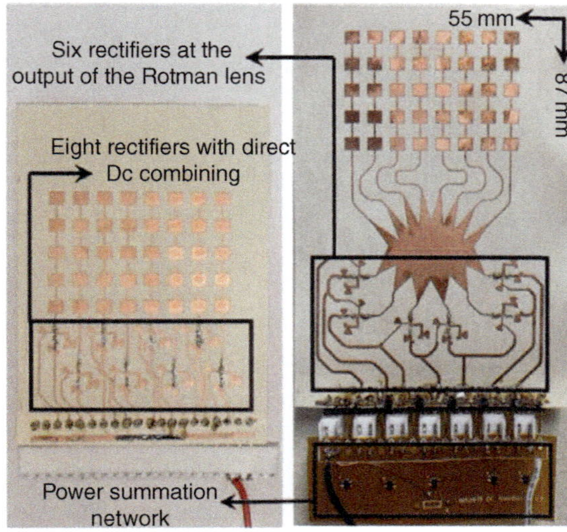

Figure 11.3 Picture of the simple rectenna design (left) and the Rotman-based rectenna (right).

by all the antennas on one end are combined internally through true-time delays and collected on the opposite end, on one of the beam ports, where rectification is conducted. A dc combination stage, based on bypass diodes, is added at the output of the rectifiers, to collect the output dc power, regardless of the active rectifier—and, therefore, the angle of arrival of the power—at that specific time. In order for us to evaluate the contribution of the Rotman lens in combining the RF power and feeding it to one rectifier, we have built a similar rectenna system based on eight antenna arrays and eight rectifiers with no Rotman lens involved as shown on the left side of Figure 11.3.

The harvested powers and output voltages of the two systems were compared as shown in Figure 11.4a, highlighting the superiority of the lens-based system, where on average 21 times more power can be harvested by adding the Rotman lens to the system. In addition to focusing the power to one port and achieving a high gain of approximately 18 dB, the lens enables a large angular coverage of 110°, visualized through its six beams and maintained under bending scenario down to a radius of 1.5″, as shown in Figure 11.4b. This flexible system is equipped with a full ground plane, and its performance is not hindered when mounted on-body or any other surface. The demonstrated results prove the suitability of this system for wearable devices and the powering of sensors placed on-body, since it is not highly dependent on the location of the power transmitter—translated through the ability of looking in six different directions—and its RF combining feature allows higher harvested powers compared to standard systems.

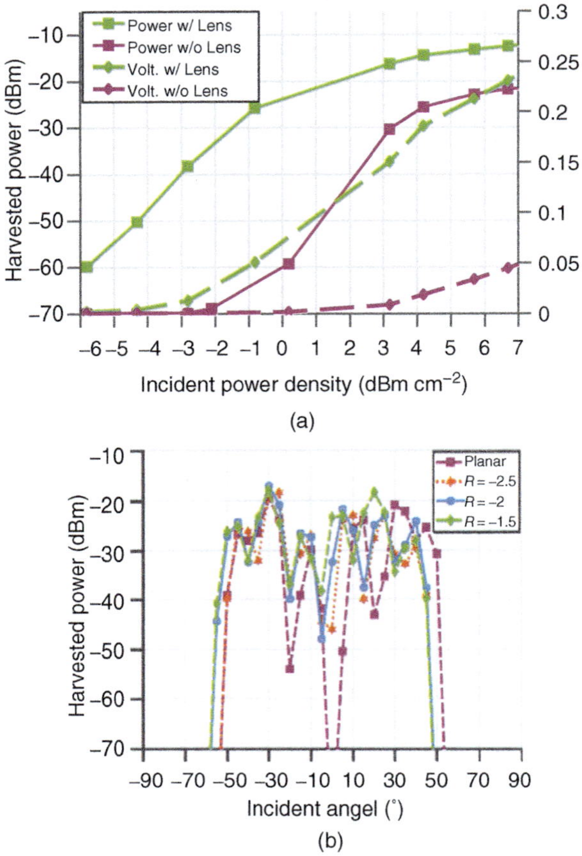

Figure 11.4 (a) Plot of the measured voltages and output powers versus incident power density for the rectenna with and without the Rotman Lens. (b) Measured harvested powers versus incidence angles for different curvatures.

11.2.2.2 Integration of W-Band Zero-Bias Diode for Harvesting Applications

Section 11.2.2.1 describes the potential of large array systems aided by the Rotman lens, and targeted for operation in the 5G bands, in improving the harvesting efficiency while offering a wide angular coverage. However, while the design and fabrication on the antenna side is still feasible up to W and G bands using additive manufacturing techniques used by our group, big challenges are faced on the rectifier side. Specifically, the rectifying elements require the fabrication and mounting of expensive Schottky diodes or of multistage CMOS millimeter-wave rectifiers. We have demonstrated in Eid et al. [3] the design of a challenging rectifier circuit at W-band based solely on inkjet-printed

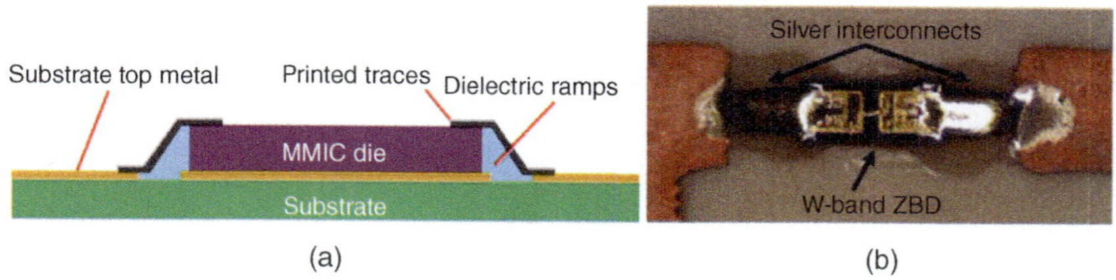

Figure 11.5 (a) Cross section of the inkjet-printed 3D interconnects. (b) Integration of the W-band ZBD ($230 \times 580\ \mu m^2$) on a flexible LCP substrate.

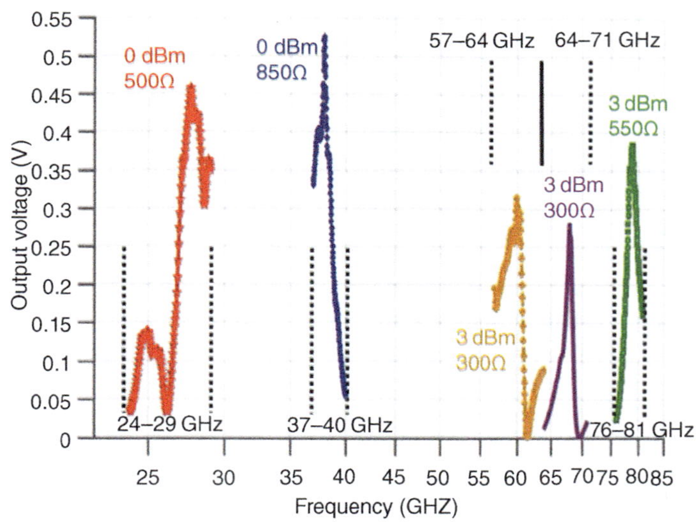

Figure 11.6 Simulated output voltages versus frequency for the five considered 5G bands at their optimal loads and input powers.

packaging. The diode used is a zero-bias detector (ZBD) from Virginia diodes. The integration of this very small die that is 230 μm wide and 580 μm long with the packaging substrate was made possible, as seen in Figure 11.5b, through an inkjet-printed die attach technique shown in Figure 11.5a—with the dielectric ramp and interconnect lines—proposed in Tehrani et al. [4], presented in more detail in the following section. The simulated output voltage of the designed rectifiers was tested over its respective band at their optimal loads and input powers, as shown in Figure 11.6. This result provides the groundwork for the exploration of millimeter-wave harvesting and its implementation for the powering of low-cost additively manufactured flexible and wearable 5G and millimeter-wave-powered motes for the IoT.

11.3 Additive Manufacturing Technologies for Low-Cost, Compact, and Wearable System

11.3.1 Wireless System Packaging for On-Body Devices

A crucial component of the wearable RF and millimeter-wave harvesting demonstrations outlined in Sections 11.2.1 and 11.2.2 is the system packaging, including the microelectronic assembly and integration technologies required to ensure efficient manufacturing and operation within a variety of dynamic environments. Two key areas of consideration with respect to wearable packages for wireless systems are miniaturization and flexibility. Miniaturization pursues the development of smaller and smaller form factors for nonintrusive integration with the body, where various individual components are integrated at the chip and package level, respectively, referred to as system-on-chip (SoC) and system-on-package (SoP) design schemes, in order to reduce physical size while achieving reduced power consumption. Additionally, flexibility targets the achievement of mechanical robustness and conformality for a variety of practical physical implementations, which is assisted through the utilization of resilient interconnection and encapsulation methodologies at both the chip and package levels. Recent developments in additive manufacturing methodologies have demonstrated their effectiveness for realizing fully printed RF sensors, passives, interconnects, and packages with applications throughout the wearable space [5, 6]. These additive techniques remove the requirement for bulky peripheral components and discrete device packages, facilitating system miniaturization and subsequently flexible, nonplanar system configurations. One such example, introduced in Section 11.2.2, presents a fully printed method for interconnecting with millimeter-wave rectifier diodes as an alternative to traditional wire and ribbon bond techniques. The 2D schematic presented in Figure 11.5a displays a side-view stack up of the printed first-level interconnects, where 3D dielectric ramps are inkjet printed with a polymer-based ink followed by the inkjet printing of metallic transitions from the circuit board to the chip utilizing a silver nanoparticle-based ink. This printed ramp configuration has been demonstrated to achieve low-loss RF interconnects with improved input/output matching for surface-mounted Ka-band (26.5–40 GHz) monolithic microwave-integrated circuits (MMICs) at the bare-die level [7].

An alternative configuration to the previously outlined surface-mounted ramp-based interconnection method is cavity embedding, where MMIC devices are placed into physical recesses within the host circuit board in order to minimize component thickness and reduce interconnect length. Traditionally, wire or ribbon bond interconnects are used to provide transitions from the circuit board to the embedded chip, which are ideally located on the same plane; however, these methods can result in limited mechanical

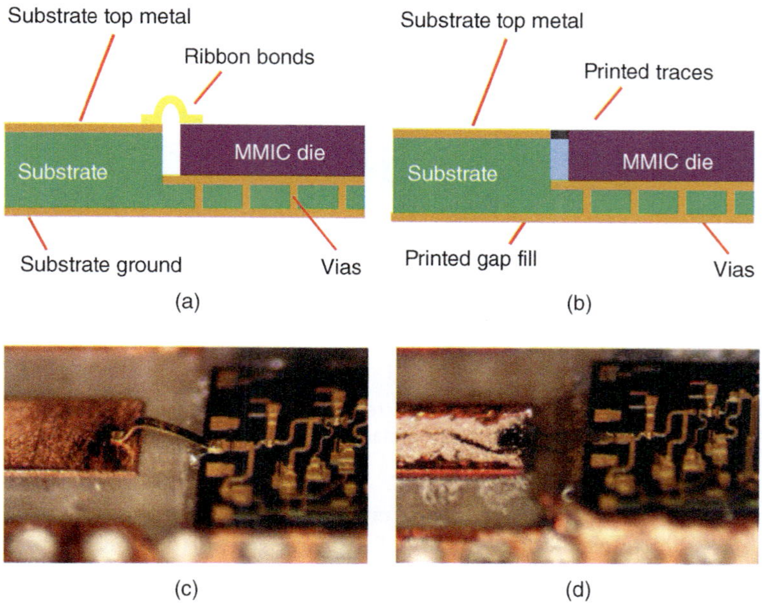

Figure 11.7 First-level interconnect configurations with MMIC devices: ribbon bonded (a) side-view schematic and (c) perspective image; inkjet printed (b) side-view schematic and (d) perspective image [8]. (*Source*: He, X., Tehrani, B. K., Bahr, R. A., et al., 2020. © IEEE.)

resiliency and RF efficiency within the millimeter-wave regime. As a promising alternative, recent efforts have demonstrated the effectiveness of utilizing inkjet-printing technology to manufacture these transitions for embedded MMIC devices operating in emerging 5G frequency bands [8]. This process includes the inkjet printing of a polymer-based gap-filling ink along with a metallic silver nanoparticle ink for the interconnect transition. Figure 11.7 presents 2D side-view schematics and perspective images of ribbon-bonded and inkjet-printed first-level interconnection methods for a Ka-band Low Noise Amplifier (LNA) MMIC. A comparison between these two assembly technologies yielded a 1—3.5 dB improvement in LNA gain for the printed configuration, in addition to improved matching throughout the Ka-band. Additionally, the presence of a printed gap-fill material has the potential to improve the mechanical reliability of the embedded module by behaving as a stress buffer between the rigid integrated circuit (IC) and flexible circuit board.

11.3.2 Energy-Autonomous System-on-Package Designs

Wearable health-monitoring devices have become a hot topic due to the consistent pursuit of a healthy lifestyle. In order to fall in the category of wearable

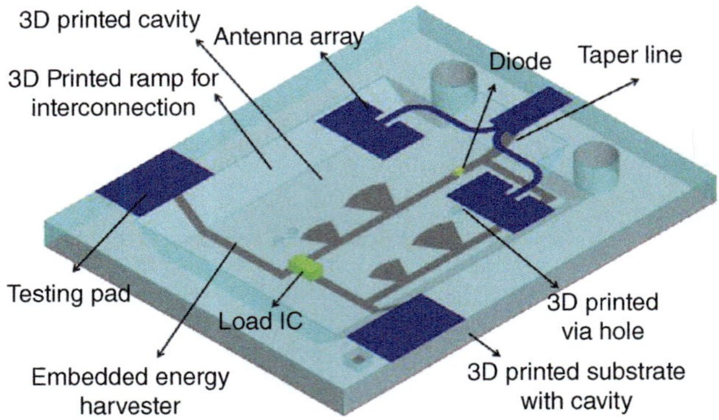

Figure 11.8 The package-integrated energy harvester with 3D printed multilayer packaging structure [9]. (*Source*: Lin, T., Daskalakis, S. N., Georgiadis, A., et al., 2019. © IEEE.)

systems, a device must meet the following criteria. The device has to be small enough, preferably power sufficient, and finally capable of communicating acquired data in real time.

One example of a wearable monitoring sensor network is the SoP design with embedded energy harvester proposed in Lin et al. [9] with circuit diagram shown in Figure 11.8. The wearable energy harvester was implemented as a power source to eliminate the need of continuously replacing and discarding batteries [10]. The 5G communication in the millimeter-wave range supports a higher data rate and reduces the size of RF components [11]. Furthermore, the EIRP allowed for 5G communication is 75 dBm [12], which opens the door for longer range energy harvesting. The additive manufacturing techniques including inkjet printing and 3D printing are helpful for fast prototyping and reducing the cost [13]. Finally, the compact SoP design with an embedded energy harvester reduces the size of a functional sensor design from a board to a single chip.

As shown in Figure 11.8, the core packaging substrate is a 3D printed flexible substrate with the cavity and ramps. The energy-harvester circuit and ICs were embedded inside the cavity. The microstrip taper line on the ramp served as the interconnection between the two layers. A photo of the fabricated system is presented in Figure 11.9a. The cavity was sealed with the same material as the core substrate, and the patch antenna array is inkjet printed on the top of the packaging as shown in Figure 11.9b. The radiation pattern of the antenna array at 26 GHz was measured as shown in Figure 11.10a. The simulated and measured output voltages under different input powers are shown in Figure 11.10b. The wireless performance test setup is shown in Figure 11.11. The system can

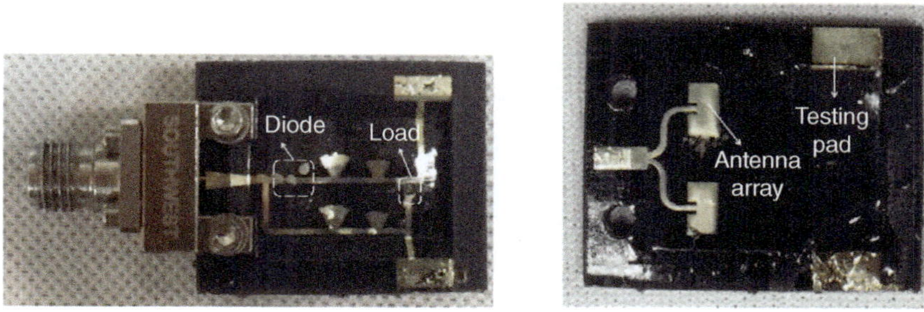

(a) (b)

Figure 11.9 (a) The package-integrated energy harvester [9]. (b) Inkjet-printed antenna array on the top of the packaging after filling the cavity with polymer [9]. (*Source*: Lin, T., Daskalakis, S. N., Georgiadis, A., et al., 2019. © IEEE.)

be turned on and is fully functional at 20 cm away from the RF source under a transmitted power of 59 dBm EIRP. The operational range can be extended to more than 1 m under 75 dBm EIRP, which is the maximum allowable transmitted power by the FCC.

11.4 Energy-Autonomous Communications for On-Body Sensing Networks

11.4.1 Energy-Autonomous Long-Range Wearable Sensor Networks

In Lin et al. [14] and Lin et al. [15], a long-range energy-autonomous on-body sensor network was proposed, and the topology is shown in Figure 11.12. The 464.5-MHz two-way talk radio was chosen to be the only power source to support the system, and thus, no batteries are required in the sensor network. The proposed wearable energy harvester shown in Figure 11.13a collects RF energy from the two-way radio and rectifies it into DC and harmonic energy. The second harmonic at 929 MHz was used as a carrier emitter to enhance the reading range of all other on-body sensor tags [16]. The DC energy was used to drive the amplifier to amplify the carrier signal and further extend the reading range of on-body sensor tags. The prototype of the backscatter sensor tag is presented in Figure 11.13b. The tag harnessed energy from the two-way radio to drive the oscillator which was used to modulate the backscattered signals. The oscillating frequency varies, depending on the resistance of the loaded ammonia sensor. The measured oscillating frequency was 50 kHz before exposure to ammonia and 7 kHz after exposure to ammonia. Thus, as shown in Figure 11.14, the

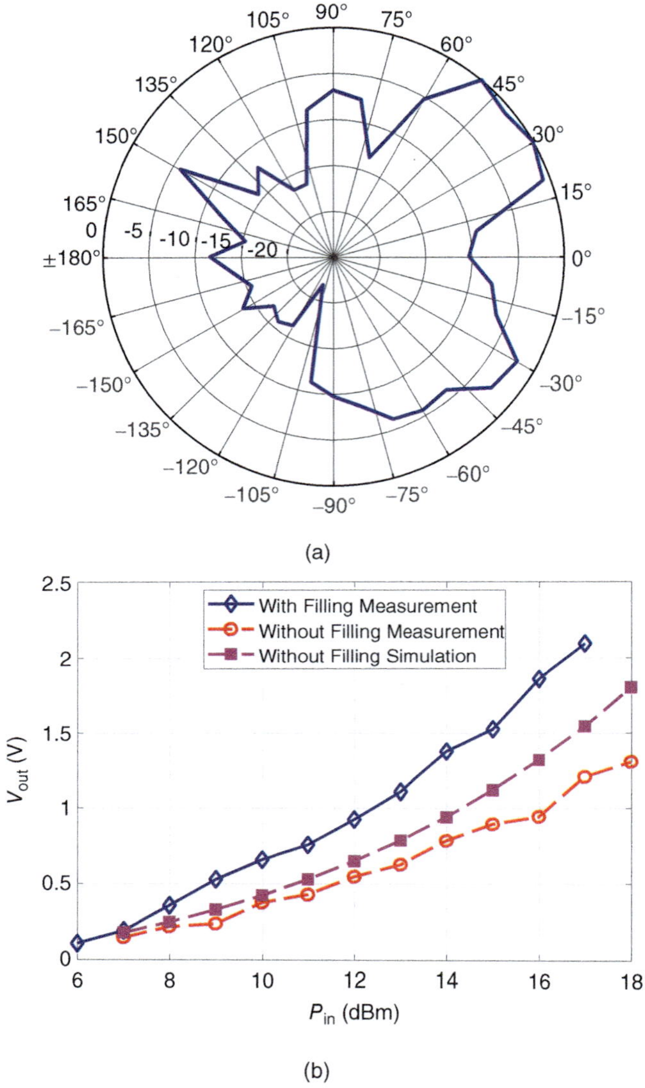

Figure 11.10 (a) Measured radiation pattern at 26 GHz for the antenna array [9]. (b) Measured and simulated output voltages with respect to different input power at 26 GHz for the embedded energy harvester [9]. (*Source*: Lin, T., Daskalakis, S. N., Georgiadis, A., et al., 2019. . © IEEE.)

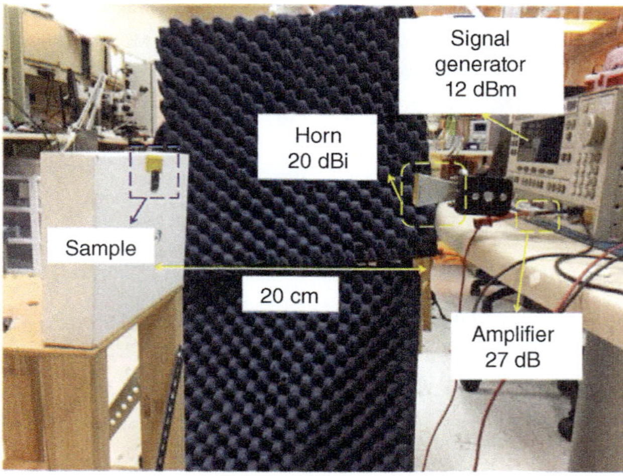

Figure 11.11 Wireless performance evaluation for the system [9]. (*Source*: Lin, T., Daskalakis, S. N., Georgiadis, A., et al., 2019. © IEEE.)

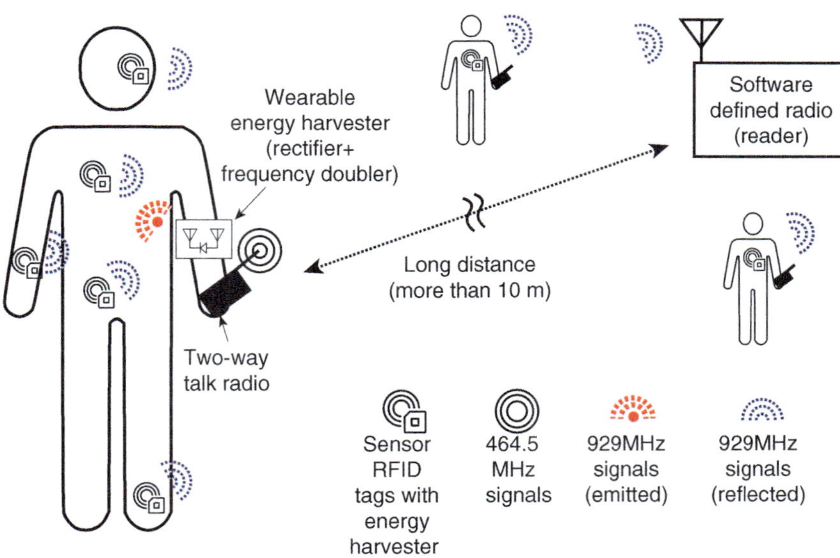

Figure 11.12 Energy-autonomous on-body sensor network [14]. (*Source*: Lin, T., Bito, J., Hester, J. G. D. et al., 2017. © IEEE.)

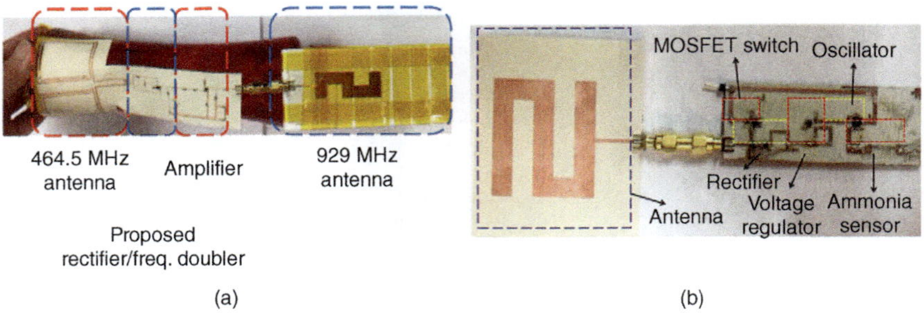

Figure 11.13 (a) Prototype of the energy-harvesting circuit [14]. (b) Prototype of the custom RFID tag with printed ammonia sensor [14]. (*Source*: Lin, T., Bito, J., Hester, J. G. D., et al., 2017. © IEEE.)

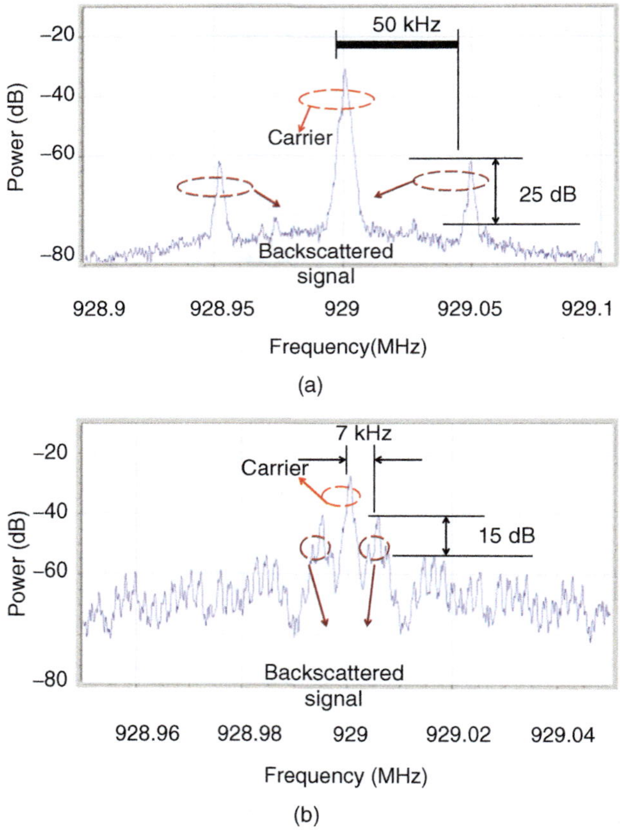

Figure 11.14 Measured results for the on-body ammonia sensor tag (a) before exposure to ammonia and (b) after exposure to ammonia [14]. (*Source*: Lin, T., Bito, J., Hester, J. G. D., et al., 2017. © IEEE.)

differences between the carrier signal and the modulated backscattered signals were 50 kHz for testing without ammonia and 7 kHz for testing with ammonia. By detecting the locations of the received backscattered signals, the presence of ammonia can be easily distinguished.

The long-range field test setup is shown in Figure 11.15a. The wearable harvester serving as the carrier emitter was placed in close proximity of the sensor tag, while the reader was at 70 m away from the carrier emitter and the sensor tag. The backscattered signals were successfully detected at 70 m

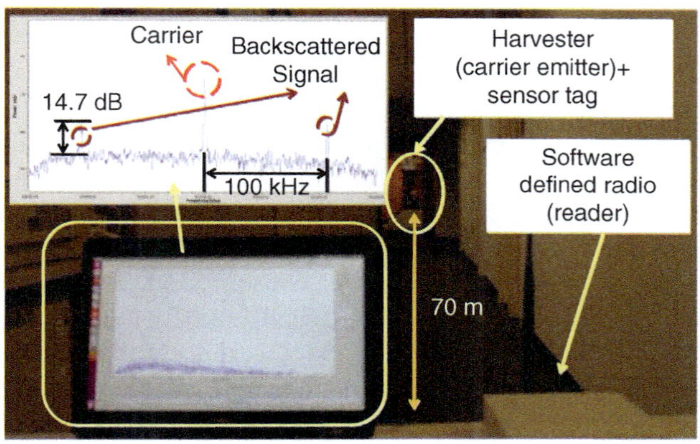

(a)

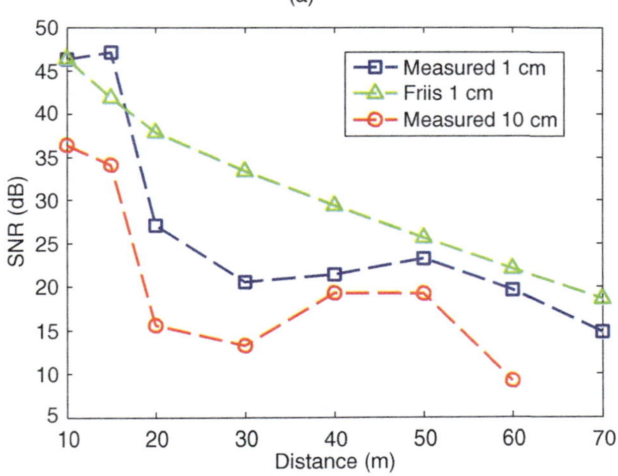

(b)

Figure 11.15 (a) Measurement setup for the long-range on-body wireless sensors [14]. (b) Measured signal-to-noise ratios at different distances [14]. (*Source*: Lin, T., Bito, J., Hester, J. G. D., et al., 2017. © IEEE.)

away as depicted in Figure 11.15a. The signal-to-noise ratio (SNR) at different tag-to-reader distances are summarized in Figure 11.15b. The "measured 1 cm" line means that the distance between the wearable harvester that generated the carrier and the sensor tag was 1 cm, while the "measured 10 cm" means that the distance was 10 cm. The theoretical results calculated using Friis transmission equation were also included for comparison, and the basic trend was the same except for some points where constructive or destructive interferences occur. Since the typically required SNR for detection is 3 dB, according to Friis equation, the maximum detection range for the proposed system is 266 m.

11.4.2 Radar and Backscatter Communications

The previous section discusses various means by which an additively manufactured wireless module may be powered. This makes up only a part of the integrated system; another factor which must be considered is the means of communication employed by the device. It is important to select an optimal means of communication that would minimize the monetary cost of system implementation as well as its total power consumption. Backscatter communication presents a unique solution in that it is easily densely implemented and presents very low start-up costs. Backscatter communication involves the modulation and reflection of an incident RF carrier. In this way, energy is only expended one way in the communication link as any information can be encoded in the reflected and modulated radio-frequency signal. Typical backscatter communication links are deployed for radio-frequency identification (RFID) applications in the UHF bands; however, there has been increasing investigation into the use of millimeter-wave frequencies due to the increased availability of bandwidth and less-stringent EIRP requirements which could allow the RFIDs to be minimized in size and operated at longer ranges. In addition, the push to use millimeter-wave frequencies enables the production of lower form factor and high-performance wireless modules. Given a dense implementation of RFID devices for medical and biomonitoring applications owing to the advent of the IoT, a proper way to simultaneously interrogate and gather useful information from an array of sensors is required. An attractive means to achieve this is through the employment of RADAR principles, specifically frequency-modulated continuous wave (FMCW). The use of FMCW RADAR enables a single reader to interrogate and gather data from a multitude of wireless modules simultaneously as well as incorporate information that would otherwise not be available or be very difficult to obtain giving the conventional RFID framework such as position and velocity. Figure 11.16 shows the architecture of a typical FMCW radar receiver. Localization information such as distance, angle of arrival, and velocity can be determined from the FMCW process in which a chirp signal is transmitted and the delayed received chirp is mixed with the original signal so that a

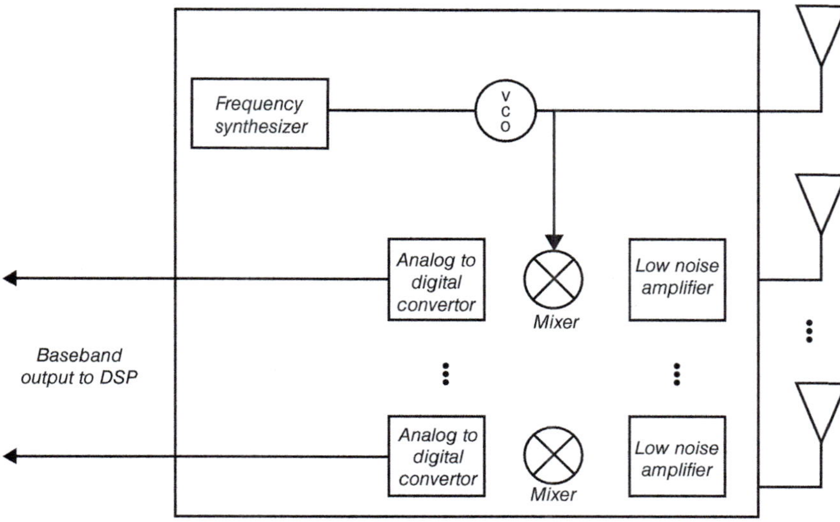

Figure 11.16 Block diagram of a MIMO FMCW reader [17]. (*Source*: Adeyeye, A. O., Hester, J., and Tentzeris, M. M., 2019. © IEEE.)

constant beat frequency is obtained which is proportional to the range of the target [18]. Angle of arrival is evaluated by taking advantage of multiple receive channels spaced half a wavelength apart so that the angle of arrival is an inverse trigonometric function of the phase difference between the channels. Finally, Doppler which contains velocity is obtained by observing the difference in phase between successive chirps in a given receive channel. The work presented in this section illustrates high-performing RFID topologies that prove to be more than suitable candidates to satisfy the exponentially increasing demand for low-power, low-cost wireless sensors and modules for use in medical applications.

11.4.2.1 FMCW Radar-Enabled Localizable Millimeter-Wave RFID

An increasing demand and need for contactless sensing particularly in the realm of biomonitoring and sensing for the detection of both stationary and moving targets has led a wide variety of investigations into how RFID technology can be incorporated to achieve this, specifically investigating the use of millimeter-wave frequency bands and the advantages that come with it as described above. In this work, a miniaturized millimeter-wave RFID tag is presented operating in the 24-GHz ISM band for spatial localization in IoT applications. The result is a low-form factor, low-power millimeter-wave RFID shown in Figure 11.17 with dimensions of $18 \times 22\,\text{mm}^2$. Evaluating the spatial location of a biosensor is of great interest and use to healthcare professionals. For example, it could be necessary to monitor a wide array of

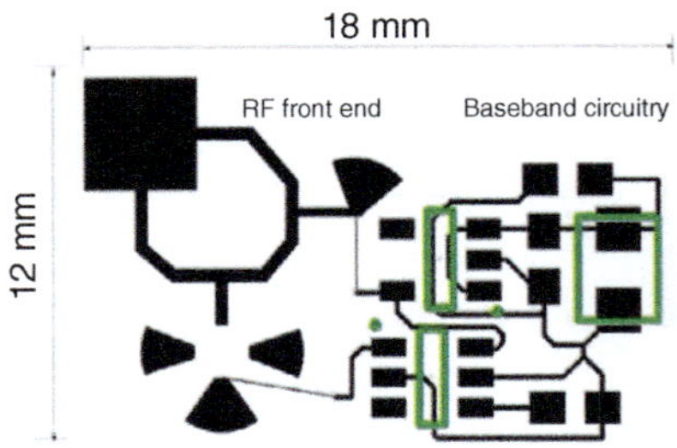

(a)

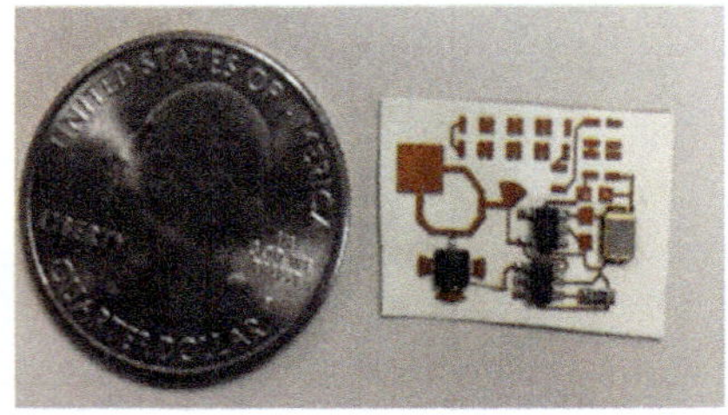

(b)

Figure 11.17 Millimeter-wave RFID tag: (a) tag design and layout and (b) fabricated prototype [17]. (*Source*: Adeyeye, A. O., Hester, J., and Tentzeris, M. M., 2019. © European Microwave Association.)

sensors across a variety of patients in a healthcare facility so it would be of paramount importance to know which sensors are producing the different sets of data. As discussed earlier, it is feasible to obtain range and angle of arrival by employing the MIMO FMCW process. A radar is used to resolve the modulated backscattered signal returned by the spatially distributed RFID tags with each tag's angular and range information encoded in the beat frequency and phase distribution across the multiple receive channels. The major advantage in using a modulated backscattering approach in conjunction with the FMCW radar shows up primarily in the SNR that can be achieved [17]. Nearby reflectors and self-interference/coupling between the TX/RX channels generate low-frequency components around DC, but in applying a modulated backscatter approach, the beat signal information can be shifted away from that cluttering and give much better SNR as shown in Figure 11.18.

11.4.3 Flexible and Deployable 4D Origami-Inspired "Smart Walls" for EMI Shielding and Communication Applications

Recently, there has been a growing trend toward the realization of "digital hospitals" through the integration of multiple wireless communication modules in various medical devices (MDs) and the physical infrastructure of the hospital to improve control, monitoring, portability, and communication between various MDs, resulting in an efficient, cost-effective, and higher quality of healthcare. However, the exponential increase in personal wireless communication devices such as cell phones, laptops, and tablets presents various challenges such as the need for electromagnetic compatibility (EMC) and electromagnetic interference (EMI) reduction between various wireless devices. Typical sources of EMI include electromagnetic waves from outside the hospital, residual magnetic-flux density at welding points in the building, conveyance systems with linear motors, the shielding within the hospital walls, and the commercial wireless devices such as cell phones, tablets, and laptops [19]. Therefore,

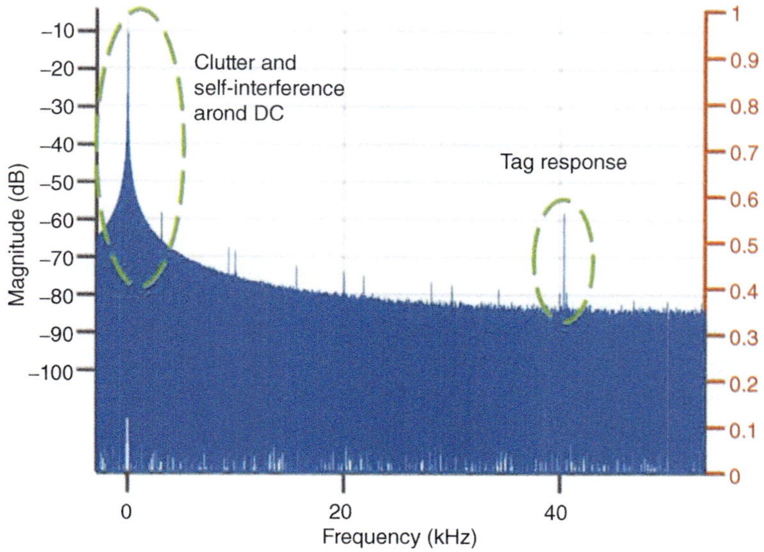

Figure 11.18 Received signal spectrum showing clutter and tag response.

comprehensive EM field measurements and realization of expensive nontunable shielding structures within the hospital walls are required to effectively eliminate EMI. Moreover, commercial wireless products are not subjected to stringent electronic instrumentation testing compared to modern MDs, making them a vital source for EMI. Hence, a lightweight and structurally strong tunable EM-shielding structure is required to block spurious EM radiations in such environments.

These problems can be addressed by realizing flexible and easily deployable frequency-selective surfaces (FSSs) with wideband tunability that can be installed within the hospital walls to block unwanted EM waves. Traditional mesh-like Faraday's cage-based shielding structures are one of the most commonly used structures that block all external EM waves. In contrast, specialized structures such as FSSs can be designed to block only the undesired frequency bands, making lightweight, cost-effective, and less prone to develop residual surface currents. These structures typically consist of an array of resonant elements etched on a rigid substrate that filter EM waves based on the size, shape, and type of the resonant elements. Traditional FSS structures are susceptible to variations in their frequency behavior due to installation errors, manufacturing tolerance, or random failures/breakages of the resonant elements. That is why it is advantageous to incorporate tunability and flexibility with such structures to account for detuning effects and improve structural integrity. Conventional techniques to realize tunability include using electronic components such as diodes, varactors, ferromagnetic materials, and microelectromagnetic systems (MEMS) switches with the resonant elements; however, these techniques tend to become expensive, laborious, and hard to realize as the overall size of the FSS structure increases.

A novel fully inkjet-printed flexible origami-inspired tunable Miura-FSS structure with an integrated thermal actuation mechanism is introduced in this section, which can realize wideband continuous range tunability by simply changing its shape, thus avoiding the use of any expensive and complicated electronic components. The Miura-Ori tessellation was used as the origami structure in this work to transform a conventional flat dipole-based FSS—inkjet-printed on a (polyester-based) heat sensitive substrate—into a 3D/4D shape-reconfigurable Miura-FSS structure. The structure facilitates a systematic change in electrical length and interelement distance between the dipole elements with folding to realize wideband resonant frequency tunability. These structures drastically simplify fabrication and tuning complexity of mechanically tuned FSS structure while facilitating flat foldability, high flexibility, and single degree of actuation, thereby improving their portability.

The unit cell of all polyester-based multilayer Miura-frequency-selective surface (MLM-FSS) structure is shown in Figure 11.19, which consists of a heat-sensitive shape-reconfigurable Miura spacer layer sandwiched between two single-layer Miura-frequency-selective surface (SLM-FSS) layers. The fabricated MLM-FSS is shown in Figure 11.21. The multilayer configuration improves the folding behavior, bandwidth, and structural strength of the overall structure, thereby allowing it to be used as the filling material in a dry wall in a sandwich configuration. A comparison of SLM-FSS and MLM-FSS under different loading conditions is shown in Figure 11.20, which clearly demonstrates the superior load handling of the latter structure. It is important to note here that the polyester-based substrate transforms from a rigid to a soft form when subjected to high temperatures (about 35°C), which facilitates the overall shape reconfiguration of the MLM-FSS structure and improves its flexibility. The two SLM-FSS layers were realized by inkjet-printing dipoles across the mountain fold lines on polyester-based substrate to ensure systematic variation in electrical length and interelement distances between the dipoles [20, 22]. Since polyester-based substrate is rigid (and brittle) at room temperature, small (2.5-mm wide) holes were etched at all vertices to avoid crack propagation and to simplify the folding process—a technique that is particularly useful for thick or 3D printed origami structures [23]. A detailed description of the fabrication process and kinematic analysis of the proposed structure was given in Nauroze and Tentzeris [21] (Figure 11.21).

The MLM-FSS with a polyester-based substrate was fabricated to evaluate its thermal response. The sample was completely folded ($\theta < 60°$) and placed in the oven. Since the polyester-based substrate is rigid at room temperature, folding the Miura structure would induce some energy in the hinges/fold

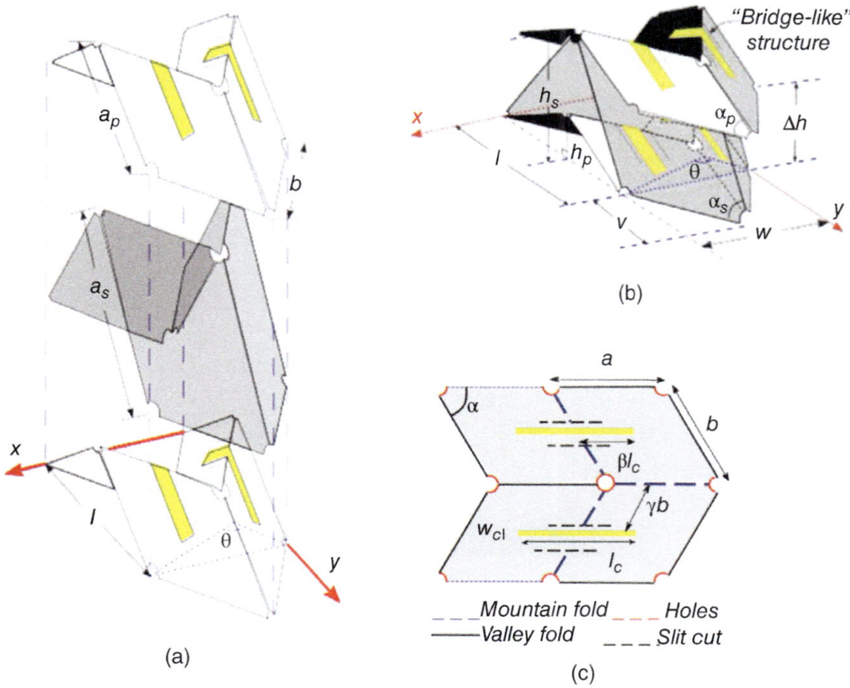

Figure 11.19 Unit cell of MLM-FSS in (a) exploded view and (b) assembled and folded configuration ($\alpha_p = 45°$). (c) Unit cell of each SLM-FSS in flat configuration ($\theta = 180°$). $b_s = b_p = b = a_p = 20$ mm. $\beta = \gamma = 0.5$, $l_c = 20$ mm, and $w_c = 2$ mm [20]. (*Source*: Modified from Nauroze, S. A., Novelino, L., Tentzeris, M. M., et al., 2017.)

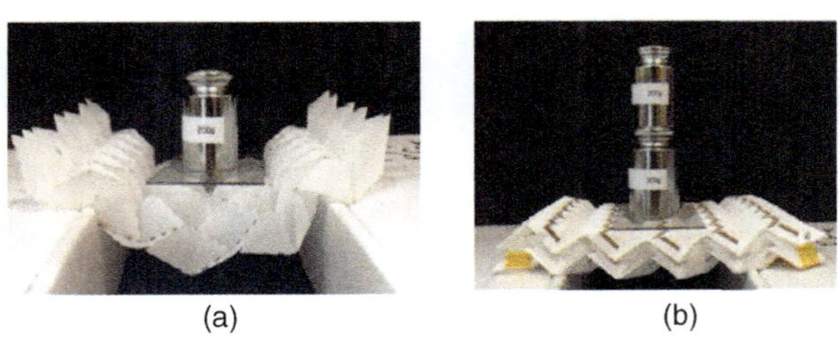

Figure 11.20 Structural response of (a) single-layer polyester-based Miura structure. (b) MLM-FSS with polyester spacer [21]. (*Source*: Nauroze, S.A. and Tentzeris, M.M., 2019. © IEEE.)

lines that tend to expand as they are released. It was observed that at room temperature, the Miura would expand slightly if released from its folded configuration. However, due to energy loss, it does not expand to its completely folded configuration. However, when the folded Miura is heated uniformly,

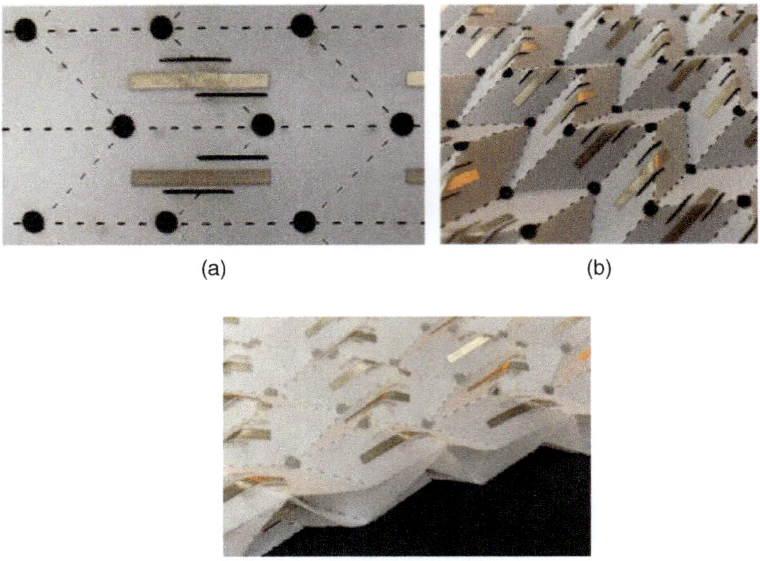

(a) (b) (c)

Figure 11.21 Fabricated SLM-FSS in (a) flat and (b) folded configuration. (c) Complete MLM-FSS structure in folded state assembled using in-line stacking configuration [20]. (*Source*: Nauroze, S.A., Hester, J. G., Tehrani, B. K., et al., 2017. © IEEE.)

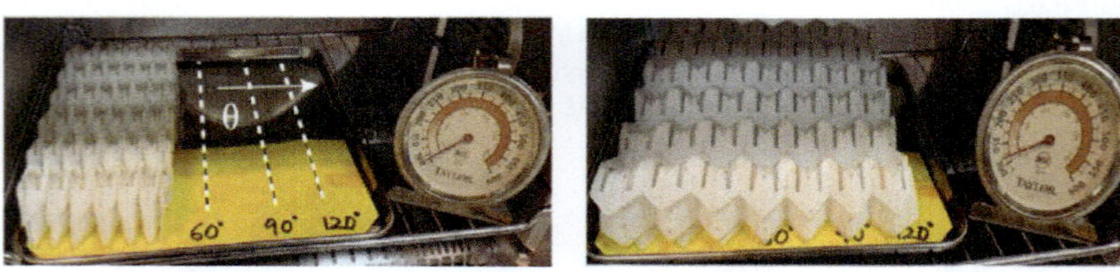

Figure 11.22 Thermal actuation of all polyester-based MLM-FSS structure with spacer layer sandwiched between two SLM-FSS structures. The marking indicates Miura extension for different values of θ [20]. (*Source*: Nauroze, S.A., Hester, J. G., Tehrani, B. K., et al., 2017. © IEEE.)

the polyester-based substrate transitions from rigid to soft state allowing the hinges/fold lines to unfold further, thus resulting in an expansion of the overall Miura structure as shown in Figure 11.22. It was observed that the polyester-based Miura FSS structures started to unfold when uniformly heated beyond 35°C in the oven and realized a completely unfolded configuration at 50°C with an unfolding rate of $\theta = 4°/°C$. While it was very difficult to

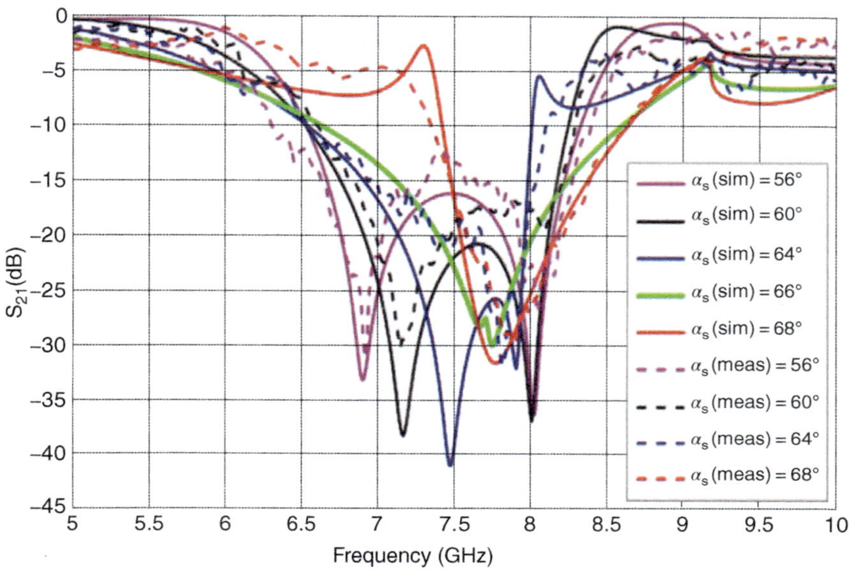

Figure 11.23 Frequency response of an MLM-FSS structure ($\theta = 90°$) for different values of internal angle (αs) of spacer layer [20]. (*Source*: Modified from Nauroze, S. A., Novelino, L., Tentzeris, M. M., et al., 2017.)

control/stop the unfolding process at a given state, the rate of Miura unfolding can be controlled by varying the temperature gradient.

The unit cell of the proposed MLM-FSS was simulated using master/slave boundary conditions in HFSS with Floquet port excitation. The simulated results were then verified experimentally using two broadband horn antennas placed facing each other with the MLM-FSS in the middle. The simulated and measured insertion loss ($S21$) of the MLM-FSS with respect to different values of αs shown in Figure 11.23 clearly indicate that at lower values of αs, the structure exhibits a broadband behavior with two distinct resonances. The lower resonance frequency is the result of the mutual coupling between the two SLM-FSS layers, while the higher frequency is the resonant frequency of the individual SLM-FSS layers. The interlayer distance increases with s, which results in shifting the coupling frequency toward the resonant frequency value. The frequency response of the proposed MLM-FSS with respect to various folding angles (θ) and angles of incidence (AoI) are shown in Figure 11.24a and b, respectively. It can be easily seen that not only the proposed structure preserves its (wideband) frequency behavior under different folding configurations and AoI, but it can also realize continuous-range tunability by simply changing its folding angle.

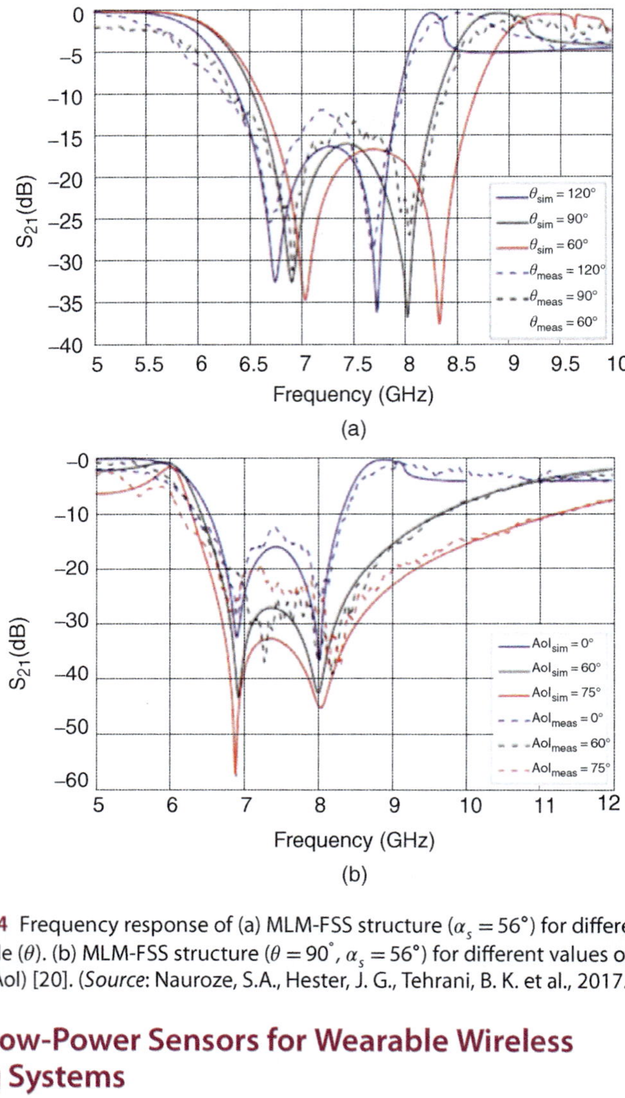

Figure 11.24 Frequency response of (a) MLM-FSS structure ($\alpha_s = 56°$) for different values of folding angle (θ). (b) MLM-FSS structure ($\theta = 90^{\circ}$, $\alpha_s = 56°$) for different values of angle of incidence (AoI) [20]. (*Source*: Nauroze, S.A., Hester, J. G., Tehrani, B. K. et al., 2017.)

11.5 Low-Power Sensors for Wearable Wireless Sensing Systems

11.5.1 Carbon-Nanomaterials-Based Fully Inkjet-Printed Gas Sensors

Wearable systems used for medical applications can greatly benefit from the ability to gather chemical exposure data of the wearer during extended amounts of time. Such capabilities open the door for an enhanced understanding of

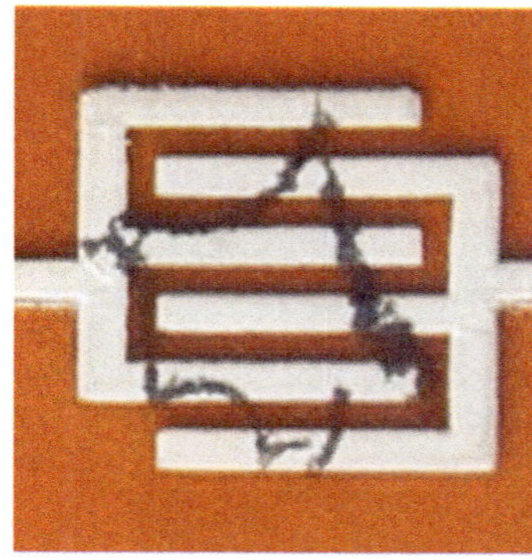

Figure 11.25 Image of a sensor fabricated using a naive ink-deposition process [28]. (*Source*: Hester, J., 2019.)

chronic illnesses, enabled by the continual gathering of longitudinal data. Inkjet printing—the most versatile additive manufacturing technology, along with aerosol jet printing—allows the rapid, tunable, and low-cost fabrication of nanomaterials-based resistometric sensors for airborne chemical analyte levels detection and monitoring. Recent efforts have demonstrated the use of thin films of nanomaterials and conductive polymers to enable the detection of gases as varied as NO2 [24], CO [25], CH4 [26], and NH3 [27]. While most of these thin-film components were not fabricated using inkjet printing, this technique can deliver an amount of precision and repeatability in the deposition of nanomaterials-carrying inks that cannot be matched by the manual deposition techniques that are usually employed in these works. An example of the consequences of this lack of control is shown in Figure 11.25.

In this figure, an optical image of a piece of polyimide substrate upon which was inkjet printed a silver-nanoparticle-based interdigitated electrode structure, followed by the deposition of a drop carbon-nanotubes ink can be seen. However, the dynamics of the drying process induce the migration of the nanotubes dispersed in the ink and cause the nonuniform deposition of the nanotubes. This pseudorandom process leads to variations of sensitivity and resistance values for these resistometric sensors by orders of magnitude, within individual batches. However, the control allowed by inkjet printing allows the adoption of another strategy. The process, shown in Figure 11.26, prints complementary arrays of droplets whose discontinuity does not allow the migration of the nanotubes suspended in the ink. These patterns are printed alternatively and dried to form a film whose uniformity is difficult to match with other deposition techniques.

Once properly deposited, this planar semiconducting and high-surface-area matrix of nanotubes can be functionalized to enhance its sensitivity to the targeted analytes. This functionalization can be conducted through wet processes

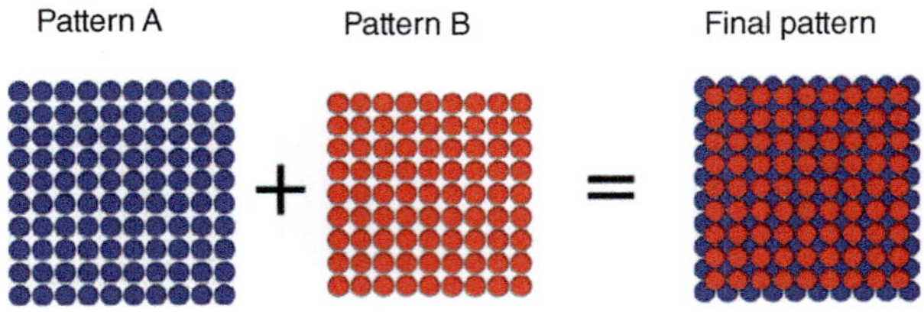

Figure 11.26 Process of the inkjet-printing technique employed to print uniform carbon-nanotube films [28]. *Source*: Hester, J., 2019.

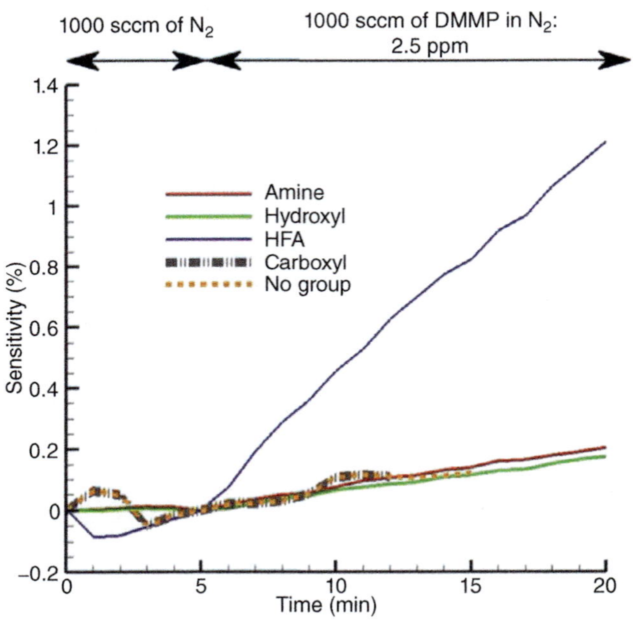

Figure 11.27 Measured sensitivity to DMMP of carbon-nanotube-based sensors with different functional groups [28]. *Source*: Hester, J., 2019 and Hester, J.G.D. and Tentzeris, M.M., 2017.)

that specifically target the surface of the nanotubes or by subsequently printing a functionalizing ink. The increases in sensitivity that can be reaped through this approach is exemplified by the measurements shown in Figure 11.27. In this specific experiment, carbon nanotubes were functionalized with a selection of functional groups ranging from amines to carboxyl groups. A hydrofluoroalcohol (HFA) stands out, displaying its ability to enhance the response of such sensors to dimethyl methylphosphonate (DMMP), a nerve agent simulant.

Using such approaches, it is possible to print arrays of nanomaterial-based sensors with varying chemical functionalizations and, therefore, different sensitivities to a range of analytes of interest. All of this can be achieved in an ultra-low-cost fashion, thereby enabling the emergence of ultra-low-power wearable electronic noses, such as the ones described in Hester [28] and Hester and Tentzeris [29].

11.5.2 Energy-Autonomous Micropump System for Wearable and IoT Microfluidic Sensing Devices

Microfluidics is a significant technique for tunable RF components and sensing methods over the past decade [30]. However, microfluidic applications remain restrictive due to the inevitable requirement for actuation forces that move fluidics inside the microchannels. Typical ways of moving fluidics include manually pressing fluidics into the channels using syringes [31], pumps [32], and electrochemically controlled capillarity [33]. All methods require a certain amount of power or voltage to drive the system which significantly limits their applications.

In order to expand the applications of microfluidics, an energy-autonomous and wearable actuation force is required. In Lin et al. [34], an energy-autonomous, flexible, and wearable micropump system was proposed. The block diagram of the proposed system is shown in Figure 11.28a, and the prototype is shown in Figure 11.28b. The broadband RF energy harvester which harnesses both near-field 464.5-MHz two-way radio and far-field UHF RFID from 850 to 950 MHz was utilized to eliminate the need for batteries. The energy harvester utilized an antenna to collect the energy from both ambient energy sources and a rectifier to output the required DC power. The DC power was used to drive the driving IC that generated the necessary waveform to activate the micropump. The micropump can be used to move any type of liquid through the microchannel, and a tunable band-stop filter was used as a demonstration.

Since we need to collect the energy from 464.5 and 850—950 MHz, a broadband behavior is necessary. One of the key elements in this system was the broadband rectifier as shown in Figure 11.29. The measured S11 under different input power levels are shown in Figure 11.30a. The measured S11 are all less than −9 dB from 300 to 1200 MHz, which covers all frequency bands of interest. The measured output powers at different frequencies are shown in Figure 11.30b. The simulated results using Advanced Design System (ADS) are also included for comparisons, and good agreements can be observed. The flat response once again proves the broadband coverage of the proposed rectifier.

Since the micropump operates based on piezoelectric principles, the periodic high-voltage waveform is required to press the liquid through the microchannel. The output voltage waveform at the output pin of the driver IC is shown in Figure 11.31a. The expected periodic high-voltage waveform can be obtained at the output pin of the driver IC. As shown in Figure 11.31a, since the two-way

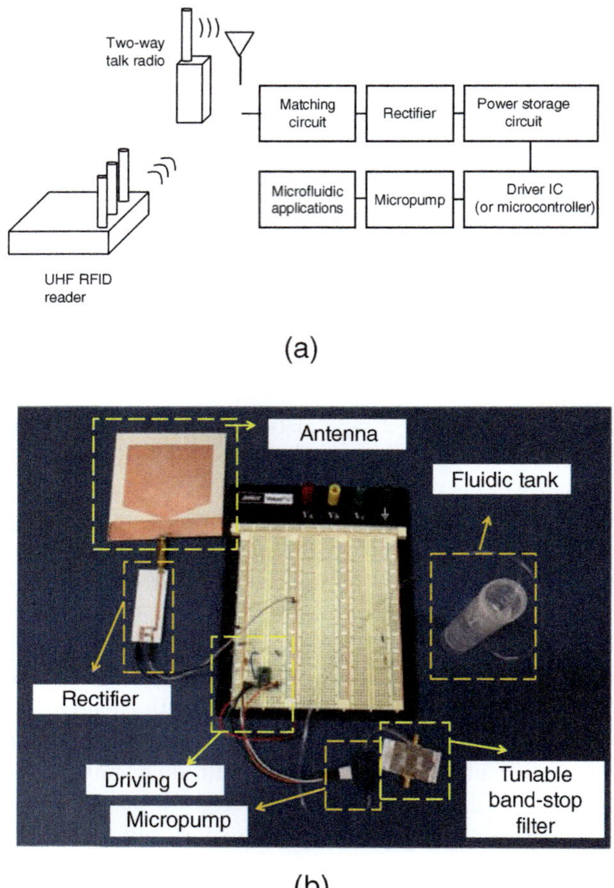

Figure 11.28 (a) Block diagram of the proposed energy-autonomous microfluidic system [34]. (b) The measurement setup of the proposed energy-autonomous microfluidic system [34]. (*Source*: Lin, T., Su, W., and Tentzeris, M.M., 2018,. © IEEE.)

talk radio can support high energy density, the IC can be turned on immediately with an output voltage of 67.2 V. The noise in the flat low-voltage area of the two-way talk radio measurement is due to the coupling between the two-way talk radio and the probing cable of the oscilloscope. Moreover, the output voltage is 10.2 V while using the UHF-charged supercapacitor.

The proposed energy harvester can acquire enough energy from either the 464.5 two-way radio or the UHF RFID reader to activate the micropump and move liquid inside the microchannel. As an example of a microfluidic application, the tunable band-stop filter, as shown in Figure 11.28b, is connected to the micropump. The measured S21 is shown in Figure 11.31b, and the stop

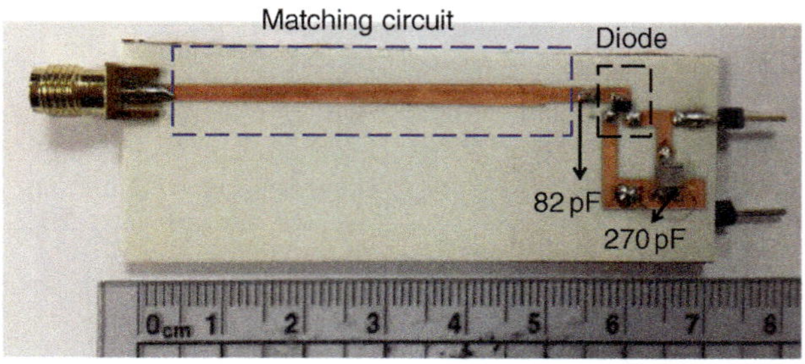

Figure 11.29 The prototype of the broadband rectifier [34]. (*Source*: Lin, T., Su, W., and Tentzeris, M.M., 2018, . © IEEE.)

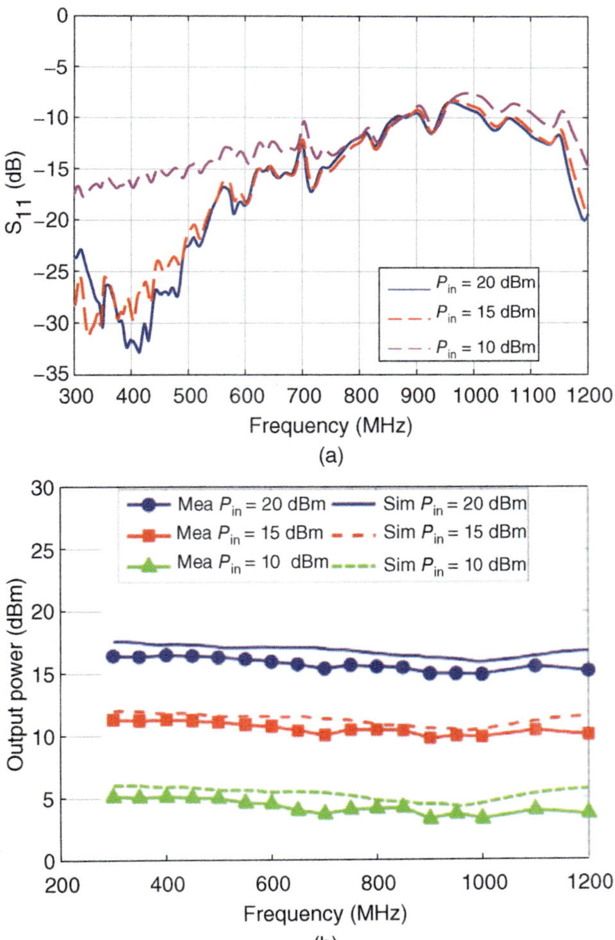

Figure 11.30 (a) Measured S_{11} of the proposed broadband rectifier [34]. (b) Measured and simulated output DC power of the proposed rectifier [34]. (*Source*: Lin, T., Su, W., and Tentzeris, M.M., 2018,. © IEEE.)

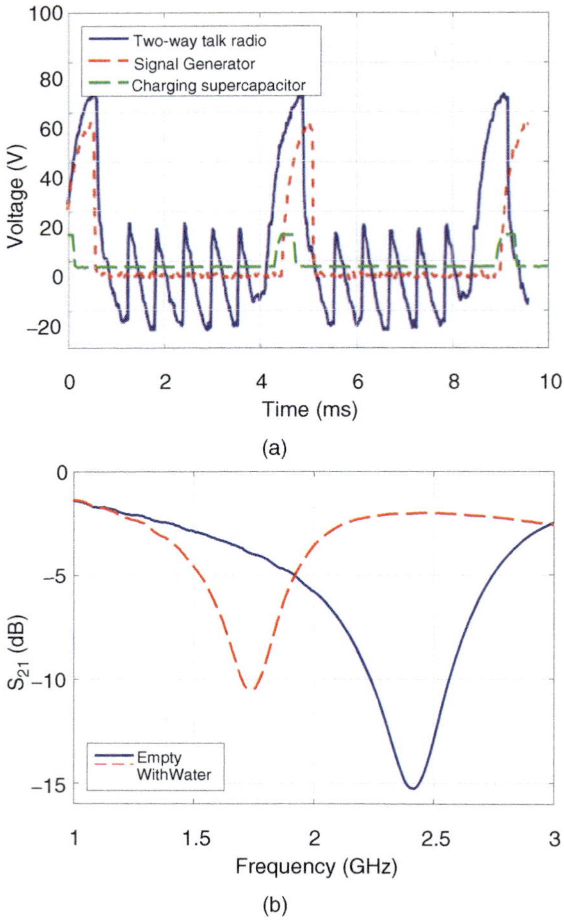

Figure 11.31 (a) Output voltage waveform at the output pin of the driver IC [34]. (b) Measured S_{21} of a liquid-tunable band-stop filter [34]. (*Source*: Lin, T., Su, W., and Tentzeris, M.M., 2018. © IEEE.)

band can be tuned by pumping the water into the microchannel using the proposed energy-autonomous micropump system.

11.5.3 Fully Inkjet-Printed Encodable Flexible Microfluidic Chipless RFID Sensor

Microfluidic systems are promising platforms for medical diagnostics and biosensing applications. Combining microfluidic channels with multiresonator chipless RFID tags can enable unprecedented capabilities for individual frequency tunability, higher accuracy, and wireless measurement. However, microfluidic channels are generally fabricated with traditional photolithography and associated techniques that are expensive, time consuming, and primarily subtractive. In order to manufacture microfluidic structures in a

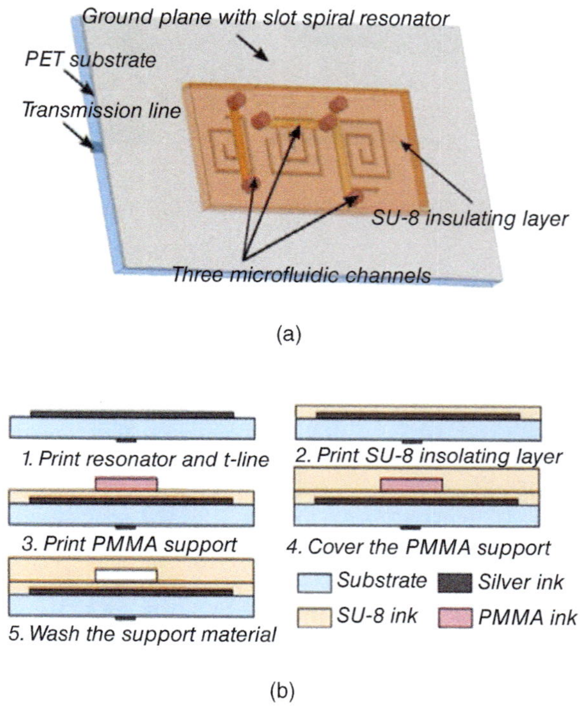

Figure 11.32 (a) The design of the proposed microfluidic RFID sensor. (b) The five-step fabrication process of the proposed microfluidic RFID sensor.

low-cost, rapid, and environmentally friendly manner, Cui et al. [35] and Su et al. [36] proposed a fully inkjet-printed encodable flexible microfluidic chipless RFID sensor.

The proposed sensor structure is shown in Figure 11.32a with three different-sized slot spiral resonators resonant at frequencies 3.4, 4.5, and 5.9 GHz. Microfluidic channels are placed in the spiral's gap between adjacent turns. By filling or removing the liquid in each channel, three resonant frequencies can be configured independently, so the RFID sensor can be "encoded" with 3bit information. The five-step fabrication process is shown in Figure 11.32b. The sensor was printed on a 125-μm-thick MELINEX ST505 PET substrate using Fujifilm Dimatix DMP-2800 inkjet-printing system (Figure 11.33).

The simulation and measurement results are shown in Figure 11.34a and b, respectively. Distilled water is used as filling liquid during measurement; when water is added to a channel, the dielectric constant on top of the resonator will change from 1 (air) to 80 (water). The increased dielectric constant will cause a resonant frequency decrement due to the increased capacitance. If the simulation and measurement matched well, the code of the RFID sensor can be defined by selectively adding or removing liquid

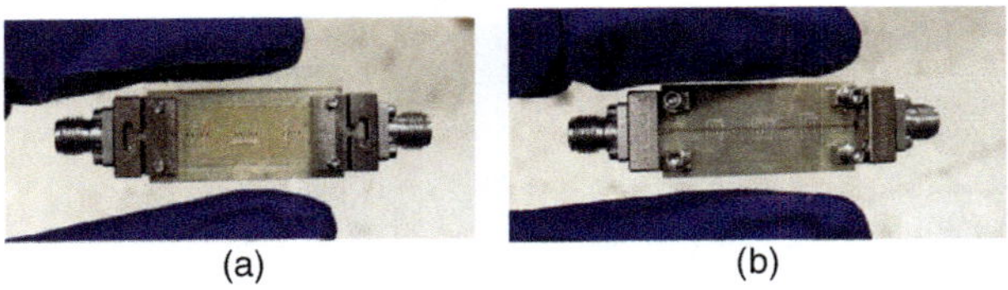

Figure 11.33 (a) Fabricated sample (front). (b) Fabricated sample (back).

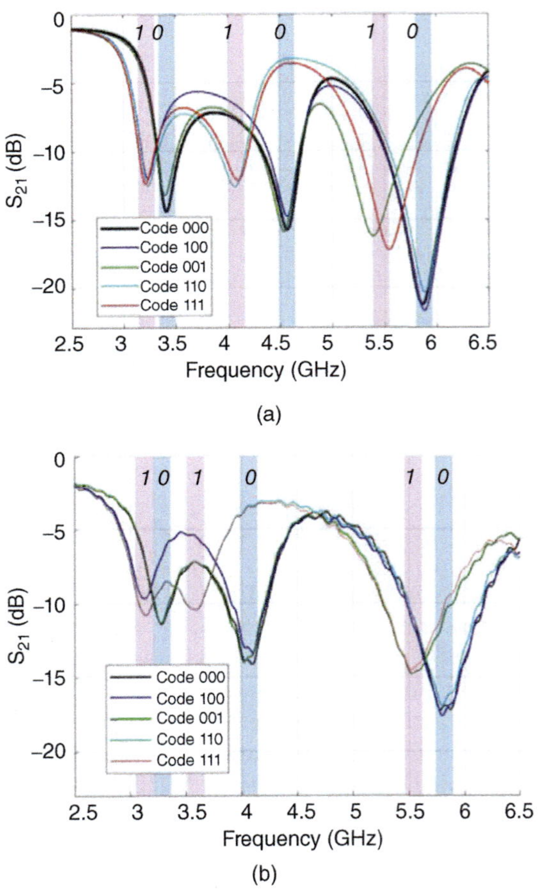

Figure 11.34 (a) Simulated insertion loss vs frequency. (b) Measured insertion loss vs frequency.

from the microfluidic channel. The frequency response can also be obtained wirelessly using cross-polarized antennas with machine-learning techniques [37]. This fully inkjet-printed microfluidic chipless RFID sensor can find applications in various areas including liquid analysis, biosensing, and medical diagnostics.

11.6 Conclusion

The projects and results succinctly presented in this chapter offer only a small preview of the veritable Cambrian explosion of innovations born during the past two decades to set the foundation for the emergence of a greatly anticipated and socially transformative offering of smart wearable health devices that will be able to monitor (among others) their users' very movements, heart beats, physical and mental activities, and chemical and physical exposure and stress levels. Technologies with these sensing and illness-predicting capabilities are, for many of them, on the cusp of the maturity levels required for market readiness. However, the printed wireless powering, packaging, wireless communications and shielding, and sensing innovations presented in this chapter are revealing what lies beyond: a future where custom-flexible wearable health devices can be printed at home or in local micromanufacturing centers to bring health monitoring to the many, where they need it and at a cost that most can afford.

References

1 Eid, A., Hester, J., Nauroze, A., et al. (2018). A flexible compact rectenna for 2.40 Hz ISM energy harvesting applications. 2018 IEEE International Symposium on Antennas and Propagation & USNC/URSI National Radio Science Meeting. IEEE, 1887–1888.
2 Eid, A., Hester, J., and Tentzeris, M.M. (2019). A scalable high-gain and large-beamwidth mm-wave harvesting approach for 5G-powered IoT. Proceedings of the 2019 IEEE MTT-S International Microwave Symposium (IMS). IEEE, 1309–1312.
3 Eid, A., Hester, J., Tehrani, B., and Tentzeris, M. (2019). Flexible w-band rectifiers for 5G-powered IoT autonomous modules. 2019 IEEE International Symposium on Antennas and Propagation and USNC-URSI Radio Science Meeting. IEEE, 1163–1164.
4 Tehrani, B.K., Cook, B.S., and Tentzeris, M.M. (2016). Inkjet-printed 3D interconnects for millimeter-wave system-on-package solutions. 2016 IEEE MTT-S International Microwave Symposium (IMS). IEEE, 1–4.
5 Eid, A., Hester, J., Fang, Y. et al. (2018). Nanotechnology-empowered flexible printed wireless electronics: a review of various applications of printed materials. *IEEE Nanotechnology Magazine* 13 (1): 18–29.
6 Eid, A., Tehrani, B., Hester, J., et al. (2018). Nanotechnology-enabled additively-manufactured RF and millimeter-wave electronics. 2018 IEEE 13th Nanotechnology Materials and Devices Conference (NMDC), IEEE, 1–4.

7 Tehrani, B.K. and Tentzeris, M.M. (2018). Fully inkjet-printed ramp interconnects for wireless ka-band MMIC devices and multi-chip module packaging. 2018 48th European Microwave Conference (EuMC), September 2018, 1037–1040.

8 He, X., Tehrani, B.K., Bahr, R.A. et al. (2020). Additively manufactured mm-wave multichip modules with fully printed "smart" encapsulation structures. *IEEE Transactions on Microwave Theory and Techniques* 68 (7): 2716–2724.

9 Lin, T., Daskalakis, S.N., Georgiadis, A., and Tentzeris, M.M. (2019). Achieving fully autonomous system-on-package designs: an embedded-on-package 5G energy harvester within 3D printed multilayer flexible packaging structures. 2019 IEEE MTT-S International Microwave Symposium (IMS), June 2019, 1375–1378.

10 Lin, T., Bito, J., and Tentzeris, M.M. (2017). Wearable inkjet printed energy harvester. 2017 IEEE International Symposium on Antennas and Propagation US-NC/URSI National Radio Science Meeting, July 2017, 1613–1614.

11 Lin, T., Raj, P.M., Watanabe, A., et al. (2017). Nanostructured miniaturized artificial magnetic conductors (AMC) for high-performance antennas in 5G, IoT, and smart skin applications 2017 IEEE 17th International Conference on Nanotechnology (IEEE-NANO), July 2017, 911–915.

12 Huo, Y., Dong, X., and Xu, W. (2017). 5G cellular user equipment: from theory to practical hardware design. *IEEE Access* 5: 13992–14010.

13 Lin, T., Bahr, R., Tentzeris, M.M., et al. (2018). Novel 3D-/inkjet-printed flexible on-package antennas, packaging structures, and modules for broadband 5G applications. 2018 IEEE 68th Electronic Components and Technology Conference (ECTC), May 2018, 214–220.

14 Lin, T., Bito, J., Hester, J.G.D. et al. (2017). On-body long-range wireless backscattering sensing system using inkjet-/3-D-printed flexible ambient RF energy harvesters capable of simultaneous DC and harmonics generation. *IEEE Transactions on Microwave Theory and Techniques* 65 (12): 5389–5400.

15 Lin, T., Bito, J., Hester, J.G., et al. (2017). Ambient energy harvesting from two-way talk radio for on-body autonomous wireless sensing network using inkjet and 3D printing. 2017 IEEE MTT-S International Microwave Symposium (IMS), June 2017, 1034–1037.

16 Kimionis, J., Bletsas, A., and Sahalos, J.N. (2014). Increased range bistatic scatter radio. *IEEE Transactions on Communications* 62 (3): 1091–1104.

17 Adeyeye, A.O., Hester, J., and Tentzeris, M.M. (2019). Miniaturized millimeter wave RFID tag for spatial identification and localization in internet of things applications. 2019 49th European Microwave Conference (EuMC), October 2019, 105–108, doi: https://doi.org/10.23919/EuMC.2019.8910740.

18 Sorrentino, R., Sbarra, E., Urbani, L., et al. (2012). Accurate FMCW radar-based indoor localization system. 2012 IEEE International Conference on RFID-Technologies and Applications (RFID-TA), November 2012, 362–368, doi: https://doi.org/10.1109/RFID-TA.2012.6404547.

19 Hanada, E., Takano, K., Antoku, Y. et al. (2002). A practical procedure to prevent electro-magnetic interference with electronic medical equipment. *Journal of Medical Systems* 26 (1): 61–65.

20 Nauroze, S.A., Hester, J.G., Tehrani, B.K. et al. (2017). Additively manufactured RF components and modules: toward empowering the birth of cost-efficient dense and ubiquitous IoT implementations. *Proceedings of the IEEE* 105 (4): 702–722. ISSN 0018-9219. doi: https://doi.org/10.1109/JPROC.2017.2658565.

21 Nauroze, S.A. and Tentzeris, M.M. (2019). A thermally actuated fully inkjet-printed origami-inspired multilayer frequency selective surface with continuous-range tunability using polyester-based substrates. *IEEE Transactions on Microwave Theory and Techniques* 67 (12): 4944–4954.

22 Nauroze, S.A., Novelino, L., Tentzeris, M.M., and Paulino, G.H. (2017). Inkjet-printed "4D" tunable spatial filters using on-demand foldable surfaces. 2017 IEEE MTT-S International Microwave Symposium (IMS), June 2017, 1575–1578, doi: https://doi.org/10.1109/MWSYM.2017.8058932.

23 Yuan, C., Wang, T., Dunn, M.L., and Qi, H.J. (2017). 3D printed active origami with complicated folding patterns. *International Journal of Precision Engineering and Manufacturing-Green Technology* 4 (3): 281–289.

24 Dua, V., Surwade, S.P., Ammu, S. et al. (2010). All-organic vapor sensor using inkjet-printed reduced graphene oxide. *Angewandte Chemie International Edition* 49 (12): 2154–2157.

25 Bittencourt, C., Felten, A., Espinosa, E.H. et al. (2006). WO 3 films modified with functionalised multi-wall carbon nanotubes: morphological, compositional and gas response studies. *Sensors and Actuators B: Chemical* 115 (1): 33–41.

26 Lu, Y., Li, J., Han, J. et al. (2004). Room temperature methane detection using palladium loaded single-walled carbon nanotube sensors. *Chemical Physics Letters* 391 (4): 344–348.

27 Jang, J., Ha, J., and Cho, J. (2007). Fabrication of water-dispersible polyaniline-poly (4-styrenesulfonate) nanoparticles for inkjet-printed chemical-sensor applications. *Advanced Materials* 19 (13): 1772–1775.

28 Hester, J. (2019). Low Cost Printed, Flexible, and Energy Autonomous Van-Atta And Carbon-Nanotubes-Based mm-Wave RFID Gas Sensors for Ultra-Long-Range Ubiquitous IoT and 5G Implementations. PhD thesis, Georgia Institute of Technology.

29 Hester, J.G.D. and Tentzeris, M.M. (2017). A mm-wave ultra-long-range energy-autonomous printed RFID-enabled van-atta wireless sensor: at the crossroads of 5G and IoT. Microwave Symposium (IMS), 2017 IEEE MTT-S International, IEEE, 1557–1560.

30 Entesari, K. and Saghati, A.P. (2016). Fluidics in microwave components. *IEEE Microwave Magazine* 17 (6): 50–75.

31 Mumcu, G., Dey, A., and Palomo, T. (2013). Frequency-agile bandpass filters using liquid metal tunable broadside coupled split ring resonators. *IEEE Microwave and Wireless Components Letters* 23 (4): 187–189.

32 Barrera, J.D. and Huff, G.H. (2014). A fluidic loading mechanism in a polarization reconfigurable antenna with a comparison to solid state approaches. *IEEE Transactions on Antennas and Propagation* 62 (8): 4008–4014.

33 Khan, M.R., Dickey, M.D., Wang, M. et al. (2015). A reconfigurable liquid metal antenna driven by electrochemically controlled capillarity. *Journal of Applied Physics* 117 (19): 194901.

34 Lin, T., Su, W., and Tentzeris, M.M. (2018). Expand horizons of microfluidic systems: an inkjet printed flexible energy autonomous micropump system for wearable and IoT microfluidic applications. 2018 IEEE/MTT-S International Microwave Symposium – IMS, 812–815.

35 Cui, Y., Su, W., and Tentzeris, M.M. (2019). Fully inkjet-printed tunable flexible microfluidic chipless RFID sensor. 2019 International Applied Computational Electromagnetics Society Symposium (ACES), 1–2.

36 Su, W., Liu, Q., Cook, B., and Tentzeris, M. (2016). All-inkjet-printed microfluidics-based encodable flexible chipless RFID sensors. 2016 IEEE MTT-S International Microwave Symposium (IMS), 1–4, doi: https://doi.org/10.1109/MWSYM.2016.7540411.

37 Jeong, S., Hester, J.G.D., Su, W., and Tentzeris, M.M. (2019). Read/interrogation enhancement of chipless RFIDs using machine learning techniques. *IEEE Antennas and Wireless Propagation Letters* 18 (11): 2272–2276, ISSN 1548-5757. doi: https://doi.org/10.1109/LAWP.2019.2937055.

12

High-Density Electronic Integration for Wearable Sensing

Shubhendu Bhardwaj, Raj Pulugurtha and John L. Volakis

Department of Electrical and Computer Engineering, Florida International University, Miami, FL, USA

12.1 Introduction

Wearable electronics integrated into clothing are of growing interest for sensing and radio-frequency (RF) communication and also for connectivity with mobile wireless devices. Indeed, the large area available in clothing is beneficial for integrating sensing electrodes, RF electronics, and antennas into a single wearable system. A future potential goal is to also employ wearable circuits for computing and communication operations while maintaining portability. Such fabric integration could also replace a need for accessories (such as smart watches) to support a large set of functionalities. In essence, the large apertures available on clothing can be leveraged to overcome size restrictions in the existing handheld devices (e.g. cell phones and PDAs). In the past decade, it has been shown that such antennas demonstrate improved connectivity by choosing appropriate placements across several locations in the body (Figure 12.1). A challenge in designing wearable RF electronics is to achieve excellent RF performance while the attire is concurrently comfortable and attractive [1]. To meet this requirement, we need electronic textile threads that have high electrical conductivity and mechanical strength [2].

12.2 Brief Comparison of Flexible Conductor Technologies

Popular approaches for making conductive surfaces on fabric substrates are using e-fiber threads and conductive ink (Figure 12.2). E-fiber-based conductive surfaces will be discussed in this chapter in the following sections; therefore, we first briefly consider the conductive ink technology. Conductive ink consists of conductive nanoparticles in a polymer binder and a solution

Antenna and Sensor Technologies in Modern Medical Applications,
First Edition. Edited by Yahya Rahmat-Samii and Erdem Topsakal.

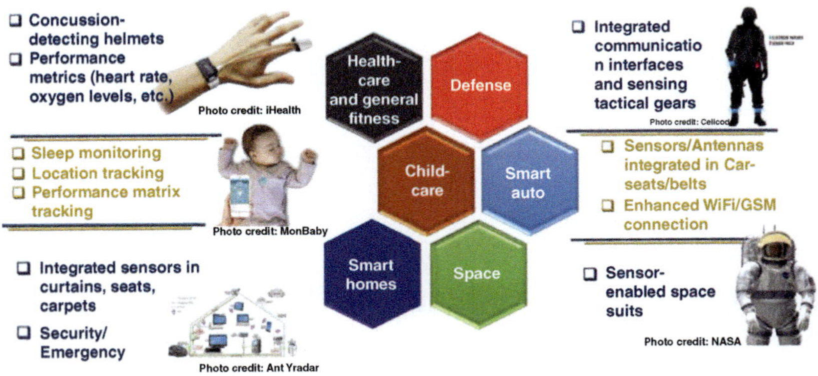

Figure 12.1 Wearable and fabric-integrated RF electronics for high-speed communications, health monitoring, and RFIDS.

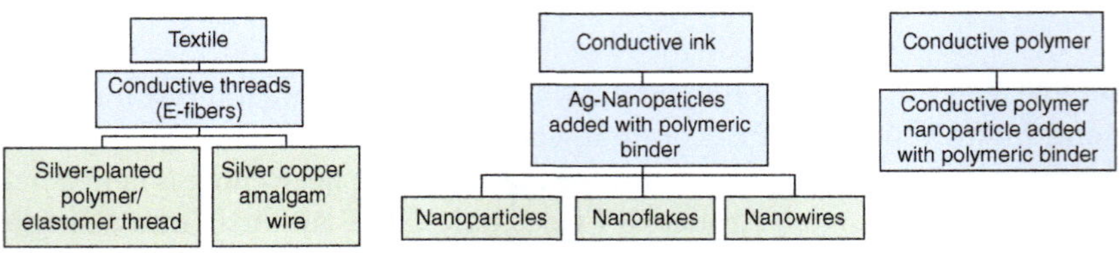

Figure 12.2 Broad classification of approaches used for developing conductive circuits on fabric substrates.

which is used for printing process and is then evaporated. The nanoparticles can be metallic [3–5] or conductive polymer [6], although conductivity of conductive polymer-based conductive inks has been shown to be two to three orders smaller than the metal nanoparticle-based inks (Table 12.1). Some other approaches are use of organometallic nanoparticles and graphene oxide and carbon nanotubes [10, 11], but their widespread use has not been noted.

A comparison of these technologies is shown in Table 12.1 by considering representative examples of conductive ink and embroidery-based conductive surfaces from recent literature. An important metric for their use in microwave applications is their ability to exhibit small conductive losses for frequencies up to 6 GHz, since most wireless communication (LTE/GSM bands) and prominently used ISM bands (2.4 and 5.8 GHz) fall in this range of frequency.

Data in Table 12.1 shows that the silver nanoparticle-based inks have superior performance over conductive polymer inks. Upon comparing the conductivity of silver nanoparticle-based inks and e-fibers, we see the highest conductivity achieved in e-fibers to be between 2×10^6 S m^{-1} and 2×10^7 S m^{-1} at 2.4 GHz [8, 9]. The transmission line loss of ~0.3 dB cm^{-1} at 3 GHz is reported showing smallest conductive losses at RF using this conductive thread technology [1, 7]. A possible reason for this advantage over conductive

Table 12.1 Comparison of loss performances of flexible conductor technologies. Metal thread technology has shown superiority for RF applications.

Technology	Materials	Conductivity	Transmission line losses
Conductive polymer	Polypyrrole (PPY) conductive polymer in PLLA and PCL polymer matrix [6]	200 to 400 $S\,m^{-1}$ (DC: 1.76 GHz)	N/A
Conductive ink	Ag nanoparticle in glycol/ethanol matrix printed in alumina substrate [3]	1.7 to $2.86 \times 10^6\,S\,m^{-1}$ (DC)	~0.5 $dB\,cm^{-1}$ at 3 GHz ~1–1.5 $dB\,cm^{-1}$ at 25 GHz
Conductive ink	Ag nanoparticle in 4-vinylphenol (PVP) [4]	0.2 to $1.2 \times 10^7\,S\,m^{-1}$ (DC)	N/A
Conductive ink	Polydimethylsiloxane (PDMS) with silver nanoparticles [5]	$10^6\,S\,cm^{-1}$ (DC)	~0.6 $dB\,cm^{-1}$ at 3 GHz
E-fiber embroidery on textile	Silver–copper amalgam thread on embroidered on fabric [7–9]	2×10^6 to $2 \times 10^7\,S\,m^{-1}$ (2.4 GHz)	~0.3 $dB\,cm^{-1}$ at 3 GHz

inks is use of continuous metallic phase in e-fibers which allows reduced conductive losses. In conductive inks, nanoparticles suspended in polymer binders may have decreased conductivity due to binder's finite resistivity. Another noteworthy technology in recent years has been use of liquid metals where antennas and devices can be embedded in elastomers [12, 13]. Antennas made from this technology have demonstrated ~90% efficiency, although fabric integration of this technology is yet to be shown.

Choice of dielectric substrates is also important for flexible RF antennas and circuits because this choice directly affects the electromagnetic loss performance as well as mechanical robustness of the flexible electronic substrates. Possible flexible substrates include liquid crystal polymer (LCP) [14], Parylene-N [15], polydimethylsiloxane (PDMS), and its ceramic composite [16]. Unlike LCP and Parylene-N, PDMS and related composites exhibit the advantages of tunable dielectric permittivity, low dielectric loss, and room temperature fabrication [4].

12.3 Review and History of E-Fiber-Based RF Technology

RF technology with e-fibers, developed over the past decade, has shown fundamental as well as application-based advancements. First report of antenna interfaces woven in wearable fabric came in 2012 where multiband antennas are reported, and performance showed copper-like losses with added flexibility features [1, 17]. Later on, the feature resolution of the embroidered structures was improved to 0.1 mm using improved fabric specifications and fabrication steps [9]. In the meantime, extensive studies have been conducted on the loss performances with changing embroidery pattern [7], ability to bear load [18], and performance under bending and twisting of RF components [19]. These point to mechanical robustness of the embroidered RF components along with flexibility and low loss performances up to 6 GHz. Following these developments, a number of antenna topologies have been proposed exploiting large areas available in cloths. For example, an ultra-wideband antenna with 67 : 1 bandwidth was reported [20] where large body area was used to allow low-frequency operation of the antennas. Flexible antennas for wireless communications [21] and for Radio Frequency Identification (RFID) tag applications [22] are some other examples of real-world applications of the technology.

Beyond antennas, more recently, e-fibers have been used to create circuits and systems for wearable applications. Noteworthy among these has been a fabric-integrated circuit for power-harvesting and power-transfer applications [8, 23]. These systems find applications in powering fitness and sensing devices worn by a user, such as a sedentary patient or a runner.

12.4 Fabrication of Conductive Flexile E-Fiber Surfaces and Loss Performance

The embroidery of e-fibers on fabric substrates is realized using computer-aided design (CAD)-based design process realized using an automated embroidery machine. These machines could be traditionally embroidery machines available from various vendors, such as Brother™. In order to create electrically conducting surfaces with small RF losses, choice of an appropriate conductive thread is crucial. Two important criteria for this choice are (i) small thread diameter required to achieve submillimeter resolution in the design features and (ii) sufficient thread strength to withstand the applied tension during the embroidery process. Generally, these two criteria are in conflict, i.e. smaller thread diameter would allow higher resolution, but thread could break during the embroidery process which deteriorates the surface finish and affects the conductivity. Ultimately, this choice is based on commercially available threads with smallest possible thickness. In this chapter, the presented RF technology is based on use of a copper-silver-based bare wire thread. Specifically, the thread consists of seven strands of Cu/Ag bare wires, each with 0.04 mm diameter, as shown in Figure 12.3. The twisting pitch of the strand is about 8 mm.

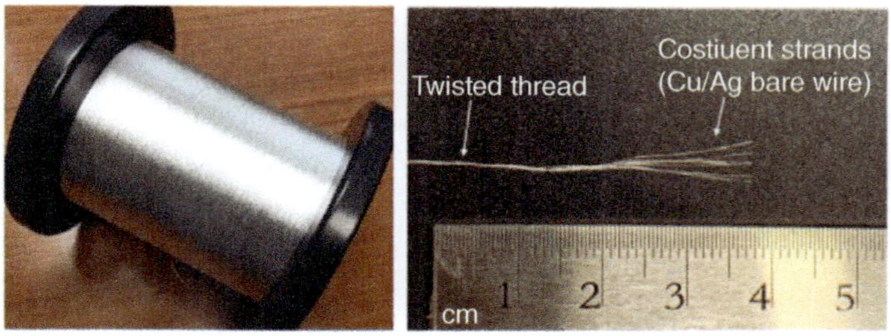

Figure 12.3 Conductive thread (or e-fiber) used for designing connections and antenna interfaces for wearable applications.

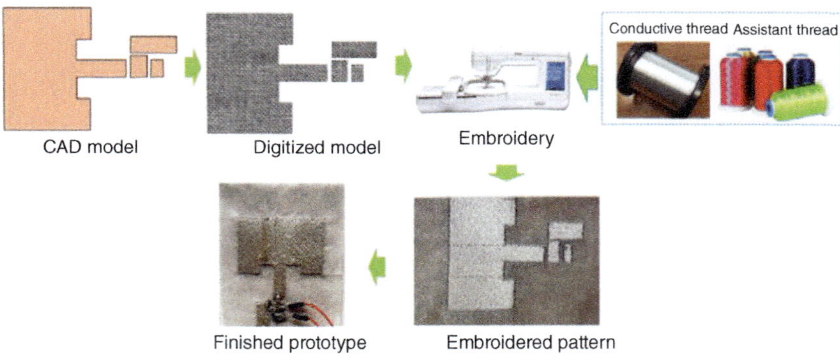

Figure 12.4 Fabrication steps for making RF devices using automated cad-based embroidery process.

The steps used for the fabrication of conductive surfaces are shown in Figure 12.4. First, a CAD model of the desired geometry is generated. This model is based on full-wave design and optimization of antenna or based on microwave circuit optimization of the transmission lines. The CAD models are then imported to a Brother^{TM} Innovis VM5100 embroidery software, where a pattern of needle paths is generated from the CAD model. The needle path patterns are fed into the embroidery machine where the pattern is embroidered on the desired fabric substrate, such as denim and organza. An assistant yarn which is a cotton/polyester thread is also used as a swing thread to support the conductive thread and is introduced from the other side of fabric. The color of the assistant thread can be chosen as per the required aesthetics or design of the clothing. The process also calls for optimization stitching density, thread tension, and thread orientation [7]. High stitching density of threads is favored for achieving high conductivity at RF. Therefore, the highest possible stitching-density setting of 14 threads per millimeter is used in the embroidery. Thread tension should be controlled to insure high precision

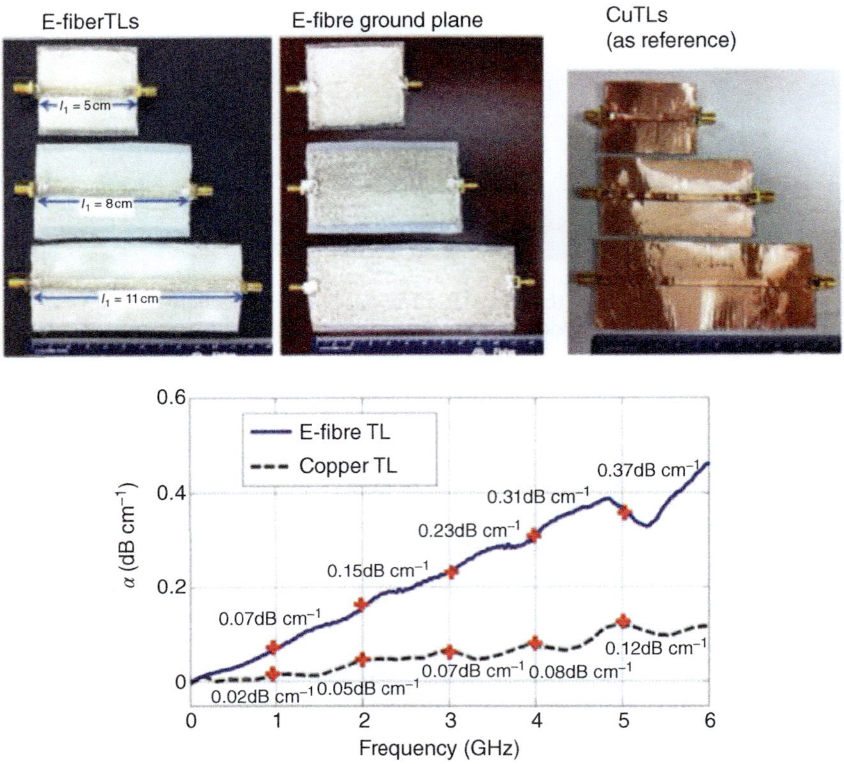

Figure 12.5 Characterization of losses by measuring losses in transmission line made from e-fiber technology [1]. (*Source:* Reprinted with Permission from Zhang, L., Wang, W., and Volakis, J.L., 2012. © IEEE.)

while also avoiding thread breakage. Considering this, a thread tension setting of 4 (out of available scale of 0–9) is used for the presented designs [8].

Loss performance of the conductive surfaces is measured by measuring losses in the transmission lines as shown in Figures 12.5 and 12.6. Figure 12.5 shows that the losses in the transmission lines made from e-fiber are in the same order as in a copper-printed transmission line. The losses increase steadily with frequency because the gaps between the threads impact the conductivity at higher frequencies. Notably, loss of 0.3 dB cm^{-1} is recorded at 3 GHz. Furthermore, in Figure 12.6 it is noted that minimum losses are obtained when the stitching pattern is along the direction of the current flow in the transmission lines. The embroidery process allows a control over stitching pattern by changing the settings in the embroidery machine. When the direction of current does not match the direction of stitching, due to lack of a single long wire along the

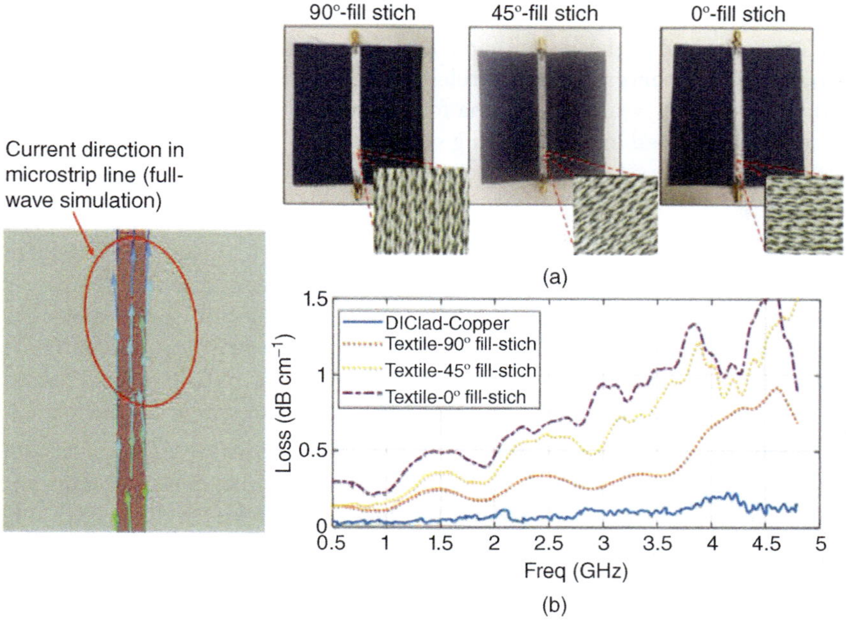

Figure 12.6 Effect of stitching pattern on the loss performance of e-fiber transmission line [7]. (*Source:* Reprinted with permission from Vital, D., Zhong, J., Bhardwaj, S., et al., 2018. © IEEE.)

current, the conductive losses are found to have increased. Investigations are also conducted to understand the effect of bending and twisting of conductive surfaces on the RF performances [5]. This investigation shows that the effect of bending and twisting of the surfaces is negligible when organza and denim substrates are used.

12.5 Antennas Using Embroidery-Based Conductive Surfaces

Ability to add conductive surfaces on textile substrates provides a unique opportunity to use clothing surfaces for integrating antenna interfaces. Antennas are generally the largest component of a communication system, and their efficiency can be increased by having a large size. Furthermore, large areas allow low-frequency antennas such as those reported in [20], which otherwise is not possible for mobile applications. Several examples of antenna integration to the daily items of clothing exist [9, 18, 20–23]. We discuss two representative examples to illustrate the performance of these antennas. The first example is dual-layer (antenna and ground plane) patch antenna for wearable power-harvesting and wireless power-transfer applications, and the second is on-body wearable antenna for wireless communication application. These are considered in the following sections.

12.5.1 Patch Antenna for Wireless Power Transfer and Harvesting

The design process of a rectangular patch antenna can be referred from basic design equations [24], but for fabric integration, a crucial unknown is the dielectric constant of the textile substrate. To determine the dielectric constant, the resonant frequency of patch antennas with varying lengths (l) made from embroidery process was measured. Then, by using the relation $l = \frac{\lambda_r}{2\sqrt{\varepsilon_r}}$, the dielectric constant of the fabric substrate could be calculated. This process was applied for the fabric substrate consisting of organza and stabilizer layers with thickness ~1.5 mm, and the effective dielectric constant was determined to be $\varepsilon_r = 2.75$. The effect of fringing fields was ignored in this estimation due to small substrate thickness [8].

The calculated dimensions of the antenna are shown in Figure 12.7. The measured reflection coefficient performance shows excellent agreement with the simulation model developed using ANSYS High Frequency Structure Simulator (HFSS) full-wave solver. In practice, we notice a decreased gain as compared to simulated values, which provides an idea of the conductivity of the surfaces as discussed next.

In order to estimate the conductivity of the surface, the conductivity in simulation model was varied till the point the measured and simulated gain values were in agreement (Figure 12.7e). For reference, we consider the simulation model with perfect electrical conductor (PEC) conductive surfaces and no dielectric losses, which shows 100% radiation efficiency and 98.2% total efficiency due to losses in the impedance mismatching. By comparing the peak gain from this simulation, i.e. 7.61 dBi, with the measured peak gain of 6.57 dBi, we calculate the total measured efficiency of the fabricated antenna to be 77.3% at 2.45 GHz. This calculation takes into account all forms of losses, i.e. dielectric losses, conductive losses, and mismatch losses at the antenna port. From the knowledge of the measured mismatch losses, we also calculate the measured radiation efficiency (which includes only dielectric and conductive losses) of the antenna to be 89.1%.

In Figure 12.7e, the peak gain for the case with conductivity $\sigma = 2.4 \times 10^6\ \mathrm{S\,m^{-1}}$ matches the peak measured gain, suggesting that fabricated surfaces should have conductivity $\sigma = 2.4 \times 10^6\ \mathrm{S\,m^{-1}}$ or better. In practice, this value should be slightly higher, since mismatch losses are higher in the measured prototype; therefore, conductor losses are overestimated in this conductivity comparison. Nevertheless, this analysis provides an approximate value of effective conductivity of the embroidered surfaces.

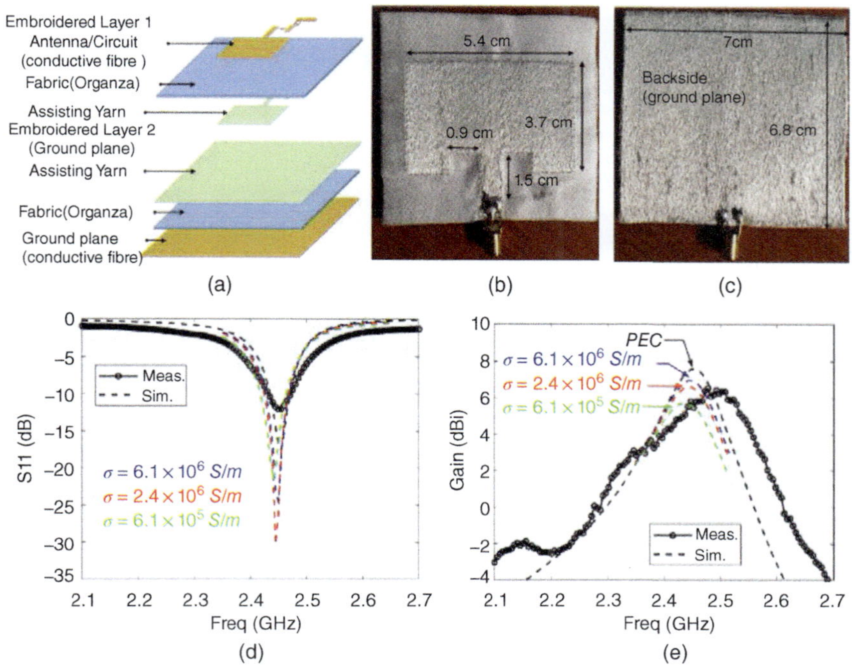

Figure 12.7 (a) Layers used in the fabrication of patch antenna for wireless power transfer application. (b) Fabricated prototype front, (c) back photos, (d) measured reflection loss performance of the antenna, and (e) gain versus frequency plot with changing conductivity levels. (*Source:* Reprinted with permission from Vital, D., Bhardwaj, S., and Volakis, J. L. 2019,. © IEEE.)

The application of this antenna will be discussed in later sections, where it will be used to collect wireless power from a distance and using on fabric rectifiers to convert the collected RF power into DC for powering wearable devices. The advantage of patch antenna is that due to conformal nature, it can align with bending surfaces without variations of the performances. Furthermore, due to the presence of ground plane under the substrate, only a small amount of power interacts with the skin.

12.5.2 Body-Worn Antenna for Wireless Communication

Pervasive application of wearable antennas is to extend the range of wireless communication, by exploiting large clothing areas. In this section, we show an example to demonstrate the applicability of this technology for communication applications. The considered antenna is shown in Figure 12.8 [1]. In this study,

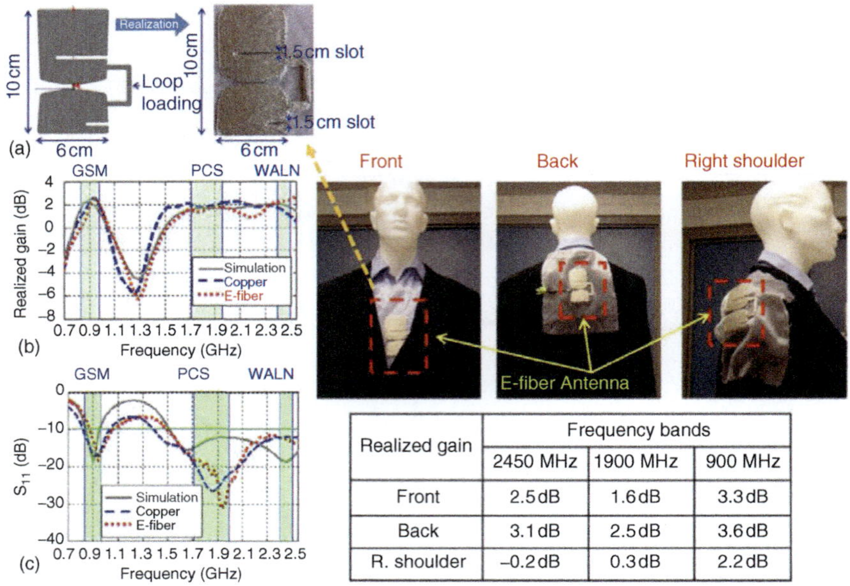

Realized gain	Frequency bands		
	2450 MHz	1900 MHz	900 MHz
Front	2.5 dB	1.6 dB	3.3 dB
Back	3.1 dB	2.5 dB	3.6 dB
R. shoulder	−0.2 dB	0.3 dB	2.2 dB

Figure 12.8 Body-worn e-fiber antenna for wearable applications. Antenna covers popular Wi-Fi and GSM bands for enhancing communication ranges of cell phones. (*Source:* Reprinted with permission from Wang, Z., Lee, L. Z., Psychoudakis, D., et al., 2014. © IEEE.)

the conductive textile surfaces are embroidered using 332-strand silver-coated AmberStrand fibers (e-fibers) [25]. The strands of the thread are made from a 10-μm-thick polymer (*p*-phenylene-2,6-benzobisoxazole (PBO)) core, coated with 2–3-μm-thick silver coating. As a result, they exhibit excellent mechanical strength, flexibility, and more importantly, low dc resistivity of 0.035 Ω/cm. To form the textile surface, hundreds of e-fibers were tightly bundled to minimize the contact loss between fibers. Subsequently, automatic embroidery was used with high-density stitching to realize the textile surfaces. The fabricated conductive textile surfaces were then used to form radiating elements (antennas) as well as ground planes and transmission lines in circuitry, as shown in Figure 12.8.

The measured gains of the antenna in popular Wi-Fi and GSM bands are shown in the table of Figure 12.8. The optimization of the antenna showed that the impedance was matched in these Wi-Fi and GSM bands. The fabricated antenna was measured and demonstrated to have a realized gain greater than 2 dBi. Furthermore, the flexibility and conformability of the antenna was shown by integrating it onto a human phantom to evaluate its body-worn antenna performances. In free space and while on body, the performance of the antenna was found equivalent to its copper counterpart.

12.6 Circuits and Systems Using Embroidery-Based Conductive Surfaces

In recent years, the e-fiber technology has been translated to implement circuits and systems, which highlights the potential of this technology for practical applications. Here, we present two such examples, where the circuits and antenna fabricated using embroidery of conductive fibers were used to develop power-harvesting circuits. In the first example, wirelessly transmitted power from a source was collected in its far field [8], whereas in the second example, RF power was transferred from a transmitter to a receiver fabric-integrated circuit using near-field power transfer modality [23]. These systems are presented in the following sections.

12.6.1 Far-Field Radio-Frequency Power Collection System on Clothing

Textile-integrated antenna and rectifier is an example of fabric integration of RF system useful for modern applications of wearable sensing devices. Such system can be used to charge supercapacitors for powering low-power sensing devices such as heart rate monitor and biochemical sensors. A prime example of biochemical sensing for health and fitness applications is sensing of cortisol level in sweat [26]. Cortisol, considered to be stress hormone, is a biomarker of psychological stress. Likewise, another example is measurement of uric acid in blood to monitor the health of a wound [26]. Another potential method for wound health monitoring is measurement of pH level. Other examples are gas sensing for early warning for personnel working in extreme conditions or sensing of vitals in patients. Many times, these sensors consume microwatt levels of power which can be easily supplied from wireless power transfer as well as power-harvesting modalities. Some examples of such low-power devices are temperature sensors with power consumption between 113 pW and 1.4 μW [27–30].

The presented system consists of an array of rectennas, where each rectenna consists of an embroidered patch antenna, which is presented in Figure 12.7, and an RF to DC rectifier. In the rectifier, the key feature is use of single diode in a resonant microstrip circuit that achieves efficiency up to 70%. These features allow minimalistic circuit and easy fabrication on a flexible fabric substrate.

Single-diode rectifiers have been used recently due to their minimalistic design and capability of achieving efficiencies beyond 50%, as shown for many rigid substrate-based designs. Having developed the antenna and rectifier elements, the 2×2 and 2×3 rectenna arrays are fabricated and tested.

Figure 12.9 shows the rectifier circuit, fabricated prototype, and measurement results for the RF–DC conversion efficiency of the proposed rectifier. Achieving high efficiencies at low input power levels (below 0 dBm) and using

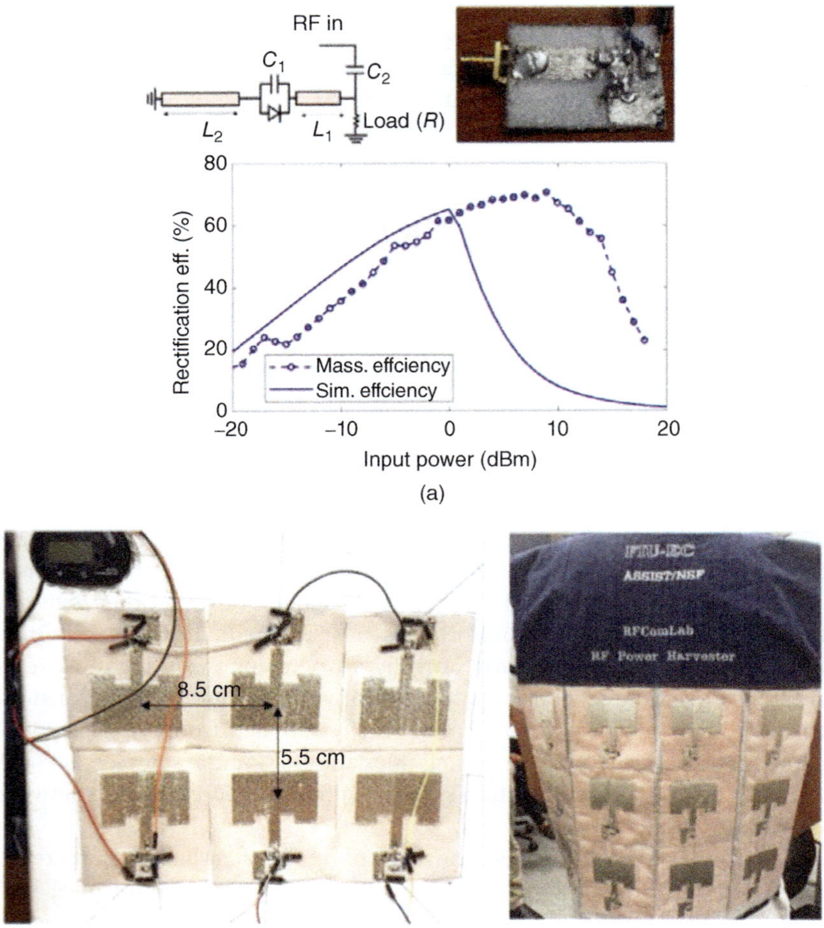

Figure 12.9 (a) On-fabric rectifier circuit [8, 25] using single diode and maximum efficiency of ~70%. (b) Power-harvesting jacket prototype. (*Source:* Reprinted with permission from Vital, D., Bhardwaj, S., and Volakis, J. L., 2019. © IEEE.)

minimal circuitry are the primary challenges for this design. The single-diode operation involves introducing a resonance in a shorted microstrip line and positioning the diode at the maxima of the resonance to convert the maximum power to DC. Since the resonance creates a standing wave where the voltage amplitude could be up to two times a propagating signal, the diodes conversion efficiency is increased. Parameters such as line lengths L_1, L_2 and capacitors C_1 and C_2 are optimized to create maximum efficiency for a provided load, with creating impedance matching with the input. Details of the optimized values can be referred from [8]. The rectifier RF to DC conversion efficiency performance shows a reasonable agreement between the simulated circuit performance from Advanced Design System (ADS) simulator and the measured performance (Figure 12.9). The noted deviation between the measured and simulated performances has been noted by researchers in the past [30] and is due to nonlinear behavior of the diode which is not modeled in the simulator.

Figure 12.10 shows the measurement results related to RF to DC conversion efficiency of the rectenna array with increasing number of elements. For this measurement, 500 mW of RF power was transmitted from a vector signal generator and a power amplifier with 30 dB gain connected to a 9-dBi gain horn antenna. At 152 cm (5 ft) from the source, a single element shows a power collection of 25 μW, which is enhanced to 55 μW, when four rectenna elements are serially connected. Although there is recorded increase in collected power

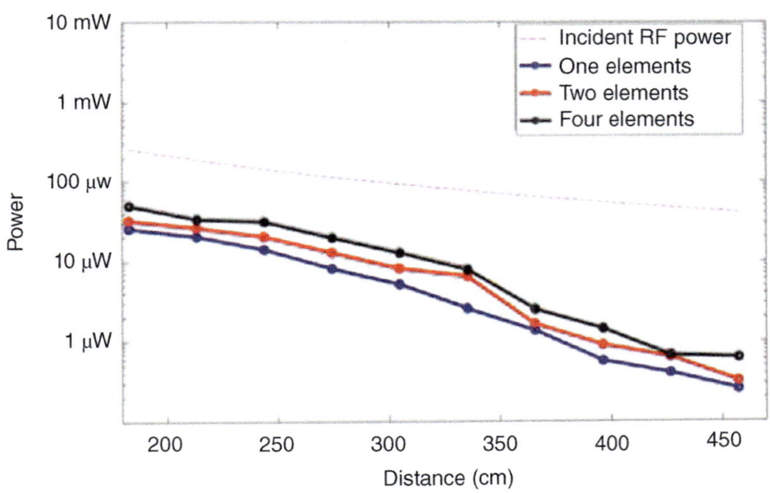

Figure 12.10 Power collection performance of the rectenna array with increasing number of elements in the array. The power received decreases as a function of distance. The total incident power in a four-element case is plotted in the dashed curve. (*Source:* Reprinted with permission from Vital, D., Bhardwaj, S., and Volakis, J. L., 2019. © IEEE.)

with increasing number of elements, the gains due to addition of elements are not linear. This is due to inherent nonlinearity of the diodes as well as required optimization of the connection configuration between the elements. Serial connection of rectenna output was employed in this setup for obtaining the output power from this system. Results related to power collection in typical Wi-Fi conditions are reported in [8].

12.6.2 Near-Zone Power Collection Using Fabric-Integrated Antennas

Similar to far-field RF power transfer, a second application of the fabric-integrated antenna and circuit is near-field wireless power transfer. Although such modality only works up to few centimeters of distance between the transmitter and the receiver, the power transfer efficiencies could be 10–80% which is significantly higher than the far-field modality. In this case, resonant antenna structures are designed to transmit RF power from the transmitter to the receiver where appropriate rectifier circuit is used for RF to DC conversion of the received RF power. The example is shown in Figure 12.11.

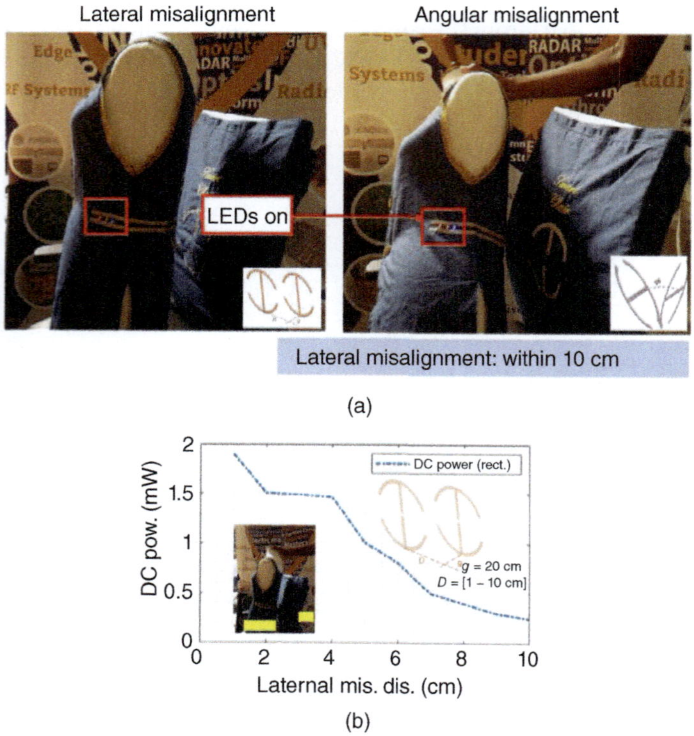

Figure 12.11 (a) Near-zone power transfer system integrated on fabric in clothing and upholstery. (b) Power transfer under misalignment.

The transmitter antenna connected to an RF source is embedded in the upholstery of a chair, while the receiver antenna and the rectifier are integrated in the clothing. The designed antennas are resonant at 360 MHz and used a unique anchor-shaped planar structure confined in an area of circle with radius 7.5 cm. This anchor-shaped antenna has been found to be resilient to misalignment as compared to simple loop antennas previously reported in [23]. The measurement setup and results are shown in Figure 12.11.

To characterize the performance of the system integration, the dress was placed at a fixed distance of 20 cm from the chair's back. The mannequin carrying the dress was moved sideways to emulate the movement of the bearer of the dress in real-world scenario. A transmitter system is composed of a Keysight MXG signal generator N5183B and Mini-circuits ZHL-20W-13+ power amplifier to transmit a total power of 1 W. The power received and rectified to DC by the receiver rectenna was measured while introducing a lateral misalignment ranging from 1 to 10 cm. As shown in Figure 12.11, the DC power of up to 2 mW was collected and used to light three LEDs, showing demonstration of the near-field power transfer application of the fabric-integrated antenna and circuits.

12.7 Voltage-Controlled Oscillator for Wound-Sensing Applications

A much-anticipated application of fabric-based electronics technology is its integration for wearable sensing devices. A use case for this is monitoring of a wound's health through smart bandages. An efficient wound-monitoring system which is integrated in dressing will allow wound monitoring without having to undress the wound, enabling continuous monitoring. Prior solutions for wound analytics research have focused on imaging-based (optical and infrared) data-collection solutions [31, 32] or smart bandages that require in situ battery [33]. In either case, the wound needs to be undressed (for taking an image or battery replacement), which ultimately limits the number of samples extracted and limits any big-data treatment of the obtained data. This suggests that even when there is increased need for solutions, none that are available can provide sufficient data for the required wound analytics. Lack of data samples effects both—treatment of the patient in question and data generated for future predictive analytics, modeling, and cost optimization.

The motivation for this work comes from a market that is worth tens of billion dollars [34], invested in the wound-care and management, much of which can be optimized by developing predictive models for time of recovery and type of medical care needed by using metadata of the patient such as age, location, type of injury, and prior history. At the center of developing such predictive models are the data collection of healing time and the effect of specific treatment approaches/medicines, among number of other critical parameters. Even with

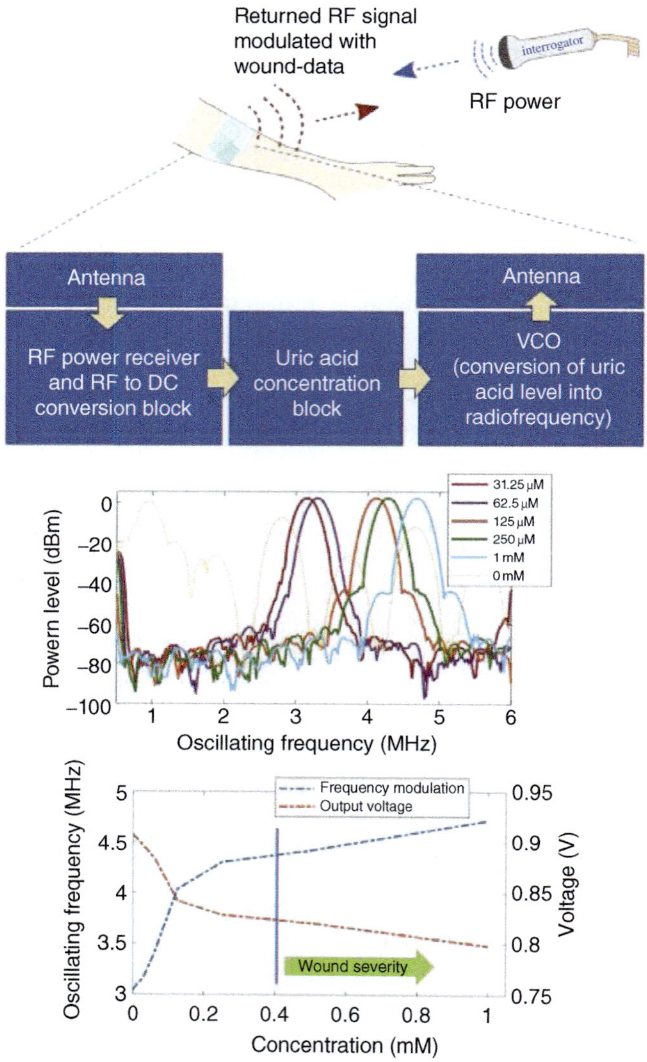

Figure 12.12 Remote wound-monitoring system using voltage-controlled oscillator (VCO)-based sensor. VCO is used to control the dc output from the sensor to an RF signal which can be transmitted back to the interrogator. (*Source:* Courtesy: Prof. Shekhar Bhansali, FIU.)

the demonstrated use of data analytics in medical-care domain, data collection for wound patients who are sedentary, and when the wounds are covered with dressing, continues to be a major challenge.

In Figure 12.12, a voltage-controlled oscillator (VCO) circuit which can convert a DC signal provided by a uric acid sensor to a unique RF frequency which can be transmitted to a remotely placed interrogator is shown. In the remarkable developments in understanding the wound electrochemistry and metabolism [24, 35, 36], it has been established that wound-healing process is associated to generation of uric acid, with its concentration decreasing over the healing period. The sensor used was three-electrode sensor dipped in a test uric acid fluid, which is a textile-based enzymatic sensor inspired from [37].

Measured results are reported in Figure 12.12. It shows the shifting of the spectral peak with changing levels of uric acid concentration. Notably, VCO causes a changing output frequency based on molar concentration levels. An important parameter is the sensitivity of modulated RF signal with changing uric acid concentration, which is calculated to be 1.5 kHz μM^{-1}. This sensitivity is adjustable by changing the ratio of resistors R_1 and R_2. The total power consumed by the sensor alone is 24 μW. The range of the sensor is found to be around the target range of 0.4 mM uric acid concentration, which is consistent with the realistic uric acid levels found in wounds [35, 38].

12.8 High-Density Integration

High-density packaging leads to increased component or functional volumetric density in the packages. Miniaturization in the system footprint and thickness, performance enhancement, and lower cost are the key drivers for high-density packaging. Package miniaturization is directly related to performance enhancement because it enables shorter interconnect lengths and improved functional integration with topology innovations and superior design rules. The key parameters that determine the functional density are package interconnect pitch, assembly interconnection pitch, via and pad dimensions, thin-film layer count, and 3D device integration. These features are illustrated in Figure 12.13. This section describes the fabrication advances that lead to such miniaturization and continuous improvement in high-density package integration.

12.8.1 Interconnect Features on Laminate Substrates

Interconnect pitch is determined by the conductor structuring or patterning techniques. These techniques are classified as subtractive, additive, and

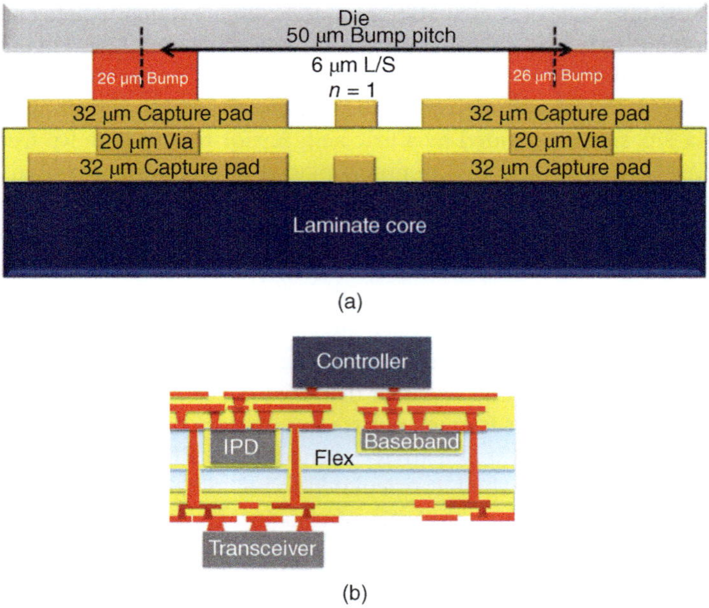

Figure 12.13 (a) Key package features of high-density integration: line/space, via/pad, bump assembly pitch; (b) 3D device integration.

semiadditive types. Subtractive patterning approaches, which are based on wet etching or laser-assisted delamination, have several processing advantages because of their simpler tool and infrastructure needs but are limited to 100–200 μm pitch when at least 10–15% tolerance is required. Semiadditive patterning (SAP) can address these limitations and is, therefore, the mainstream interconnect technology for package substrate fabrication. In SAP process, polymer lamination is performed, typically with a vacuum laminator, followed by polymer curing. A copper seed layer with a thickness of 0.2 μm is uniformly deposited through electroless plating or sputtering. Adhesion of electroless copper to polymer is improved by prior roughening of the polymer surface using a permanganate chemical etch to create mechanical anchor sites. The wet chemical etch also cleans the residual polymer in the via locations that land on the underneath copper pads. This is extremely critical to improve the via yield. Photoresist patterning and copper plating through the patterned photoresist are then performed, followed by the removal of the photoresist and the underneath seed layer to yield high-precision copper patterns. Leading fabricators manufacture substrates with 10–12 μm lines and spaces using

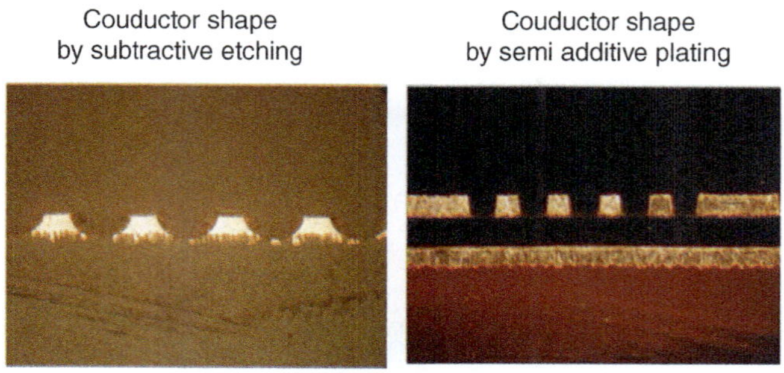

Figure 12.14 Subtractive vs. semiadditive patterning. SAP leads to sharp features with lower undercut because of the minimal seed-layer etch than subtractive patterning where the whole metal layer needs to be etched. (*Source:* Courtesy of Hidetaka Uno, DuPont MRC Dryfilm Co. Ltd.)

SAP on traditional organic laminate substrates. Unlike subtractive patterning, where a thick copper foil is etched off from the undesired areas to form circuit patterns, SAP yields better dimensional and copper sidewall control because only the seed layer is etched. This is because SAP avoids the long etching and lateral undercut that is usually prevalent during subtractive etching. The comparison is illustrated in Figure 12.14.

It is critical to note that single-layer features described so far are not the only key metrics for package densities. When multiple wiring layers are required, the package density is also limited by the via capability, and layer-to-layer dimensional control from the alignment capabilities, via-pad shifts from polymer curing strains, and warpage. The challenges that need to be solved to achieve fine lines and spaces are highlighted in Figure 12.15. For the best multilayered feature capability, it is important to provide dimensionally stable cores with high Tg, smooth surfaces, and also optimal coefficient of thermal expansion (CTE) for both die- and board-side assembly reliability. Semirigid high-glass-transition (Tg) organic laminates provide enough dimensional stability for layer-to-layer registration. By utilizing glass cores or other inorganic cores with superior dimensional stability, features of less than 2 μm can be achieved for digital packaging and less than 10 μm for RF structures with high impedance control. Several processing challenges were addressed to realize this key milestone. These include advances in chemically amplified dry-film photoresists for large-area panel-scale lithography, adhesion improvement between copper and dielectric films without invoking surface roughness techniques, advanced seed-layer removal with anisotropic etching kinetics, and fine via formation with ultraviolet laser ablation.

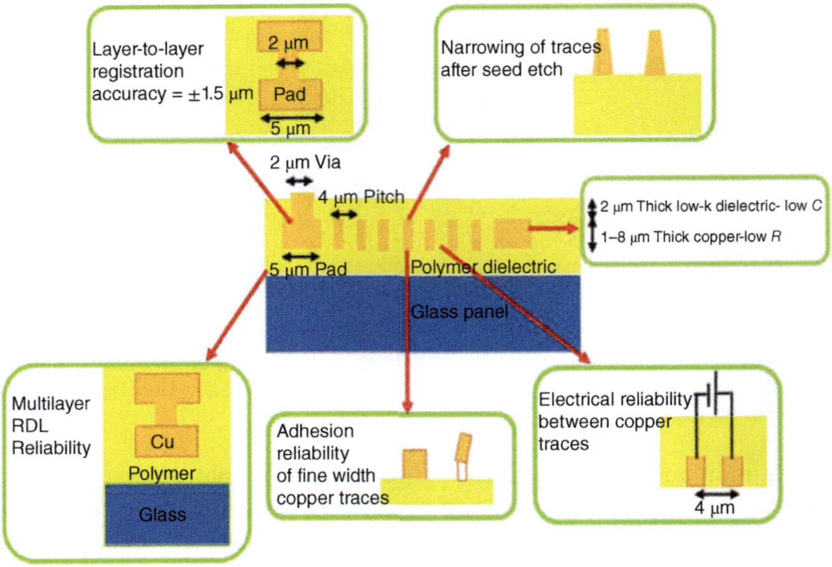

Figure 12.15 Challenges with fine lines and spaces on package substrates. (*Source:* Courtesy of Chandra Nair, Intel.)

As illustrated through Table 12.1, inorganic core packaging with glass in 2D and 3D is emerging as an emerging solution for high-performance and ultraminiaturized modules with simultaneous reduction in both X–Y and Z directions. Glass combines the benefits of ceramic, organic, and silicon. This is because glass provides many advantages such as ultrathinness, ultralow electrical loss, silicon-like dimensional stability for precise and fine-pitch circuits, high stiffness, high Tg, high surface smoothness, and adjustable CTE. Moreover, it is superior to silicon for RF applications because it enables high-Q RF components due to its high resistivity for ultralow loss. Compared to organics, glass enables precision circuitry with finer design ground rules because of its dimensional stability, and ability to process with ultrathin and low-loss buildup organic or inorganic dielectrics, without process-compatibility issues. Recent advances have demonstrated reliable and through pin vias (TPVs) in glass with double-side assembly of active and passive components with ultrashort interconnections [39, 40]. In addition to these, glass as a packaging substrate appears to be a perfect solution for its cost-effectiveness through panel-scale manufacturability [41, 42].

12.8.2 Interconnects on Flex Substrates

Flexible packaging starts with thin thermoplastic substrates. Polyimide is the most widely used substrate for flexible packaging because of its high elongation to failure, strength, chemical stability, and adequate electrical properties. LCP and Teflon are the other classes of widely used flexible substrates. LCP and polyimides show high tensile strength of 200 MPa and CTE of 20 ppm C^{-1} and less. These materials feature stable and excellent electrical properties such as low loss tangent of 0.002–0.004 till 110 GHz. LCP is stable in extreme humidity because of its low moisture absorption and also resistant to chemical environments.

Interconnects for flexible packaging are created by either additive or subtractive patterning. With additive manufacturing, silver inks are the most common sources of conductors, while copper pastes are emerging as a low-cost alternative to silver. Sintering at 200–220°C for 15–30 minutes is known to achieve conductivities of above 10^7 S m^{-1} with nanosilver pastes and inks. On the other hand, copper sinters at a higher temperature and needs an inert atmosphere to form sintered low-resistance interconnects. The processing challenges with copper pastes are addressed with innovations in nanoparticle synthesis having size of less than 100 nm, bimodal mixing to increase densification at lower temperatures, and more importantly by creating surface passivation to protect copper oxidation. With these innovations, copper pastes that can be sintered at 200–260°C are developed to achieve conductivities higher than 10^7 S m^{-1}.

The achievable feature sizes of silver or copper traces on flexible substrates are limited by the additive printing techniques. Screen printing, inkjet printing, and aerosol jet printing are the common metallization approaches. The key process steps are: (i) polymer surface treatment to improve metal-polymer wetting and adhesion, (ii) printing, and (iii) thermal treatment to achieve bulk conductivity. Aerosol jet printing and microdispensing techniques are known to give <10 μm lines/spaces, while screen-printing techniques achieve about 50 μm dimensions. Commonly used inkjet printing achieves intermediate dimensions that reach 25 μm. The process features of various techniques are compiled in Table 12.2. Inkjet-printed silver on polyimide flex substrates is sintered at temperatures of even up to 300°C to achieve above 60% of the bulk silver conductivity. Multiple wiring layers are also achieved with via drilling and conductive-paste via fill.

12.8.3 Device Assembly

Assembly on flex substrates is accomplished with multiple options such as solders, isotropic conductive adhesives, or anisotropic conducting films (ACFs). Solders provide high conductivity and reliable interconnects on traditional substrates but require high-temperature processing and surface-finish requirements that are not compatible with printed silver traces. Several innovations such as laser soldering or photonic soldering are emerging to address the high-temperature requirements of solders. In order to address the limitations of solders, active devices are assembled with alternative options

Table 12.2 Comparison of substrate technology capabilities with semiadditive patterning.

	LTCC	Laminates	Si or glass cores
Substrate thickness (μm)	>500	>300	<150
Feature size with 5% precision (μm)	100	40–50	<10
Through-via diameter and pitch (μm/μm)	100/300	100/300	25/50
Through-thickness variation (μm)	>25	>10	0.5–1
Die assembly pitch (μm)	60–150	60–150	20–50
Panel size (metric for cost) (μm)	150–200	510	510

LTCC, low-temperature cofired ceramics.

such as conductive silver adhesives or copper pastes. This assembly approach is compatible with printed silver or copper traces on the flex substrates and gold surface finish on the die pads. Conductive adhesives result in higher bump resistances. Assuming 1 mΩ cm resistivity, a 100-μm-thick bump with 100×100 μm area interconnect results in 100 mΩ of resistance as opposed to 10 mΩ of resistance with solders. After including the interfacial barrier resistance, the net resistance of conducting adhesive films can be much higher. However, with conductivities of less than 0.1 mΩ cm that are recently demonstrated with conductive adhesives, much lower resistances can be achieved.

For ACF-based assembly process, the film with conducting nanoparticles is sandwiched between the die and package surfaces to be connected. Under heat and pressure, conductive particles become trapped between the two conductive surfaces and bridge them, creating an electrical path. Because of the anisotropy in conductivity, ACF materials do not have to be selectively applied and can cover the entire bonding area. This eliminates the need for patterning. No underfilling step is required in this process as the ACF itself acts as an underfill. In ACF bonding, Au, Ni-Au, or Cu bumps are typically applied onto the device pads. Harder bumps are typically preferred over conventional solders to trap the conductive particles. ACFs are also compatible with fine-pitch applications using fine fillers that are of a few nanometers in size.

Ramp interconnections-based assembly technologies entirely rely on additive manufacturing and are recently developed by nScrypt and other groups, an example of which is shown in [43]. The chip is attached to the substrate, with active face up, using printable die-attach materials. A ring of polymer is then printed around the chip to build a ramp (hence referred to as printed ramp interconnections), along which Ag ink is run from the bonding pads on the chip to the substrate. These printed interconnections have been demonstrated

Table 12.3 Comparison of interconnect technologies with additive manufacturing.

Additive manufacturing processes		Resolution (line width)	Viscosity (Pa s)	Write speed	Complex curvature printing
Large-area paste printing	Screen printing	30–50 μm thickness: 12 μm or thicker (depending on emulsion thickness)	1–50	0.15–0.25 $m\,s^{-1}$	No
Droplet	Inkjet	25–200 μm	<0.01	0.3 $mm^3\,s^{-1}$ (single nozzle) 0.25–8 $m\,s^{-1}$	Moderate
	Aerosol jet	10–150 μm thickness: 10 nm–5 μm	<2.5	0.25 $mm^3\,s^{-1}$ (single nozzle) 0.2 $m\,s^{-1}$	Excellent
Flow	Micropen	100 μm	<1000	50 $mm^3\,s^{-1}$	Excellent
Tip	AFM	12 nm line width 5 nm spatial resolution	Macromolecules, (e.g. thiol) or nanoparticles	0.2–5 $\mu m\,s^{-1}$	Limited

Courtesy: Billyde Brown, Georgia Tech.

to perform similar to standard bond wires at high frequencies. All processing is carried out a low temperature, below 200°C. The routing layers are built along with the interconnections, reducing the number of process steps and eliminating the need for precise alignment during chip placement. Various assembly options are compiled in Table 12.3. Printed adhesives are emerging as a key option for interconnecting low-temperature sensing electronics with the analog, processing, and communication electronics. Fan-out interconnect technology, in conjunction with wafer or die thinning to less than 50 μm, is emerging as the ultimate solution to seamless connect devices with the interconnect fabric. In this approach, die-to-package interconnects are formed during the package substrate fabrication processes. This approach is discussed more in the following section.

12.8.4 3D Packaging

Providing double-side device assembly in a package and stacking of such packages is the next major innovation in high-density packaging. A comparison

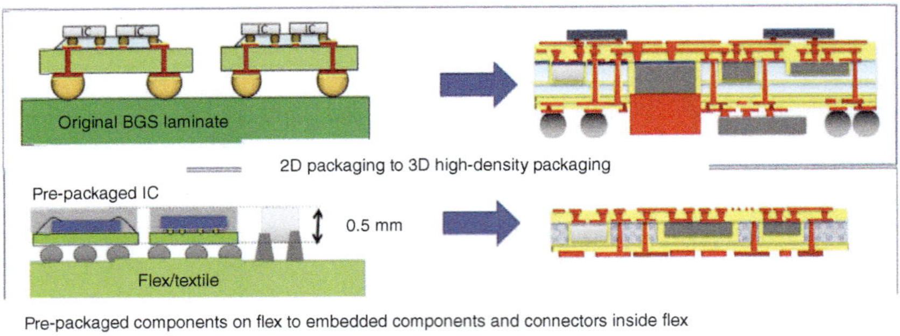

Figure 12.16 Emerging 3D high-density packaging architectures compared to existing 2D packages.

of traditional 2D packages and recent 3D packages is shown in Figure 12.16. Technology comparisons are shown in Table 12.4. In high-performance computing, the key architecture to enable this is the 2.5D interposer that supports high logic-memory bandwidth between the processor and stacked memory modules that are assembled side by side. This will also become the mainstream approach for emerging high-performance computing for artificial intelligence (AI) big-data processing. In mobile computing, the key package architecture is based on the embedded processor chip in the package, followed by stacking of the memory chip on the top. Such architecture, now prevalent in smartphones, is illustrated in Figure 12.16 (right, top; with Apple's A10 processor). In the 5G applications, a key 3D architecture that is now widely utilized by IBM, Intel, Qualcomm, and others is the backside transceiver IC assembly on a high-density substrate that supports antenna arrays, beam-forming circuits, controller ICs, power and ground layers, and the associated routing layers to support the system functions in the package. Double-side assembly leads to 2X reduction in the X–Y dimensions. More important benefit from double-side assembly is the reduction in the interconnect length from several millimeters to tens of microns. However, this approach imposes constraints on the die and interconnect thickness if Ball Grid Assembly (BGA) is utilized. It also creates thermal design constraints. The back side of the die is directly cooled by the embedded heat slugs in the printed circuit board (PCB), onto which the die is attached.

Fan-out packaging is perceived as the next major breakthrough in high-density packaging. In this approach, the devices are assembled onto a temporary carrier, followed by planar molding into 12-inch wafers. Fan-out packaging eliminates the use of wire bonding and therefore, suppresses the major part of signal losses and also reduces the footprint of the high-pin-count die. Standard back-end-of-the-line (BEOL) processes or SAP techniques are

Table 12.4 Comparison of assembly technologies on flex substrates.

Assembly type	Performance	Assembly process
Solder • High temp. E.g. An–Ag–Cu • Low temp. E.g. Sn–Bi	• High conductivity • Self-alignment • High current handling	• High reflow temp (<260°C) • Gold surface finish with Ni barrier (or organic solderability and preservatives) • Not compatible with printed traces
Isotropic conductive adhesive • Silver epoxy • Silver nanoflakes • Silver elastomer	• Higher bump resistance • Pitch limited by printing	• Printed bumps (e.g. stencil printing) • Low-temperature assembly
Anisotropic conductive films • Epoxy films with Au-shell particles	• No alignment needed • Acts as inbuilt underfill	• Higher resistance • Cross-talk between bumps causes higher RF losses
Ramp interconnections	• High inductance from long interconnects • Design flexibility	• Epoxy ramps • Printed silver adhesives
Fan-out connections	• Lowest parasitic • Thinnest packages • Ideal for THz and mm wave	• Via on IC pads • Printed vias and conductor traces

utilized to create high-density routing layers. In another emerging variation of fan-out packaging that is adapted by substrate or board manufacturers or OSAT (Outsourced Semiconductor Assembly and Test) companies, active components are assembled into panels (of up to 510 mm × 510 mm), followed by formation of interconnects. The key feature of fan-out packaging is that the interconnects are directly formed onto the IC pads. Hence, soldering or conductive adhesives are not needed for off-chip interconnections. Fan-out packaging, however, comes with several process penalties. Die-shift and die-placement errors cause major issues in the subsequent lithographies and substantially reduce the reticle size for step-and-repeat pattern.

12.8.5 Applications of High-Density Packaging in RF and Sensing

Low substrate loss is a key packaging metric for RF applications. RF packaging traditionally evolved with low-temperature cofired ceramic (LTCC) substrates.

The primary reason is the superior properties of LTCC, such as low dielectric loss, low moisture absorption, high reliability based on hermetic nature of ceramics, high thermal stability, and ability to form complex 3D multilayered circuits [44, 45]. LTCC technology started to migrate to organic laminate packaging because of its lower cost and higher component density from fine-line multilayered wiring. Supply-chain readiness, lower cost, and adequate low-loss performance have driven most end users toward adapting organic laminates for 5G substrates. Conventional RF substrates utilize low-loss epoxy laminates, while advanced RF packages utilize organic substrates such as LCP [46], hydrocarbon ceramic, and polytetrafluoroethylene (PTFE) [47, 48] because of their large-area low-cost manufacturing infrastructure cost and low dissipation factor [49]. Organic substrates that are ~0.3–0.6 mm thick form the preferred platform for today's modules, with up to two metal layers on each side of the core. The lines and spaces are approaching 15–20 μm with vias of 100 μm in leading-edge RF substrates [49], although 40–50 μm lines are most commonly used to maintain the required tolerance. Selected passive components are embedded inside the laminate substrate. Laminate panels have lower elastic modulus and poor dimensional stability during thermal processing. This results in a need to have large capture pads, limiting the wiring density. Package substrate RDL is fabricated using a sequential approach which requires curing of polymer dielectric (typically around 200°C) for every layer, and the dimensional instability of laminate core panel causes the capture pads to shift from their original location in the RDL. Thus, capture pads larger than the diameter of microvias are required to land the microvia, severely restricting the space available for routing copper lines to connect the die bumps. The current organic laminate panels require 25-μm diameter capture pads to land 10-μm microvia diameters [44].

As described earlier, 3D packages with transceiver ICs on the backside and antenna arrays along the top surface are the most prevalent 5G package architectures, as illustrated by the IBM's antenna array package in Figure 12.17a. Multilayered organics with flip-chip ICs on the backside and antenna arrays on the top, connected through vias, is illustrated through a recent product by Qualcomm in Figure 12.17b. Four 2×4 antenna arrays (three are shown in the figure, while the fourth one is on the backside) are shown in the figure. Each array is $13\,\text{mm} \times 26\,\text{mm}$, with two transceiver chips, one driving the dual polarization antennas and the other driving the differential polarization antennas [52]. Intel has reported a stack up that consists of an organic copper-clad laminate (CCL)-prepreg core for antenna implementation, trace routing, a flip-chip radio frequency IC (RFIC) module that is responsible to quad-feed the antenna where each port is responsible for one band and polarization, and ball-grid array balls for connection to a main PCB, along with conformal shielding [52]. The package size is $30\,\text{mm} \times 15\,\text{mm} \times 1.5\,\text{mm}$, with 1500 connections for each transceiver IC supporting an 8×4 patch antenna array

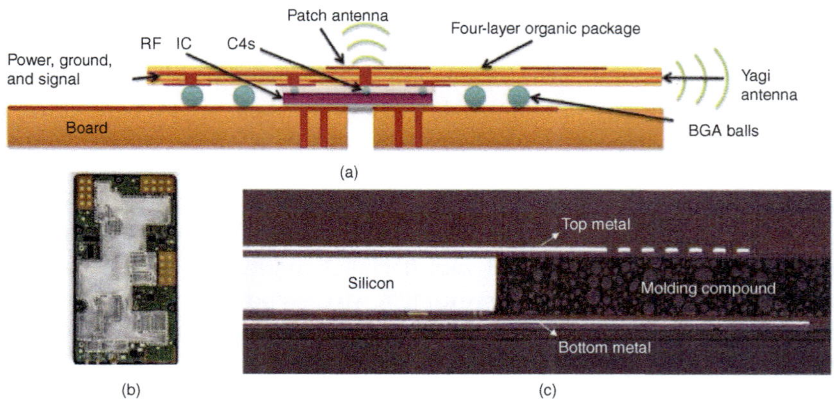

Figure 12.17 5G millimeter-wave antenna modules with backside-assembled RF ICs: (a) IBM's switched beam antenna in package [50, 51]. (*Source*: Gu, X., Liu, D., Baks, C., et al., 2017 and 2019.) (b) Qualcomm's antenna array modules [52], (*Source*: Dunworth, J., Ku, B.-H., Ou, Y.C. et al., 2018 © IEEE.) and (c) fan-out packaging and embedded components from TSMC [53]. (*Source:* Tsai, C.H., Hsieh, J.-S., Liu, M., et al., 2013. © IEEE.)

to support linear dual polarization with 20 dB isolation and dual-frequency antennas. A fan-out embedded wafer level ball (eWLB) with SiGe-BiCMOS technology and integrated fan-out (InFO) with embedded millimeter-wave ICs were demonstrated by Infineon Technologies and Taiwan semiconductor company (TSMC), respectively [53, 54]. In one such approach by TSMC, RDL in the bottom feeds the slot-coupled patch antennas on the top side. Wafer fan-out packaging technologies are developed to address the interconnect power losses from solder bumps and long substrate traces. TSMC's antenna array with embedded transceiver ICs showed a gain of 14.7 dBi with 10 mm ICs, as illustrated in Figure 12.17c [53]. The power divider (3.5 dB loss), coupler (4.1 dB), and balun (4.1 dB) show substantial improvement of 20–36% in loss compared to the on-chip counterparts.

12.8.6 High-Density RF Flex Packaging

Flexible packaging is predominantly driven by the integration of sensors, communication, and power functions. These packages do not support large data processing as the computing is performed outside the package. Therefore, the lines/spaces, layer count, and device integration requirements are much relaxed. The packages typically support lines/spaces of above 100 μm and typically two layers. The key innovation, however, is in the heterogeneous integration of sensing, processing, and communication functions using low-cost conformal flexible, wearable, or on-skin packaging materials. One key innovation is in the integration of sensing functions in textiles, bandages, or other flex substrates with the incorporation of electrochemical and sensing electrodes with the respective biological recognition layers and encapsulants. These electrical functions are created with smart conductive threads that can be interwoven with any wound or fabric dressing. These sensors are utilized to monitor pH, temperature, oxygenation, inflammation or wound status, glucose, urea, cortisol levels, or other health monitors. Other than health tracking, wireless sensors are also used for smart cities, structural health monitoring, security, and broadly all Internet of Things (IoT) applications.

Power functions are embedded with flexible batteries and supercapacitors that are charged with a power-harvesting or wireless power-transfer interface. This topic is described in detail in Section 12.8.7. The electronic communication interface is integrated as a detachable or permanent layer on the top in order to provide the power, signal processing, and communications to the internal reader. A schematic description of a smart bandage as a wound-monitoring and therapeutic device can be referred from [33].

12.8.7 Hybrid Flex Sensor-Processing-Communication Systems

A hybrid combination of these technologies is ideal for gaining the optimal performance, cost, and integration benefits from the multiple technologies such as bandage, fabric or textile, flex, and rigid substrate integration. For example, power-harvesting and communication antenna can be embedded in the wearable textiles such as jackets, benefitting from their large areas, while the active devices for processing and controller functions along with communications are embedded in the high-density flex or rigid packages. The sensing functions are integrated as fabric or bandage patches on the skin with compliant electrodes. The key to enable these distributed functions is the development of smart, flexible, and remateable or permanent connectors between different subsystems. Connectors between rigid devices and flexible package interfaces are a key reliability concern. The key to address this reliability concern is to delocalize the strain or deformation from the sensitive interface to other regions along the interconnect so that the interfaces only undergo elastic deformation instead of the plastic deformation. Flexible connectors that utilize various interconnect options such as conductive adhesives, plastically deformably metal joints, and compliant mechanically interlocking metal interconnect structures are being developed to address this need.

References

1 Zhang, L., Wang, Z., and Volakis, J.L. (2012). Textile antennas and sensors for body-worn applications. *IEEE Antennas and Wireless Propagation Letters* 11: 1690–1693.

2 Wang, Z., Zhang, L., and Volakis, J.L. (2013). Textile antennas for wearable radio frequency applications. *Textiles and Light Industrial Science and Technology (TLIST)* 2 (3): 105–112.

3 Chiolerio, A., Cotto, M., Pandolfi, P. et al. (2012). Ag nanoparticle-based inkjet printed planar transmission lines for RF and microwave applications: considerations on ink composition, nanoparticle size distribution and sintering time. *Microelectronic Engineering* 97: 8–15.

4 McKerricher, G., Perez, J.G., and Shamim, A. (2015). Fully inkjet printed RF inductors and capacitors using polymer dielectric and silver conductive ink with through vias. *IEEE Transactions on Electron Devices* 62 (3): 1002–1009.

5 Chen, Z., Xi, J., Huang, W., and Yuen, M.M.F. (2017). Stretchable conductive elastomer for wireless wearable communication applications. *Scientific Reports* 7 (1): 1–8.

6 Boutry, C.M., Chandrahalim, H., and Hierold, C. (2012). RF conductivity of biodegradable conductive polymers used for a new generation of partially/fully resorbable wireless implantable sensors. Proceedings of the IEEE International Conference on Micro Electro Mechanical Systems (MEMS), 2012, 468–471.

7 Vital, D., Zhong, J., Bhardwaj, S., and Volakis, J.L. (2018). Loss-characterization and guidelines for embroidery of conductive textiles. 2018 IEEE Antennas and Propagation Society International Symposium and USNC/URSI National Radio Science Meeting, APSURSI 2018 - Proceedings, 2018, 1301–1302.

8 Vital, D., Bhardwaj, S., and Volakis, J.L. (2020). Textile based large area RF-power harvesting system for wearable applications. *IEEE Transactions on Antennas and Propagation* 68 (3): 2323–2331.

9 Kiourti, A., Lee, C., and Volakis, J.L. (2016). Fabrication of textile antennas and circuits with 0.1 mm precision. *IEEE Antennas and Wireless Propagation Letters* 15: 151–153.

10 Cummins, G. and Desmulliez, M.P.Y. (2012). Inkjet printing of conductive materials: a review. *Circuit World* 38 (4): 193–213.

11 Zhou, Y., Bayram, Y., Du, F. et al. (2010). Polymer-carbon nanotube sheets for conformal load bearing antennas. *IEEE Transactions on Antennas and Propagation* 58 (7): 2169–2175.

12 So, J.-H., Thelen, J., Qusba, A. et al. (2009). Reversibly deformable and mechanically tunable fluidic antennas. *Advanced Functional Materials* 19 (22): 3632–3637.

13 Li, X., Kjellander, B.K.C., Anthony, J. et al. (2009). Azeotropic binary solvent mixtures for preparation of organic single crystals. *Advanced Functional Materials* 19 (22): 3610–3617.

14 Vyas, R., Rida, A., Bhattacharya, S., and Tentzeris, M.M. (2007). Liquid Crystal Polymer (LCP): the ultimate solution for low-cost RF flexible

electronics and antennas. IEEE Antennas and Propagation Society, AP-S International Symposium (Digest), 2007, 1729–1732.

15 Sharifi, H., Lahiji, R.R., Lin, H.C. et al. (2009). Characterization of parylene-N as flexible substrate and passivation layer for microwave and millimeter-wave integrated circuits. *IEEE Transactions on Advanced Packaging* 32 (1): 84–92.

16 Koulouridis, S., Kiziltas, G., Zhou, Y. et al. (2006). Polymer-ceramic composites for microwave applications: fabrication and performance assessment. *IEEE Transactions on Microwave Theory and Techniques* 54 (12): 4202–4208.

17 Volakis, J.L., Zhang, L., Wang, Z., and Bayram, Y. (2012). Embroidered flexible RF electronics. 2012 IEEE International Workshop on Antenna Technology, iWAT 2012, 2012, 8–11.

18 Zhong, J., Kiourti, A., Sebastian, T. et al. (2017). Conformal load-bearing spiral antenna on conductive textile threads. *IEEE Antennas and Wireless Propagation Letters* 16: 230–233.

19 Vital, D., Bhardwaj, S., and Volakis, J.L. (2019). Bending and twisting tests for RF performances of textile transmission lines. 2019 IEEE International Symposium on Antennas and Propagation and USNC-URSI Radio Science Meeting, APSURSI 2019 - Proceedings, 2019, 2173–2174.

20 Lee, C.W., Papantonis, D., Kiourti, A., and Volakis, J.L. (2017). Body-worn 67:1 bandwidth antenna using 3 overlapping dipole elements. 2017 11th European Conference on Antennas and Propagation, EUCAP 2017, 2017, 1557–1558.

21 Wang, Z., Lee, L.Z., Psychoudakis, D., and Volakis, J.L. (2014). Embroidered multiband body-worn antenna for GSM/PCS/WLAN communications. *IEEE Transactions on Antennas and Propagation* 62 (6): 3321–3329.

22 Shao, S., Kiourti, A., Burkholder, R.J., and Volakis, J.L. (2015). Broadband textile-based passive UHF RFID tag antenna for elastic material. *IEEE Antennas and Wireless Propagation Letters* 14: 1385–1388.

23 Vital, D., Bhardwaj, S., and Volakis, J.L. (2019). Misalignment resilient, near field wireless power transfer (WPT) antennas using anchor shape. 2019 IEEE International Symposium on Antennas and Propagation and USNC-URSI Radio Science Meeting, APSURSI 2019 - Proceedings, 2019, 1795–1796.

24 Dargaville, T.R., Farrugia, B.L., Broadbent, J.A. et al. (2013). Sensors and imaging for wound healing: a review. *Biosensors and Bioelectronics* 41 (1): 30–42.

25 Wang, Z., Zhang, L., Bayram, Y., and Volakis, J.L. (2012). Embroidered conductive fibers on polymer composite for conformal antennas. *IEEE Transactions on Antennas and Propagation* 60 (9): 4141–4147.

26 Sekar, M., Pandiaraj, M., Bhansali, S. et al. (2019). Carbon fiber based electrochemical sensor for sweat cortisol measurement. *Scientific Reports* 9 (1) Article number: 403: 1–8.

27 Deng, F., He, Y., Li, B. et al. (2015). Design of an embedded CMOS temperature sensor for passive RFID tag chips. *Sensors (Switzerland)* 15 (5): 11442–11453.

28 Wang, H. and Mercier, P.P. (2017). Near-zero-power temperature sensing via tunneling currents through complementary metal-oxide-semiconductor transistors. *Scientific Reports* 7 (1) Article number: 4427: 1–8.

29 Souri, K., Chae, Y., Thus, F., and Makinwa, K. (2014). A 0.85V 600nW all-CMOS temperature sensor with an inaccuracy of ±0.4°C (3s) from -40 to 125°C. Digest of Technical Papers - IEEE International Solid-State Circuits Conference, 2014, vol. 57, 222–223.

30 Law, M.K. and Bermak, A. (2009). A 405-nW CMOS temperature sensor based on linear MOS operation. *IEEE Transactions on Circuits and Systems II: Express Briefs* 56 (12): 891–895.

31 ARANZ Medical. Imaging/Photography for Clinical Trials & Research | ARANZ Medical [Online]. www.aranzmedical.com (accessed 22 December 2019).

32 Bowling, F.L., Paterson, J., and Ndip, A. (2013). Applying 21st century imaging technology to wound healing: an Avant-Gardist approach. *Journal of Diabetes Science and Technology* 7 (5): 1190–1194.

33 Mostafalu, P., Tamayol, A., Rahimi, R. et al. (2018). Smart bandage for monitoring and treatment of chronic wounds. *Small* 14 (33): 1703509.

34 MarketsandMarkets. Wound Care Market Worth $24.8 Billion by 2024 - Exclusive Report by MarketsandMarkets™ [Online]. https://www.prnewswire.com/news-releases/wound-care-market-worth-24-8-billion-by-2024--exclusive-report-by-marketsandmarkets-300921596.html (accessed 22 December 2019).

35 Fernandez, M.L., Upton, Z., Edwards, H. et al. (2012). Elevated uric acid correlates with wound severity. *International Wound Journal* 9 (2): 139–149.

36 Fernandez, M.L., Upton, Z., and Shooter, G.K. (2014). Uric acid and xanthine oxidoreductase in wound healing. *Current Rheumatology Reports* 16 (2): 396.

37 Umasankar, Y., Mujawar, M., and Bhansali, S. (2018). Towards biosensor enabled smart bandages for wound monitoring: approach and overview. Proceedings of IEEE Sensors, 2018, vol. October 2018.

38 Filanovsky, M.G., Sukhdeo, K., and McNamara, M.C. (2015). Ulcerated tophaceous gout. BML Case Reports, bcr2015210707, 2015.

39 Sato, Y., Sitaraman, S., Sukumaran, V. et al. (2013). Ultra-miniaturized and surface-mountable glass-based 3D IPAC packages for RF modules. Proceedings - Electronic Components and Technology Conference, 2013, 1656–1661.

40 Min, J., Wu, Z., Pulugurtha, M.R. et al. (2016). Modeling design fabrication and demonstration of RF front-end module with ultra-thin glass substrate for LTE applications. Proceedings - Electronic Components and Technology Conference, 2016, vol. August 2016, 1297–1302.

41 Sukumaran, V., Kumar, G., Ramachandran, K. et al. (2014). Design, fabrication, and characterization of ultrathin 3-D glass interposers with through-package-vias at same pitch as tSVs in silicon. *IEEE Transactions on Components, Packaging and Manufacturing Technology* 4 (5): 786–795.

42 Sukumaran, V., Bandyopadhyay, T., Sundaram, V., and Rao, T. (2012). Low-cost thin glass interposers as a superior alternative to silicon and organic interposers for packaging of 3-D ICs. *IEEE Transactions on Components, Packaging and Manufacturing Technology* 2 (9): 1426–1433.

43 Tehrani, B.K., Cook, B.S., and Tentzeris, M.M. (2016). Inkjet-printed 3D interconnects for millimeter-wave system-on-package solutions. IEEE MTT-S International Microwave Symposium Digest, 2016, vol. August 2016.

44 Zhu, L.Z., Wei, X.B., Wang, P. et al. (2011). Compact LTCC module for WLAN RF front-end. 2011 International Conference on Computational Problem-Solving, ICCP 2011, 2011, 387–389.

45 Sakhnenko, S., Orlenko, D., Vorotnikov, B. et al. (2009). Ultra-low-profile small-size LTCC Front-End Module (FEM) for WLAN applications based on a novel diplexer design approach. IEEE MTT-S International Microwave Symposium Digest, 2009, 609–612.

46 Yang, K., Pinel, S., Kim, I.K., and Laskar, J. (2006). Millimeter-wave low-loss integrated waveguide on liquid crystal polymer substrate. IEEE MTT-S International Microwave Symposium Digest, 2006, 965–968.

47 Mohamed, I. and Sebak, A.R. (2018). Broadband transition of substrate-integrated waveguide-to-air-filled rectangular waveguide. *IEEE Microwave and Wireless Components Letters* 28 (11): 966–968.

48 Peng, X., Chen, J., Tang, H. et al. (2015). Broadband and low-loss rectangular waveguide to substrate integrated waveguide transition with fin line. 2015 IEEE MTT-S International Microwave Symposium, IMS 2015, 2015.

49 Kazemi, R., Fathy, A.E., Yang, S., and Sadeghzadeh, R.A. (2012). Development of an ultra wide band GCPW to SIW transition. RWW 2012 - Proceedings: IEEE Radio and Wireless Symposium, RWS 2012, 2012, 171–174.

50 Gu, X., Liu, D., Baks, C. et al. (2019). Development, implementation, and characterization of a 64-element dual-polarized phased-array antenna module for 28-GHz high-speed data communications. *IEEE Transactions on Microwave Theory and Techniques* 67 (7): 2975–2984.

51 Gu, X., Liu, D., Baks, C. et al. (2017). A multilayer organic package with 64 dual-polarized antennas for 28GHz 5G communication. IEEE MTT-S International Microwave Symposium Digest, 2017, 1899–1901.

52 Dunworth, J., Ku, B.-H., Ou, Y.-C. et al. (2018). 28 GHz phased array transceiver in 28nm bulk CMOS for 5G prototype user equipment and base stations. IEEE MTT-S International Microwave Symposium Digest, 2018, vol. June 2018, 1330–1333.

53 Tsai, C.H., Hsieh, J.-S., Liu, M. et al. (2013). Array antenna integrated fan-out wafer level packaging (InFO-WLP) for millimeter wave system applications. Technical Digest - International Electron Devices Meeting, IEDM, 2013.

54 Thai, T., Dalmia, S., Hagn, J. et al. (2019). Novel multicore PCB and substrate solutions for ultra broadband dual polarized antennas for 5G millimeter wave covering 28GHz & 39GHz range. Proceedings - Electronic Components and Technology Conference, 2019, vol. May 2019, 954–959.

13

Coupling-Independent Sensing Systems with Fully Passive Sensors

Siavash Kananian, George Alexopoulos and Ada Poon

Department of Electrical Engineering, Stanford University, Stanford, CA, USA

13.1 Introduction

Contactless sensing and data telemetry enable a wide range of applications. For example, early detection and diagnosis of diseases through simple checkups and remote diagnostics on handheld devices at home eliminate the need for excessive visits to healthcare providers. In hospitals, wireless, handheld tracking of these same diagnostics allows for greater mobility during in-patient stay. Furthermore, tracking of environmental variables, such as temperature, pressure, humidity, and more, can enable cost- and energy-efficient remote monitoring of infrastructure and inventory conditions in smart cities, warehouses, and markets. Specifically, it can allow for improved safety in the food chain, where contamination can happen in many stages of production and transportation, by providing consumers and businesses with a noninvasive, yet convenient way to monitor possible food spoilage and deterioration. Additionally, it can provide for the capability of fruit ripeness determination in smart agriculture, aiding the farming industry in timing of harvests and transportation. Finally, remote sensing can enable many other applications, such as gesture detection and touchless control of devices in consumer electronics and medical procedures.

A *complete* and *practical* sensing system requires simultaneous innovations in both the reader and the sensor; current solutions have only managed to achieve one, pairing either simple sensors with bulky readers containing highly sophisticated front and back ends or simple readers with prohibitively complex and costly sensors that inhibit widespread remote sensing (Figure 13.1).

The first major requirement, therefore, is a *practical* reader that is ultra-low-power, simple, and potentially handheld or wearable; this solution should rely on simple measurement techniques in order to eliminate the need for bulky and expensive parts. Next, the system should employ sensors that

Antenna and Sensor Technologies in Modern Medical Applications,
First Edition. Edited by Yahya Rahmat-Samii and Erdem Topsakal.

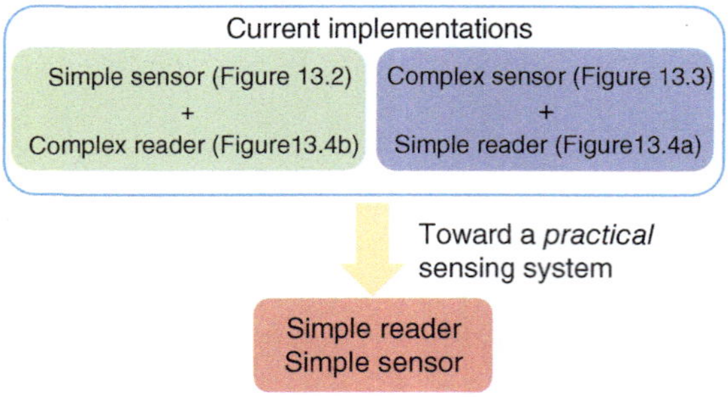

Figure 13.1 Current implementations of sensing systems and the path toward more practical sensing systems.

have *low complexity, cost,* and *power consumption.* Finally, such a system must be *robust,* avoiding the need for frequency, distance, and orientation optimization in order to achieve efficient power and/or data transfer.

Fully passive sensors in this chapter refer to sensors consisting only of an RLC tank; an inductor coil is used to communicate the measurement of the sensor, a capacitive and/or a resistive element whose value changes in response to a parameter such as pressure, humidity, and pH. Examples of such sensors are shown in Figure 13.2 [1–3]; such sensors provide information through features in their impedance profile, offering a considerably lower price and complexity compared to their active counterparts. Examples of active sensors are shown in Figure 13.3 [4, 5]. Such sensors require a power source either in the form of a battery (Figure 13.3a), posing size and replacement concerns, or in the form of inefficient wireless energy-harvesting techniques (Figure 13.3b), necessitating a power-hungry reader (Figure 13.4a). Figure 13.3c shows the block diagram of an active (or active/passive) sensor, which in comparison to its passive counterparts, shown in Figure 13.2d, requires more building blocks. On the other hand, while passive sensors traditionally require an asymmetric link with a complex reader to compensate for their lack of versatility (Figure 13.4b,c), they can be made disposable, biodegradable, and stretchable; and do not require an explicit power source.

In order to extract measurements from fully passive sensors, electromagnetic far- or near-field interrogation techniques are commonly used. In the former, a radio transmits an interrogation signal and listens for a specific reflection pattern at the resonant frequency of the sensor (Figure 13.4b). This approach suffers from a two-way propagation path loss ($\propto R^4$, where R is the separation between the sensor and the reader), necessitating a high transmitted power and dynamic range. Although far-field interrogation provides an extended range, it is not well suited for ultra-low-power, handheld applications. Near-field techniques bypass these propagation-related issues by instead relying on magnetic coupling (traditionally) between the reader and the sensor; while the maximum operating distance is more limited, the more complex aspects of antenna

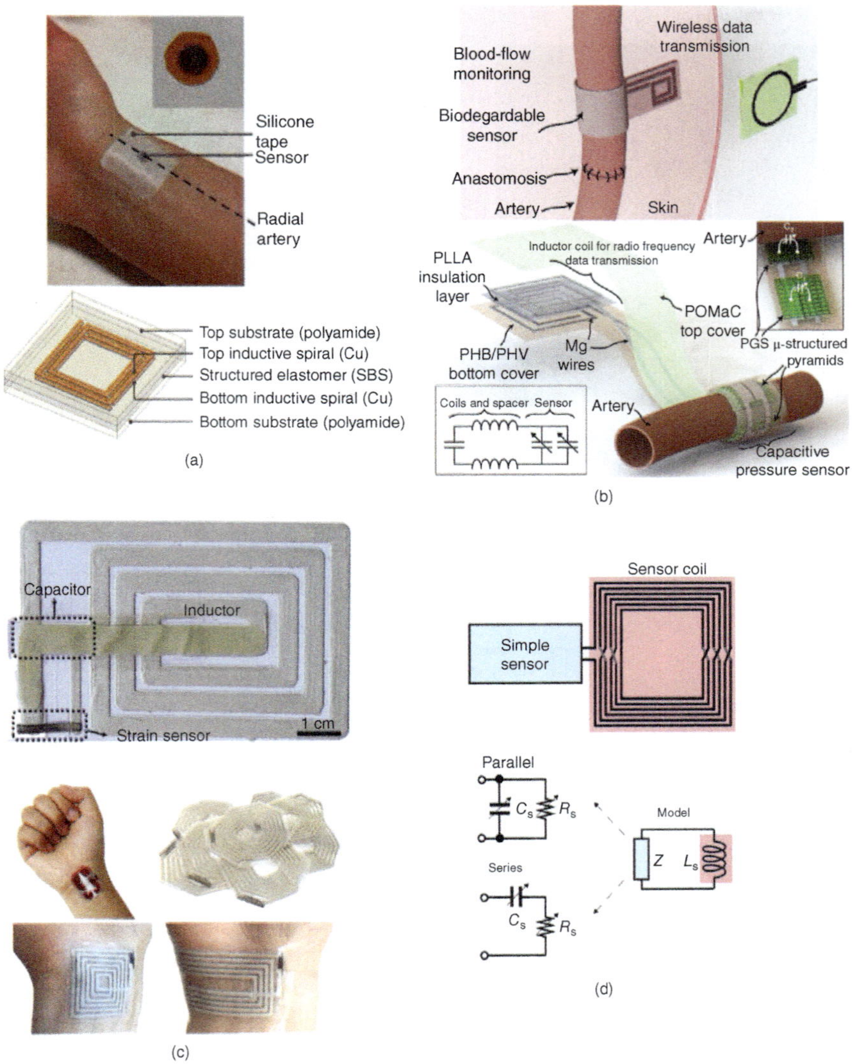

Figure 13.2 (a–c) Examples of fully passive (simple) sensors in the literature. (d) Electrical model of a fully passive sensor, consisting of a capacitive and/or resistive element whose value changes in response to a sensing parameter. (*Source*: Chen, L.Y., Tee, BC., Chortos, A.L., et al., 2015. © Springer Nature; Boutry, C.M., Beker, L., Kaizawa, Y., et al., 2019; and Niu, S., Matsuhisa, N., Beker, L., et al., 2019. © 2019 Springer Nature.)

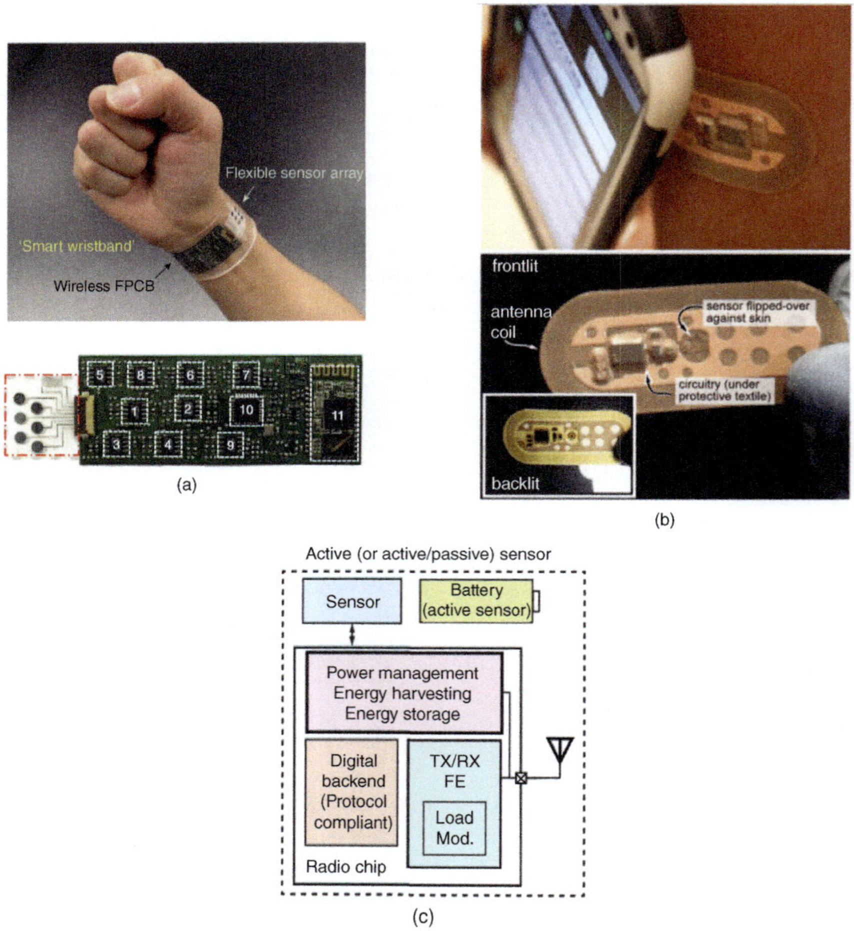

Figure 13.3 Examples of more complex sensors (active or active/passive) in the literature with (a) an active sensor running on a LiPo battery [4] (*Source*: Gao, W., Emaminejad, S., Nyein, H., et al., 2016. Reproduced with permission from Nature. Springer Nature.) and (b) an active/passive sensor using RFID-based energy harvesting [5]. (*Source*: Rose, D. P. et al., 2015. Reproduced with permission from IEEE.) (c) Generic block diagram of an active or active/passive sensor. Active sensors require a battery, while active/passive sensors rely on energy harvesting from an external RF signal. Such sensors consist of a protocol compliant transmitter (TX), receiver (RX), and front end (FE), as well as a digital backend to handle protocol-related processing. Load (or backscatter) modulation is commonly employed in RFID systems in which mismatched loads are used to reflect the incident RF signal back with a certain modulation (amplitude and/or phase).

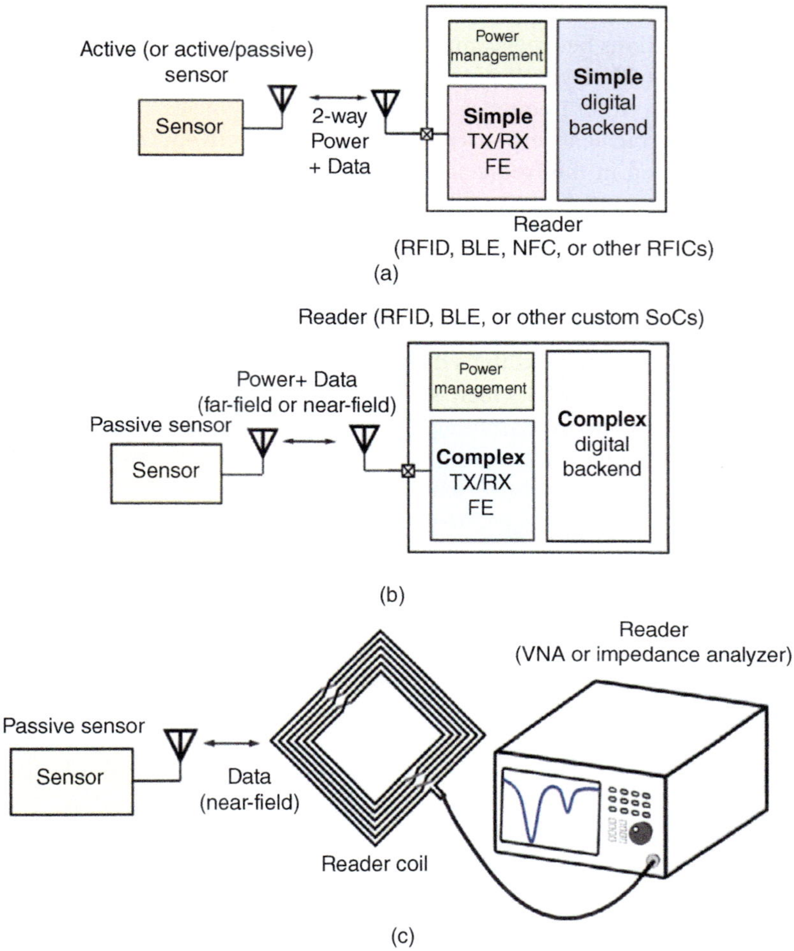

Figure 13.4 (a) Sensing system based on active sensors: the reader is relatively simple, yet the sensor is costly and complex. Passive sensor interrogation techniques: (b) using RFID or other legacy radios, requiring a protocol compliant sensor and (c) using bulky analyzers. Passive sensors and near-field reader methods provide reduced cost and complexity at the expense of robustness compared to active/passive (sensors with energy harvesting) and active (battery-powered) sensors and far-field reader methods; the goal is to maintain the low cost and complexity of near-field and passive methods while combining them in an intelligent manner to dramatically improve robustness.

design, optimization, and implementation are instead replaced by magnetic coupling considerations between simple, typically planar inductive coils.

Currently, near-field magnetically coupled techniques provide sensor measurements based on either frequency or time-domain responses, which rely on the steady state or transient response of the sensor, respectively. In the former, sensing is performed in the frequency domain through the measurement of some features of the impedance profile (or its variants, such as reflection coefficient) of the coupled system using either bulky and expensive lab equipment like a vector network analyzer (VNA) (Figure 13.4c) or a custom-designed radio front end with complex baseband receiver (RX) and frequency-swept transmitter (TX) [6–8] (Figure 13.4b); for example, as will be seen later, the phase of the input impedance will simply exhibit a dip at the resonant frequency of the sensor [9, 10]. This technique offers high SNR and large dynamic range [11]; nevertheless, the major issue in examining impedance profiles is the dependence of the mutual inductance (or coupling factor, k) on coil geometry, separation distance, alignment, and relative orientation. For this reason, this technique requires fixed orientation and spacing between coils [12], which is impractical or infeasible in many applications. Some methods address this k-dependence of the sensor readout using other properties of the impedance; they do, however, require a high-quality factor (Q) sensor and higher power consumption and more complex reader [13, 14]. Time-domain approaches, on the other hand, are based on time gating; in other words, perturbing the sensor with a pulse and recording its damped oscillations [15–18]. In these approaches the perturbing action and sensor readout must occur in nonoverlapping cycles, requiring a T/R switch. Additionally, the received signal typically has small amplitude and short duration, calling for front-end amplification and higher sampling rates [18, 19]. The goal, therefore, of this chapter, is to introduce a set of new methods for a complete and practical sensing system that can provide repeatable measurements irrespective of coupling strength variations.

The chapter is organized as follows.

- First, a distinction will be made between *forced* (or controlled) oscillating systems, which require an external source to tune or sweep the amplitude and/or frequency of oscillation, and *self-oscillating* systems that can reach a steady-state oscillation on their own.
- Next, the respective measurement methods of such systems will be discussed, starting with those using a nonresonant primary. Then, methods that add either a forced resonator or oscillator to the reader will be detailed; as the forced reader is tuned across a frequency range, changes in the frequency response are monitored as a means of sensing.
- These controls will then be replaced by an oscillator that will allow for *self-oscillating* capability such that the reader does not need to be forced to provide a steady-state oscillation; in this case, measurements of changes in

either the amplitude or frequency of oscillation allow for sensor readout. Such systems offer more flexibility and less complexity as they do not rely on lab equipment such as a VNA or impedance analyzer or, for that matter, other power-hungry and complex custom-designed solutions, to directly characterize the input impedance profile and observe the resonant frequency.

- We provide a system-by-system comparison for the reader in terms of both sensitivity of the system to small coupling strengths and complexity of measurement. A high sensitivity to small coupling strengths is desirable as it enables measurements from smaller sensors; we, however, show that this can come at the cost of either requiring multiple sweeps and extra resonators/oscillators or exhibiting high measurement sensitivity to inaccuracies/errors in tuning; this comparison will aid the reader in understanding the various performance-complexity trade-offs of these near-field, passive sensing systems.
- We finally conclude with some future directions in this area including more real-time approaches that preclude the need for tuning/sweeping and sensing using other different sensor modalities.

13.2 Forced vs. Self-Oscillating Near-Field Readout

In terms of methods for exciting/energizing sensors, readout techniques for near-field passive sensors can be categorized into forced and self-oscillating approaches. In the former, the reader is forced to oscillate at a certain frequency, for example, using a VNA, an impedance analyzer, or a signal generator. Once the sensor is placed in the measurement range of the reader, the frequency or time-domain response of the coupled system, which is related to the resonant frequency of the sensor, is measured. As will be discussed later, the measured parameter, related to the resonant frequency of the sensor, can be the frequency and/or impedance profile (phase or real part of the impedance) of the coupled sensor–reader system or the amplitude of damped oscillations.

In the self-oscillating approach, a negative resistance is embedded in the reader. The nonlinear behavior of this negative resistance turns the system into an oscillator, which does not require an external excitation to operate and perform the sensor readout. The frequency or amplitude of these oscillations will then be measured and used to perform sensor readout. In some implementations, a frequency sweep is performed, similar to the forced oscillation approach. These techniques do not require an explicit signal source, namely a VNA or impedance analyzer, and, as a result, allow for more practical sensing. The parameter which is measured and is related to the resonant frequency can be the frequency of oscillations, frequency variations during a frequency

Table 13.1 Summary of the existing fully passive sensing techniques based on near-field magnetic coupling.

	Measured parameters		
	Amplitude	**Frequency**	**Impedance phase**
Forced oscillations	Amplitude peaking (Section 13.3.1a)	Diabolic point (Section 13.3.2a)	Phase-dip method (Section 13.3.1a)
	Step response (Section 13.3.1b)	$\mathcal{PT}$-symmetric (Section 13.3.2b)	Reflection coefficient (Section 13.3.1a)
		Exceptional point-locking (Section 13.3.2c)	
Self-oscillating	Grid-dip meter (Section 13.3.3b)	$\mathcal{PT}$-symmetric (Section 13.3.3a)	—
		Exceptional point-locking (Section 13.3.3c)	

sweep, or the amplitude of oscillations. Table 13.1 summarizes the existing techniques.

Figure 13.5a provides an analogy between an ideal resonator circuit and an ideal mechanical mass-spring system (in the absence of friction). In such a system, either a periodic external force with frequency ω can force the mass-spring system to resonate at a certain steady-state frequency (forced oscillation), or an impulse force can initiate steady-state oscillation at the resonant frequency of the system (self-oscillating). Regardless, the mass-spring system resonates with a certain displacement and resonant frequency similar to the voltage (or current) amplitude and resonant frequency in the ideal resonator circuit; the difference lies in whether the resonator must be continuously excited (forced oscillation) or only initially excited (self-oscillating).

Without loss of generality, for the rest of this chapter we assume that a resonator consists of either a parallel or series RLC circuit and that both cases may be considered to be equivalent. A circuit exhibiting loss (positive resistance) will be referred to as a resonator, whereas a circuit exhibiting gain (negative resistance) will be referred to as an oscillator. This chapter focuses on four main reader architectures, and the details of each of these approaches are shown in Figure 13.5. These will consist of a forced nonresonant reader, a forced resonator reader, a forced oscillator reader, and a self-oscillating reader; the higher order techniques discussed in Sections 13.3.2c and 13.3.3c will merely be extensions of these architectures. The sensed parameter in the techniques mentioned

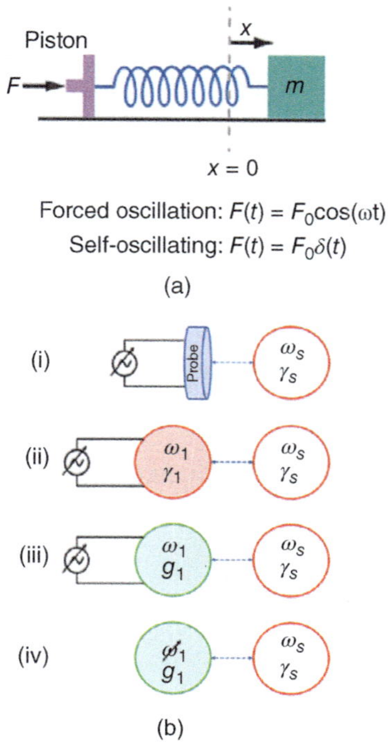

Figure 13.5 (a) Mechanical mass-spring analogy indicating the behavior of a forcing term on resonator system operation. A resonator system requiring a periodic forcing term to oscillate at a certain steady-state frequency undergoes *forced* oscillation at a certain frequency, whereas a resonator system simply requiring a finite-time, *initial* forcing term to resonate at a certain steady-state frequency (resonant frequency, ω_0) undergoes a *self-oscillating* behavior. (b) Systems with the various reader architectures that this chapter will focus on: (i) forced nonresonant probe reader, (ii) forced resonator reader, (iii) forced oscillator reader, and (iv) self-oscillating reader; both the forcing mechanism (external, equipment such as a VNA and impedance analyzer) and the self-oscillating reader are frequency swept, and coupling (blue, dashed arrows) between the reader and sensor is assumed to be magnetic. Green circles represent oscillators, whereas red circles represent resonators; reader circles have a fill to further distinguish them from sensor circles (no fill). Henceforth, the subscript *s* will denote properties of the sensor, whereas numerical subscripts will denote properties of the reader.

in Table 13.1 and Figure 13.5 can be a capacitance, a resistance, combination of the two, and/or coupling strength.

13.3 Readout Techniques

13.3.1 Forced Oscillation Techniques with Nonresonant Primary

a) Steady-state measurement

The simplest way of performing readout on a fully passive sensor is by means of inductive coupling, in which case the coupled system forms an impedance transformer. The primary side of the transformer can be a single inductor (non-resonant) or a tuned *LC* tank (resonant). For now, we consider the former, and address the latter in the rest of this section.

The circuit in Figure 13.6 is a possible implementation of Figure 13.5b–i, where a sensor is coupled to the readout coil [13, 14]. The input impedance,

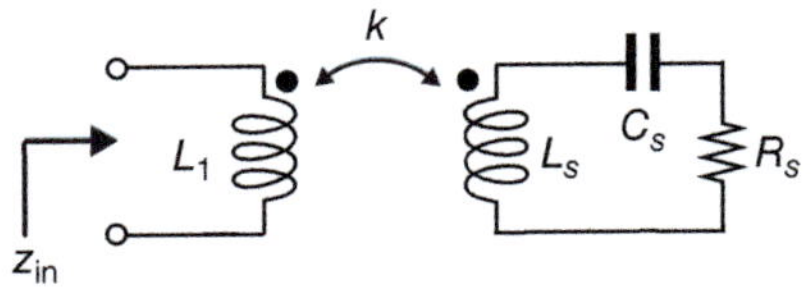

Figure 13.6 Series sensor readout with a nonprimary reader coil and the impedance seen from the reader coil.

as seen from the reader coil, can be written as

$$Z_{\text{in}} = j\omega L_1 + \frac{\omega^2 k^2 L_1 L_s}{R_s + \frac{1}{j\omega C_s} + j\omega L_s}. \tag{13.1}$$

From this, the real and imaginary parts of the impedance are given by

$$Re\{Z_{\text{in}}\} = \omega L_1 k^2 Q_s \left(\frac{\frac{\omega}{\omega_s}}{1 + Q_s^2 \left(\frac{\omega}{\omega_s} - \frac{\omega_s}{\omega} \right)^2} \right), \tag{13.2a}$$

$$Im\{Z_{\text{in}}\} = \omega L_1 \left(1 + k^2 Q_s^2 \frac{1 - \left(\frac{\omega}{\omega_s} \right)^2}{1 + Q_s^2 \left(\frac{\omega}{\omega_s} - \frac{\omega_s}{\omega} \right)^2} \right), \tag{13.2b}$$

where $Q_s = \frac{1}{R_s}\sqrt{\frac{L_s}{C_s}}$ is the quality factor of the sensor. As shown in [13, 20–24], the phase of the input impedance exhibits a dip at

$$\omega_{\varphi,\text{min}} \approx \left(1 + \frac{k^2}{4} \right) \omega_s \tag{13.3}$$

for $Q_s \gg 1$ and small k. As suggested by Equation (13.3), $\omega_{\varphi,\,\text{min}}$ is a function of the coupling strength, k. The value of the dip is calculated in [20] as $\Delta\varphi = \tan^{-1}(k^2 Q_s)$. Therefore, not only does this approach require a large quality factor in the sensor to achieve a sharper dip [23], but it is also not accurate for large k. Figure 13.7 illustrates the phase of the input impedance for $k = 0.1$ to 1 vs. frequency, suggesting that the measurements of ω_s will be heavily dependent on the value of k. This phase dip is usually measured with a network or impedance analyzer [21–25], and the measurement needs to be done at a certain fixed, optimized distance such that k is both not too large and not too small for accurate measurement of ω_s, as a very small k will result in a very small $\Delta\varphi$ (Figure 13.7). As a result, the phase dip technique does not provide a robust measurement.

In order to provide a more robust measurement of ω_s the authors of [13, 14, 26, 27] have proposed measurement of the real part of the input impedance vs.

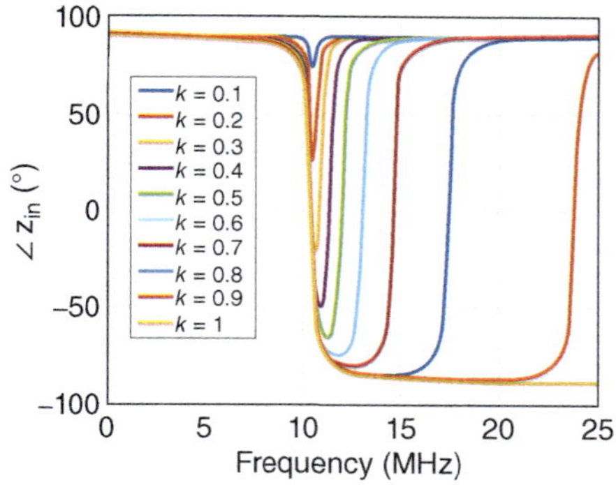

Figure 13.7 Dependence of the phase dip on the coupling strength for $k = 0.1$ through $k = 1$ in steps of 0.1; as k increases, the sharpness of the peak disappears.

frequency. As shown in [13, 14, 26], the real part of the impedance exhibits a peak at

$$\omega_{\max} = \frac{2Q_s}{\sqrt{4Q_s^2 - 2}}\omega_s \Bigg|_{Q_s \gg 1} \approx \left(1 + \frac{1}{4Q_s^2}\right)\omega_s, \tag{13.4}$$

which, unlike Equation (13.3), does not depend on k. Therefore, if the real part of the input impedance is measured vs. frequency, the peak frequency will be close to the sensor resonant frequency, that is, $\omega_{\max} \approx \omega_s$ for $Q_s \gg 1$; for example, $Q_s = 5$ results in an error of 1% in ω_s. For $Q_s \gg 1$ at $\omega_{\max}$, the authors of [13, 14, 26] show that $Re\{Z_{\text{in, max}}\} \approx \omega_s L_1 k^2 Q_s$. The behaviors of the real part and the phase and of the input impedance are illustrated in Figure 13.8a,b,

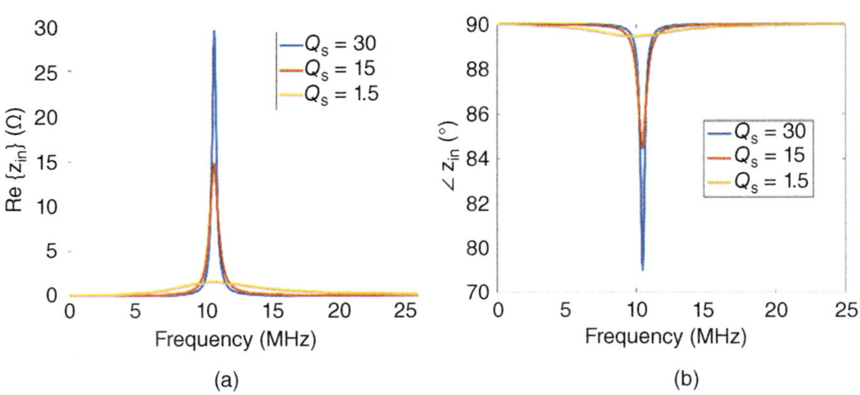

Figure 13.8 (a) Real part of the impedance and (b) phase dip with varying Q_s for the series sensor resonator, $L_1 = L_2 = 2.3\ \mu\text{H}$, $C_1 = C_2 = 100$ pF, $k = 0.08$.

respectively. It can be shown that for a parallel sensor configuration, the real part of the input impedance and its phase still exhibit similar peaking and dipping behavior as its series counterpart.

First proposed by Lizon-Martinez et al. [26] and also implemented in [13, 14, 27], the measurement of ω_{max} is based on obtaining the frequency response of the coupled system by injecting a frequency-swept current at the input, as shown in Figure 13.9a. This approach is based on coherent demodulation of the voltage across the primary coil and requires a mixer, synthesizer, analog front end, and other digital blocks. Although relatively complex, this work achieves relative errors of 0.02, 2, and 4% in measuring ω_s, Q, and k. However, as suggested in [25], no characterization of the error due to variations in the distance between the sensor and the reader are reported in [13, 14]. Figure 13.9b shows the implemented system, and Figure 13.9c shows the hardware prototype in [14], with the analog mixed-signal blocks required to perform sensing.

Using a similar principle, Chen et al. [1] has implemented an algorithm based on the input reflection coefficient. A power reflection distortion (PRD) quantity is defined as

$$\text{PRD}(\omega) = |\Gamma_{\text{in}}^2(\omega)|_{\text{without sensor}} - |\Gamma_{\text{in}}^2(\omega)|_{\text{with sensor}}, \tag{13.5}$$

which is maximized near the sensor's resonant frequency, similar to the peak frequency derived by the authors of [13, 14] in Equation (13.4). This can be explained by noting that, at the peak frequency, the imaginary part is approximately zero [13, 14] and the impedance is mostly resistive. As argued by Chen et al. [1], power absorption depends on the medium in which the sensor is placed and is sensitive to lossy environments such as human tissue. To overcome this issue, Chen et al. [1] has introduced another parameter, referred to as group-delay distortion (GDD) defined by

$$\text{GDD}(\omega) = \left.\frac{\partial\angle\Gamma_{\text{in}}}{\partial\omega}\right|_{\text{without sensor}} - \left.\frac{\partial\angle\Gamma_{\text{in}}}{\partial\omega}\right|_{\text{with sensor}}. \tag{13.6}$$

The peak frequency of GDD is given by Chen et al. [1] as

$$\text{argmax}_{\omega}[\text{GDD}(\omega)] = \omega_{\text{max}} \approx \left(1 + \frac{1}{8Q_s^2}\right)\omega_s. \tag{13.7}$$

A Q_s of 5 gives an error of 0.5% between the peak frequency and the sensor resonant frequency, while Q_s above 50 reduces this error to below 0.005%. Although independent of k, both the PRD and GDD methods rely on taking measurements and manipulation of the phase of the reflection coefficient using a VNA (Figure 13.10), an impractical requirement for handheld applications. Additionally, a calibration phase is required to determine the reference spectrum in the absence of the sensor, and the algorithm to find ω_{max} is implemented on a computer.

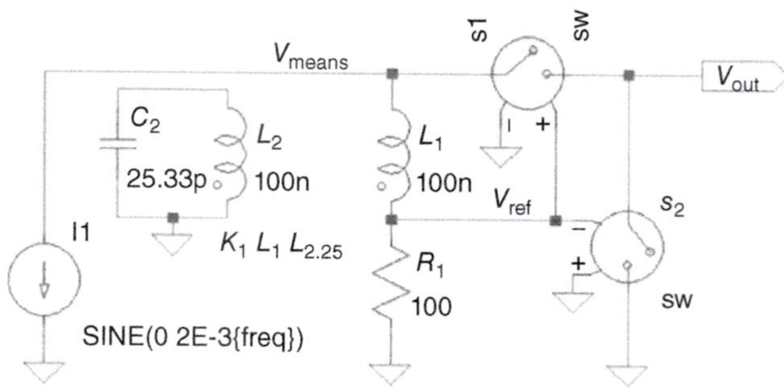

(a)

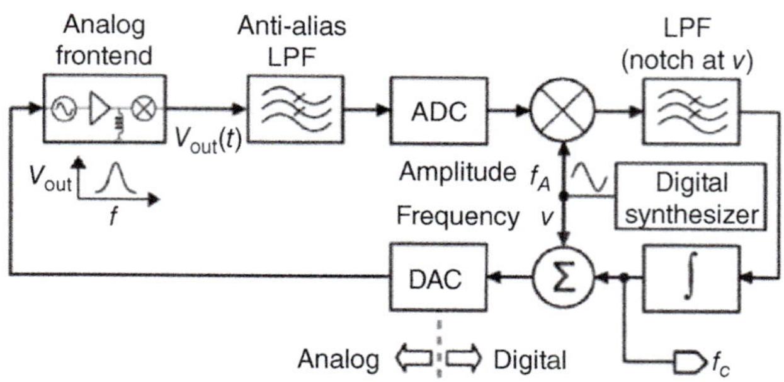

(b)

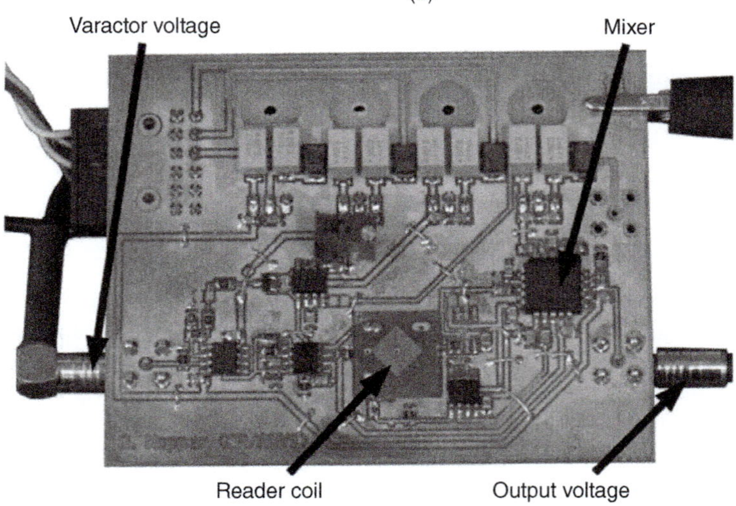

(c)

Figure 13.9 (a) The conceptual schematic of the reader in [14]. (b) Block diagram of the system including analog front end with inductively coupled sensor and digitally implemented extremum-seeking control [14]. (c) Prototype of the system in (b). *Source:* Nopper, R., Has, R., and Reindl, L., 2011. Reproduced with permission from IEEE.

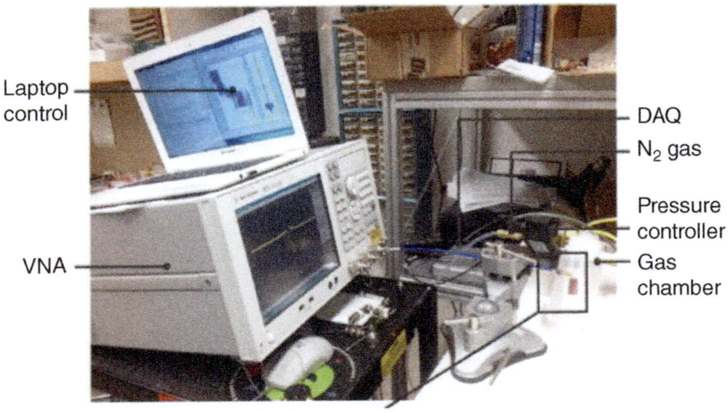

Figure 13.10 The measurement setup used in [1] involving the use of a VNA for GDD measurement. (*Source*: Chen et al. [1], Reproduced with permission from Nature Communications.)

Numerous other readout techniques have also been developed using the topology in Figure 13.5b–i for frequency-domain measurement. For example, Pichorim and Abatti [28] employs three coils, two of which form anti-Helmholtz coils to excite the sensor using one coil and make measurements on the others. Shown in Figure 13.11, this method is based on making three measurements at three different input frequencies and using the measured signal to calculate ω_s and Q_s. Compared to the method used by the authors of [1, 13, 14, 26, 27] which relies on continuous frequency sweeps, the method employed by Pichorim and Abatti [28] dramatically reduces the number of sweeps; nevertheless, the implemented system is still complicated, requiring three reader coils, three bandpass filters (with enough selectivity), and an external excitation source and signal processing to extract the sensor parameters by solving a system of equations.

b) Transient measurement

Transient techniques are based on perturbing the sensor with a pulsed excitation, modulated or unmodulated, and measuring the damped response of the sensor when the excitation is off. First proposed and implemented by Farrar et al. [29] and later by Joy et al. [30], the basic principle is depicted in Figure 13.12. It is instructive to derive an expression for the damped oscillations of V_1, the voltage across the primary coil in Figure 13.12a. To this end, we model the excitation signal by a single pulse of width τ and, for simplicity, we assume an unmodulated waveform (employed in [31] for sensor measurement). An ideal current source is assumed in this analysis with the knowledge that the input pulse with zero rise and fall time will cause an infinitely large voltage on the primary inductor (delta function); however, in a

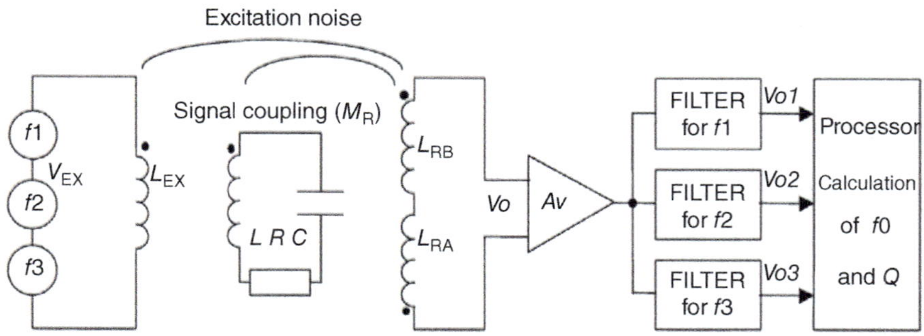

Figure 13.11 Block diagram of the sensing method based on using three measurements to solve a system of three equations and three unknowns [28]. (*Source*: Pichorim, S.F. and Abatti, P.J., 2008. © IEEE.)

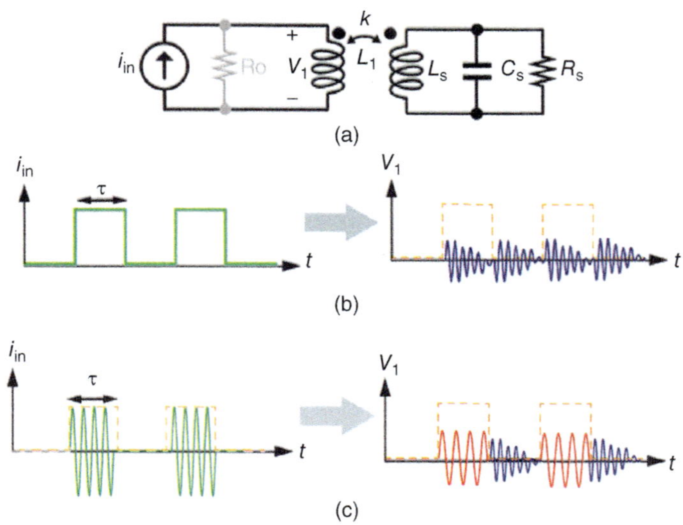

Figure 13.12 (a) Schematic of the parallel sensor configuration with pulsed current input. The transient response (damped oscillations) is obtained using either (b) an unmodulated or (c) a modulated pulse input. For series configuration, a voltage input should be used.

practical scenario the finite output resistance of the current source and finite rise and fall times of the input pulse will limit this voltage.

The input pulse can be written in the Laplace domain as

$$I_{in}(s) = \frac{1}{s}(1 - e^{-s\tau}) \tag{13.8}$$

with the input impedance for the parallel sensor given by

$$Z_{in}(s) = sL_1 + \frac{\omega^2 k^2 L_1 L_s (R_s C_s s + 1)}{s^2 L_s C_s R_s + sL_s + R_s}. \tag{13.9}$$

Noting that we seek the voltage across the primary inductor, we write $V_1(s) = I_{\text{in}}(s) \times Z_{\text{in}}(s)$, arriving at

$$V_{\text{in}}(s) = L_1(1 - e^{-s\tau}) + \frac{1}{s}\frac{\omega^2 k^2 L_1 L_s (R_s C_s s + 1)}{s^2 L_s C_s R_s + s L_s + R_s}(1 - e^{-s\tau}) \tag{13.10}$$

which can be rewritten as

$$V_{\text{in}}(s) = \left(L_1 + \frac{A}{s} + \frac{Bs + C}{s^2 L_s C_s R_s + s L_s + R_s}\right)(1 - e^{-s\tau}) \tag{13.11}$$

using partial fraction decomposition.

The constants A, B, and C may be solved by equating Equation (13.11) to Equation (13.10), which is left to the reader. However, we make an important observation from Equation (13.11) that the oscillatory behavior is determined by the third term which contains a second-order denominator. Assuming $L_1 = L_s$ and $\omega_s = \frac{1}{\sqrt{L_s C_s}}$, without loss of generality, the poles for this term which determine the behavior of damped oscillations are given by

$$p_{1,2} = -\frac{\omega_s}{2Q_s} \pm j\omega_s\sqrt{1 - \frac{1}{4Q_s^2}}, \tag{13.12}$$

where $Q_s = \frac{R_s}{Z_s}$ for the configuration used in Figure 13.12a, and $Z_s = \sqrt{\frac{L_s}{C_s}}$. Therefore, the frequency of the damped oscillations, ω_d, is simply given by

$$\omega_d = \omega_s\sqrt{1 - \frac{1}{4Q_s^2}}, \tag{13.13}$$

which for a large Q_s is approximately equal to ω_s. Figure 13.13a and b shows two examples of the damped oscillations ($Q_s = 14, 70$) in the time domain for $k = 0.2, 0.5$. A higher Q_s results in a longer signal duration, simplifying the measurement.

The same derivation may be completed for a modulated pulse, in the form of $i_{\text{in}}(t) = [u(t) - u(t - \tau)]\cos(\omega_{\text{ex}} t)$ for example, where ω_{ex} is the excitation frequency. In this case, the response will include both the forced oscillation frequency and the damped one when the excitation is on; however, when the excitation is turned off, only the damped oscillations will be present. During the on time, the excitation waveform will be dominant, and the damped response cannot be measured; when the excitation is off however, sensor measurement can be performed. Figure 13.13c and d shows two examples of the damped oscillations in the time domain with a modulated input current for $k = 0.2, 0.5$. A higher Q_s results in a better SNR and a longer signal duration. Employing the modulated excitation signal is more common since the current induced in

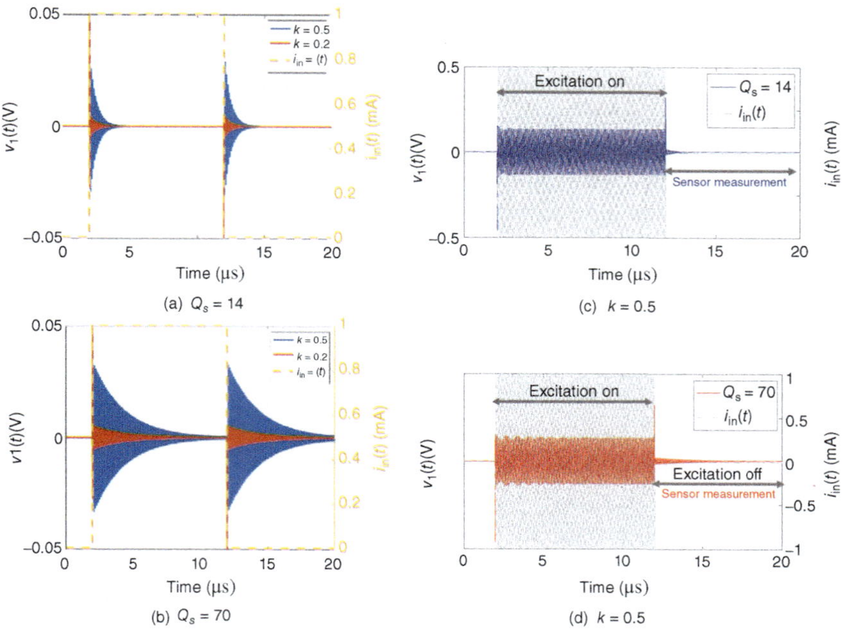

Figure 13.13 (a, b) The voltage across L_1 for $k = 0.2$, $k = 0.5$ and $Q_s = 14$, $Q_s = 70$ for an unmodulated input pulse. (c, d) The voltage across L_1 for $k = 0.5$ and $Q_s = 14$, $Q_s = 70$ for a modulated input signal at 11 MHz. Circuit values are $L_1 = L_s = 2.3$ μH, $C_s = 120$ pF, $R_s = 2\ k\Omega$ ($Q_s = 14$), $R_s = 10\ k\Omega$ ($Q_s = 70$), and $\omega_s = 2\pi(9.58\text{ MHz})$.

the sensor is maximized when the resonant frequencies of the excitation signal and the sensor are the same [17].

It should be noted that although Equation (13.13) does not exhibit any dependence on the coupling strength, k, the amplitude of the signal is strongly affected by k, as can be seen from Equation (13.10) as well as Figure 13.13. Therefore, depending on the sensitivity and noise of the reader circuitry, in order for the amplitude of oscillation and hence its frequency to be measurable, a larger coupling between the sensor and reader is desirable. From Equation (13.12), the decaying response of the sensor has an exponential envelope with a time constant of

$$\tau_d = \frac{2Q_s}{\omega_s} = 2\frac{R_s\sqrt{\frac{C_s}{L_s}}}{\frac{1}{\sqrt{L_sC_s}}} = 2R_sC_s. \tag{13.14}$$

This suggests that if the either R_s or C_s is known, the decay rate can be used to find the other. Measuring the envelope of the signal does not need the same resolution and sampling rate as measuring the damped oscillations; however, the measurement window is still limited.

The main issue with transient response technique is the short duration of the damped oscillations, which, as shown in Figure 13.13 and predicted by Equation (13.14), is proportional to the quality factor. The short duration of the pulse calls for high sampling rate for the analog front end. Additionally, the magnitude of the received signal is small, necessitating front-end amplification [32], requiring a high-resolution, complex, and costly reader [25]. The sensor response can be picked up either by a different coil than the excitation coil [30, 32] or on the same coil, provided that proper isolation measures have been taken by means of a T/R switch, to prevent the excitation signal from damaging or desensitizing the receiver front end [33].

It is important to note that the measurement accuracy in both steady-state and transient techniques depends on the value of Q_s where the measurement error is on the order of $\frac{\omega_s}{Q_s^2}$ from the actual sensor resonant frequency. Another major limitation of nonresonant primary systems arises from the parasitic resonance of the primary coil. The resonant primary causes interference in the measurement of both of the above techniques, causing a shift in the measured resonant frequency [34, 35]. Figure 13.14a depicts the percentage of the deviation in the measured frequency, ω_m, from ω_s as a function of k, due to parasitic capacitance, C_{par}, in the reader assuming $Q_s \to \infty$. To tackle this, Demori et al. [36] proposes a negative capacitance circuit to cancel the parasitic capacitance of the primary coil and avoid interference (Figure 13.14b).

13.3.2 Forced Oscillation Techniques with Resonant Primary

In order to overcome the limitations associated with nonresonant primaries, other techniques have sought to sharpen spectral features while employing resonance in the reader circuit as illustrated in Figure 13.5b-ii and -iii. The previous impedance approach used to analyze the nonresonant reader systems is overly burdensome once the system contains more than one resonator. Instead, such a system of coupled resonators or oscillators can be linearized and analyzed more conveniently in the steady state using the principles of coupled mode theory (CMT) summarized in [37]. We now briefly review CMT. We begin by examining the relationships of the following four key parameters based on the circuits in Figure 13.15:

1. Resonant amplitude, assuming time harmonic dependence $e^{i\omega t}$,
   $a_i = \sqrt{\frac{C_i}{2}}|V_i|e^{i\omega t} = \sqrt{\frac{L_i}{2}}|I_i|e^{i\omega t}$. Note that this resonant amplitude is related to the square root of the electromagnetic energy stored in an individual resonator, $|a_i|^2 = \frac{C_i}{2}|V_i|^2 = \frac{L_i}{2}|I_i|^2$.

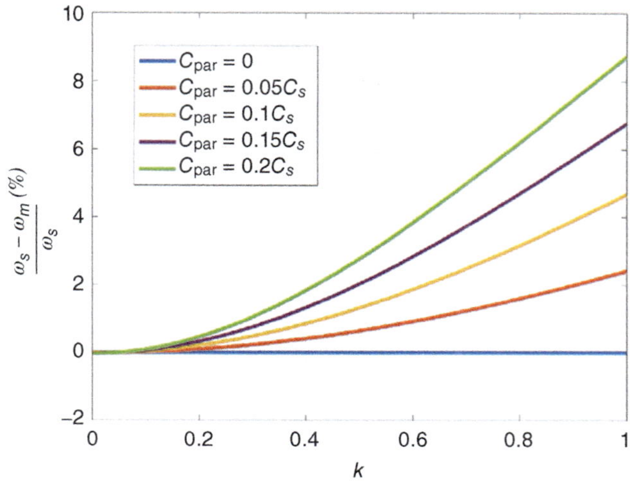

(a)

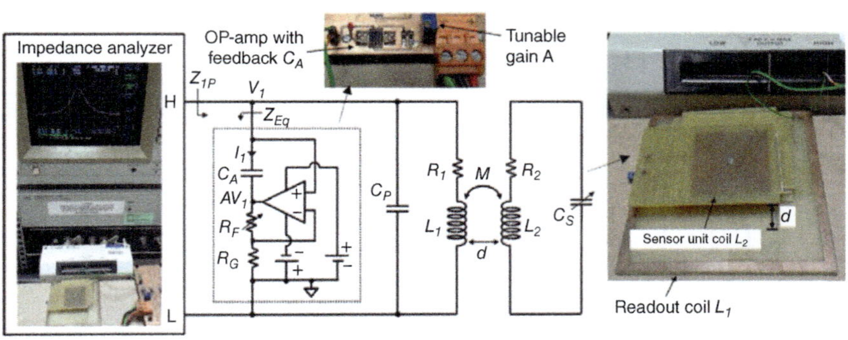

(b)

Figure 13.14 (a) Percentage deviation in the measured frequency, ω_m, from actual sensor resonant frequency, ω_s, as a function of *k* due to parasitic resonance in the primary. (b) Block diagram of the readout system, negative capacitance circuit for parasitic capacitance compensation connected to the readout coil L_1, and pictures of the prototype and experimental setup in [36]. (*Source*: Demori, M., Baù, M., Ferrari, M., et al., 2018. Reproduced with permission from Elsevier.)

2. Resonant frequency, $\omega_i = \frac{1}{\sqrt{L_i C_i}}$; typically controlled by varying the capacitance of a resonant circuit (*LC* tank).
3. Loss rate, related to the resistance in the resonator (or oscillator). The definition of the loss rate depends on the configuration of the *LC* circuit; for a parallel circuit configuration (Figure 13.15a), $\gamma_i = \frac{1}{2R_i C_i} = \frac{\omega_i}{2Q_i}$, where

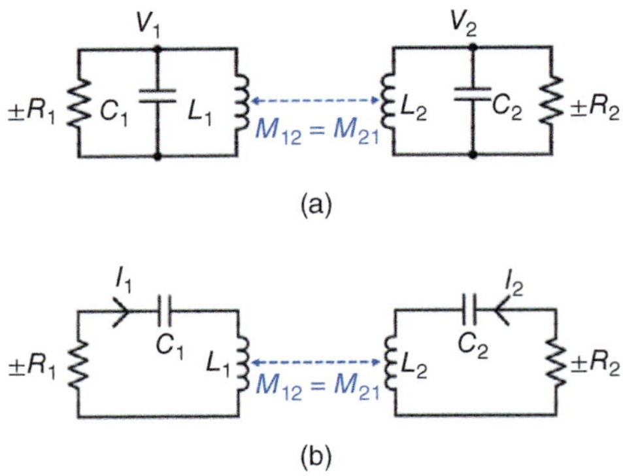

Figure 13.15 (a) Parallel and (b) series magnetically coupled resonators. The individual circuit components, $\pm R_i$, C_i, and L_i, set the resonant frequencies, ω_i, as well as the gain/loss rates, g_i or γ_i. The resonant amplitudes, a_i, are determined by the voltage or current on each resonator tank circuit, V_i or I_i.

Q_i is the quality factor of the parallel circuit, and for series configuration (Figure 13.15b), $\gamma_i = 2R_iC_i = \frac{2}{Q_i\omega_i}$, where Q_i is the quality factor of the series circuit. In a resonator, $\gamma_i > 0$ due to loss (positive resistance), whereas in an oscillator where $R_i < 0$, $\gamma_i < 0$ signifying gain; we may, therefore, introduce the gain rate as $g_i = -\gamma_i$ such that $g_i > 0$ in an oscillator.

4. Coupling rate between resonators i and j, $\kappa_{ij} = \frac{\omega_j M_{ij}}{2\sqrt{L_iL_j}}$; typically, $L_i = L_j = L$ and $\kappa_{ij} = \frac{\omega_j M_{ij}}{2L}$, where $M_{ij} = k_{ij}\sqrt{L_iL_j}$.

The time evolution for such linear systems may be defined using a general differential equation; for the case of two resonators or oscillators ($n = 2$), this equation may be written as

$$\frac{\mathrm{d}}{\mathrm{d}t}\begin{bmatrix} a_1 \\ a_2 \end{bmatrix} = \begin{bmatrix} i\omega_1 - \gamma_1 & -i\kappa_{12} \\ -i\kappa_{21} & i\omega_2 - \gamma_2 \end{bmatrix}\begin{bmatrix} a_1 \\ a_2 \end{bmatrix} = H\begin{bmatrix} a_1 \\ a_2 \end{bmatrix}. \tag{13.15}$$

This matrix H is known as the effective Hamiltonian [38–40]. The Hamiltonian is symmetric in the sense that, due to reciprocity, we can assume $\kappa_{12} = \kappa_{21} = \kappa$. A fundamental assumption of this method (that also allows for equivalence of series and parallel resonators) is that the normalized coupling rate is small $\left(\frac{\kappa_{12}}{\omega_{1,2}} \ll 1\right)$; arbitrarily large coupling factors require the use of nonlinear dynamics and the Liouvillian formalism [41–43] and are not the subject of this chapter. For an oscillator, a gain rate, g_1 and/or g_2, will be used in the Hamiltonian, whereas for a resonator, a loss rate, γ_1 or γ_2, will be used in the Hamiltonian. We now proceed to examine the three most common cases found in the literature: (i) two resonators, (ii) one resonator and one oscillator, and (iii) more than two resonators/oscillators.

a) Resonating reader and resonating sensor

We first study the case of two resonators with resonant frequencies, ω_1 and ω_s, and loss rates, γ_1 and γ_s (Figure 13.5b-ii); the Hamiltonian dynamics for such a system are given by Equation (13.15). The eigenfrequencies (or modes) of the system can be calculated from the Hamiltonian matrix by solving the characteristic equation $\det(H - i\omega I) = 0$.[1] The characteristic equation in this case is given by

$$[i(\omega_1 - \omega) - \gamma_1][i(\omega_s - \omega) - \gamma_s] + \kappa^2 = 0. \tag{13.16}$$

Equation (13.16) exhibits two possible roots for ω corresponding to the system's two modes. We define a frequency split parameter as the real part of the difference between the eigenfrequency (given by the roots of the characteristic equation), denoted by ω_m, and the sensor resonant frequency, ω_s; this parameter is given by $\Delta\omega = Re\{\omega_m - \omega_s\}$. The maximum $\Delta\omega$ achievable by this two-resonator system occurs when the coupled resonators operate about a diabolical point (DP) [44, 45], that is, when $\omega_1 = \omega_s$ and $\gamma_1 = \gamma_s$. Under this scenario, these eigenfrequencies (or modes) are given by

$$\omega_{m1,2} = \omega_s \pm \kappa + i\gamma_s \tag{13.17}$$

and

$$|\Delta\omega| = \kappa. \tag{13.18}$$

The frequency response in this case is plotted in Figure 13.16a for $\gamma_s = \gamma_1 = 0.01\omega_s$. The presence of a sensor in this coupled, lossy resonator system therefore generates a nonzero frequency split regardless of the coupling rate between the reader and the sensor (Figure 13.16b); hence, the sensor is theoretically detectable in the presence of any coupling ($\kappa > 0$) to the reader. However, the major limitation of this method is the reduced sharpness in the spectral features caused by the loss rate-induced nonzero imaginary part of the eigenfrequency ($Im\{\omega_{m1,2}\} = \gamma_s$) as seen from Figure 13.16a. Figure 13.16b shows that while $\Delta\omega$ should theoretically be distinguishable for all $\kappa > 0$, the imaginary part of the eigenfrequencies broadens the spectral effect of the eigenfrequencies, preventing the split from being recognizable for small κ, as illustrated by Figure 13.16a.

Note that the frequency splitting behaviors introduced earlier are directly related to the resonant frequency of the sensor, ω_s, and therefore provide a direct sensing mechanism. For the coupled resonant systems in the rest of this chapter, $\Delta\omega$ will ultimately be determined by the characteristics of the individual resonators and the respective coupling rates between each resonator. Forced techniques will rely on sweeping the reader frequency across a spectrum by tuning the reader's capacitance; for a certain frequency, ω_{reader}, corresponding to specific system properties, the system will have a certain eigenfrequency, and $\Delta\omega$ will achieve its maximal response. For every point in the spectrum, ω_{reader},

1 These eigenfrequencies also correspond to the poles of the transfer function taken when the reader is connected to a waveguide through a port for excitation and measurement.

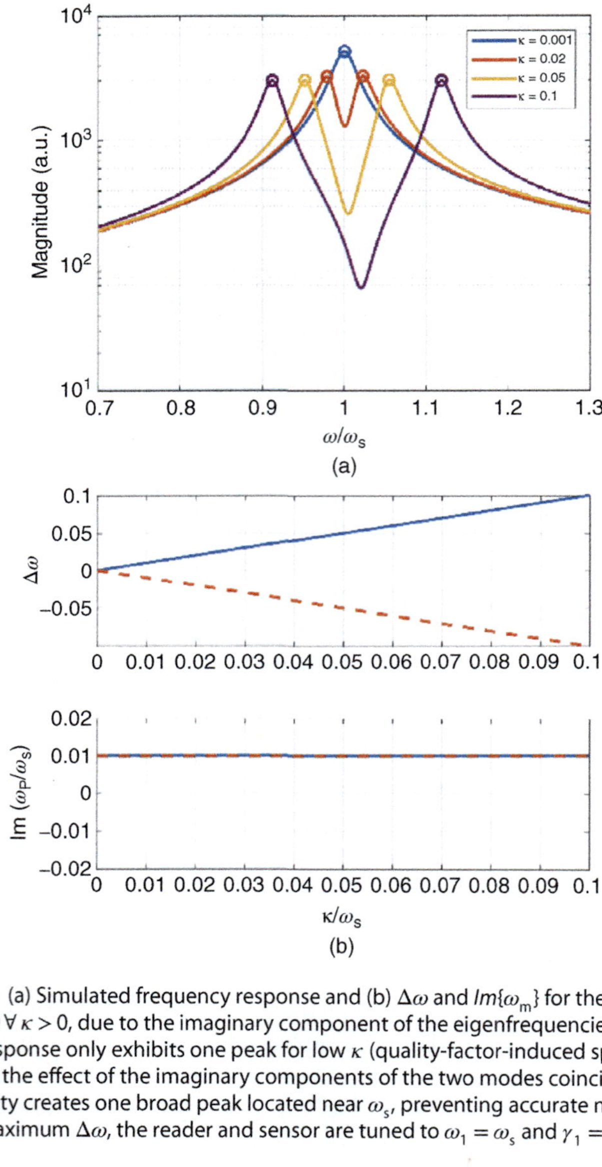

Figure 13.16 (a) Simulated frequency response and (b) $\Delta\omega$ and $Im\{\omega_m\}$ for the DP system. While $\Delta\omega > 0 \; \forall \; \kappa > 0$, due to the imaginary component of the eigenfrequencies, the frequency response only exhibits one peak for low κ (quality-factor-induced spectral broadening); the effect of the imaginary components of the two modes coinciding in such close proximity creates one broad peak located near ω_s, preventing accurate measurement of $\Delta\omega$. For maximum $\Delta\omega$, the reader and sensor are tuned to $\omega_1 = \omega_s$ and $\gamma_1 = \gamma_s$, where $\frac{\gamma_s}{\omega_s} = 0.01$.

the gain and loss rates will be controllable and equalized via manual or automatic tuning. In general, the techniques in this section will seek to maximize $\Delta\omega$ vs. κ and to ensure the presence of a $\Delta\omega$ across the largest possible range of κ.

b) Oscillating reader and resonating sensor

In order to improve the sharpness of spectral features, the reader resonator may be replaced by an oscillator (Figure 13.5b-iii). The oscillator provides a gain rate equal to the loss rate in magnitude; if the oscillator and resonator frequencies are balanced, this is known as a $\mathcal{PT}$-symmetric arrangement where, ideally, the gain rate and the loss rate exactly cancel, resulting in purely real eigenfrequencies. In general, the Hamiltonian dynamics for this coupled oscillator and resonator system are given by substituting a gain rate for the loss rate, in other words $g_1 = -\gamma_1$, into Equation (13.15). In this case, the characteristic equation of this system is given by

$$[i(\omega_1 - \omega) + g_1][i(\omega_s - \omega) - \gamma_s] + \kappa^2 = 0. \tag{13.19}$$

The maximum $\Delta\omega$ achievable by this system occurs when the coupled resonators operate about an exceptional point (EP) [41–47] under $\mathcal{PT}$-symmetric conditions; this is when $\omega_1 = \omega_s$ and $g_1 = \gamma_s$. Under this scenario, the eigenfrequencies and $\Delta\omega$ are given by

$$\omega_{m1,2} = \omega_s \pm \sqrt{\kappa^2 - \gamma_s^2} \tag{13.20a}$$

$$|\Delta\omega| = \sqrt{\kappa^2 - \gamma_s^2}. \tag{13.20b}$$

The frequency response in this case is plotted in Figure 13.17a for $\gamma_s = g_1 = 0.01\omega_s$. These results present two characteristics. First, $\Delta\omega$ is only real above a minimum coupling rate equal to the loss rate in the sensor ($\kappa_{min} = \gamma_s$); below this point, often referred to as the *broken* phase, $\Delta\omega$ is zero and cannot be measured (Figure 13.17b). Second, above this minimum coupling rate, the eigenfrequencies are entirely real, allowing for lossless resonance; for higher coupling rates, it can be seen that this oscillator–resonator combination exhibits $\Delta\omega \cong \kappa$ as in the DP case. The issue of the minimum coupling rate may be overcome by ensuring that the loss rate is very small. The sensor's resistance may either be sufficiently chosen to ensure a low loss rate, or it may not be used at all. In the latter scenario, the loss rate is simply defined by the finite Q of the inductor. In practice, these techniques allow for normalized coupling rates (κ/ω_s) smaller than 0.01 [41–47].

The measurement approach for a typical, forced $\mathcal{PT}$-symmetric system is that employed by the authors of [43, 46]. A VNA is connected to the

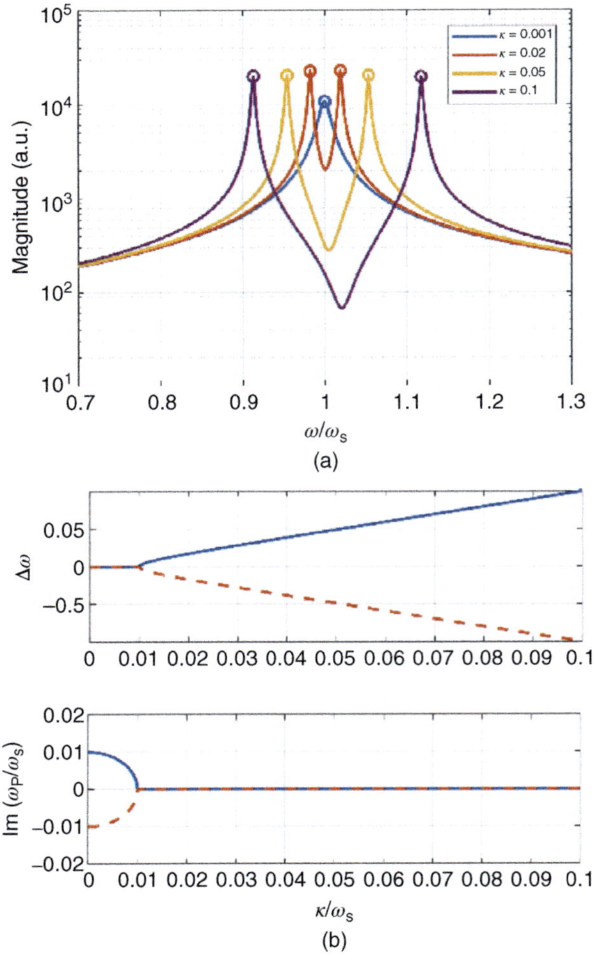

Figure 13.17 (a) Simulated frequency response and (b) $\Delta\omega$ and $Im\{\omega_m\}$ for $\mathcal{PT}$-symmetric system; note that $\Delta\omega > 0$ only for $\kappa > \gamma_s$. Now, due to the fact that the gain rate perfectly cancels the loss rate ($Im\{\omega_{m1,2}\} = 0$), the two eigenfrequencies are visible as peaks in the squared magnitude in the frequency response for $\kappa > \gamma_s$; for $\kappa < \gamma_s$, a singular peak persists, once again preventing accurate measurement of $\Delta\omega$. For maximum $\Delta\omega$, these resonators will be tuned to $\omega_1 = \omega_s$ and $g_1 = \gamma_s$, where $\frac{\gamma_s}{\omega_s} = 0.01$.

reader oscillator. The VNA forces a signal onto the coupled system and measures the reflection spectrum over a certain frequency range. At the frequencies matching the eigenfrequencies, the dip in the reflection spectrum is the strongest. As the VNA measures across the frequency spectrum, the capacitance and the negative resistance of the reader are constantly tuned (Figure 13.18a and b) in order to ensure that $\omega_1 = \omega_s$ and $g_1 = \gamma_s$; at this point, the dip in the reflection spectrum is the deepest, and the sensor frequency may be detected from the known ω_1. Figure 13.18c and Equation (13.20) show that in comparison to the nonresonant method (Equation (13.1)), the $\mathcal{PT}$-symmetric system can achieve much more noticeable and measurable $\Delta\omega$, especially above the minimum coupling rate; the frequency split in the $\mathcal{PT}$-symmetric case is proportional to κ compared to κ^2 in the nonresonant primary case (Equation (13.1)). While $\Delta\omega$ of the $\mathcal{PT}$-symmetric system can provide for accurate measurement of a sensor's frequency above the minimum coupling rate, the frequency split becomes insignificant below that rate (Figure 13.18c, top right panel). In order to overcome this, the following section explores forced, higher order ($n > 2$) systems.

c. Higher order resonator/oscillator combinations

Recent efforts to enhance frequency split have sought to add further degrees of freedom in the form of extra resonators. In general, an $n \times n$ Hamiltonian of such a system will exhibit n eigenfrequencies which, depending on the exact resonator configuration, can enhance $\Delta\omega$.

One such attempt introduces a third, lossless LC resonator ($\gamma_2 = 0$) into a $\mathcal{PT}$-symmetric setup as an intermediate coupling stage, in essence boosting the coupling rate between the reader oscillator and the sensor resonator (Figure 13.19a) [48]. In order to ensure strict $\mathcal{PT}$-symmetry, the oscillator and two resonators must satisfy the condition $\omega_1 = \omega_2 = \omega_s$; under this condition, frequency split is enhanced compared to the case without the intermediate resonator (Figure 13.19b) [48]. The main result of this three-resonator system is that it exhibits nonzero $\Delta\omega$ for significantly lower $\kappa = \frac{1}{2\sqrt{2}}$ than the two-resonator system[2]; in fact, the authors note that for a system with $n = 5$ resonators, this may be improved to $\kappa = \frac{1}{2\sqrt{3}}$ [48]. The measurement is identical to that of the forced $\mathcal{PT}$-symmetric system with the intermediary resonator simply inserted at the appropriate coupling distance between the reader oscillator and the sensor resonator.

Another attempt takes advantage of EP enhancement due to a perturbation by a sensor [46]. In a concept well known to the optics community, two resonators operating at an EP are sensitive to weak perturbations, ε; this perturbation is further enhanced in an nth-order system by $\varepsilon^{1/n}$ [45, 49, 50]. This concept is exploited by Dong et al. [44] where a coupled oscillator–resonator system is perturbed by weak coupling to a third, sensor resonator (Figure 13.20a). The authors show that further coupling to a third

2 In this reference, the authors use $\gamma_i = \frac{1}{2R_iC_i}$ for series resonators, equivalent to the parallel definition at the beginning of this section; they also operate the system at a constant $\kappa = 0.35$ (defining $\kappa = k$) while varying γ_s.

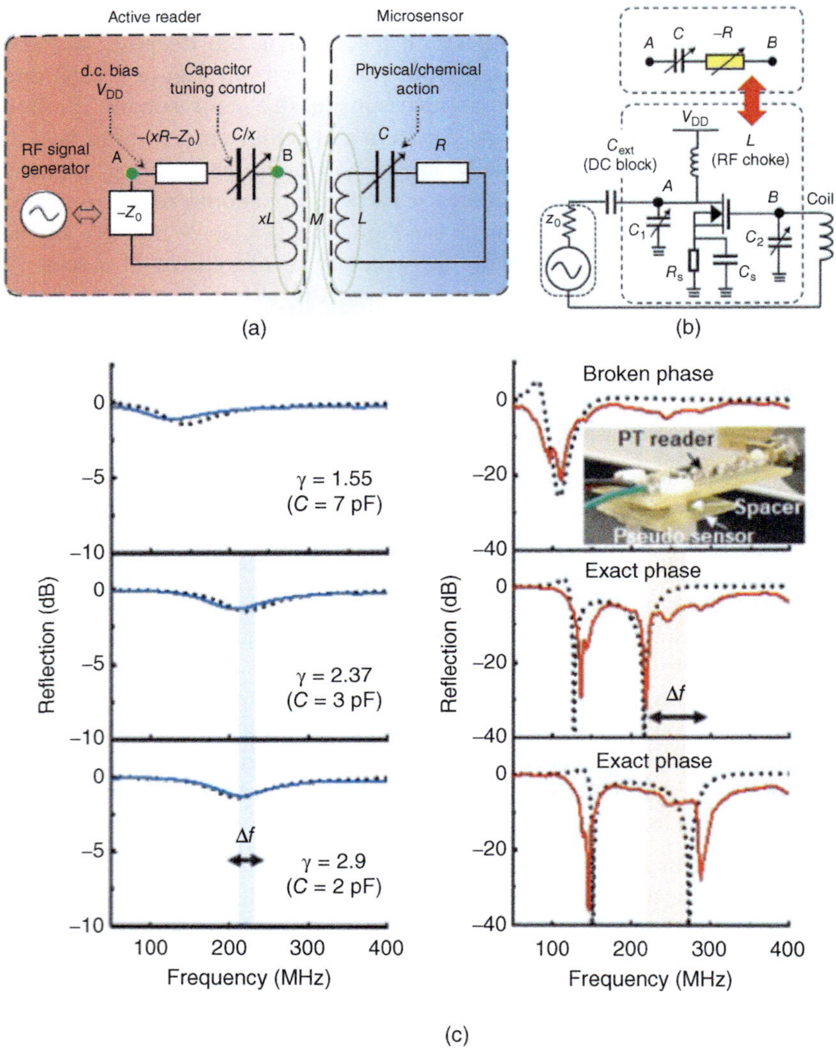

Figure 13.18 (a) Forced $\mathcal{PT}$-symmetric system from Chen et al. [46]. Typical systems such as those in [43] assume that $L_{reader} = L_{sensor}$ and simply tune the reader capacitance and negative resistance to achieve $\omega_1 = \omega_s$ and $g_1 = \gamma_s$. In [46], however, an appropriate scaling factor, *x*, is provided for the case where the reader and the sensor coils must be severely mismatched for applications in implantable systems (i.e. a small sensor coil); this scaling factor ensures that the theoretical results from Sakhdari, et al. [43] remain identical for such a system. (*Source*: Chen, P.-Y., Sakhdari, M., Hajizadega, M., et al., 2018. © Springer Nature.) (b) Negative resistance implementation from Sakhdari et al. [43] using a Colpitts oscillator that also implements the reader capacitance; note that the negative resistance provided by the reader accounts for the negative resistance provided by the VNA. (c) Reflection spectrum measurements comparing a system with a nonresonant reader to the left and the $\mathcal{PT}$-symmetric system to the right; in the *exact* phase ($\kappa > \gamma_s$), strong reflection dips are evident and easily measurable in the $\mathcal{PT}$-symmetric case. (*Source:* Sakhdari, M., Hajizadegan, M., Li, Y., et al., 2018. © IEEE.)

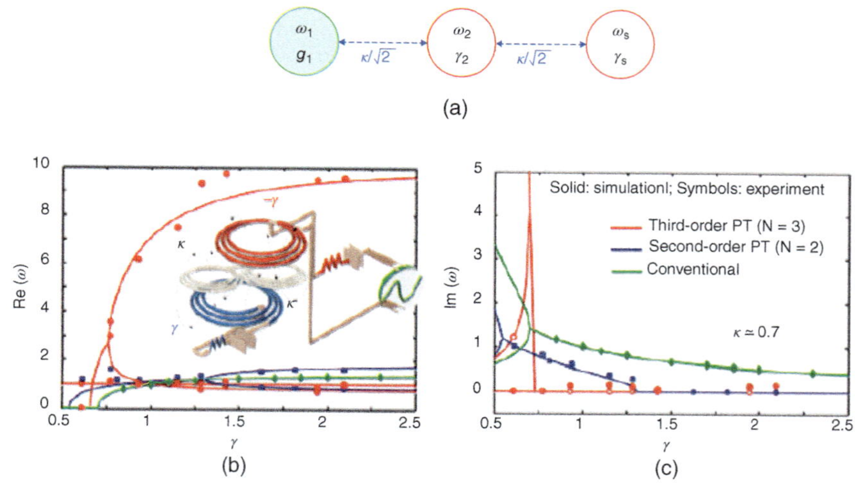

Figure 13.19 (a) System implementation of three coupled resonators, a reader oscillator with a gain rate, an intermediary resonator with negligible loss rate ($\gamma_2 \to 0$), and a sensor resonator with a loss rate (forcing mechanism omitted for simplicity); for maximum $\Delta\omega$, this system is tuned to $\omega_1 = \omega_2 = \omega_s$ and $g_1 = \gamma_s$. This is essentially a $\mathcal{PT}$-symmetric system with an intermediary, coupling-rate-boosting resonator (see footnote 2 for explanation of author's notation). (b) Real and imaginary parts of the resulting eigenfrequencies compared to the $\mathcal{PT}$-symmetric and DP systems [48]. (*Source:* Chen, P.-Y., 2018. © IEEE.)

resonator produces a $\kappa^{2/3}$ perturbation (Figure 13.20b and c). Assuming $\kappa_{12} = \kappa_{21} = \mu$ and $\kappa_{13} = \kappa_{31} = \kappa_{23} = \kappa_{32} = \kappa$, the Hamiltonian describing the system is

$$\frac{\mathrm{d}}{\mathrm{d}t}\begin{bmatrix} a_1 \\ a_2 \\ a_s \end{bmatrix} = \begin{bmatrix} i\omega_1 + g_1 & -i\mu & -i\kappa \\ -i\mu & i\omega_2 - \gamma_2 & -i\kappa \\ -i\kappa & -i\kappa & i\omega_s - \gamma_s \end{bmatrix}\begin{bmatrix} a_1 \\ a_2 \\ a_s \end{bmatrix}. \tag{13.21}$$

The oscillator and the resonator are forced to operate at the EP where their coupling rate is identical to the gain/loss rates; in other words, these are $\mathcal{PT}$-symmetric resonators that are forced to operate at $\kappa_{12} = g_1 = \gamma_2$ and $\omega_1 = \omega_2$. In this case, the characteristic equation is given by

$$(\omega_2 - \omega)^2[i(\omega_s - \omega) - \gamma_s] - 2i\kappa^2((\omega_2 - \omega) + \mu) = 0. \tag{13.22}$$

The frequency response in this case is plotted in Figure 13.20b for $g_1 = \gamma_2 = \mu = 0.2\omega_s$ and $\gamma_s = 0.01\omega_s$. Assuming $\omega_1 = \omega_2 = \omega_s$ and $\mu \gg \gamma_s$, using a Newton–Puiseux expansion, the eigenfrequencies may be approximated as [44]

$$\omega_{m,n} \approx \omega_s + 2^{\frac{1}{3}} e^{\frac{i2\pi n}{3}} \mu^{\frac{1}{3}} \kappa^{2/3} \tag{13.23}$$

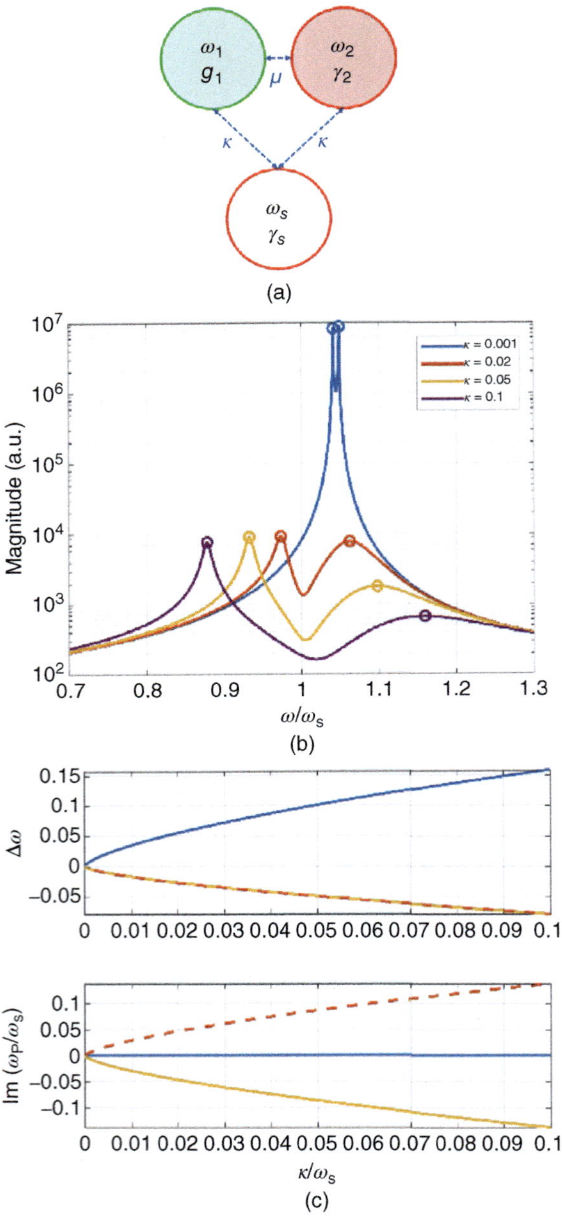

Figure 13.20 (a) System implementation of three coupled resonators, a reader oscillator with a gain rate, a reader resonator with a loss rate, and a sensor resonator with a loss rate (forcing mechanism omitted for simplicity); for maximum $\Delta\omega$, these resonators will be tuned to $\omega_1 = \omega_2 = \omega_s$ and $g_1 = \gamma_2$. The reader oscillator and resonator are essentially a $\mathcal{PT}$-symmetric system coupled at the EP, $\mu = \gamma_2$. (b) Simulated frequency response. (c) $\Delta\omega$ and $Im\{\omega_m\}$ for the EP system; note that $\Delta\omega > 0, \forall\, \kappa > 0$, $\frac{\mu}{\omega_s} = 0.2$, and $\frac{\gamma_s}{\omega_s} = 0.01$. Now, due to operation at this EP, the eigenfrequencies are visible for even low κ compared to the $\mathcal{PT}$-symmetric system and $\Delta\omega \propto \kappa^{2/3}$ (upper solid curve).

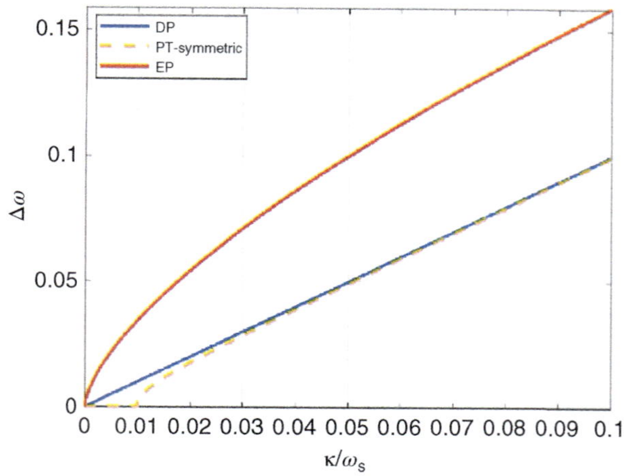

Figure 13.21 $\Delta\omega$ vs. κ dependence for all three systems discussed in this section; $\frac{\mu}{\omega_s} = 0.2$ for the EP system and $\frac{\gamma_s}{\omega_s} = 0.01$ for the $\mathcal{PT}$-symmetric system. The DP system achieves a nonzero $\Delta\omega \, \forall \, \kappa > 0$; however, the imaginary parts of its eigenfrequencies prevent sharp spectral features. On the other hand, the EP system presents a clear advantage in frequency splitting but at the expense of requiring an extra resonator and precise tuning for operation at the EP.

where $n = 1, 2, 3$, suggesting three possible eigenfrequencies. Finally, the dependence of $\Delta\omega$ on κ is

$$\Delta\omega \propto \kappa^{2/3}. \tag{13.24}$$

The dependence of $\Delta\omega$ on $\kappa^{2/3}$ is superior to two-resonator approaches but requires an additional resonator and nontrivial, precise control of the coupled $\mathcal{PT}$-symmetric components at the EP; a final comparison of the three resonator/oscillator combinations from this section is shown in Figure 13.21. In general, a larger number of resonators, $n > 3$, would provide even better $\Delta\omega$ vs. κ performance; however, it is postulated that operation at such higher order EPs eventually becomes dominated by noise [44, 45, 51–54].

Measurements in a forced EP system require four separate tuning/sweeping operations along with an initialization tuning procedure. Once again, a VNA must be connected to the reader oscillator, forcing a signal on the coupled system and measuring the reflection spectrum over a certain frequency range (first sweep). An initialization tuning procedure is required to ensure that $\omega_1 = \omega_2$ for strict operation at the EP by adjusting the reader capacitances; in order to match the sensor frequency for maximum $\Delta\omega$, these capacitances are then swept across a frequency range in unison (second sweep), with a VNA making a spectral measurement at each frequency point. Typically, in order to properly establish operation at the EP, γ_2 is swept (through the reader resonator's resistance, R_2) to make sure that the maximum $\Delta\omega$ occurs at $\gamma_2 = \mu$ (third sweep). Alignment at the EP must be incredibly precise; therefore, while sweeping γ_2, a tuning operation is required to ensure strict equalization of γ_1 and γ_2 in the reader oscillator and resonator (first tuning).

13.3.3 Self-Oscillating Techniques

The forced $\mathcal{PT}$-symmetric system assumed that the oscillator contained a linear negative resistance that is manually tunable to precisely accomplish $g_1 = \gamma_s$. While the use of forced oscillations with linear negative resistance greatly simplifies the system analysis, the extra tuning steps required to precisely match the gain rate to the loss rate add unnecessary complexity to its implementation; additionally, the requirement of a forced/external oscillation further burdens the system. In a bid to overcome these issues, other approaches have instead sought to take advantage of the automatic or *self-oscillating* techniques.

The basis of these approaches is in nonlinear compressive gain implemented through a resonator coupled with a nonlinear amplifier (voltage or current-saturating topologies). These topologies, initialized either by an initial condition on the oscillator's capacitance or even electronic noise, use positive feedback to grow an oscillation, eventually reaching steady state when saturated. During system operation, these topologies can adapt, on their own, to any changes in the system's parameters such as gain/loss rates, g_i and γ_i, individual resonant frequencies, ω_i, and coupling rates, κ_{ij}. After a transient period induced by changes to these parameters, the oscillator will allow the system to settle at a new steady-state operating point with a new resonant amplitude and frequency. It is in this sense that such systems may now be described as self-oscillating as they require neither an external equipment to force an oscillation frequency or amplitude nor precise tuning of the now nonlinear gain rate. They instead settle on a gain rate that suits the system's characteristics and results in a balance between the effective loss and gain rates. This steady-state gain rate is henceforth referred to as the saturated gain.

The exact topology of the nonlinear compressive oscillator varies between individual works. Some methods rely on negative impedance converters, in which, as mentioned before, an operational amplifier exhibits a negative input impedance through positive feedback (Figure 13.22a and b) [41, 42, 47]. Alternatively, simple transistor schemes have also been implemented to present a negative resistance, such as variants of the Colpitts oscillator (Figure 13.18b) used in [43, 46, 48] or the widely implemented cross-coupled pair (Figure 13.22c) which, unlike the Colpitts oscillator, can exhibit a negative resistance, $R = -2/g_m$, that, to first order, is independent of the operating

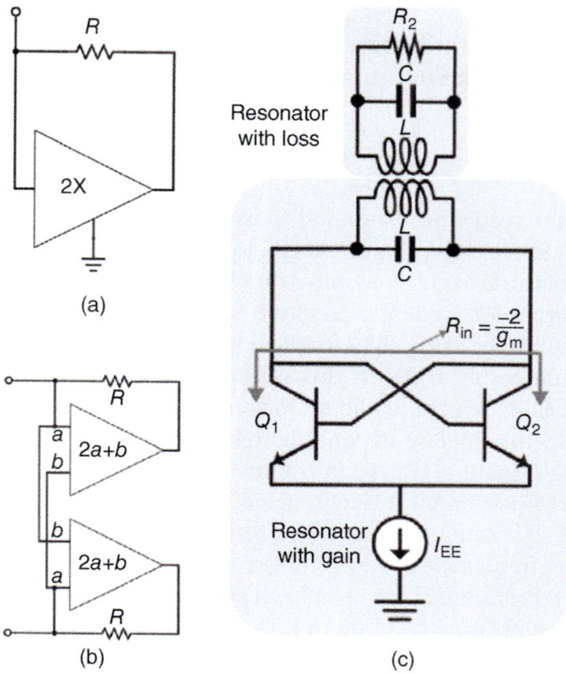

Figure 13.22 (a) Amplifier with positive resistive feedback for negative impedance conversion; the generic amplifier in this figure may be implemented using an op-amp-based noninverting amplifier. (b) Floating, two-terminal negative impedance converter similar to [41]; the generic amplifiers in this figure may be implemented using op-amp-based summing amplifiers and inverting buffers [41]. (*Source*: Modified from Schindler, J., Lin, Z., Lee, J.M. et al., 2012.) (c) Cross-coupled pair negative resistance structure interfaced with both the frequency-tunable reader oscillator and coupled resonator in a $\mathcal{PT}$-symmetric system; transistors Q_1 and Q_2 are assumed to be identical.

frequency and has negligible input capacitance, mainly determined by the device parasitics [55, 56]. These nonlinear circuits, combined with an LC tank, form the reader oscillator that self-oscillating techniques will exploit. In order to further understand these techniques, this section first examines the effect of the nonlinear gain rate in self-oscillating $\mathcal{PT}$-symmetric systems for both frequency and amplitude sensing before finally proceeding to self-oscillating higher order techniques.

a. Self-oscillating $\mathcal{PT}$-symmetric systems for frequency measurement

Now assuming a nonlinear gain in Equation (13.19), the characteristic equation may be rewritten as

$$-(\omega_1 - \omega)(\omega_s - \omega) + ig_1(\omega_s - \omega) - i\gamma_s(\omega_1 - \omega) - g_1\gamma_s + \kappa^2 = 0. \quad (13.25)$$

Equation (13.25) can be decomposed into a purely real and a purely imaginary part. In order for the system to present purely real eigenfrequencies, the nonlinear gain, g_1, will saturate to a value that forces the imaginary part to zero. The solutions are

$$g_1 = \gamma_s \frac{\omega_1 - \omega}{\omega_s - \omega}. \tag{13.26}$$

Note that if the reader oscillator and sensor resonator have identical LC resonant frequencies, $\omega_1 = \omega_s$, Equation (13.26) reduces to $g_1 = \gamma_s$, matching the requirements of the forced $\mathcal{PT}$-symmetric system; in fact, the frequency split in this self-oscillating $\mathcal{PT}$-symmetric system is identical to that of the externally forced system with the same eigenfrequencies as Equation (13.20a).

An interesting result arises in this self-oscillating system if $\omega_1 \neq \omega_s$. This frequency-imbalanced case, while no longer strictly $\mathcal{PT}$-symmetric, can still exhibit real eigenfrequency if equivalent loss and gain rates are balanced. By substituting Equation (13.26) into Equation (13.25), the eigenfrequencies and their corresponding saturated gains may be numerically solved for (Figure 13.23). As can be seen, the saturated gains corresponding to the individual eigenfrequencies are no longer equal (denoted by g_{1a} and g_{1b} in (Figure 13.23)). From the classic feedback systems analysis, we note that only the eigenfrequency corresponding to the lowest gain will exist in steady state as it has the highest loop gain. Therefore, from Figure 13.23a, one can conclude that the eigenfrequency corresponding to g_{1a} will be stable for all cases as it has the lowest gain. The eigenfrequency corresponding to g_{1b} can only exist for the $\mathcal{PT}$-symmetric system, in which case $g_{1a} = g_{1b}$ (both eigenfrequencies exhibit the lowest gain). For $\omega_1 > \omega_s$, the eigenfrequency corresponding to the lowest gain has a value, ω_h, larger than both ω_1 and ω_s, whereas for $\omega_1 < \omega_s$, the eigenfrequency corresponding to the lowest gain has a value, ω_l, smaller than both ω_1 and ω_s.

The difference is that g_1 does not need to be constantly tuned; in fact, measurements of $\Delta\omega$ may now be made by sweeping the reader capacitance over a frequency range and measuring the steady-state frequency of oscillation in the reader oscillator. Because the system is self-oscillating, this steady-state frequency corresponds directly to one of the eigenfrequencies in Figure 13.23b; when a system parameter is changed, the steady-state oscillation frequency automatically adjusts to a new value corresponding to that exact condition. In practice, this effect has been observed as a frequency jump from the lower to the higher parallel resonant frequency (real eigenfrequency) when ω_1 is swept and the sensor is close enough to the reader [13], which can be seen as the jump from the lower to the upper branch of the $\mathcal{PT}$-symmetric system when $\omega_1 = \omega_s$ (Figure 13.23b). This presents another interesting sensing opportunity. A similar approach based on sweeping the resonant frequency of the reader is used in [44] for sensing in the EP-locked system.

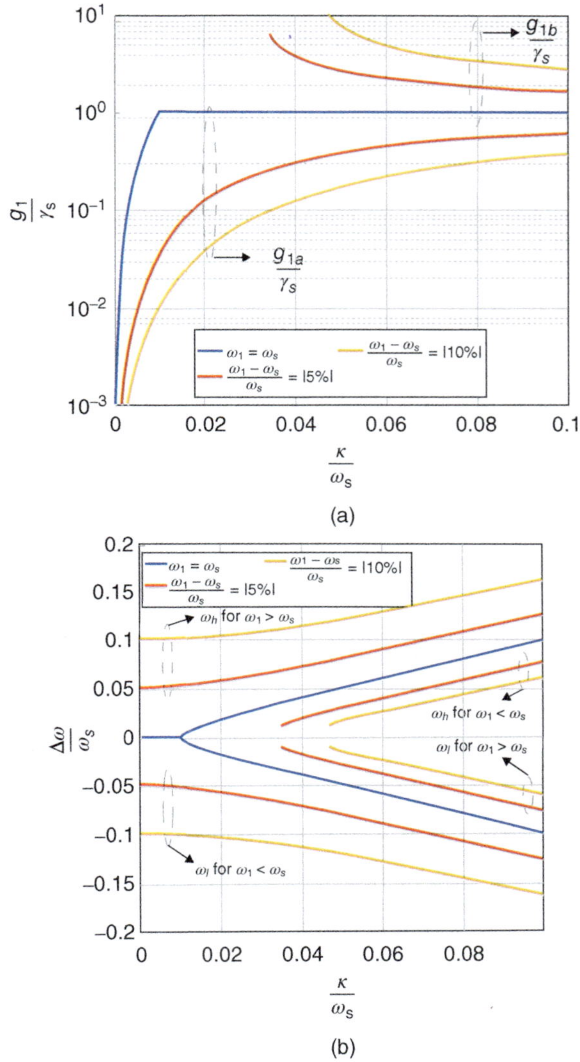

Figure 13.23 (a) Ratio between saturated gain rates and loss rates for the $\mathcal{PT}$-symmetric and frequency-imbalanced case, $\omega_1 \neq \omega_s$; g_{1a} is the saturated gain corresponding to the mode with the lowest gain rate (stable mode), whereas g_{1b} is the saturated gain corresponding to the mode with the highest gain rate (unstable mode). (b) Purely real eigenfrequencies for the $\mathcal{PT}$-symmetric and frequency imbalanced case, $\omega_1 \neq \omega_s$; for $\omega_1 < \omega_s$, the system oscillates at the lower eigenfrequency, ω_l, corresponding to g_{1a}, whereas for $\omega_1 > \omega_s$, the system oscillates at the higher eigenfrequency frequencies, ω_h, corresponding, again, to g_{1a}. For this figure, $\frac{\gamma_s}{\omega_s} = 0.01$.

b. Self-oscillating $\mathcal{PT}$-symmetric systems for amplitude measurement

This section describes one of the earliest measurement techniques for fully passive LC resonators, the grid-dip technique, which was developed in the 1920s [57, 58], applicable to both a resonant and nonresonant primary. It is based on forming a self-oscillating circuit using the reader and the sensor by balancing the loss present in the system, either due to the limited quality factor of the passives or an explicit resistance used for sensing.

As previously mentioned, when the loss rate is balanced with an equal gain rate, the reader and sensor resonators form an oscillator. When oscillations reach a steady state, the amplitude and frequency of oscillations can be used to perform sensor measurements. The grid-dip technique takes advantage of the amplitude of oscillations. A simplified schematic of the grid-dip meter is shown in Figure 13.24a[3], where the transistor provides the required negative resistance in the form of a Pierce oscillator [55, 56]. In this circuit (parallel configuration), the effective quality factor of the reader resonator, $Q_{\mathrm{eff},1}$, which is given by

$$Q_{\mathrm{eff},1} = \frac{\omega_{\mathrm{m}}}{2g_{1a}} \tag{13.27}$$

determines the amplitude of oscillation [13, 55, 56]. In Equation (13.27), g_{1a} is the gain rate corresponding to the stable eigenfrequency which is required to balance the total loss in the system reflected from the sensor. When $\omega_1 = \omega_{\mathrm{s}}$, this system turns into a $\mathcal{PT}$-symmetric system, with the previously derived expressions for the self-oscillating frequency (or real eigenfrequency), ω_{m}, and saturated gain, g_1.

We observe from Figure 13.23a that g_{1a} is maximized for the $\mathcal{PT}$-symmetric case when $g_{1a} = \gamma_{\mathrm{s}}$, and for any other case when $\omega_1 \neq \omega_{\mathrm{s}}$, $\frac{g_{1a}}{\gamma_{\mathrm{s}}}$ drops below unity for a constant γ_{s} at the same κ. This observation suggests that when $\mathcal{PT}$-symmetry is achieved, $\frac{g_{1a}}{\gamma_{\mathrm{s}}}$ is maximized, and as a result, $Q_{\mathrm{eff},1}$ is minimized. In order to better understand this, Figure 13.24b illustrates $\frac{g_{1a}}{\gamma_{\mathrm{s}}}$ vs. normalized frequency difference between the sensor and the reader for different κ.

A lower $Q_{\mathrm{eff},1}$ corresponds to lower amplitudes of oscillations [13, 55, 56]. In a grid-dip meter therefore, the primary resonant frequency is swept, until the minimum amplitude of oscillations, at which point $\omega_1 = \omega_{\mathrm{s}}$, is detected (Figure 13.24c). First employed for biosensing in [60, 61], this principle forms the basis for many works in the literature [62–65].

This technique is very popular in the amateur radio (HAM radio) community and is widely employed as benchtop equipment, for example, Amtron UK402 (http://www.radiomanual.info/schemi/ACC_instrument/Amtron_UK402_Grid-dip_user.pdf). The first implementations, such as the 955-acorn tube in 1953 [59] or the APX-6 1296MHz grid-dip meter in 1967, relied on vacuum tubes [60]; however, soon after transistors became ubiquitous, JFET transistors were employed, in the Amtron UK402 for example http://www.radiomanual.info/schemi/ACC_instrument/Amtron_UK402_Grid-dip_user.pdf. Traditionally, the grid-dip meter is equipped with several (five or six) of interchangeable coils that can be inserted according to the frequency range

3 Not all details of a grid-dip meter circuit are shown in Figure 13.24a for the sake of clarity. For a more detailed diagram, the reader is referred to schematics in [58–60].

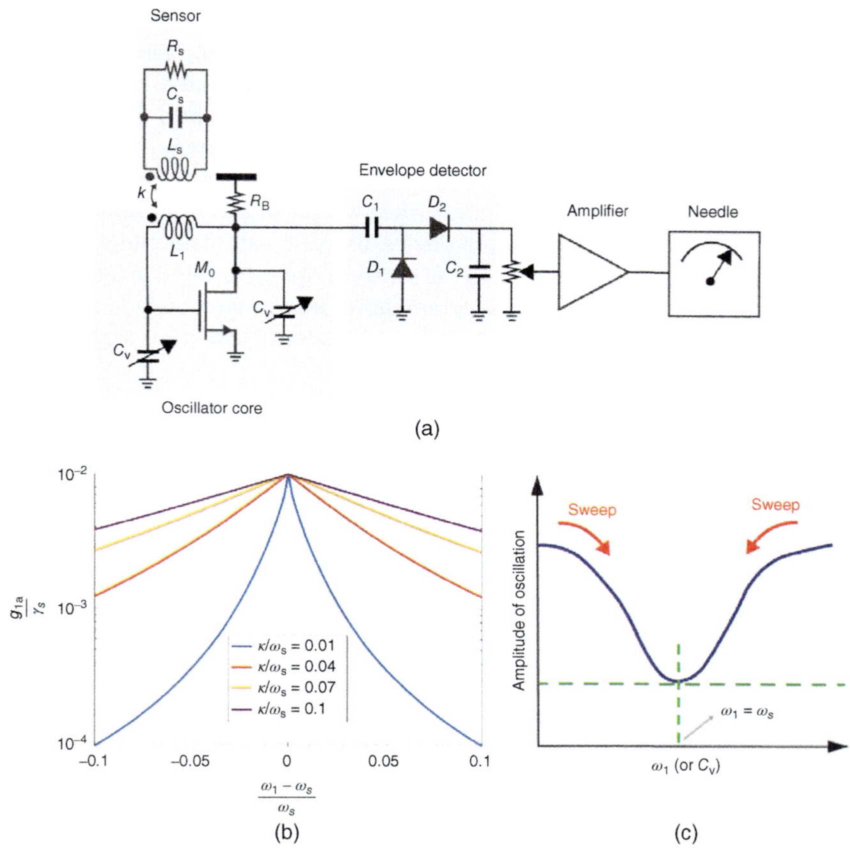

Figure 13.24 (a) The simplified schematic of a grid-dip meter. (b) The ratio of $\frac{g_{1a}}{\gamma_s}$ vs. normalized frequency difference between the sensor and the reader for different κ; here, $\frac{\gamma_s}{\omega_s} = 0.01$, and g_{1a} is the saturated gain corresponding to the stable mode. (c) Conceptual plot of the variations in the amplitude of oscillations vs. ω_1.

of interest. A dial on the device changes the capacitance embedded inside the grid-dip meter and is attached across the coil. In order to make a measurement of an *LC* tank with unknown resonant frequency wirelessly, the user first has to pick the right external coil, depending on the range of the resonant frequency of the unknown coil, and plug it into the grid-dip meter. The user should then turn the dial, which sweeps the resonant frequency of the reader, or the grid-dip meter. When the resonant frequencies of the sensor and the reader are equal, the needle on the meter jumps to a higher position on the scale, completing the measurement (http://www.radiomanual.info/schemi/ACC_instrument/Amtron_UK402_Grid-dip_user.pdf).

Although very popular, this technique suffers from a number of disadvantages. The original implementation in the form of a benchtop lab equipment is impractical for handheld sensing applications. The variants of this system in the literature are still often bulky, require complex circuitry, or have high power consumption. More importantly, similar to the other frequency-domain techniques discussed thus far, this technique fundamentally relies on frequency sweeps, which can be time-consuming. The sweep can be done either manually by the user, as with the benchtop device, or using automatic tuning with a closed-loop control system to lock to the sensor frequency. This can limit sensing in cases where variations in the parameter of interest are much faster than the reader sweep rate. Therefore, this technique does not lend itself to real-time sensing.

c. Self-oscillating higher order techniques for frequency measurement

The self-oscillating concept may also be applied to the EP system. If we assume a nonlinear gain in Equation (13.21), the equations for the real and imaginary parts of the characteristic equations of (13.15) may be rewritten as [44]

$$(\omega - \omega_s)^2(g_1 - \mu - \gamma_s) + (\kappa^2 + \mu\gamma_s)(\mu - g_1) = 0 \tag{13.28a}$$

$$(\omega - \omega_s)^3 - (\omega - \omega_s)[(\mu + \gamma_s)(\mu - g_1) + 2\kappa^2] + 2\kappa^2\mu = 0. \tag{13.28b}$$

The nonlinear gain, g_1, will saturate to a value that allows for the system to present purely real eigenfrequencies. The solutions can be found from Equation (13.28b) as

$$g_1 = -\frac{(\omega - \omega_s)^3 - (\omega - \omega_s)[\mu(\mu + \gamma_s) + 2\kappa^2] + 2\kappa^2\mu}{(\omega - \omega_s)(\mu + \gamma_s)}. \tag{13.29}$$

The real eigenfrequencies can be calculated by substituting Equation (13.29) into (13.28a). From this, the saturated gains and the eigenfrequencies may be numerically solved as shown in Figure 13.25a and b, respectively. All of these eigenfrequencies are purely real, yet, once again, in steady state, the system will settle on only the eigenfrequency with the lowest saturated gain rate.

The dependence of the eigenfrequencies (and therefore $\Delta\omega$) on the coupling between the sensor and the reader oscillator and resonator combination retains its $\kappa^{2/3}$ dependence, though the exact value of the frequency split is somewhat reduced (compared to Figure 13.26) for larger κ. Much like the linear concept, the nonlinear EP system still requires the initialization tuning procedure along with a frequency sweep and a tuning of the reader loss rate, γ_2, to ensure that the system is operated precisely at the EP ($\omega_1 = \omega_2 = \omega_0$, $g_1 = \gamma_2 = \mu$). However, nonlinear operation removes the need to also tune

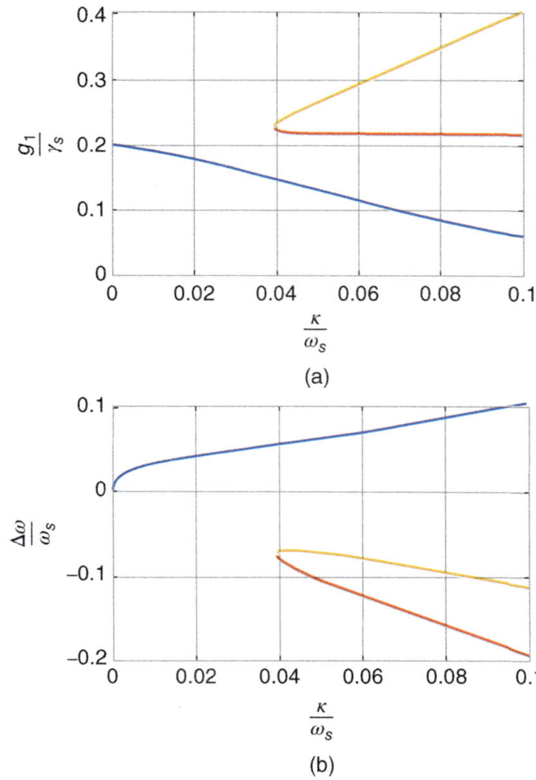

Figure 13.25 (a) Saturated gain rates, g_1, vs. coupling rate and (b) the corresponding frequency split, $\Delta\omega$; for these plots, the reader oscillator/resonator combination is operated at $\frac{\mu}{\omega_s} = \frac{\gamma_2}{\omega_s} = 0.2$, $\omega_1 = \omega_2$, and the sensor is assumed to have a loss rate of $\frac{\gamma_s}{\omega_s} = 0.01$. The eigenfrequency corresponding to the lowest saturated gain (blue lines) ultimately emerges as this results in the highest loop gain.

the gain rate due to the self-oscillating capability of the nonlinear negative resistance mechanism. Instead, the reader capacitances are swept in unison with the self-oscillating frequencies of the reader oscillator and resonator measured by an oscilloscope; at each frequency point, the reader resonator's resistance is swept to ensure that the system is operating at an EP so that when $\gamma_2 = \mu$, the maximal $\Delta\omega$ may be measured. While the number of sweeping/tuning operations is high, the increased sensitivity of $\Delta\omega$ to κ is still evident, especially for lower coupling rates, as shown in Figure 13.26a; this allows the detection and measurement of the resonant frequency of sensors that are very weakly coupled to the reader system. Additionally, the authors have shown the ability to detect the presence of two different sensors operating at different frequencies during the same frequency sweep as long as the frequencies are adequately spaced apart (Figure 13.26b).

The move toward higher order systems will only intensify in the search for more degrees of freedom, larger frequency split for robust operation, and more.

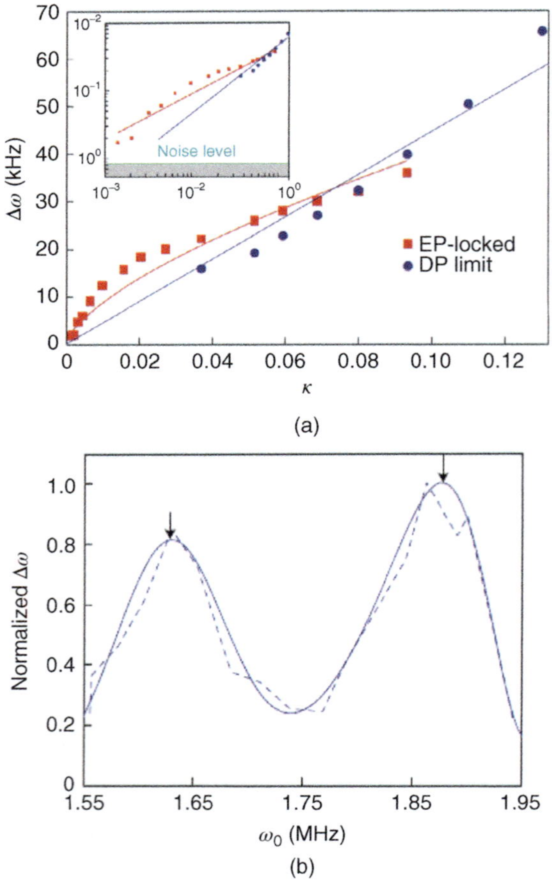

Figure 13.26 (a) Measured (discrete points) and curve-fit (solid lines) reader frequency split, $\Delta\omega$, as a function of coupling rate, κ, for both the EP and DP systems from [44]; the EP-locked system is fit with a $\kappa^{2/3}$ dependence, while the DP system is fit with a κ dependence. (b) Experimental (dashed lines) and Gaussian-fitted (solid lines) reader frequency split in the presence of two sensors with frequencies spaced 0.3 MHz apart showing the ability to sense two distinct sensors (fourth-order system) as long as their resonant frequencies are sufficiently far apart. (*Source*: Dong, Z., Li, Z., Yang, F., et al., 2019. Reproduced with permission from Nature.)

While the analysis methods discussed in this section are still valid, the system dynamics for a system with general n resonators or oscillators will become significantly more complex:

$$\frac{\mathrm{d}}{\mathrm{d}t}\begin{bmatrix} a_1 \\ a_2 \\ \vdots \\ a_{n-1} \\ a_n \end{bmatrix} = H \begin{bmatrix} a_1 \\ a_2 \\ \vdots \\ a_{n-1} \\ a_n \end{bmatrix} = \begin{bmatrix} i\omega_1 - \gamma_1 & -i\kappa_{12} & \ldots & -i\kappa_{1,n-1} & -i\kappa_{1,n} \\ -i\kappa_{21} & i\omega_2 - \gamma_2 & & -i\kappa_{2,n-1} & -i\kappa_{2,n} \\ \vdots & & \ddots & \vdots & \\ -i\kappa_{n-1,1} & -i\kappa_{n-1,2} & \ldots & i\omega_{n-1} - \gamma_{n-1} & -i\kappa_{n-1,n} \\ -i\kappa_{n,1} & -i\kappa_{n,2} & & -i\kappa_{n,n-1} & i\omega_n - \gamma_n \end{bmatrix} \begin{bmatrix} a_1 \\ a_2 \\ \vdots \\ a_{n-1} \\ a_n \end{bmatrix}. \tag{13.30}$$

This Hamiltonian will still be symmetric ($\kappa_{ij} = \kappa_{ji}, \forall\, i, j$), and, just like the second- and third-order systems, the nth-order system will exhibit n possible eigenfrequencies. Such systems could incorporate many oscillators

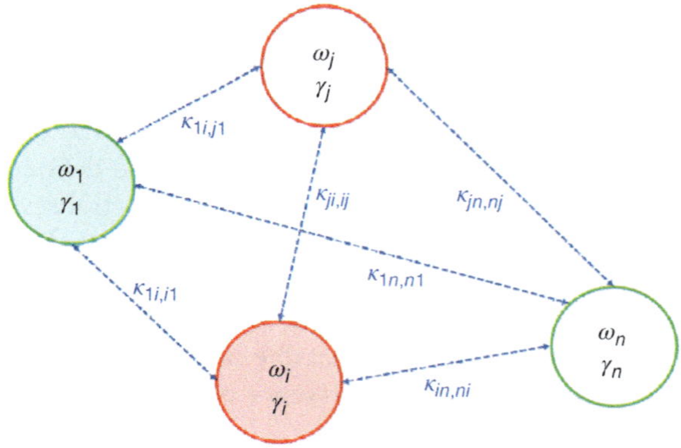

Figure 13.27 System of n coupled oscillators and resonators, each with a distinct resonant frequency. Due to reciprocity, the coupling rates between any two oscillators or resonators are symmetric, that is $\kappa_{ij} = \kappa_{ji}$, $\kappa_{jn} = \kappa_{nj}$, etc.

and resonators to allow for more intermediary coupling stages or to lower the overall effective loss rate, more numerous perturbations to further enhance spectral features, etc. (Figure 13.27). Newer applications will also require further types of information such as distance and orientation from multiple sensors, mandating the use and thorough understanding of higher order systems.

13.4 Comparison of the State of the Art

Now that the sensing methods in the literature have been introduced, it is useful to compare and contrast their pros and cons. Depending on the application of the sensing system, one or more performance metrics may prove crucial. For example, to realize a practical sensing solution for handheld applications, complexity, robustness, and cost of the sensing system are important. As mentioned earlier, passive sensors provide a solution that minimizes cost and complexity and does not require power to operate, leaving the reader as the main bottleneck; this is the focus of this section. We now introduce some of the important performance metrics based on the literature.

a. κ-Sensitivity

κ-Sensitivity measures the sensitivity of the spectral response of the reader with respect to its coupling to the sensor. A high κ-sensitivity in the reader is desirable because it means that small perturbations due to the presence of the sensor can cause a large enough and measurable spectral response in the reader (in other words provide sufficient signal-to-noise ratio).

The aforementioned nonresonant methods all achieve a κ-sensitivity of $\mathcal{O}(\kappa^2)$. This means that smaller sensors for which $\kappa \ll 1$ will have insignificant spectral response in the reader and cannot be measured with high accuracy, precision, and robustness. Nevertheless, in each case, the spectral response of the reader is different. For example, the authors of [13, 14, 26, 27] rely on the measurement of the peak frequency of the real part of the impedance (Figure 13.5b-iii), in which case, the spectral response of the reader is defined as the real part of the input impedance, given by Equation (13.2a). In the phase dip approach, the spectral response can be defined as the phase of the input impedance, whereas in [1], GDD is the spectral response.

The basis of measurement in systems such as the DP, $\mathcal{PT}$-symmetric, and EP versions is a change in the resonant frequency; therefore, the spectral response in these cases is the frequency split. In these three cases, the frequency split of the system is directly relatable to changes in some measurable parameter in the sensor, for example, presence of new particles and changes in dimensions [49, 66, 67].

In DP sensing, where only the eigenvalues coalesce, the κ-sensitivity is proportional to the coupling rate, i.e. $\mathcal{O}(\kappa)$ [44, 45]. The κ-sensitivity of the $\mathcal{PT}$-symmetric system, in which both eigenvalues and eigenvectors coalesce, is derived as $\sqrt{\kappa^2 - \gamma_s^2} \approx \mathcal{O}(\kappa)$.

The grid-dip measurement based on amplitude measurement follows the same basic principle as the $\mathcal{PT}$-symmetric system and therefore exhibits the same κ-sensitivity. Higher order EPs result in a higher κ-sensitivity, theoretically $\mathcal{O}\left(\kappa^{\frac{2}{n}}\right)$ for an nth-order EP [45, 49, 50]. It is shown in [53] that operation at the EP will result in enhanced sensitivity and amplification of the sensor's perturbations but simultaneously increases the noise as well, leaving the SNR unchanged.

The system in [44] operates at the EP of an oscillator and a resonator together forming the reader, and a third resonator (the sensor) acts as the perturbation to the system. The EP system entails complexity in implementation and results in relatively long sweeps, nonetheless, achieving a better κ-sensitivity of $\mathcal{O}\left(\kappa^{\frac{2}{3}}\right)$, (Equation (13.24)).

b. Effect of mismatches on κ-sensitivity

Some of the sensing systems rely on sweeping the frequency of the reader resonator/oscillator to perform readout of the sensor's resonant frequency. The ultimate readout accuracy is therefore determined by the minimum frequency step of the sweeping. For example, if the minimum frequency step is such that $\omega_1 \pm n\Delta_{\min} \neq \omega_s$, where n is an integer and $\Delta_{\min}$ is the minimum frequency step, when ω_1 is swept, it will never be equal to ω_s. In this case, the κ-sensitivity of the sensing system is also affected as the system will no longer be operating at the required conditions. Obviously, while a higher frequency step may alleviate this concern, this requires a more complex reader sweeping circuitry and is more time intensive. Gain/loss equality is another condition that is required for the operation of some systems: in DP, $\gamma_1 = \gamma_s$, in $\mathcal{PT}$-symmetric, $g_1 = \gamma_s$, and in EP, $g_1 = \gamma_2$. If these conditions are not met, operation with the expected κ-sensitivity cannot be achieved. This occurs when the gain step, $\Delta_{\gamma,\min}$, is not fine enough such that $|\gamma_1| \pm n\Delta_{\gamma,\min} \neq \gamma_s$ (for DP or $\mathcal{PT}$-symmetric) or $g_1 \pm n\Delta_{\gamma,\min} \neq \gamma_2$ (for EP). This becomes specifically problematic for the forced oscillation scenarios where gain (or loss) needs to be manually swept to assure this equality because the resistance or capacitance which determines the gain/loss rates has finite resolution. In self-oscillating systems, this issue is not of concern since the nonlinear resistance will automatically adjust (with infinitesimally small resolution) to the required value.

In addition to these, the EP-locked system requires that $\mu = \gamma_2$. This mandates an extra step compared to the DP and $\mathcal{PT}$-symmetric systems especially in the case of [44] because sensing is based on sweeping the resonant frequency of the EP-locked reader. At each step of sweeping, $C_1 = C_2$ changes, as will g_1 and γ_2; however, the nonlinear resistance will always guarantee that $g_1 = \gamma_2$. Nevertheless, because μ is fixed in order to guarantee $\mu = \gamma_2$, R_2 needs to be retuned. This suggests that if $\gamma_2 \pm n\Delta_{\gamma_2,\min} \neq \mu$, operation at EP cannot be achieved. Table 13.2 summarizes the sources of errors in DP, $\mathcal{PT}$-symmetric, and third-order EP systems and also defines errors which can result in κ-sensitivity degradation.

We first derive the frequency split and the imaginary part of the eigenfrequencies in each of the three cases given the mismatches introduced in Table 13.2 and then compare the effects on the κ-sensitivity.

DP system: The frequency split is given by

$$\Delta\omega = Re\left\{\frac{1}{2}(\omega_s - \omega_1) + \frac{i}{2}(\gamma_s + \gamma_1) \pm \frac{1}{2}\sqrt{[(\omega_1 - \omega_s) + i(\gamma_1 - \gamma_s)]^2 + 4\kappa^2}\right\}. \tag{13.31}$$

Using the error definitions in Table 13.2, we write

$$\Delta\omega = Re\left\{-\frac{\varepsilon_1}{2}\omega_s + i\gamma_s\left(1 - \frac{\varepsilon_2}{2}\right) \pm \kappa\sqrt{\frac{(\varepsilon_1\omega_s + i\varepsilon_2\gamma_s)^2}{4\kappa^2} + 1}\right\}. \tag{13.32}$$

Comparing Equation (13.32) with (13.18) suggests that $|\Delta\omega| \neq \kappa$ due to the errors resulting from frequency and loss mismatch.

$\mathcal{PT}$-symmetric system: The frequency split is given by

$$\Delta\omega = Re\left\{\frac{1}{2}(\omega_s - \omega_1) + \frac{i}{2}(\gamma_s - g_1) \pm \frac{1}{2}\sqrt{[(\omega_1 - \omega_s) - i(g_1 + \gamma_s)]^2 + 4\kappa^2}\right\}. \tag{13.33}$$

Table 13.2 Sources of errors in DP, $\mathcal{PT}$-symmetric, and third-order EP systems along with error definitions.

Method	Required conditions	Errors
DP	$\omega_1 = \omega_s$	$\varepsilon_1 = 1 - \frac{\omega_1}{\omega_s}$
	$\gamma_1 = \gamma_s$	$\varepsilon_2 = 1 - \frac{\lvert\gamma_1\rvert}{\gamma_s}$ a)
$\mathcal{PT}$-symmetric	$\omega_1 = \omega_s$	$\varepsilon_1 = 1 - \frac{\omega_1}{\omega_s}$
	$g_1 = \lvert\gamma_1\rvert = \gamma_s$	$\varepsilon_2 = 1 - \frac{\lvert\gamma_1\rvert}{\gamma_s}$ a)
EP ($n = 3$)	$\omega_1 = \omega_s$ b)	$\varepsilon_1 = 1 - \frac{\omega_1}{\omega_s}$
	$g_1 = \lvert\gamma_1\rvert = \gamma_2$	$\varepsilon_2 = 1 - \frac{\lvert\gamma_1\rvert}{\gamma_s}$ a)
	$\mu = \gamma_2$	$\varepsilon_3 = 1 - \frac{\gamma_2}{\mu}$
	$\omega_1 = \omega_2$ c)	$\varepsilon_4 = 1 - \frac{\omega_1}{\omega_2}$

a) Note $g_1 = -\gamma_1$; therefore, the definition of ε_2 is equivalent for all three systems.
b) This error assumes $\omega_1 = \omega_2$, but $\omega_s \neq \omega_1$.
c) This error models the mismatch between the resonant frequencies of the EP reader oscillator and resonator.

Using the error definitions in Table 13.2, we write

$$\Delta\omega = Re\left\{-\frac{\varepsilon_1}{2}\omega_s + \frac{i}{2}\varepsilon_2\gamma_s \pm \kappa\sqrt{\frac{\left[\varepsilon_1\omega_s - 2i\gamma_s\left(1 - \frac{\varepsilon_2}{2}\right)\right]^2}{4\kappa^2} + 1}\right\}. \quad (13.34)$$

Equation (13.34) suggests that $Im\{\omega_m\} \neq 0$, which means that the eigenfrequencies now have a nonzero imaginary part. A nonzero imaginary part results in either a growing or decaying oscillation, depending on its sign. However, if a nonlinear system is employed to implement the negative resistance, it will automatically adjust its value such that the total loss and gain are balanced, and the nonzero imaginary part will be accounted for. The system is therefore no longer $\mathcal{PT}$-symmetric ($\omega_1 \neq \omega_s$); nevertheless, this frequency-imbalanced system can still exhibit two real modes whose frequency split is given by the real part of Equation (13.34). Recall that in the absence of gain and frequency mismatch, $|\Delta\omega| = \sqrt{\kappa^2 - \gamma_s^2}$. Therefore, in the $\mathcal{PT}$-symmetric scenario, the error term resulting from the gain and frequency mismatch will reduce its accuracy, or equivalently κ-sensitivity, as predicted by Equation (13.34).

EP-locked system: In this case, an oscillator and resonator with resonant frequencies of ω_1 and ω_2 are coupled in the $\mathcal{PT}$-symmetric manner and locked at the EP. For the EP-locked *reader*, the reader-only frequency split is approximately given by

$$\Delta\omega = Re\left\{-\frac{\varepsilon_1}{2}\omega_s + \frac{i}{2}\varepsilon_2\gamma_s \pm \kappa\sqrt{\frac{\varepsilon_1^2\omega_s^2 - 4i\gamma_s\varepsilon_1\omega_s\left(1 - \frac{\varepsilon_2}{2}\right)}{4\kappa^2} + \varepsilon_2 + 2\varepsilon_3}\right\}. \tag{13.35}$$

An additional error term resulting from $\mu \neq \gamma_2$ is present in Equation (13.35) compared to Equation (13.34). If the reader is actually locked *at* the EP, $\Delta\omega = 0$, in the absence of the sensor.

Next, we evaluate the effect of the unlocked reader on the κ-sensitivity of the EP-locked reader–sensor system (triple resonator). Compared to the previously derived modes and required gain for the special case of the locked reader–sensor frequency, here, we consider the most general case when ω_1, ω_2, and ω_s are not necessarily equal. The required gain is now

$$g_1 = -\frac{(\omega_1 - \omega)(\omega_2 - \omega)(\omega_s - \omega) - (\gamma_2\gamma_s + \kappa^2)(\omega_1 - \omega) - \mu^2(\omega_s - \omega) - 2\mu\kappa^2 - \kappa^2(\omega_2 - \omega)}{\gamma_2(\omega_s - \omega) + \gamma_s(\omega_2 - \omega)}. \tag{13.36}$$

The real eigenfrequencies can be found by solving for ω in Equation (13.37) after substituting g_1 from Equation (13.36)

$$\gamma_s[(\omega_1 - \omega)(\omega_2 - \omega) + \gamma_2 g_1] - (\omega_s - \omega)[g_1(\omega_2 - \omega) - \gamma_2(\omega_1 - \omega)] + g_1\kappa^2 - \mu^2\gamma_s - \kappa^2\gamma_2 = 0. \tag{13.37}$$

For the special case $\omega_1 = \omega_2 = \omega_s$ and $\mu = \gamma_2$, Equations (13.36) and (13.37) will collapse to Equations (13.28a) and (13.28b), respectively; Equations (13.36) and (13.37) can also be used to evaluate the effect of mismatch between the two reader resonators ($\omega_1 \neq \omega_2$).

Comparison: Now, we compare these three systems considering all of these mismatches. The ideal frequency split for each system is summarized in Table 13.3.

Table 13.3 Ideal frequency split of DP, $\mathcal{PT}$-symmetric, and third-order EP systems.

Method	Ideal frequency split
DP	$\lvert\Delta\omega\rvert = \kappa$
$\mathcal{PT}$-symmetric	$\lvert\Delta\omega\rvert = \sqrt{\kappa^2 - \gamma_s^2}$
EP ($n = 3$)	$\lvert\Delta\omega\rvert = 2^{\frac{1}{3}}\mu^{\frac{1}{3}}\kappa^{\frac{2}{3}}$

We first plot the effect of frequency mismatch between the sensor and reader (ε_1) on the κ-sensitivity of the frequency split. To this end, we define the change in κ-sensitivity, Δ, as the magnitude of the difference between the κ-sensitivity values in the presence of the errors and the ideal κ-sensitivity normalized by ω_s. Since the expression for the modes is not straightforward in the presence of the mismatches for the EP-locked system, we solve for the modes using MATLAB numerically. To this end, we substitute $\omega_1 = \omega_2$ in Equations (13.36) and (13.37). Δ as a function of ε_1 (assuming all other error terms equal to zero) is shown in Figure 13.28, which reveals that the EP-locked system has the largest degradation in κ-sensitivity in the presence of ε_1. Figure 13.28 also suggests that the $\mathcal{PT}$-symmetric system achieves a lower Δ for medium ranges of κ compared to its DP counterpart; however, as κ grows, their performance become similar. Additionally, the performance gap between the EP-locked system and the other two systems reduces with larger values of κ.

Next, we evaluate the effect of ε_2 on κ-sensitivity. The results are shown in Figure 13.29, where Δ vs. ε_2 is plotted for the three systems (assuming all other error terms equal to zero). A general observation from Figure 13.29 is that all three systems are more robust to ε_2 compared to the frequency mismatch, ε_1. Additionally, the EP-locked system remains the most sensitive to ε_2, followed by the $\mathcal{PT}$-symmetric and DP systems, respectively.

The EP-locked method also relies on $\mu = \gamma_2$. The effect of this mismatch, ε_3, is shown in Figure 13.30a, suggesting that the EP-locked system is not highly sensitive, and even with $\varepsilon_3 = 5\%$ the κ-sensitivity remains higher than the DP and $\mathcal{PT}$-symmetric systems. Next, we examine the robustness of the EP-locked system against the mismatch between the two reader resonators, that is when $\omega_1 \neq \omega_2$ ($\varepsilon_4 \neq 0$) but assume $\omega_1 = \omega_s$ and plot the κ-sensitivity in Figure 13.30b; as can be seen, the EP-locked reader is very sensitive to the accuracy of the frequency match between ω_1 and ω_2. A mismatch as small as 1% between the two frequencies ($\varepsilon_4 = 1\%$), for example, results in a roughly 20 dB degradation in κ-sensitivity.

Figure 13.30b also suggests that for the EP-locked system to maintain its κ-sensitivity advantage over the $\mathcal{PT}$-symmetric and DP systems, a higher

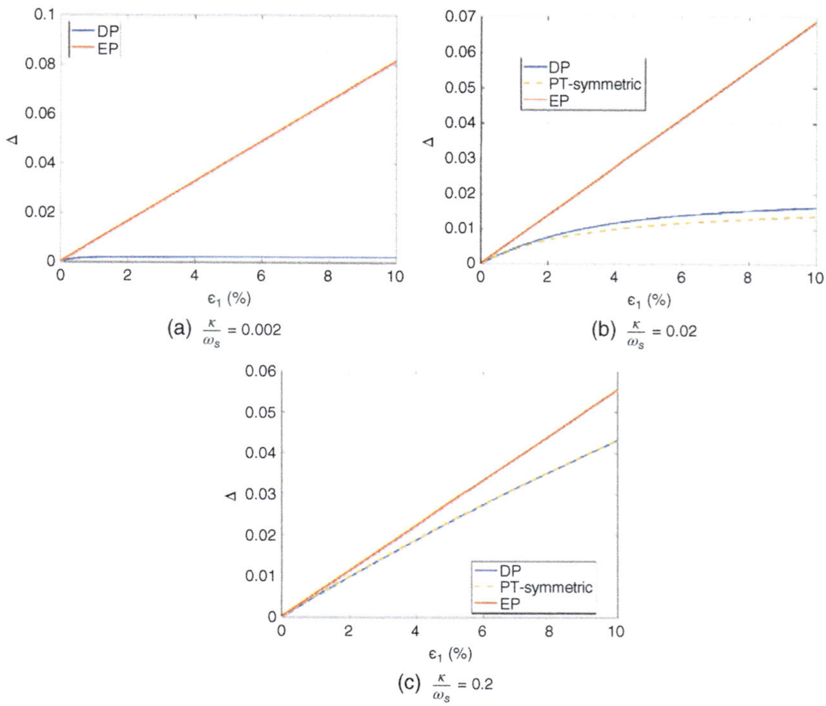

Figure 13.28 Change in κ-sensitivity, Δ (the magnitude of the difference between κ-sensitivity in the presence of errors and its ideal value normalized by ω_s) for DP, $\mathcal{PT}$-symmetric, and EP-locked systems at different coupling rates for ε_1 in the range of 0–10% ($\varepsilon_2 = \varepsilon_3 = \varepsilon_4 = 0$). The EP-locked system exhibits the highest Δ and therefore is the most sensitive to ε_1. As κ increases, the sensitivity to ε_1 reduces. In the DP and $\mathcal{PT}$-symmetric systems, $\frac{\gamma_s}{\omega_s} = 0.01$, and for the EP-locked system, $\frac{\gamma_s}{\omega_s} = 0.01$ and $\frac{\mu}{\omega_s} = \frac{\gamma_2}{\omega_s} = 0.2$. For $\frac{\kappa}{\omega_s} = 0.002$, the response of the $\mathcal{PT}$-symmetric system is omitted since this is below the minimum coupling rate $\left(\frac{k_{\min}}{\omega_s} = \frac{\gamma_s}{\omega_s} = 0.01\right)$.

complexity is required, e.g. the frequency sweep resolution for locking ω_1 to ω_2 must be fine enough to allow for relative errors well below even 0.5%; for example, a locking resolution of better than 0.05% ($\varepsilon_4 < 0.05\,\%$) is required (Figure 3 in [44]). Additionally, as explained before, the EP-locked approach may require up to four sweeps, depending on whether a self-oscillating approach or forced approach is employed.

Table 13.4 summarizes our findings and compares sensitivity and complexity for all of the methods discussed in this chapter.

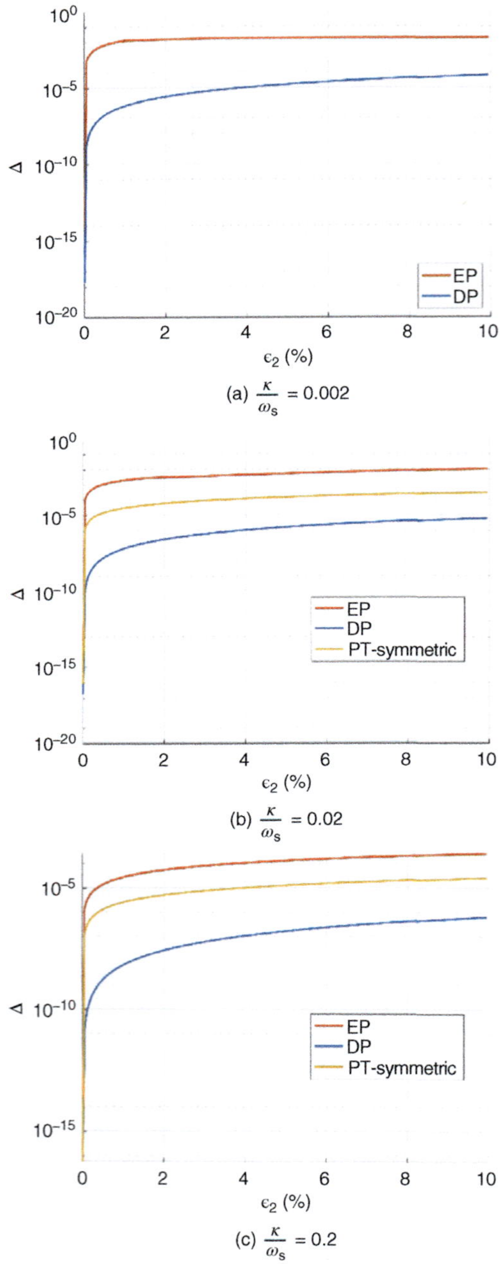

Figure 13.29 Change in κ-sensitivity, Δ, vs. ε_2 at different coupling rates in the range of 0–10% ($\varepsilon_1 = \varepsilon_3 = \varepsilon_4 = 0$). The EP-locked system exhibits the highest Δ and is therefore the most sensitive to ε_2. As κ increases, the sensitivity to ε_2 reduces. In the DP and $\mathcal{PT}$-symmetric systems, $\frac{\gamma_s}{\omega_s} = 0.01$, and for the EP-locked system, $\frac{\gamma_s}{\omega_s} = 0.01$ and $\frac{\mu}{\omega_s} = \frac{\gamma_2}{\omega_s} = 0.2$. For $\frac{\kappa}{\omega_s} = 0.002$, the response of the $\mathcal{PT}$-symmetric system is omitted since this is below the minimum coupling rate $\left(\frac{k_{\text{min}}}{\omega_s} = \frac{\gamma_s}{\omega_s} = 0.01\right)$.

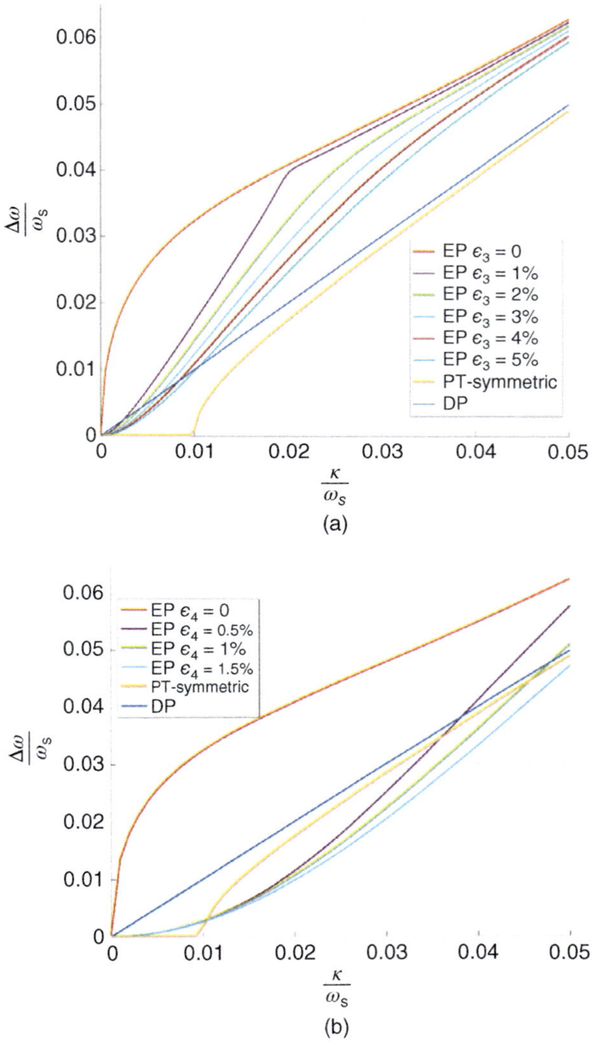

Figure 13.30 (a) Comparison between the κ-sensitivity of the perfectly matched EP-locked reader ($\varepsilon_1 = \varepsilon_2 = \varepsilon_3 = \varepsilon_4 = 0$) and the mismatched case where $\mu \neq \gamma_2$ ($\varepsilon_3 \neq 0$, $\varepsilon_1 = \varepsilon_2 = \varepsilon_4 = 0$) vs. DP and $\mathcal{PT}$-symmetric scenarios with $\varepsilon_1 = \varepsilon_2 = 0$. In the DP and $\mathcal{PT}$-symmetric systems, $\frac{\gamma_s}{\omega_s} = 0.01$, and for the EP-locked system, $\frac{\gamma_s}{\omega_s} = 0.01$ and $\frac{\mu}{\omega_s} = \frac{\gamma_2}{\omega_s} = 0.2$. (b) Comparison between the κ-sensitivity of the perfectly matched EP-locked reader ($\varepsilon_1 = \varepsilon_2 = \varepsilon_3 = \varepsilon_4 = 0$) and the mismatched case where $\omega_1 \neq \omega_2$ ($\varepsilon_4 \neq 0$, $\varepsilon_1 = \varepsilon_2 = \varepsilon_3 = 0$) vs. DP and $\mathcal{PT}$-symmetric scenarios with $\varepsilon_1 = \varepsilon_2 = 0$. In the DP and $\mathcal{PT}$-symmetric systems, $\frac{\gamma_s}{\omega_s} = 0.01$, and for the EP-locked system, $\frac{\gamma_s}{\omega_s} = 0.01$ and $\frac{\mu}{\omega_s} = \frac{\gamma_2}{\omega_s} = 0.2$.

Table 13.4 Comparison between sensing systems.

Method	Excitation type	κ-sensitivity	Mismatch sources	Mismatch sensitivity	Number of sweeps[a)]	Number of resonators + oscillators
Nonresonant primary	Forced	κ^2	—	—	2	1
DP	Forced	κ	2	Low	1	2
$\mathcal{PT}$-symmetric	Forced	$\sqrt{\kappa^2 - \gamma_s^2}$	2	Low	Up to 3	2
	Self-oscillating				1	
EP ($n = 3$)	Forced	$\kappa^{\frac{2}{3}}$	4	Medium	Up to 4	3
	Self-oscillating				2	
Higher order	Forced	$\propto \kappa^{\frac{2}{n}}$	$>n$	High	Up to n	n
($n > 3$)	Self-oscillating				Up to $n - 2$	

a) Per sensor measurement.

13.5 Conclusion

Near-field, passive sensing systems offer a low-complexity, cost-effective, and versatile solution for many sensing applications. With the advantage of minimal complexity compared to passive RFID and NFC sensors, the fully passive sensors covered in this chapter rely only on capacitive or resistive sensors along with an inductor coil for inductive coupling. Inductive coupling has several advantages for sensor measurements over its far-field counterparts which rely on two-way path loss, suffering from higher power consumption. The major limitation of some of the discussed near-field techniques is in the requirement of bulky and expensive lab equipment to perform sensor measurement, making them impractical for realistic sensing scenarios.

Another important aspect in the implementation of practical sensing system is the sensing rate, e.g. how fast the readout is performed. The sensing rate proves crucial in some applications, especially those dealing with parameters that vary rapidly. This limits the number of frequency steps in the frequency sweep, for example, and calls for real-time techniques, establishing an essential benchmark for forced and self-oscillating systems. Currently available methods all require at least one frequency sweep and/or further tuning to adjust sensitive parameters for operation under a specific set of conditions. The ultimate system will be able to take advantage of a few measurement points instead of a full spectral sweep, allowing for real-time operation.

More recent efforts in fully passive sensor telemetry have focused on using higher numbers of resonators in more clever ways. In this chapter, we already saw systems with two resonators and one oscillator first used as intermediary coupling-rate boosters [46] and then as a way to *bias* the system at an EP where a purely real frequency split may be enforced for arbitrary coupling rates. The latter concept was even used to sense two different *perturbing* sensors operating at distinct frequencies. With more resonators, these opportunities may be further expanded by capitalizing on the additional available degrees of freedom. Introducing higher degrees of freedoms (more resonators) in these EP-locked systems, however, will increase the sensitivity of the system to mismatches. Although the EP-locked system achieves a higher κ-sensitivity, it loses this advantage in the presence of mismatches in the reader frequencies and requires higher complexity in the implementation of the reader.

While this chapter focused on capacitive sensing, other efforts are also beginning to tackle resistive sensing using $\Delta\omega$ to measure changes in the loss rate, instead of translating the loss rate to a resistance ($\gamma \propto R$ or $1/R$) [43]; this currently still requires the use of a VNA. Making such sensing mechanisms more practical by obviating the need for such bulky lab equipment is another direction that must be pursued.

References

1 Chen, L.Y., Tee, B.C., Chortos, A.L. et al. (2015). Continuous wireless pressure monitoring and mapping with ultra-small passive sensors for health monitoring and critical care. *Nature Communications* 5: 5028.
2 Boutry, C.M., Beker, L., Kaizawa, Y. et al. (2019). Biodegradable and flexible arterial-pulse sensor for the wireless monitoring of blood flow. *Nature Biomedical Engineering* 3: 47–57.
3 Niu, S., Matsuhisa, N., Beker, L. et al. (2019). A wireless body area sensor network based on stretchable passive tags. *Nature Elecronics* 2: 361–368.
4 Gao, W., Emaminejad, S., Nyein, H. et al. (2016). Fully integrated wearable sensor arrays for multiplexed in situ perspiration analysis. *Nature* 529: 509–514.
5 Rose, D.P. et al. (2015). Adhesive RFID sensor patch for monitoring of sweat electrolytes. *IEEE Transactions on Biomedical Engineering* 62 (6): 1457–1465.
6 Lonsdale, A. and Lonsdale, B. (2002). Apparatus and method for interrogating a passive sensor. US Patent: 6,765,493, 20 July 2002.
7 Salpavaara, T., Verho, J., Kumpulainen, P., and Lekkala, J. (2005). Wireless interrogation techniques for sensors utilizing inductively coupled resonance circuits. *Procedia Engineering* 5: 216–219.
8 Salpavaara, T., Verho, J., Kumpulainen, P., and Lekkala, J. (2011). Readout methods for an inductively coupled resonance sensor used in pressure garment application. *Sensors and Actuators A: Physical* 172 (1): 109–116.

9 Radosavljevic, G.J., Zivanov, L.D., Smetana, W. et al. (2009). A wireless embedded resonant pressure sensor fabricated in the standard LTCC technology. *IEEE Sensors Journal* 9 (12): 1956–1962.

10 Garcia-Canton, J., Merlos, A., and Baldi, A. (2007). High-quality factor electrolyte insulator silicon capacitor for wireless chemical sensing. *IEEE Electron Device Lett.* 28 (1): 27–29.

11 Babu, A. and George, B. (2018). An efficient readout scheme for simultaneous measurement from multiple wireless passive LC sensors. *IEEE Transactions on Instrumentation and Measurement* 67 (5): 1161–1168.

12 Escobedo, P., Martínez-Olmosa, A., Fernández-Salmerón, J. et al. (2018). Compact readout system for chipless passive LC tags and its application for humidity monitoring. *Sensors and Actuators A: Physical* 280: 287–294.

13 Nopper, R., Niekrawietz, R., and Reindl, L. (2010). Wireless readout of passive LC sensors. *IEEE Transactions on Instrumentation and Measurement* 59 (9): 2450–2457.

14 Nopper, R., Has, R., and Reindl, L. (2011). A wireless sensor readout system—circuit concept, simulation, and accuracy. *IEEE Transactions on Instrumentation and Measurement* 60 (8): 2976–2983.

15 Demori, M., Mehedi, M., Marco, B., et al. (2017). Passive LC sensor label with distance-independent contactless interrogation. Proceedings of the IEEE SENSORS, Glasgow, UK.

16 Baù, M., Ferrari, M., and Ferrari, V. (2017). Analysis and validation of contactless time-gated interrogation technique for quartz resonator sensors. *Sensors* 17 (6): 1264.

17 Joy, J., Kroh, J., Ellis, M. et al. (2007). Communicating with implanted wireless sensor. US Patent 7,245,117, 17 July 2007.

18 Zhang, J. et al. (2018). Feature extraction for robust crack monitoring using passive wireless RFID antenna sensors. *IEEE Sensors Journal* 18 (15): 6273–6280.

19 Zhang, C. et al. (2015). An LC-type passive wireless humidity sensor system with portable telemetry unit. *Journal of Microelectromechanical Systems* 24 (3): 575–581.

20 Baldi, A., Choi, W., and Ziaie, B. (2003). A self-resonant frequency-modulated micromachined passive pressure transensor. *IEEE Sensors Jour.* 3 (6): 728–733.

21 Garcia-Canton, J., Merlos, A., and Baldi, A. (2007). High-quality factor electrolyte insulator silicon capacitor for wireless chemical sensing. *IEEE Electron Device Letters* 28 (1): 27–29.

22 Chen, P., Rodger, D.C., Saati, S. et al. (2008). Microfabricated implantable parylene-based wireless passive intraocular pressure sensors. *Journal of Microelectromechanical Systems* 17 (6): 1342–1351.

23 Harpster, T.J., Stark, B., and Najafi, K. (2002). A passive wireless integrated humidity sensor. *Sensors and Actuators A: Physical* 95 (2/3): 100–107.

24 Harpster, T., Hauvespre, S., Dokmeci, M., et al. (2000). A passive humidity monitoring system for in-situ remote wireless testing of micropackages. Proceedings of the IEEE Thirteenth Annual International Conference on Micro Electro Mechanical Systems, Miyazaki, Japan, 335–340.

25 Huang, Q., Dong, L., and Wang, L. (2016). LC passive wireless sensors toward a wireless sensing platform: status, prospects, and challenges. *Journal of Microelectromechanical Systems* 25 (5): 822–841.

26 Lizon-Martinez, S., Giannetti, R., Rodriguez-Marrero, J.L., and Tellini, B. (2005). Design of a system for continuous intraocular pressure monitoring. *IEEE Transactions on Instrumentation and Measurement* 54 (4): 1534–1540.

27 Sajeeda and Kaiser, T.J. (2006). Passive telemetric readout system. *IEEE Sensors Journal* 6 (5): 1340–1345.

28 Pichorim, S.F. and Abatti, P.J. (2008). A novel method to read remotely resonant passive sensors in biotelemetric systems. *IEEE Sensors Journal* 8 (1): 6–11.

29 Joy, J., Kroh, J., Ellis, M., Allen, M., and Pyle, W. (2007). Communicating with implanted wireless sensor. US Patent 7245117, 17 July 2007.

30 Farrar, J.T., Berkley, C., and Zworykin, V.K. (1960). Telemetering of intraenteric pressure in man by an externally energized wireless capsule. *Science* 131: 1814.

31 Wei, Q., Wang, Y., Chen, D., Chen, J., and Wang, J. (2016). A novel method based on RF detection enabling wireless and passive LC sensing. Proceedings of the 2016 IEEE SENSORS, Orlando, FL, 1–3.

32 Sauer, S., Marschner, U., Adolphi, B. et al. (2012). Passive wireless resonant galfenol sensor for osteosynthesis plate bending measurement. *IEEE Sensors Journal* 12 (5): 1226–1233.

33 Xu, M. (2019). Wireless LC sensor reader. US Patent 10307067, 4 June 2019.

34 Demori, M., Baù, M., Ferrari, M., and Ferrari, V. (2018). Interrogation techniques and interface circuits for coil-coupled passive sensors. *Micromachines* 9 (9): pii: E449.

35 Chen, Y. (2013). Scalable wireless monitoring systems with passive sensors for biomedical applications. PhD thesis, Department of Electrical Engineering, Stanford University, Stanford, CA.

36 Demori, M., Baù, M., Ferrari, M., and Ferrari, V. (2018). Electronic technique and circuit topology for accurate distance-independent contactless readout of passive LC sensors. *AEU - International Journal of Electronics and Communications* 92: 82–85.

37 Haus, H.A. (1984). Coupling of modes – resonators and couplers. In: *Waves and Fields in Optoelectronics* (ed. N. Holonyak). Englewood Cliffs: Prentice-Hall, ch. 7.

38 Bender, C.M. (2007). Making sense of non-Hermitian Hamiltonians. *Reports on Progress in Physics* 70 (6): 947–1018.

39 Bender, C.M. and Boettcher, S. (1998). Real spectra in non-Hermitian Hamiltonians having $\mathcal{PT}$ symmetry. *Physical Review Letters* 80 (24): 5243–5246.

40 Bender, C.M., Berry, M.V., and Mandilara, A. (2002). Generalized $\mathcal{PT}$ symmetry and real spectra. *Journal of Physics A: Mathematical and General* 35 (31): L467–L471.

41 Schindler, J., Lin, Z., Lee, J.M. et al. (2012). $\mathcal{PT}$-symmetric electronics. *Journal of Physics A: Mathematical and Theoretical* 45 (44): 444029.

42 Schindler, J. (2013). $\mathcal{PT}$-symmetric electronics. MS thesis, Department of Physics, Wesleyan University, Middletown, CT.

43 Sakhdari, M., Hajizadegan, M., Li, Y. et al. (2018). Ultrasensitive, parity-time-symmetric wireless reactive and resistive sensors. *IEEE Sensors Journal* 18 (23): 9548–9555.

44 Dong, Z., Li, Z., Yang, F. et al. (2019). Sensitive readout of implantable microsensors using a wireless system locked to an exceptional point. *Nature Electronics* 2: 335–342.

45 Ozdemir, S.K., Rotter, S., Nori, F., and Yang, L. (2019). Parity-time symmetry and exceptional points in photonics. *Nature Materials* 18: 783–798.

46 Chen, P.-Y., Sakhdari, M., Hajizadegan, M. et al. (2018). Generalized parity-time symmetry condition for enhanced sensor telemetry. *Nature Electronics* 1: 297–304.

47 Assawaworrarit, S., Yu, X., and Fan, S. (2017). Robust wireless power transfer using a nonlinear parity-time-symmetric. *Nature Letters* 546: 387–390.

48 Chen, P.-Y. (2018). High-order parity-time-symmetric electromagnetic sensors. Proceedings of the International Conference on Electromagnetic in Advanced Applications, Cartagena de Indias, Colombia (10–14 September 2018).

49 Chen, W., Özdemir, Ş.K., Zhao, G. et al. (2017). Exceptional points enhance sensing in an optical microcavity. *Nature* 548: 192–196.

50 Hodaei, H., Hassan, A.U., Wittek, S. et al. (2017). Enhanced sensitivity at higher-order exceptional points. *Nature* 548: 187–191.

51 Langbein, W. (2018). No exceptional precision of exceptional-point sensors. *Physical Review A* 98 (2): 023805.

52 Chen, C., Jin, L., and Liu, R.-B. (2019). Sensitivity of parameter estimation near the exceptional point of a non-Hermitian system. *New Journal of Physics* 21: 083002.

53 Zhang, M., Sweeney, W., Hsu, C.W. et al. (2019). Quantum noise theory of exceptional point amplifying sensors. *Physical Review Letter* 123 (18): 180501.

54 Lau, H.-K. and Clerk, A.A. (2018). Fundamental limits and non-reciprocal approaches in non-Hermitian quantum sensing. *Nature Communications* 9: 4320.

55 Razavi, B. (2001). Oscillators: cross-coupled oscillator. In: *Design of Analog CMOS Integrated Circuits* (ed. K.T. Kane), 499–501. New York: McGraw-Hill, ch. 14, sec. 14.3.1.

56 Razavi, B. (2011). *RF Microelectronics (2nd Edition) (Prentice Hall Communications Engineering and Emerging Technologies Series)*, 2e. Upper Saddle River: Prentice Hall Press.

57 Chen, A. (1963). Passive telemetering system feasibility study. MS thesis, Department of Electrical Engineering, University of California at Berkeley, Berkeley, CA.

58 Tranter, J. (2013). *Classic Heathkit Electronic Test Equipment*. Jeff Tranter.

59 The Technical Journal of the Television-Radio Trade. (1953). vol. 22.

60 73 Amateur Radio Magazine (June 1967).

61 Collins, C.C. (1967). Miniature passive pressure transensor for implanting in the eye. *IEEE Transactions on Biomedical Engineering* BME-14 (2): 74–83.

62 Mackay, R.S. (1965). Telemetering from within the body of animals and man: endoradiosondes. In: *Biomedical Telemetry* (ed. C. Caceres), 148–189. New York: Academic Press.

63 Coosemans, J., Catrysse, M., and Puers, R. (2004). A readout circuit for an intra-ocular pressure sensor. *Sensors and Actuators A: Physical* 110 (1–3): 432–438.

64 Carvajal, M.A., Escobedo, P., Martínez-Olmos, A., and Palma, A.J. (2020). Readout circuit with improved sensitivity for contactless LC sensing tags. *IEEE Sensors Journal* 20 (2): 885–891.

65 Butler, J.C., Vigliotti, A.J., Verdi, F.W., and Walsh, S.M. (2002). Wireless passive resonant circuit, inductively coupled, inductive strain sensor. *Sensors and Actuators A: Physical* 102 (1/2): 61–66.

66 Zhu, J., Ozdemir, S.K., Xiao, Y.-F. et al. (2010). On-chip single nanoparticle detection and sizing by mode splitting in an ultrahigh-Q microresonator. *Nature Photonics* 4: 46–49.

67 He, L., Özdemir, S.K., Zhu, J. et al. (2011). Detecting single viruses and nanoparticles using whispering gallery microlasers. *Nature Nanotechnology* 6: 428–432.

14

Wireless and Wearable Biomarker Analysis

Shuyu Lin, Bo Wang, Ryan Shih, and Sam Emaminejad

Interconnected and Integrated Bioelectronics Lab (I^2BL), Department of Electrical and Computer Engineering, University of California, Los Angeles, CA, USA

14.1 Introduction

Recent advances in wearable and wireless sensors have provided unprecedented opportunities for (semi)continuous monitoring of personal health. The proliferation of these sensors and the accumulation of the collected physiologically relevant information can be adapted to applications ranging from personal fitness and nutrition monitoring to clinical diagnostics [1]. To date, most wearable medical devices focus on detection and tracking of physical signals (e.g. physical activity and vital signs) using physical sensors. Some notable examples include heart rate, electrodermal activity, electrocardiography, and muscle oxygen saturation [2–4]. However, physical signals are not the only source of physiologically relevant data. Chemical signals accessible through various biofluids (e.g. endogenous biomarker molecules and xenobiotics) can also provide valuable insights into personal health and disease status, which can enable various applications including general health monitoring (e.g. fitness and nutrient monitoring), drug tracking (e.g. drug compliance, pharmacokinetics, and pharmacodynamics), and disease diagnosis. Compared to traditional lab-based chemical tests, wearable chemical sensing modalities are more accessible and can enable real-time data acquisition and analysis. The significant increase in temporal data acquisition frequency (e.g. from one sample per year in the annual body check to one sample per hour for a (semi)continuous monitoring wearable sensor) presents a high potential to transform the current practices in health care and to catalyze the transition from traditional reactive medicine to preventive and personalized medicine.

While blood is the gold-standard biofluid for accessing the body's chemical information, the invasive nature of its sampling process (and its subsequent risk of infection and tissue damage) renders it unsuitable for wearable applications

Antenna and Sensor Technologies in Modern Medical Applications,
First Edition. Edited by Yahya Rahmat-Samii and Erdem Topsakal.

designed for the general population. To access analytes in a noninvasive or minimally invasive manner, alternative biofluids may be targeted instead, including interstitial fluid (ISF), saliva, sweat, and tears [5, 6]. Each of these candidates has been shown to have distinct advantages and limitations:

1. ISF: Analyte concentration in ISF is highly correlated with blood (nearly 1 : 1 for most analytes), which has been demonstrated in the case of glucose monitoring [7]. However, sampling ISF can be challenging as it does not have a naturally existing secretion pathway.
2. Saliva: Wearable saliva monitoring was also demonstrated [8]. While saliva is easy to access, the analyte concentration in saliva is prone to the influence of meal intake.
3. Tears: Sampling tears can be extremely challenging and may cause irritation [9].

In this chapter, we specifically focus on sweat because of its unique potential for (semi)continuous chemical signal monitoring. Sweat shares analyte partitioning pathway with blood and can be accessed noninvasively on the skin surface with minimal user intervention. Within this context, here we present: (i) categories of analytes in sweat and their "real-life" application; (ii) chemical sensing interfaces for target analyte quantification; (iii) biofluid sampling approaches to access sweat; (iv) microfluidic interfaces for biofluid manipulation on body, and (v) peripheral electronics for data acquisition and wireless transmission. Importantly, it is worth noting that while this chapter focuses specifically on sweat, the framework presented can be generalized to biomarker analysis efforts for other biofluids.

14.2 Sweat-Based Biomarkers

The rich diversity of biomarkers present in sweat can be broadly classified according to physical and chemical properties. Of significant interest are metabolites, electrolytes, steroids, proteins, and xenobiotics.

14.2.1 Metabolites

One class of biomarkers is metabolites (compounds that are produced from or used in biochemical reactions within the body). These biomarkers can provide insights about naturally occurring dynamic processes inside the human body, which is especially critical in periodic/continuous monitoring scenarios. Of note, glucose and lactate are some of the most-studied metabolites because of their importance in diabetes management and sepsis or lactic acidosis. A common procedure among diabetics for measuring blood glucose is the standard finger-prick method, which requires that the individual punctures the skin to sample blood. The blood is subsequently analyzed with enzyme-electrode strips inserted into an electronic reader [10]. However, this approach is inherently invasive and represents a severe inconvenience to individuals who often will test their serum glucose levels multiple times a day [11]. Wearables and wireless sensors can monitor physiological changes in glucose noninvasively and continuously represent a significant improvement and would likely foster improved compliance and disease management. Lactate also holds clinical significance. While correlation between sweat and blood lactate can be confounded by lactate generation by sweat glands, lactate concentration in sweat can still be utilized as an indicator of pressure ischemia and tissue perfusion [12].

14.2.2 Electrolytes

Soluble ionic salts make for strong electrolytes, which are compounds that can conduct electricity through a fluid. Of the electrolytes found in sweat, perhaps the most physiologically relevant electrolytes are sodium, potassium, and chloride. Sodium is especially important because it is one of the primary factors that influence the body's water content and volume status. Detection of abnormally low (hyponatremia) or high (hypernatremia) serum sodium levels can thus provide profound clinical insights. For example, a hyponatremic individual may have a low serum sodium level due to increased water consumption. If severe enough, this can manifest as water intoxication, and rapid progression without intervention can result in coma or death [13]. Inappropriate serum sodium levels can also be indicative of heart failure, renal failure, and inappropriate secretion of arginine vasopressin [14]. In all cases, if correlations between serum and sweat levels were established, earlier detection could improve outcomes, and noninvasive wearable detection could facilitate convenient and constant monitoring. Potassium is also an important biomarker because its serum level reflects the risk of cardiac arrhythmias. Normal cells have a high intracellular potassium content, while the extracellular environment typically has a low potassium concentration. If the balance is disrupted and excessive potassium is present in the blood (hyperkalemia), this can lead to pathological cardiac activity that can be fatal. Fortunately, recent work has demonstrated that the collection of stimulated sweat potassium correlates with serum levels [15]. Additionally, sweat chloride has been reported as an indicator of cystic fibrosis (CF) [16–18]. Thus, while the exact biomarker partitioning still remains unknown, sweat potassium could be used as a clinical diagnostic metric.

14.2.3 Steroids

Steroids, such as steroid hormones, constitute another category of biomarkers including testosterone, estrogen, and cortisol. Due to the low molecular weight and high lipophilicity, their concentrations in sweat and blood are speculated to be highly correlated [5]. With widespread regulatory functions in the body, steroids such as testosterone and estrogen contribute to growth and development, sexual health, and muscle/bone metabolism [19, 20]. Noninvasive monitoring of these compounds could then detect hormonal inadequacies at an early stage. Total and free testosterone, for example, have been shown to be substantially lowered in obese males, indicating potential links to hypothalamo–hypophyseal–gonadal axis malfunction [21]. Similar inadequacies with testosterone and estrogen have been noted in both males and females (hypogonadism) [22]. Early identification of individuals with these conditions in prepubescent stages allows for maximal treatment with hormone replacement therapy, making accurate detection of reduced sex steroid levels a beneficial goal for wearable and wireless sensors. Cortisol is also of clinical significance due to its role as a "stress hormone" that regulates gluconeogenesis, immune suppression, and metabolic processes (among others) [23, 24]. As a biomarker with so many functions, it holds wide utility as a potential target for identifying health issues such as hyperglycemia, immunocompromised state, and Cushing's disease [25]. A simple biomarker detection platform using wireless wearable sensors could quickly identify elevated cortisol levels, which would provide preliminary cause for appropriate intervention and additional diagnostics.

14.2.4 Proteins

Electrolytes, metabolites, and hormones are physically smaller compared to proteins, which make up a small fraction of sweat (only 20% of proteins found in plasma were found in eccrine sweat with much lower concentration level) [26]. This is because plasma substances must pass through multiple layers of tissue in order to reach the skin (these include capillary endothelium, the interstitium, and epithelial stratifications with additional layers of connective and adipose tissues). While larger proteins and peptides encounter these barriers and are mostly repelled, smaller proteins may appear in sweat. If reproducible correlates with plasma levels are identified, they can provide useful clinical feedback regarding health status. Of particular interest to medical professionals is the finding that eccrine sweat can contain inflammatory cytokines [27]. This could indicate an ongoing infection or other inflammatory response, which could be treated appropriately.

14.2.5 Xenobiotics

While many biomarkers of interest are endogenous compounds produced or recycled in the body, exogenous substances that enter the body (such as prescription medications and illicit drugs) also hold value in the context of wearables and wireless sensors. For example, caffeine's effects as a central nervous system stimulant have been well documented, and concerns over caffeine-induced health problems have focused on cardiovascular defects such as heart failure, hypertension, and arrhythmias. Current recommendations suggest that caffeine consumption be limited to 600 mg day^{-1} (preferably less) [28]. While this is not an issue for most individuals, continuous monitoring with the aid of wearable sensors may assist in controlling intake for those with a caffeine addiction [29]. Similar monitoring would also benefit the tracking of drug dosage over time. For patients particularly liable for forgetting to take medications as scheduled, a wearable sensor that tracks the drug's pharmacokinetics and gives real-time reminders when the dosage becomes too low would be an effective solution. Nearly identical platforms could be employed to monitor illicit drug levels without the need for urine or blood samples [30].

14.3 Wearable Chemical Sensing Interfaces

Compared with wearable physical sensors, which aim to track the user's vital signs and mobility, wearable chemical sensors are designed for monitoring of chemical markers (analytes) continuously and obtaining comprehensive information about the individuals' health and wellness at the molecular level [1, 31]. To target a biomarker precisely, specific characteristics of ideal chemical sensors include:

1. Low limit of detection and high sensitivity. While the precise partitioning mechanism of biomarkers into biofluids is unknown, these molecules are often significantly diluted compared to the concentrations in blood. It naturally follows that an ideal sensor will be sensitive to these low levels.
2. High selectivity to the target biomarker(s) with minimal interference of biofluid matrix. Due to the myriad of compounds present in any biofluid, it is imperative that a sensor selectively targets the biomarker(s) of interest without being influencing by other molecules and biofluid conditions (e.g. pH and ionic strength).
3. Long-term operational and storage stability. As wearable sensors are envisioned to operate for continuous monitoring applications, they must be able to function predictably over relatively long periods of time with minimal degradation. This property also extends to storage stability, which has obvious importance for commercial products.
4. The convenience of application and maintenance during use. While biomarker sensor research has primarily focused on developing robust sensing platforms, convenient sensor applications, user comfort, and ease of maintenance/removal are necessary requirements for commercial products. For some, the ergonomic performance may even be of equal importance to the sensor's scientific potency.

5. Capacity for integration within data-collection infrastructure. Most relevant for Internet-of-Thing (IoT) networks, sensors must be easily integrated with electronic devices that can convert sensed signals into useful data. These data could then be analyzed in real time or secured in cloud storage for larger data sets.

Various signal transduction mechanisms can be leveraged to facilitate chemical sensing, including electrochemical [32], optical [33], and mechanical [34]. Among those mechanisms, electrochemical sensing methodology (chemical-to-electrical signal transduction) appears to be promising for wearable applications because of its ease of integration with electronics for signal process/transduction and eliminating user intervention. Therefore, the majority of the reported wearable sensors employed electrochemical methods aiming for a sample-to-answer manner.

Targeting for the selective and sensitive measurement of desired biomarkers, recognition elements (e.g. selective membrane, enzyme, antibody, or nucleic acid) are usually immobilized onto the surface of a transducer (e.g. metal electrodes or transistors), which can convert analyte–receptor interactions into a measurable signal. To this end, the electrochemical analysis approaches, such as amperometry, voltammetry, and open circuit potential (OCP), can be tailored toward the detection of specific analytes in various concentration ranges and biofluids. In this chapter, we discuss electroenzymatic, ion-selective, bioaffinity-based, synthetic receptor-based sensors, and recognition element-free sensors in detail. For each type, we first discuss the nature of recognition followed by complete sensor construction and physical examples existing in a wearable format.

14.3.1 Electroenzymatic Sensors

Electroenzymatic sensors have been widely employed in wearable sensing platforms, due to their relatively simple design and the availability of commercialized enzyme products. Driven by the need for the management of diabetes, personal blood glucose monitors, such as glucose strips and continuous glucose monitoring systems (CGMS), are arguably the most successful commercialized electroenzymatic sensors. In these devices, enzymes serve as highly specific biorecognition elements (due to their active sites' complex and naturally selected 3D structures) to target molecules even in complex biofluids.

Glucose and lactate are two popular sweat analytes in many reported wearable sensing platforms due to their great clinical significance and relatively high concentration levels in sweat (e.g. micromolar to millimolar). Recently, He et al. reported a wearable sweat analysis patch based on a silk fabric-derived carbon textile for simultaneous detection of multiple biomarkers, including glucose and lactate, which were monitored by electroenzymatic sensors

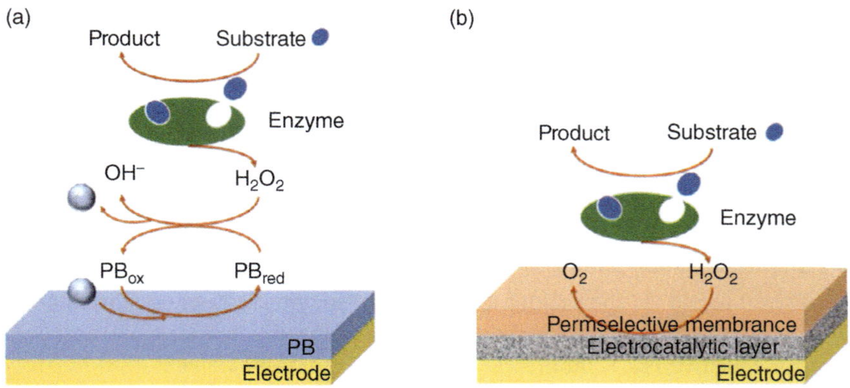

Figure 14.1 Schematic diagram of electroenzymatic sensor. (a) A Prussian blue (PB)-mediated sensor. (b) A mediator-free sensor.

constructed via immobilization of glucose and lactate oxidases by chitosan, respectively (detection range: glucose, 50–150 μM; lactate, 5–15 mM). Amperometric methods were employed for the detection with an applied potential of −0.2 V for lactate and 0.65 V for glucose (versus Ag/AgCl). The responses of glucose sensors did not show significant change after different bending cycles, and they were stable over four weeks. The accuracy of the glucose sensor was validated by comparing the readout from a sweat analysis patch with that of liquid chromatography–mass spectrometry data (HPLC-MS) [35]. Additionally, Emaminejad et al. used a glucose enzymatic sensor, constructed on a flexible polyethylene terephthalate (PET) substrate, to validate the physiological utility of sweat glucose by tracking the concentration elevation after glucose consumption. The sensing interface was fabricated on a gold electrode surface with Prussian blue (PB) as a mediating layer and glucose oxidase as the biorecognition element [36] (Figure 14.1a). The sensors were further coupled with a miniaturized iontophoresis interface for sweat extraction and in situ analysis. In addition to glucose and lactate, Heikenfeld et al. demonstrated a wearable sweat alcohol-sensing platform, utilizing alcohol oxidase as the biorecognition element and amperometry as electrochemical method, which can stimulate and collect sweat and continuously measure sweat ethanol concentrations. The system determined that sweat alcohol is correlated with blood ethanol, which provides further impetus for studies in wearables and sweat analysis [37].

As we can see, the aforementioned enzymatic sensors all utilized amperometry as the electroanalysis method and enzymes (e.g. oxidases) as biorecognition elements. The amperometric sensors rely on measuring the change in current (proportional to the analyte concentration change) with a constant potential applied between the working and reference electrodes. The current change is caused by the electrooxidation/-reduction of hydrogen peroxide (H_2O_2), which is an electroactive by-product of oxidase-based enzymatic reactions. For example, glucose oxidase can facilitate glucose consumption in the presence of oxygen and produce H_2O_2 as a by-product. In that regard, selective and sensitive measurement of the H_2O_2 is crucial for high-performance oxidase-based enzymatic sensors.

However, the optimal working potential for H_2O_2 electroanalysis is usually around 0.6–0.7 V, which would electrooxidize other naturally existing electroactive species (e.g. ascorbic acid and uric acid), and therefore may mask the desired signal. In the majority of wearable enzymatic sensors, a mediating layer (e.g. PB) was often incorporated to reduce the working potential to ~0 V for selective H_2O_2 monitoring. However, Emaminejad et al. [38] recently demonstrated that the use of PB for H_2O_2 analysis has fundamental challenges:

1. The susceptibility of the sensor response to ionic-level variations. For example, potassium ions are often required to participate in the PB-based electron-transfer reaction for charge balance. Accordingly, the sensor response is prone to potassium concentration changes.
2. The poor operational stability. The framework of PB (Fe–CN–Fe), which is responsible for catalytic capability, is prone to degradation at neutral pH (e.g. attach by OH^-) [39].

To this end, the authors provided an alternative sensor development methodology without utilizing the mediating layers. The sensing interface leveraged the high electrocatalytic capability of a platinum–carbon nanotube hybrid layer, the permselective nature of a polymer membrane [40], and the biocatalytic capability of an enzyme layer (Figure 14.1b). This methodology was proved in the context of constructing wearable glucose, lactate, and choline sensors, which were selective against a wide panel of interferents. The results showed great potential for the methodology to be employed in the development of wearable electroenzymatic sensors.

14.3.2 Ion-selective Sensing Interfaces

Sweat contains several important electrolytes, which can be monitored by ion-selective electrodes (ISEs). The sensing interface is constructed by depositing a membrane (e.g. containing sodium ionophore X or calcium ionophore) onto an electrode surface [41, 42]. Since only one ionic species is allowed to pass into the membrane, electrical potential buildup across the membrane reflects the concentration of the respective ion, which can be measured by potentiometric methods. According to the Nernst equation, the output voltage signals are logarithmically related to the concentration of the target ions in the solution.

ISEs have been successfully demonstrated for the analysis of electrolytes in a wearable format, including sodium (Na^+), potassium (K^+), and chloride (Cl^-). Emaminejad et al. [36] demonstrated a sweat analysis wristband, which can extract sweat on demand and analyze electrolytes in situ. The system was deployed for tracking the chloride levels in cystic fibrosis patients and healthy subjects, where the CF patients showed elevated levels. The authors used electrodeposited poly(3,4-ethylenedioxythiophene) polystyrene sulfonate (PEDOT:PSS) as the ion–electron transducer for the potential drift minimization. In addition, Nyein et al. [43] developed a wearable platform for simultaneous monitoring of calcium (Ca^{2+}) and pH (H^+) in sweat. Calcium ionophore II (ETH 129) was included in the calcium sensors, and polyaniline-based pH sensor was fabricated based on electrodeposition of aniline. The results showed that calcium concentration increases with decreasing pH, which may provide insight into primary hyperparathyroidism or the presence of kidney stones.

14.3.3 Bioaffinity-based Sensors

Wearable ion-selective and electroenzymatic sensors are generally used to target biomarkers in the micromolar–millimolar concentration range. Unfortunately, this significantly limits the applicability of wearable chemical sensors for the detection of low-concentration biomarkers (e.g. submicromolar range). Affinity-based electrochemical sensors, such as electrochemical aptamer-based (EAB) sensors and immunosensors, may provide a solution to this problem. Immunoassays are already quite popular for biomedical applications. Electrochemical immunosensors are antibody-based biosensors for the detection of target biomarkers, such as drugs and hormones. For example, Jang et al. [44] reported an antibody-based cortisol sensor, where the antibody was embedded in a polymer layer (here, poly(styrene-co-methacrylic acid)) formed on the remote gate of a transistor. The sensing interface showed a limit of detection of 1 ng mL^{-1} in artificial sweat.

Another promising option may be EAB sensors, which utilize structure-switching nucleic acid aptamers as biorecognition elements. An aptamer is a short and single-stranded DNA or RNA sequence that captures desired targets with high affinity (also known as artificial bioreceptor). A thiol-terminated aptamer can be immobilized onto gold electrode surfaces via self-assembly. Redox-active molecules, such as methylene blue (MB) and ferrocene, could be covalently linked to the other end of the aptamer as signal reporters. The EAB sensors provide a reagentless and substrate-specific biomarker detection platform. The binding of the target molecule to its respective aptamer induces the aptamer conformational changes, which leads to the spatial changes of the signal reporters and alters the charge transfer rate (Figure 14.2). This process

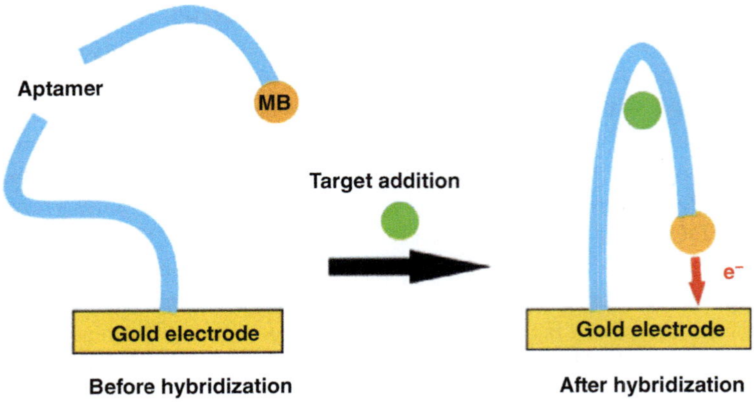

Figure 14.2 Schematic diagram of an electrochemical aptamer-based sensor.

can be probed by a variety of voltammetric methods, such as square wave voltammetry.

For example, Soh et al. [45] demonstrated EAB-based continuous cocaine monitoring in a microfluidic channel. Plaxco et al. [46] developed an EAB-based platform for real-time measurement of small molecules (e.g. doxorubicin, kanamycin, gentamicin, and tobramycin) in awake animals. In another study, the researchers used EAB sensors for continuous measurements in the circulatory systems of living animals [47]. All the works achieved precise molecular measurements at a clinically relevant concentration range. More importantly, the EAB sensors can function properly in human whole blood for several hours with high sensitivity and specificity, which is encouraging for medical applications [48].

14.3.4 Synthetic Receptor-based Chemical Sensors

Biological receptors, such as enzymes, antibodies, and aptamers, often have limited reproducibility and stability during the sensor fabrication process and measurement. Therefore, synthetic receptors (e.g. molecularly imprinted polymers, or MIPs) may offer a promising alternative. A typical MIP preparation procedure includes polymerization of the selected monomers by light or heat in the presence of a target analyte called the template. When the template is eluted, the structure is left with precisely molded cavities that can act as artificial structural receptors (Figure 14.3). Compared to biological receptors, MIPs are more stable in various conditions (e.g. pH, pressure, and temperature) and can function in organic solvents. For example, Parlak et al. reported a molecularly selective nanoporous membrane-based wearable sensing interface on styrene–ethylene–butylene–styrene (SEBS) substrate for the detection of cortisol. The polymeric membrane was formed by the mixture of cortisol (template), methacrylic acid (monomer), ethylene glycol

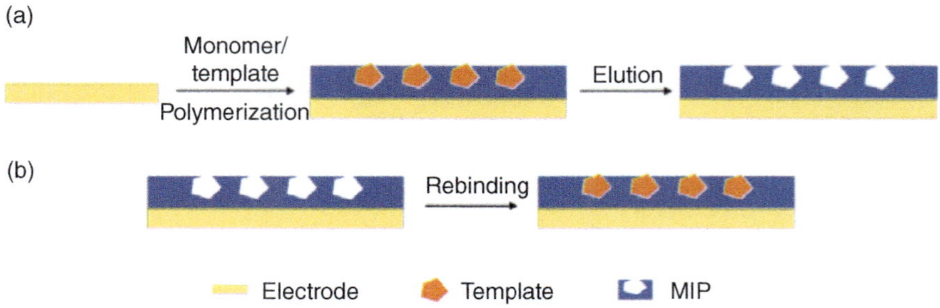

Figure 14.3 Schematic diagram of (a) fabrication and (b) application of molecularly imprinted polymers.

methacrylate (cross-linker), and azobisisobutyronitrile (initiator) with the aid of UV treatment. After template elution, the membrane with molecular memory was coupled with organic electrochemical transistors (OECTs) for signal transduction. Specifically, the molecularly imprinted polymer-based membrane was deposited on the channel materials (here, PEDOT:PSS) of the organic transistors. The fabricated device was used for both ex situ and on-body sweat cortisol measurements [24].

14.3.5 Recognition Element-free Sensors

Another class of wearable sensors is based on carbon electrodes, which are suitable for the detection of various endo-/exogenous electroactive species (such as caffeine, ascorbic acid, and uric acid) using pulse voltammetric methods such as differential pulse voltammetry (DPV). In these devices, electroactive molecules with distinct chemical structures are oxidized or reduced, displaying fingerprint peaks at different voltage positions. For example, Tai et al. [49] presented a wearable platform for the detection of caffeine based on the DPV method. Sweat caffeine levels were monitored under various conditions, such as with different caffeine dosages and different measurement times after caffeine intake. The device utilized a carbon working electrode modified with carbon nanotubes and Nafion layers. Additionally, Yang et al. [50] reported a laser-engraved graphene sensor for uric acid and tyrosine detection. Levels of uric acid in sweat were reported to be correlated with that in serum. The results showed that uric acid could be considered as a potential biomarker for gout management.

14.4 Biofluid Accessibility

To have access to the molecular-level information, a reliable biofluid sampling interface with minimal user intervention needs to be devised and integrated

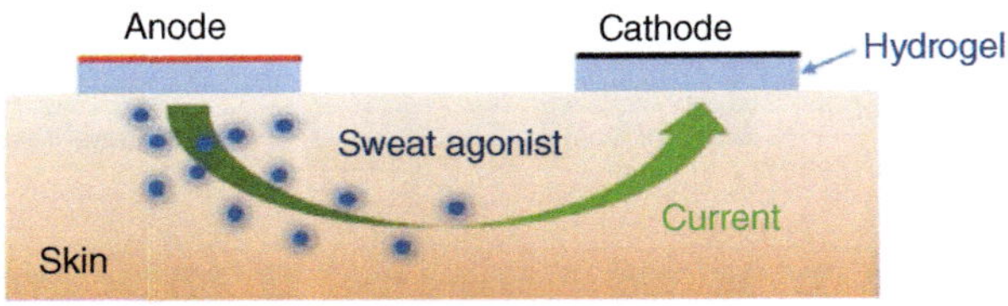

Figure 14.4 Schematic for iontophoresis-based sweat induction.

within the wearable sensing platforms. In the context of wearable chemical sensing systems targeting sweat, exercise is widely utilized for sweat generation [51, 52]. However, while it can be particularly useful in some specific scenarios (e.g. monitoring of athletic performance), sweat monitoring based on exercise may not be suitable for large-scale deployment or for general population monitoring. The requirement for intensive physical activity makes it unrealistic to be used among the neonatal and elderly populations. In that regard, alternative methods of accessing sweat in sedentary settings are required. One such alternative is iontophoresis. Iontophoresis is widely used to stimulate local sweat secretion at a selected site and involves the delivery of stimulatory agonists (e.g. pilocarpine) to the sweat glands with the aid of minimal levels of electrical current [53]. As illustrated in Figure 14.4, an iontophoresis sweat induction module consists of a pair of electrodes (connected with an external current source) and agonist-embedded hydrogel patches (interfacing electrodes and skin). By miniaturizing the required components in a small footprint, iontophoresis-based sweat induction and analysis can be performed in a wearable format without user intervention [36]. Repeated and prolonged iontophoresis-based sweat stimulation can be further achieved by adjusting the agonist type and iontophoresis operation setting [54, 55].

In addition to the active sweat stimulation methods, biomarkers in sweat can also be accessed by the naturally occurring/background perspiration. Due to the low natural perspiration rate, instead of sampling liquid-form sweat, a sampling reservoir is usually needed to facilitate analyte partitioning and collection from sweat glands [56]. Emaminejad et al. [57] demonstrated a thin hydrogel interface for reliable sampling of naturally perspired analytes, which was further integrated for in situ biomarker analysis.

14.5 Microfluidic Interfaces

To facilitate reliable wearable biomarker analysis, a microfluidic interface is essential for biofluid sampling and storage, which can further serve as the foundation of biofluid manipulation. By adopting the widely exploited lab-on-a-chip-based microfluidic manipulation techniques into a wearable setting, complex analytical assays can be performed on-body.

14.5.1 Types of Microfluidic Interfaces

Various interfaces have been developed for wearable biomarker monitoring applications, including absorbent pads, silicone elastomer-based 2D microfluidic housings, and tape-based 3D microfluidic housings. Absorbent pads were used to interface skin and sensor directly in the early sweat sensor prototypes [51, 58]. The water-absorbance feature of the material makes it effective for sweat sampling and manipulation. However, this interface has fundamental challenges, including contamination (from residues of old samples) and lack of sensor protection.

To overcome these challenges, conformal microfluidic modules that are flexible, compact, and scalable need to be integrated in wearable sensing systems. Microfluidic interfaces based on silicone elastomer-based material (e.g. ecoflex, polydimethylsiloxane (PDMS)) allow for conformal contact to the human body because they have similar elastic properties to those of the skin [59]. As illustrated in Figure 14.5, the fabrication process of traditional PDMS-based microfluidic devices includes (i) silicon wafer cleaning, (ii–iv) photolithograph to transfer the designed pattern onto the silicon wafer and to create a resist-based PDMS mold. (v) PDMS microfluidic channel fabrication, and (vi) device assembly. Rogers et al. [52] have demonstrated silicone elastomer-based epidermal microfluidic devices with superior mechanical properties for sweat collection, manipulation, and biomarker

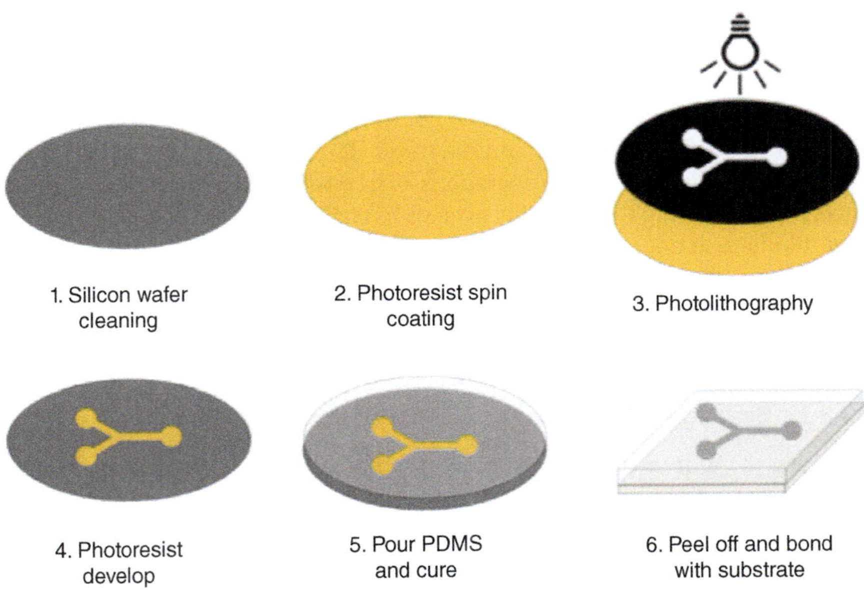

Figure 14.5 Schematic of PDMS-based microfluidic device fabrication.

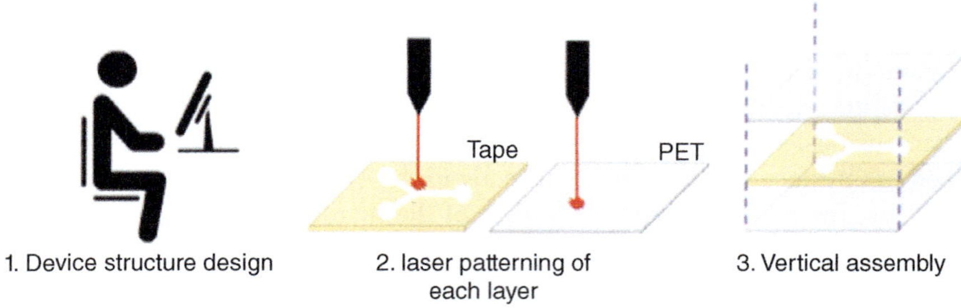

Figure 14.6 Schematic of tape-based microfluidic device fabrication.

analysis. The standard cleanroom-based fabrication scheme renders silicone elastomer-based microfluidic modules with high resolution, accuracy, and scalability [60]. However, this method also has disadvantages as it is time consuming and comes at high cost due to the heavy involvement of resource-intensive facilities. Also, the conventional bottom-up methodology of cleanroom-based fabrication constrains the microfluidic module spatially to two dimensions, which inherently limits its versatility for bioanalytical operations.

An alternative microfluidic interface for wearable application is the tape-based 3D microfluidic housing, which leverages laser cutting and vertical assembly of thin layers of tape-based substrates (Figure 14.6) [61, 62]. For device fabrication, the laser cutter can be programmed at the software level (by computer-aided design, or CAD) to rapidly define microfluidic features such as biofluid collection interface, microchannels, and vertical interconnect accesses (VIAs). By leveraging the adhesive property of the substrates and precise positioning of microfluidic VIAs, the 2D-patterned layers can simply be stacked to form leak-free, multilayered 3D architectures. Furthermore, to deliver a diverse set of operations, electrode-patterned layers can be incorporated during the assembly process to facilitate electrochemical sensing and biofluid actuation functionalities, which will effectively increase the versatility and quantity of bioanalytical operations. A diverse set of wearable bioanalytical applications was demonstrated using this low cost, CAD-3D fabrication scheme [63].

14.5.2 Biofluid Manipulation in Microfluidic Interfaces

Utilizing the aforementioned fabrication scheme, augmented with dedicated structure and material design, a variety of biofluid manipulation applications can be realized in a wearable format. One such application is the sweat sampling device. To collect sweat in the microfluidic module, the pressure readily accumulated in sweat glands (up to ~70 kPa) can continuously push secreted sweat into the microfluidic channel [52, 64]. Capillary effect and osmotic pressure were also demonstrated to improve the sampling efficiency. Heikenfeld et al. [65] devised a hex wick microfluidic structure with superhydrophilic surface, which achieved the collection of ultralow sample volumes (<100 nL). Zhang et al. [66] demonstrated a superhydrophobic–superhydrophilic microarray for effective sweat collection at predefined analytical sites. Velev et al. integrated high-saline-concentration hydrogel disks into the microfluidic channel. The osmotic pressure created by the concentration difference can thus be used to drive fluid into the channel [67].

Routing sweat into the designated channel or chamber is a foundation to realize multiplexed biomarker analysis and/or complex analytical assays. Wearable microfluidic valving systems based on different mechanisms have been exploited by Rogers's group. For example, capillary bursting valves were incorporated in the epidermal microfluidic devices, with the bursting pressure adjusted by different structure designs. Accordingly, the sampled biofluid can be guided into channels with different bursting pressure passively in a sequential manner [68]. Similar function was also realized by embedding a superabsorbent polymer (SAP) at the outlet of the assay chamber. When sweat reached the outlet and was absorbed by the SAP material, the valve would close due to the expansion of the SAP, thereby guiding the sample to the next reservoir. This sequential filling behavior can effectively prevent backflow and cross-contamination of sweat samples [69]. By utilizing punch valves and suction pumps, Rogers et al. [70] demonstrated a resettable microfluidic sweat collector, which is useful for dehydration monitoring.

Besides the passive fluid manipulation, on-demand active fluid control (e.g. programmable manipulation of fluid flow) can create new degrees of freedom to implement a broad range of critical auxiliary operations. For example, an addressable wearable microfluidic valve was demonstrated, which operates based on the shrinkage and expansion of a thermo-responsive hydrogel to permit/block fluid flow [71]. Accordingly, addressable biofluid compartmentalization can be realized to enable isolation of old and new samples and sample incubation for implementation of advanced assays. Besides, electrofluidic-based techniques can be useful in biofluid actuation, given their small footprint and electronic programmability. Accordingly, alternating current electrothermal (ACET) flow-based actuation techniques are particularly suitable as they have been proven to be effective in manipulating fluids with high conductivity (which is usually the case for biofluid). The ACET flow arises from a nonuniform temperature gradient. Specifically, by applying an AC voltage across a pair of coplanar electrodes, a nonuniform electric field, followed by a temperature gradient profile, is established inside the microfluidic channel. This temperature gradient effectively produces gradients in permittivity and conductivity. The interaction of the electric field with these gradient profiles results in a body force acting on the fluid, which was utilized for wearable autonomous active biofluid actuation (e.g. mixing and pumping) [72].

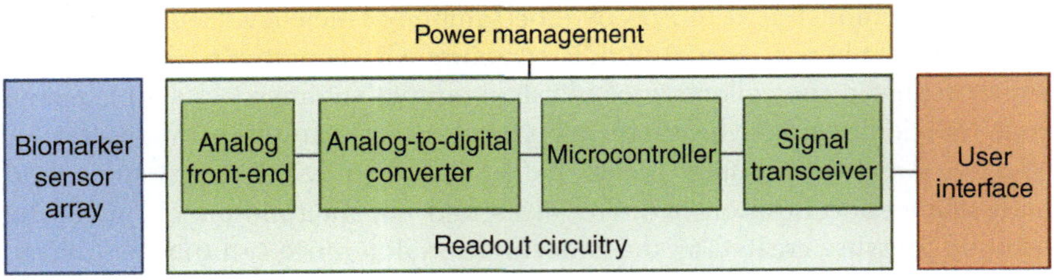

Figure 14.7 Block diagram of electronic interface for wearable chemical sensing applications.

14.6 Electronic and Wireless Integration

To effectively extract the biomarker sensing information and mitigate the confounding factor of external noise (e.g. body motion and electromagnetic interference), wireless signal processing electronics need to be integrated in situ to interface the biomarker sensor for real-time signal readout and to transmit the acquired signal to the user interface (Figure 14.7). One such typical electronic circuitry consists of (i) an analog front end for excitation signal generation, sensor readout amplification, and noise filtration, (ii) an analog-to-digital converter to enable digital signal processing, (iii) a preprogrammed microcontroller with calibration algorithm (e.g. sensor calibration, pH, temperature, and sweat rate correction), and (iv) a signal transceiver module (e.g. Bluetooth and near field communication, NFC).

One key component in the readout circuitry that needs to be custom-tailored is the analog front end. Among different front ends, the potentiostat circuit is widely adopted in wearable chemical sensing applications to facilitate electrochemical measurements. To fulfill the requirement of different electrochemical sensing methods, the function of the circuit needs to be customized accordingly [73]. For example, for amperometric and voltammetric sensors, the circuit measures the current through the working electrode, which is held at a fixed potential. The potential on the reference electrode is set to a constant value (for amperometric), a bidirectional ramp voltage (for cyclic voltammetry), or a differential pulse potential waveform (potential pulses superimposed upon a staircase waveform, for DPV). The sensor-rendered current readout is acquired by implementing a transimpedance stage to convert the current signal into a voltage. On the other hand, for potentiometric sensors, the generated signal is essentially the voltage difference between the working electrode and the reference electrode. To this end, a voltage buffer can be used to interface the respective electrodes, followed by a differential amplifier to implement instrumentation amplification.

The realization of the aforementioned electronic functions necessitates the miniaturization of bulky and power outlet-connected lab instruments (e.g. potentiostat). To this end, at the research level, commercially available components can be integrated on a printed circuit board (PCB) in a modular fashion. This methodology takes advantage of low costs and convenient prototyping. Emaminejad et al. [51] demonstrated a multiplexed biomarker sensing circuitry consisting of more than 10 chips, which allow for sensing across five different measurement channels. A problem that accompanies such integration, however, is the large size of the developed circuit board (beyond centimeter scale), as a panel of discrete chips and peripherals are required to realize the required functionalities. To overcome this drawback and provide conformal skin contact, ideally the readout circuitry needs to be fabricated on a flexible substrate (e.g. flexible PCB). Xu et al. [74] demonstrated a framework for the construction of a novel flexible circuitry for wearable applications, which enclosed all the electronic components in the silicone elastomer matrix and interconnected via free-floating connectors. By leveraging the low modulus of the elastomer, stretchable conformal contact with skin was realized. In the future, the required electronic functionalities can be integrated into application-specific integrated circuits (ASICs), which will effectively miniaturize the system by more than one order of magnitude.

Power management is also essential in constructing a wearable sensing system. To power the circuitry, a miniaturized rechargeable battery is widely used. Inductively coupled wireless power transfer has also been demonstrated to be a promising approach [75]. Besides delivery from external sources, the required energy can also be harvested on-body. For example, biofuel cells can be utilized to harvest electrical energy from metabolites present in biofluids (via their electrochemical reaction) [76]. Flexible thermoelectric materials and devices can also be leveraged to collect human body-heat energy in a wearable format [77]. Piezoelectric, triboelectric, or electromagnetic devices can be utilized to harvest biomechanical energy from human motion (e.g. foot strike and joint motion) [78]. NFC modalities have also been adapted to wearable chemical sensing applications, which eliminates the use of external power source [79–81]. However, the application of NFC is limited to a short distance between the wearables and user interface. The requirement for the user to bring the readout devices near the sensors will make autonomous operation challenging.

References

1 Heikenfeld, J., Jajack, A., Rogers, J. et al. (2018). Wearable sensors: modalities, challenges, and prospects. *Lab on a Chip* 18 (2): 217–248.

2 Yeo, J.C. and Lim, C.T. (2016). Emerging flexible and wearable physical sensing platforms for healthcare and biomedical applications. *Microsystems & Nanoengineering* 2: 16043.

3 Seshadri, D.R., Li, R.T., Voos, J.E. et al. (2019). Wearable sensors for monitoring the internal and external workload of the athlete. *NPJ Digital Medicine* 2 (1): 1–18.
4 Trung, T.Q. and Lee, N. (2016). Flexible and stretchable physical sensor integrated platforms for wearable human-activity monitoringand personal healthcare. *Advanced Materials* 28 (22): 4338–4372.
5 Heikenfeld, J., Jajack, A., Feldman, B. et al. (2019). Accessing analytes in biofluids for peripheral biochemical monitoring. *Nature Biotechnology* 37 (4): 407–419.
6 Kim, J., Campbell, A.S., de Ávila, B.E.-F., and Wang, J. (2019). Wearable biosensors for healthcare monitoring. *Nature Biotechnology* 37 (4): 389–406.
7 Bantle, J.P. and Thomas, W. (1997). Glucose measurement in patients with diabetes mellitus with dermal interstitial fluid. *Journal of Laboratory and Clinical Medicine* 130 (4): 436–441.
8 Kim, J., Imani, S., de Araujo, W.R. et al. (2015). Wearable salivary uric acid mouthguard biosensor with integrated wireless electronics. *Biosensors and Bioelectronics* 74: 1061–1068.
9 Kim, J., Kim, M., Lee, M. et al. (2017). Contact lenses for wireless ocular diagnostics. *Nature Communications* 8 (1): 1–8.
10 Kim, J., Campbell, A.S., and Wang, J. (2018). Wearable non-invasive epidermal glucose sensors: A review. *Talanta* 177: 163–170.
11 Lee, W.C., Smith, E., Chubb, B., and Wolden, M.L. (2014). Frequency of blood glucose testing among insulin-treated diabetes mellitus patients in the United Kingdom. *Journal of Medical Economics* 17 (3): 167–175.
12 Derbyshire, P.J., Barr, H., Davis, F., and Higson, S.P.J. (2012). Lactate in human sweat: a critical review of research to the present day. *The Journal of Physiological Sciences* 62 (6): 429–440.
13 Farrell, D.J. and Bower, L. (2003). Fatal water intoxication. *Journal of Clinical Pathology* 56 (10): 803–804.
14 Mydlík, M., Derzsiová, K., and Frank, K. (2013). Differential diagnosis and treatment of hyponatremia. *Vnitrni Lekarstvi* 59 (6): 478–481.
15 Vairo, D., Bruzzese, L., Marlinge, M. et al. (2017). Towards addressing the body electrolyte environment via sweat analysis: pilocarpine iontophoresis supports assessment of plasma potassium concentration. *Scientific Reports* 7 (1): 11801.
16 Farrell, P.M., White, T.B., Ren, C.L. et al. (2017). Diagnosis of cystic fibrosis: consensus guidelines from the Cystic Fibrosis Foundation. *The Journal of Pediatrics* 181: S4–S15.
17 Gibson, L.E. and Cooke, R.E. (1959). A test for concentration of electrolytes in sweat in cystic fibrosis of the pancreas utilizing pilocarpine by iontophoresis. *Pediatrics* 23 (3): 545–549.

18 Gonzalo-Ruiz, J., Mas, R., de Haro, C. et al. (2009). Early determination of cystic fibrosis by electrochemical chloride quantification in sweat. *Biosensors and Bioelectronics* 24 (6): 1788–1791.

19 Wang, C., Swerdloff, R.S., Iranmanesh, A. et al. (2000). Transdermal testosterone gel improves sexual function, mood, muscle strength, and body composition parameters in hypogonadal men. *The Journal of Clinical Endocrinology & Metabolism* 85 (8): 2839–2853.

20 Cauley, J.A. (2015). Estrogen and bone health in men and women. *Steroids* 99: 11–15.

21 Mogri, M., Dhindsa, S., Quattrin, T. et al. (2013). Testosterone concentrations in young pubertal and post-pubertal obese males. *Clinical Endocrinology* 78 (4): 593–599.

22 Richard-Eaglin, A. (2018). Male and female hypogonadism. *Nursing Clinics* 53 (3): 395–405.

23 Kinnamon, D., Ghanta, R., Lin, K.-C. et al. (2017). Portable biosensor for monitoring cortisol in low-volume perspired human sweat. *Scientific Reports* 7 (1): 13312.

24 Parlak, O., Keene, S.T., Marais, A. et al. (2018). Molecularly selective nanoporous membrane-based wearable organic electrochemical device for noninvasive cortisol sensing. *Science Advances* 4 (7): eaar2904.

25 Jia, M., Chew, W.M., Feinstein, Y. et al. (2016). Quantification of cortisol in human eccrine sweat by liquid chromatography–tandem mass spectrometry. *Analyst* 141 (6): 2053–2060.

26 Raiszadeh, M.M., Ross, M.M., Russo, P.S. et al. (2012). Proteomic analysis of eccrine sweat: implications for the discovery of schizophrenia biomarker proteins. *Journal of Proteome Research* 11 (4): 2127–2139.

27 Dai, X., Okazaki, H., Hanakawa, Y. et al. (2013). Eccrine sweat contains IL-1α, IL-1β and IL-31 and activates epidermal keratinocytes as a danger signal. *PloS One* 8 (7): e67666.

28 Turnbull, D., Rodricks, J.V., Mariano, G.F., and Chowdhury, F. (2017). Caffeine and cardiovascular health. *Regulatory Toxicology and Pharmacology* 89: 165–185.

29 Budney, A.J. and Emond, J.A. (2014). Caffeine addiction? Caffeine for youth? Time to act! *Addition* 109: 1771–1772.

30 Gambelunghe, C., Rossi, R., Aroni, K. et al. (2013). Sweat testing to monitor drug exposure. *Annals of Clinical & Laboratory Science* 43 (1): 22–30.

31 Bandodkar, A.J., Jeerapan, I., and Wang, J. (2016). Wearable chemical sensors: present challenges and future prospects. *ACS Sensors* 1 (5): 464–482.

32 Bakker, E. and Telting-Diaz, M. (2002). Electrochemical sensors. *Analytical Chemistry* 74 (12): 2781–2800.

33 McDonagh, C., Burke, C.S., and MacCraith, B.D. (2008). Optical chemical sensors. *Chemical Reviews* 108 (2): 400–422.

34 Lavrik, N.V., Sepaniak, M.J., and Datskos, P.G. (2004). Cantilever transducers as a platform for chemical and biological sensors. *Review of Scientific Instruments* 75 (7): 2229–2253.

35 He, W., Wang, C., Wang, H. et al. (2019). Integrated textile sensor patch for real-time and multiplex sweat analysis. *Science Advances* 5 (11): eaax0649.

36 Emaminejad, S., Gao, W., Wu, E. et al. (2017). Autonomous sweat extraction and analysis applied to cystic fibrosis and glucose monitoring using a fully integrated wearable platform. *Proceedings of the National Academy of Sciences of the United States of America* 114 (18): 4625–4630.

37 Hauke, A., Simmers, P., Ojha, Y.R. et al. (2018). Complete validation of a continuous and blood-correlated sweat biosensing device with integrated sweat stimulation. *Lab on a Chip* 18 (24): 3750–3759.

38 Cheng, X., Wang, B., Zhao, Y. et al. (2019). A mediator-free electroenzymatic sensing methodology to mitigate ionic and electroactive interferents' effects for reliable wearable metabolite and nutrient monitoring. *Advanced Functional Materials* 30: 1908507.

39 Koncki, R. (2002). Chemical sensors and biosensors based on Prussian blues. *Critical Reviews in Analytical Chemistry* 32 (1): 79–96.

40 Wen, X., Wang, B., Huang, S. et al. (2019). Flexible, multifunctional neural probe with liquid metal enabled, ultra-large tunable stiffness for deep-brain chemical sensing and agent delivery. *Biosensors and Bioelectronics* 131: 37–45.

41 Yang, Y. and Gao, W. (2019). Wearable and flexible electronics for continuous molecular monitoring. *Chemical Society Reviews* 48 (6): 1465–1491.

42 Bandodkar, A.J. and Wang, J. (2014). Non-invasive wearable electrochemical sensors: a review. *Trends in Biotechnology* 32 (7): 363–371.

43 Nyein, H.Y.Y., Gao, W., Shahpar, Z. et al. (2016). A wearable electrochemical platform for noninvasive simultaneous monitoring of Ca^{2+} and pH. *ACS Nano* 10 (7): 7216–7224.

44 Jang, H.-J., Lee, T., Song, J. et al. (2018). Electronic cortisol detection using an antibody-embedded polymer coupled to a field-effect transistor. *ACS Applied Materials & Interfaces* 10 (19): 16233–16237.

45 Swensen, J.S., Xiao, Y., Ferguson, B.S. et al. (2009). Continuous, real-time monitoring of cocaine in undiluted blood serum via a microfluidic, electrochemical aptamer-based sensor. *Journal of the American Chemical Society* 131 (12): 4262–4266.

46 Arroyo-Currás, N., Somerson, J., Vieira, P.A. et al. (2017). Real-time measurement of small molecules directly in awake, ambulatory animals. *Proceedings of the National Academy of Sciences of the United States of America* 114 (4): 645–650.

47 Ferguson, B.S., Hoggarth, D.A., Maliniak, D. et al. (2013). Real-time, aptamer-based tracking of circulating therapeutic agents in living animals. *Science Translational Medicine* 5 (213): 213ra165–213ra165.

48 Xiao, Y., Lubin, A.A., Heeger, A.J., and Plaxco, K.W. (2005). Label-free electronic detection of thrombin in blood serum by using an aptamer-based sensor. *Angewandte Chemie International Edition* 44 (34): 5456–5459.
49 Tai, L.C., Gao, W., Chao, M. et al. (2018). Methylxanthine drug monitoring with wearable sweat sensors. *Advanced Materials* 30 (23): 1707442.
50 Yang, Y., Song, Y., Bo, X. et al. (2019). A laser-engraved wearable sensor for sensitive detection of uric acid and tyrosine in sweat. *Nature Biotechnology*: 1–8.
51 Gao, W., Emaminejad, S., Yin, H. et al. (2016). Fully integrated wearable sensor arrays for multiplexed in situ perspiration analysis. *Nature* 529 (7587): 509–514.
52 Koh, A., Kang, D., Xue, Y. et al. (2016). A soft, wearable microfluidic device for the capture, storage, and colorimetric sensing of sweat. *Science Translational Medicine* 8 (366): 366ra165–366ra165.
53 Carter, E.P., Barrett, A.D., Heeley, A.F., and Kuzemko, J.A. (1984). Improved sweat test method for the diagnosis of cystic fibrosis. *Archives of Disease in Childhood* 59 (10): 919–922.
54 Simmers, P., Li, S.K., Kasting, G., and Heikenfeld, J. (2018). Prolonged and localized sweat stimulation by iontophoretic delivery of the slowly-metabolized cholinergic agent carbachol. *Journal of Dermatological Science* 89 (1): 40–51.
55 Simmers, P., Yuan, Y., Sonner, Z., and Heikenfeld, J. (2018). Membrane isolation of repeated-use sweat stimulants for mitigating both direct dermal contact and sweat dilution. *Biomicrofluidics* 12 (3): 34101.
56 Ohshima, Y., Shimizu, H., Yanagishita, T. et al. (2008). Changes in Na+, K+ concentrations in perspiration and perspiration volume with alternating current iontophoresis in palmoplantar hyperhidrosis patients. *Archives of Dermatological Research* 300 (10): 595–600.
57 Lin, S., Wang, B., Zhao, Y. et al. (2020). Natural perspiration sampling and in situ electrochemical analysis with hydrogel micropatches for user-identifiable and wireless chemo/biosensing. *ACS Sensors* 5 (1): 93–102.
58 Yin, H., Nyein, Y., Gao, W. et al. (2016). A wearable electrochemical platform for noninvasive simultaneous monitoring of Ca^{2+} and pH. *ACS Nano* 10 (7): 7216–7224.
59 Liu, Y., Pharr, M., and Salvatore, G.A. (2017). Lab-on-skin: a review of flexible and stretchable electronics for wearable health monitoring. *ACS Nano* 11 (10): 9614–9635.
60 Qin, D., Xia, Y., and Whitesides, G.M. (2010). Soft lithography for micro-and nanoscale patterning. *Nature Protocols* 5 (3): 491.
61 Nath, P., Fung, D., Kunde, Y.A. et al. (2010). Rapid prototyping of robust and versatile microfluidic components using adhesive transfer tapes. *Lab on a Chip* 10 (17): 2286–2291.

62 Walsh, D.I. III, Kong, D.S., Murthy, S.K., and Carr, P.A. (2017). Enabling microfluidics: from clean rooms to makerspaces. *Trends in Biotechnology* 35 (5): 383–392.
63 Lin, H., Zhao, Y., Lin, S. et al. (2019). A rapid and low-cost fabrication and integration scheme to render 3D microfluidic architectures for wearable biofluid sampling, manipulation, and sensing. *Lab on a Chip* 19 (17): 2844–2853.
64 Zhao, F.J., Bonmarin, M., Chen, Z.C. et al. (2020). Ultra-simple wearable local sweat volume monitoring patch based on swellable hydrogels. *Lab on a Chip* 20 (1): 168–174.
65 Twine, N.B., Norton, R.M., Brothers, M.C. et al. (2018). Open nanofluidic films with rapid transport and no analyte exchange for ultra-low sample volumes. *Lab on a Chip* 18 (18): 2816–2825.
66 He, X., Xu, T., Gu, Z. et al. (2019). Flexible and superwettable bands as a platform toward sweat sampling and sensing. *Analytical Chemistry* 91 (7): 4296–4300.
67 Shay, T., Dickey, M.D., and Velev, O.D. (2017). Hydrogel-enabled osmotic pumping for microfluidics: towards wearable human-device interfaces. *Lab on a Chip* 17 (4): 710–716.
68 Choi, J., Kang, D., Han, S. et al. (2017). Thin, soft, skin-mounted microfluidic networks with capillary bursting valves for chrono-sampling of sweat. *Advanced Healthcare Materials* 6 (5): 1601355.
69 Kim, S.B., Zhang, Y., Won, S.M. et al. (2018). Super-absorbent polymer valves and colorimetric chemistries for time-sequenced discrete sampling and chloride analysis of sweat via skin-mounted soft microfluidics. *Small* 14 (12): 1703334.
70 Reeder, J.T., Xue, Y., Franklin, D. et al. (2019). Resettable skin interfaced microfluidic sweat collection devices with chemesthetic hydration feedback. *Nature Communications* 10 (1): 1–12.
71 Kuwayama, K. and Tsujikawa, K. (2013). Time-course measurements of caffeine and its metabolites extracted from fingertips after coffee intake: a preliminary study for the detection of drugs from fingerprints. *Analytical Bioanalytical Chemistry* 405: 3945–3952. https://doi.org/10.1007/s00216-012-6569-3.
72 Lin, H., Hojaiji, H., Lin, S. et al. (2019). A wearable electrofluidic actuation system. *Lab on a Chip* 19 (18): 2966–2972.
73 Nazari, M.H., Mazhab-Jafari, H., Leng, L. et al. (2012). CMOS neurotransmitter microarray: 96-channel integrated potentiostat with on-die microsensors. *IEEE Transactions on Biomedical Circuits and Systems* 7 (3): 338–348.
74 Huang, Z., Hao, Y., Li, Y. et al. (2018). Three-dimensional integrated stretchable electronics. *Nature Electronics* 1 (8): 473.

75 Nguyen, C., Kota, P., Nguyen, M. et al. (2015). Wireless power transfer for autonomous wearable neurotransmitter sensors. *Sensors* 15 (9): 24553–24572.

76 Bandodkar, A.J. and Wang, J. (2016). Wearable biofuel cells: a review. *Electroanalysis* 28 (6): 1188–1200.

77 Bahk, J.-H., Fang, H., Yazawa, K., and Shakouri, A. (2015). Flexible thermoelectric materials and device optimization for wearable energy harvesting. *Journal of Materials Chemistry C* 3 (40): 10362–10374.

78 Choi, Y.-M., Lee, M.G., and Jeon, Y. (2017). Wearable biomechanical energy harvesting technologies. *Energies* 10 (10): 1483.

79 Bandodkar, A.J., Gutruf, P., Choi, J. et al. (2019). Battery-free, skin-interfaced microfluidic/electronic systems for simultaneous electrochemical, colorimetric, and volumetric analysis of sweat. *Science Advances* 5 (1): eaav3294.

80 Kim, J., Banks, A., Cheng, H. et al. (2015). Epidermal electronics with advanced capabilities in near-field communication. *Small* 11 (8): 906–912.

81 Steinberg, M.D., Kassal, P., Kereković, I., and Steinberg, I.M. (2015). A wireless potentiostat for mobile chemical sensing and biosensing. *Talanta* 143: 178–183.

Appendix A

Antennas and Sensors for Medical Applications: A Representative Literature Review

Lingnan Song and Yahya Rahmat-Samii

Department of Electrical and Computer Engineering, University of California, Los Angeles, CA, USA

A.1 Purpose and Scope of the Chapter

Advanced wireless diagnosis and treatment technologies have recently and rapidly moved from largely a vision of science fiction to widely spreading consumer and clinical products. Large numbers of research and literature are published in different journals and conferences each year on the development of antennas and sensors of various health-care applications. This chapter presents a representative literature review on the recently developed antenna and sensor technologies for advanced medical applications. A block diagram summarizing the subtopics included in this review chapter is shown in Figure A.1. The antenna-related topics are broken into three subsections according to their operating mechanisms: medical imaging antennas and coils, wireless telemetry antennas for implantable and ingestible devices, and microwave ablation antennas for localized tumor treatments. The discussion on sensor technologies consists of mechanical, electrical, optical, and chemical sensing devices. For each of the subtopics, we present the basic system-level physics, followed by the state of the art with representative literature, general outlooks for current challenges, and potential solutions in each field. This review not only serves as an introductory platform for new researchers to the fields but also benefits experienced researchers by broadening their views among various related topics. Various chapters of this book provide in-depth discussions with additional references, detailing the topics briefly covered in this appendix.

Antenna and Sensor Technologies in Modern Medical Applications,
First Edition. Edited by Yahya Rahmat-Samii and Erdem Topsakal.

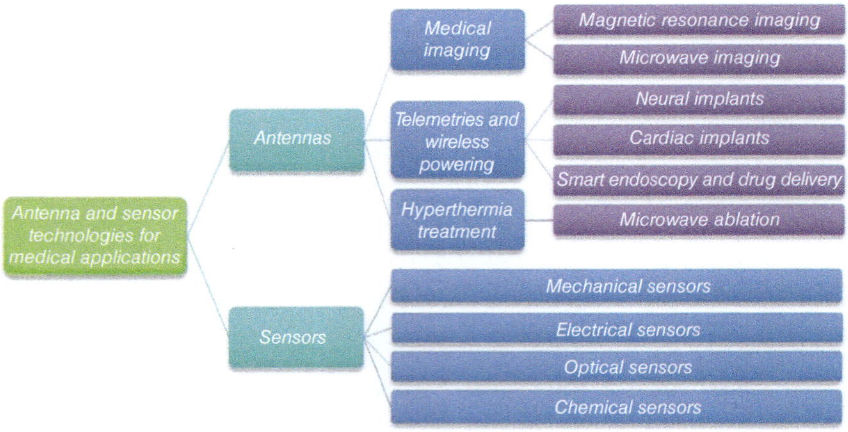

Figure A.1 Scope of organization of the chapter. Various topics of biomedical antennas and sensors are briefly included with representative literatures.

A.2 Antennas for Wireless Diagnosis and Treatment

A.2.1 Medical Imaging

A.2.1.1 RF Coil for Magnetic Resonance Imaging

Magnetic resonance imaging, known as MRI, is a powerful and noninvasive imaging technique that has played and will continue to play a significant role in the medical imaging community. The radio-frequency (RF) coil is the important component of the MRI system by which the MRI signal is stimulated and received from the scanned tissue.

In this section, a brief review on MRI RF coils and their recent advance is given from the perspective of an RF coil design engineer. The section starts from introducing the basic principles of MRI and concepts associated with MRI RF coils. Then, the current state-of-the-art transmit and receive RF coil designs are discussed. The section concludes with examples of the novel technologies, approaches, and current advances in the field of MRI RF coils.

Basic Principles of MRI and MRI RF Coil Design. MRI technique is based on the phenomenon of nuclear magnetic resonance (NMR). Certain atomic nuclei (those with odd number of protons such as ^{1}H, ^{13}C, ^{19}F, and ^{23}N), when placed in a static magnetic field, will present one of the two possible states with opposite magnetic spin states, one has a lower energy level with the spin aligned in the direction of the magnetic field, and the other has a higher energy level with the spin aligned in the opposite direction of the magnetic field. The energy difference between the two states is proportional to the strength of the applied magnetic field states. Therefore, when the nuclei in the applied static magnetic field are excited with RF electromagnetic pulse generated by transmitting (TX)

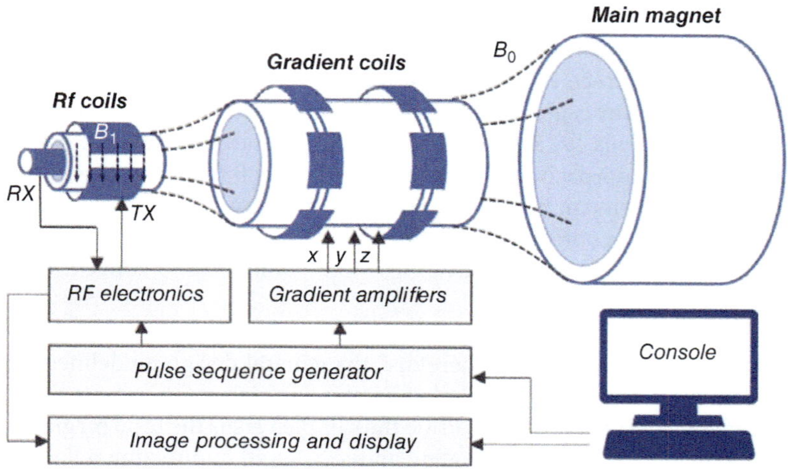

Figure A.2 The basic components of any MRI system: The main magnet produces the B_0 field, necessary to align the spins and achieve equilibrium. Gradient coils enable image encoding in the *x*, *y*, and *z* directions. The RF coil excites the aligned momentum and receives an RF signal back from the sample [1]. (*Source*: Gruber, B., Froeling, M., Leiner, T., et al., 2018. © John Wiley & Sons.)

RF coil, some nuclei in the lower energy state will flip the spin and jump to the higher energy state. Immediately after the excitation, the excess nuclei in the higher energy state will recover the equilibrium by emitting electromagnetic fields which are collected by the receiving (RX) RF coil. The basic components of any MRI system are illustrated in Figure A.2 [1]. The main magnet produces the static B_0 field to align the spin of atoms and achieve equilibrium. The TX coils generate the B_1 field, which is perpendicular to the B_0 field, at the Larmor Frequency ω_r, with ω_r depending on the type of nucleus and the B_0 field strength. The TX and RX coils are separately designed in general to individually optimize for each function. When the TX coil is active, the RX coil has to be off-resonance, in order to prevent the potential damage on RX electronics due to TX leakage.

TX and RX Coils: State of the Art. Based on the homogeneity of the produced B_1 field, the types of RF coils can be distinguished into volume coils [2, 3] and surface and array coils [4, 5]. Volume coils are typically cylindrical shaped and completely encompass the anatomy of interest. They could generate highly homogeneous RF excitation across the entire sample volume. Surface coils are in general designed for a localized high signal-to-noise ratio (SNR) close to the surface of the patient's body. Their different characteristics make them suitable for different modes of operations (TX or RX).

For TX RF coils, the primary design focus is to generate a homogeneous B_1 field that excites the spin in the sample. The increased homogeneity of the transmit field increases the received signal and results in better imaging quality or improved scan time. Birdcage coils [2, 6], saddle-shaped coils [3], solenoid coils [7], and Helmholtz coils [8] are some of the representative types of TX coil designs. The recent approach of parallel transmit RF coil (pTX) increases the homogeneity of the transmit field by breaking down the transmit field into multiple regions and each controlled by a separate transmit channel and TX coil element, also creating spatial degrees of freedom comparing to conventional birdcage coils [9].

For RX coils, the basic goal is to achieve the highest possible SNR within the volume of interest of the sample. Therefore, the general design guidelines for RX coils include (i) optimizing the coil geometry for higher filling factor (the ratio of magnetic field energy stored inside the sample versus the total magnetic energy stored by the RX coil), (ii) reducing ohmic loss and minimizing reflected power with improved impedance matching, and (iii) making the RX coil more conformal to the sample of testing. Kumar et al. [10] have summarized the simulated optimal radii of a surface coil loop and the corresponding measured SNR limits for various target depths of interest at 1, 1.5, 3, 7, and 9.4 T. To further improve the system SNR, parallel imaging (PI) technique has been introduced, which utilizes coil array with accelerated data acquisition [9, 11, 12]. Wiesinger et al. [13] have presented a theoretical investigation for the ultimate SNR of PI systems.

One additional concern for array coils is that each element of the array should be properly decoupled from each other [14], since the mutual couplings generate coupled modes and result in splitting in the resonant spectrum. Strategies to remove the effects of mutual coupling include but are not limited to (i) adjusting the overlap of adjacent coil elements to a certain value so that the shared flux between adjacent coils becomes ideally zero (Figure A.3), (ii) using low impedance preamplifier to isolate coupling between nonadjacent elements [15], (iii) inserting ladder capacitor network to decouple both the adjacent and nonadjacent elements [16], and (iv) designing wide-band decoupling network based on phased-array theory [17]. With that said, the development of novel decoupling methods to position more receiver channels closely around the sample remains a hot topic in the current MRI society.

Recent Advances in MRI RF Coils. One recent development on MRI coil design involves the utilization of metamaterial or metasurface. In [18], mushroom-type electromagnetic bandgap (EBG) metasurfaces are employed to improve decoupling in array coils for 7 T MRI. The SNR enhancement for 1.5 T MRI with wire-array metasurfaces is also reported by Slobozhanyuk et al. [19]. The artificially designed electromagnetic properties of metamaterial facilitate novel MRI coil developments, particularly for ultrahigh field MRI with improved resolution and reduced scanning time. Another patient-oriented

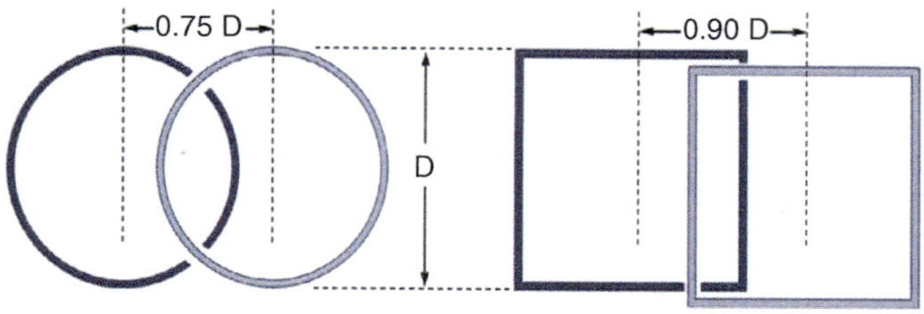

Figure A.3 Adjacent coil coupling can be almost removed with the critical overlap, which depends on the coil geometry. As two special cases of critical overlap, the centers of the circular loops are separated by about 0.75 of their diameters, and square loops by about 0.9 of length.

approach is the development of flexible [20–22] or stretchable [23] RX coil elements, aiming at an improved SNR and comfort of patients. These adaptive coils also need retuning and rematching techniques due to the change of coil shape and size [24].

A.2.1.2 Antennas for Microwave Imaging

Classification and Principles of Microwave Imaging. Microwave sensing and imaging (MSI) is an imaging method based on nonionizing electromagnetic signals operating over the frequency range covering hundreds of MHz to tens of GHz. Hassan and El-Shenawee [25] presented a performance comparison of the different imaging techniques on cancer detection in terms of sensitivity, specificity, and accuracy. Comparing to other widely used imaging techniques, such as X-rays, magnetic resonance imaging (MRI), computed tomography (CT), etc., microwave imaging overcomes the disadvantages such as false indications, low-resolution scans, higher cost, and patient discomfort [26].

The principle of the MSI relies on the inherent contrast between the dielectric properties (relative permittivity and conductivity) of various organs and tissues, due to their difference in water content. A malignant tissue usually presents different electrical properties than the surrounding normal and healthy tissues, which can be differentiated in the image for diagnosing purpose. During the MSI scan, the human body to be imaged is surrounded by several transmit and receive antennas. Each transmit antenna illuminates the body with the microwave signal at a time. The scattered signal by the targeting region of tissue is collected by all the receive antennas, as illustrated by Figure A.4. The scattered fields are then processed by an iterative algorithm for image reconstruction of the biological tissue [27, 28].

Based on the operating mechanisms and target applications, MSI can be classified into quantitative and qualitative imaging technologies. Quantitative imaging maps the relative dielectric constant and conductivity for the tissue within a target region of measurement. The algorithms are usually based on solving inverse scattering problems. Qualitative imaging technology is

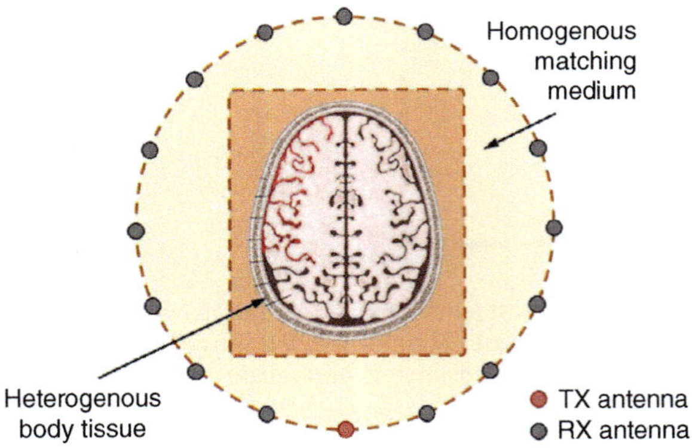

Figure A.4 Basic setup for microwave imaging in a two-dimensional case when one antenna (TX) transmits the signal, and all other antennas (RX) are in receiving mode.

implemented with similarities to radar systems [29]. It differentiates the malignant tissues from the normal tissues based on their scattering properties. As for various applications, respiration and heart-beat detection [30], imaging brain for strokes and cerebral edema [31], breast cancer [32, 33], and bone and joint tissue imaging [34] have been well investigated in the literatures.

Recent Advances in Microwave Imaging Antennas. The design and fabrication of high-performance antennas present significant challenges in the implementation of all categories of microwave imaging. Typical design requirements that have been considered in the literature are wide impedance bandwidth with high efficiency, high directivity, and small size. Under these concerns, ultra-wideband (UWB) antennas are commonly preferred with their unique features of high data rates, small interference, low-cost designs, and low power spectrum density [35]. Representative antenna topologies being used include monopoles [36, 37], microstrip patches [38], bowtie antennas [39], Vivaldi antennas [40], and horn antennas [41, 42]. Antennas with wearable clinical interfaces are also proposed to improve the comfort of patients during long-term microwave monitoring [43].

Another design challenge for microwave imaging antennas is to increase the number of antenna elements in order to relax the nonuniqueness and the ill posedness of nonlinear inverse problems to some extent. However, the number of antennas in an MSI system is limited by the size of antenna elements and the potential issue of mutual coupling between antenna elements, which introduces error in the measurements. A calibration process to remove some of these errors is suggested in [44], by avoiding the frequencies where the coupling is large enough to prevent successful imaging in a wideband measurement setup. The design of antennas with a minimal mutual coupling is one of the future research directions. Some decoupling techniques have been investigated to this end [45, 46].

A.2.2 Telemetries and Wireless Powering

Today, there are a few regulated frequency bands assigned for biotelemetry or bioimplants, including the Medical Device Radiocommunications Service (MedRadio) band from 401 to 406 MHz; the Industrial, Scientific, and Medical (ISM) bands from 433.1 to 434.8 MHz, 868 to 868.6 MHz, 902.8 to 928 MHz, and 2.4 to 2.5 GHz; and the Wireless Medical Telemetry Services (WMTS) bands from 608 to 614 MHz, 1395 to 1400 MHz, and 1427 to 1427.5 MHz [47, 48]. Higher frequency bands up to millimeter-wave range are not well regulated so far but are still under active investigation for research purpose. The maximum RF exposure level is well regulated by standards including the specific absorption rate (SAR) and maximum permissible exposure (MPE) [49].

A.2.2.1 Neural Implants

The development of long-lasting neural interfaces with the capability to safely monitor neuropotentials has been a crucial task toward understanding the brain activities and brain disease treatments. And, as understanding of the brain functionalities continues to improve, there is also the demand for dynamically modulating the nervous system for therapeutic or monitoring purposes [50, 51] and eventually realizing a closed-loop neural sensing and stimulating system (Figure A.5).

From an engineering perspective, there are three major design challenges for the wireless neural interface: size, power, and data rate [53]. A desirable

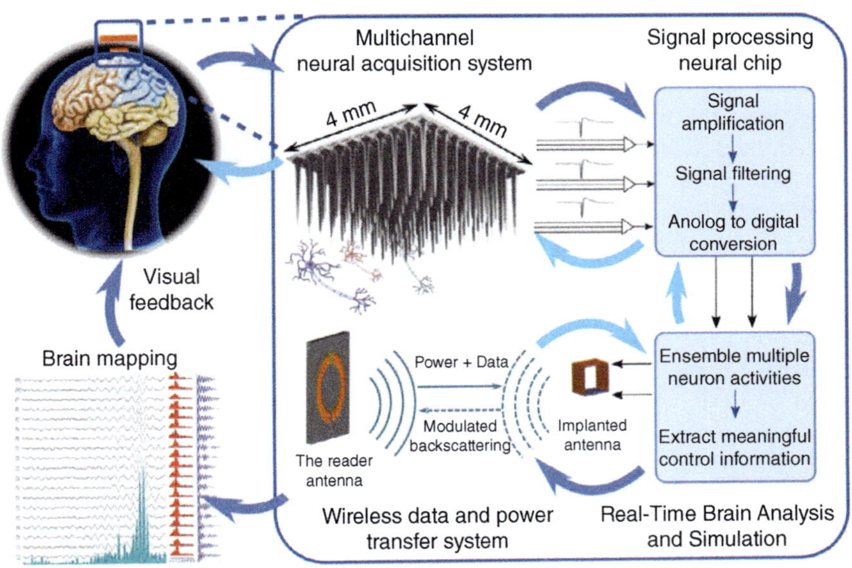

Figure A.5 A schematic of general brain sensing and stimulating system [52]. (*Source*: Song, L. and Rahmat-Samii, Y., 2017. © IEEE.)

neural implant system should be highly miniaturized to minimize the damage to brain tissues and possible complications. With the advance of modern integrated circuits, the size limitation of implanted neural sensing systems typically lies in the size of the antenna. A chronic implanted system needs to be batteryless and wirelessly powered. Wireless inductive coupling is probably the most promising approach for wireless powering. However, one major implication of the small size is the reduced amount of power available for electronic circuits. Limited by safety regulations and the electromagnetic characteristics of brain tissue, maximum amount of power available is on the order of $10\,\mu W\,mm^{-2}$[54]. On the other hand, the required data capacity is relatively large. To capture the waveform of a neural spike from a single electrode, a sampling rate of 15–20 $kSample\,s^{-1}$ at 5–10 bits of resolution, equivalent up to 200 kbps of data rate, is required. For an electrode array with 10 channels, it corresponds to data capacity on the order of Mbps [55].

The selection of optimal operating frequency reflects the trade-offs among those concerns. Today, there are only very few frequency bands regulated for biotelemetry or bioimplants, including the MICSs band from 402 to 405 MHz and the ISM bands from 433.1 to 434.8 MHz, 868 to 868.6 MHz, 902.8 to 928 MHz, and 2.4 to 2.5 GHz [47, 48]. Higher frequency bands up to millimeter-wave range are not well regulated so far but are still under active investigation for research purpose. Choosing a higher frequency gives benefits to increased data capacity and ease of antenna miniaturization, with the sacrifice of reduced power efficiency due to tissue absorption. Poon et al. [56] and Leelatien et al. [57] provide thorough discussions on the optimal frequency for wireless powered implants through dispersive biological tissue. It has been shown that the optimal frequency that trades-off received power and tissue absorption lies in the GHz range.

Generally, there are two types of solutions that are extensively studied and utilized, inductive link with magnetic coil antennas and RF link with electrically small planar antennas. Advanced electromagnetic numerical techniques are often utilized to model and design these implanted antennas [58].

Near-Field Inductive Links. In the first case, two coil antennas are inductively coupled in near-field region. As magnetic radiators, they typically present high magnetic field other than high electric field, which brings benefit on absorption level and enables a higher transmit power compliant with safety standards. These types of links are simple to implement and miniaturize (could be designed to occupy only a few cubic millimeter space), within a narrow frequency band since they are typically much smaller than the order of wavelength at the frequency of operation. Matching to capacitive chip impedance is relatively easy to achieve with coil antennas since they are inherently inductive. In [59] the analytical analysis of inductively coupled link with loop antennas is presented. In [60] it has been derived that when two coils are separated by a distance D, choosing the transmit coil with radius $\sqrt{2}D$ results in the optimized mutual inductance, as the transmit coil encloses

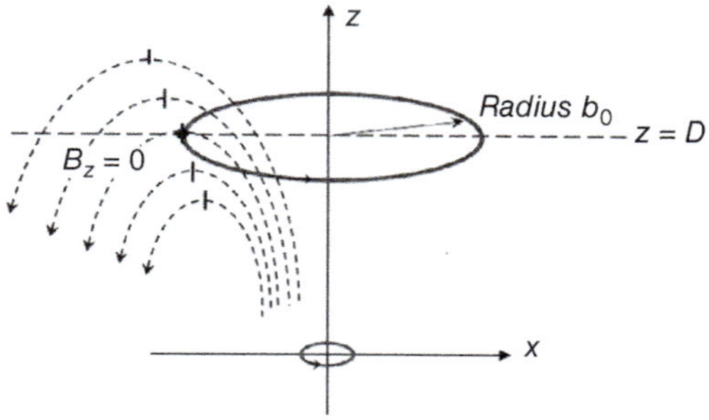

Figure A.6 Radius of primary coil b_o for maximum mutual inductance is determined by the point where the magnetic flux density in the z-direction is zero ($B_z = 0$). The optimum primary coil radius b_o is found as $\sqrt{2}D$, where D represents the vertical distance between the primary and secondary coils. The secondary coil is assumed to be much smaller than the primary coil and well aligned with the primary coil within the x–y plane [60]. (*Source*: Modified from Pichorim, S.F. and Abatti P.J., 2004.)

the maximum positive magnetic flux. Several design variations could help improve the link efficiency and bandwidth performance, e.g. designing 3D coil structure [52, 61, 62], inserting ferromagnetic core, and segmenting the loop [63]. Though their achievable bandwidth is limited to a few MHz, many state-of-the-art neural implant systems are still using coil antennas to establish wireless communication [64–66], due to their ease of on-chip integration.

Far-Field RF Telemetries. Comparing to near-field inductive link, communications via far-field RF telemetry have advantages of longer distances and higher data rates [67]. Planar inverted-F antennas (PIFAs) have recently been presented as a promising candidate for brain-implanted biotelemetries, with the advantages in miniaturization and bandwidth enhancement [68, 69] compared to other planar types of antennas. Many proposed designs could achieve size reduction to a few square centimeter area and bandwidth of 10s to 100s of MHz, at the MICS or ISM frequency bands (Figure A.6).

There are several well-recognized miniaturization methods for planar type of antennas. Using high-permittivity dielectric substrate/superstrate helps reduce the effective wavelength and therefore reduce the dimensions of implantable antennas [70]. Commercially available high-frequency laminate boards provide relative dielectric constant as high as 10.2, resulting in a size reduction by around three times. Using PIFAs inherently shrink the size of antenna from half to quarter wavelength. Using meandered or spiraled line [71] in PIFAs or slot antennas [72, 73] could help reduce the area of occupation for the planar antenna by lengthening the current path. In [74], stacked layers are employed in implanted PIFA for further miniaturization purpose. Reactive loading or metamaterial-based miniaturization techniques [75] have also been explored. The differential planar antenna design has been investigated to be compatible with the differential IC input for noise rejection [76] (Figure A.7).

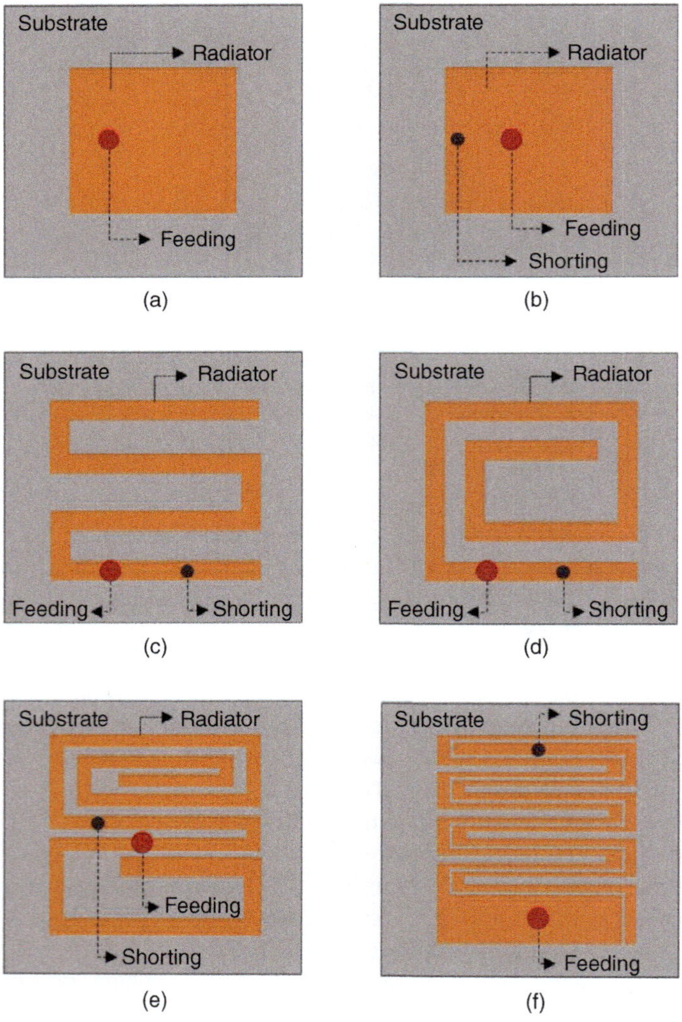

Figure A.7 A few variations of planar antennas for implanted applications [68, 77]. PIFA topologies inherently reduce the resonant length of microstrip patch antenna from half wavelength to quarter wavelength. With the implementation of spiral or meander lines, the size of antenna can be further reduced. (*Source*: Liu, C., Guo, Y.-X., et al., 2016 and Kim J. and Rahmat-Samii, Y., 2004.)

A.2.2.2 Cardiac Implants

Implantable cardiac devices have become a huge market. Over 250 000 new pacemakers and over 100 000 cardioverter defibrillators (ICDs) are implanted each year. These commercial pacemakers and defibrillators, however, still rely on nonrechargeable batteries, and periodic surgeries are needed every 5–8 years due to the battery lifetime [78]. Development of long-lasting and fully implantable pacemakers and implantable cardioverter defibrillators (ICDs) remains a big challenge. Another application that is drawing attention is the continuous heart pressure-volume (PV) monitoring for preventing congestive heart failure (CHF). It relies on development of micro-sized implantable cardiac monitoring systems.

Cardiac implants typically require a longer range for power and data transfer, as the link is across the chest and requires a distance of at least 3–5 cm. To enable fully implanted cardiac implants, wireless powering or energy harvesting techniques need to be implemented. In [79], the authors analyzed the power budget for operating a typical cardiac implant at the implantation depth of 5 cm under the safety constraints, through a combination of inductive and radiative coupling in the midfield regime. In [80], researchers demonstrated a permanent pacemaker system that harvests power from the heartbeat. Various antenna topologies have been investigated for cardiac implants applications, including conformal spiral antenna [81], stent-shaped antenna [82], and on-chip dipole antenna [83].

A.2.2.3 Wireless Capsule Endoscopy and Wireless Drug Delivery

Conventionally, visualization of the human gastrointestinal (GI) tracts, upper small intestine, and colon for diagnostic purposes relies on optical fiber endoscopy, which could induce discomfort among patients due to the large diameter flexible cables needed to withstand the push force. Fortunately, with the rapid progress of semiconductor and RF technologies, wireless capsule endoscopy has arisen as a new approach to address the problems with flexible wire endoscopy [84]. Besides diagnostic functionalities, development of wireless capsule endoscopy also enables controllable drug delivery that would allow clinicians to release an appropriate amount of a drug at specific sections of the GI tract [85–87]. It is generally achieved by navigating the capsule toward the targeted location and actuating the control unit to release drug through microneedles [88].

The size of the capsules is typically around 10 mm in diameter and 20–30 mm in length (one widely used standard is $11 \times 26\,\text{mm}^2$). Typically, a wireless capsule endoscopy consists of an imaging system, localization system [89], light-emitting diodes (LEDs), battery, an ultralow power transceiver, and a highly integrated antenna that is packaged into the pill-shaped capsule [90]. Bidirectional communication is required for sending out the detected signal or image and receiving control signals outside human body (Figure A.8).

The research efforts toward compact and high-performance antennas for wireless endoscope system have recently aroused in antenna society. Many antenna designs have been proposed for these capsule devices based on MICS or WMTS frequency bands [92–94]. The use of impulse-based UWB communication has also been explored aiming at improved data rate, higher

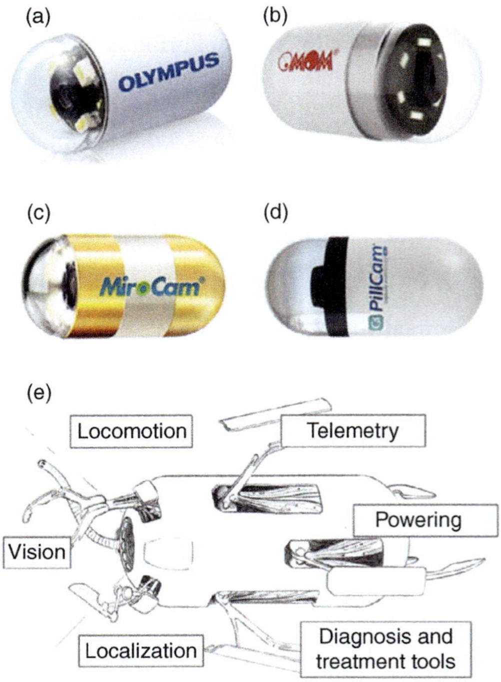

Figure A.8 Representative wireless endoscopy systems. (a) EndoCapsule (*Source*: Olympus Corporation); (b) OMOM capsule (*Source*: Chongqing Jinshan Science & Technology); (c) MiroCam (*Source*: INTROMEDIC); and (d) PillCam (*Source*: ©2020 MEDTRONIC), with an example of system architecture in (e) [91]. (*Source:* Ciuti, G., Caliò, R., Camboni, D., et al., 2016. © Springer Nature.)

image quality, and reduced power consumption, since they can transmit images at a high data rate without any power-consuming image-compression algorithms [95, 96]. One crucial constraint for capsule antennas is the miniaturization due to the limiting space. Therefore, spiral or helical antennas [92, 97, 98], meander dipole or loop antennas [99, 100], and conformal wrapped antennas [92, 101] are widely used in capsule antenna designs.

Since the location and orientation of the capsule system vary as it passes through the GI tract, polarization diversity is needed to address the antenna polarization mismatch. A comparative study on linearly polarized (LP) and circularly polarized (CP) capsule antennas is given in [102], focusing on the issues of link efficiency, bandwidth, and SAR, proving the advantages of using CP antenna over LP ones for wireless capsule devices. Many CP antenna designs are proposed accordingly [103, 104], with the CP radiation generated from helix topology or shaped loading stub. In [92, 105], orientation-insensitive antennas have been proposed with three orthogonal current paths implemented by bending meander dipole arms. A recent study in [106] proposed using multi-polarization antenna over CP antenna in maintaining robustness of the communication link, since an axial ratio for CP antenna is especially sensitive to the antenna location and orientation.

As well as other wireless medical devices, power shortage is one of the major challenges for designing wireless smart endoscopy. The use of battery is acceptable in most cases; however, it is not suitable for systems with complex functionalities (including high-quality image acquisition, motor control or locomotion and drug release, and LED illumination). In [107], the use of magnetic resonance-wireless power transferring has been investigated aiming at the optimal power link efficiency in midfield region. In [108], the use of multi-coil mutual inductance, mutual capacitance, and relative polarity are implemented for enhanced power transfer efficiency.

A.2.3 Microwave Ablations for Localized Tumor Treatment

Microwave ablation has emerged as a minimally invasive treatment method in clinical use, for various types of unresectable tumors in the lung, liver, and kidney. It is typically achieved with an interstitial antenna delivering high-level microwave power up to a few tens of watts from the generator to the target region, to elevate local temperature and destruct cancerous tissue. Comparing to thermal ablation based on other energy sources (e.g. laser and ultrasound), microwave ablation enables heating of larger tissue volume.

A microwave ablation system consists of ablation antenna or applicator, cooling system, and imaging guidance system tailored to specific clinical application. Most current microwave ablation systems in clinical use operate at 915 MHz and 2.45 GHz, which fall within the ISM bands and exhibit reasonable penetration depth and less cable heating. The use of higher frequency has been explored in [109, 110], in which electromagnetic and thermal simulations at discrete frequencies up to 26 GHz are performed. It has been shown that although using higher frequency results in smaller antenna size and more localized spherical SAR pattern, the cable heating became a problematic issue. The antenna return loss is affected by temperature [111]. In addition, the SAR pattern does not accurately predict ablation performance due to the effect of thermal diffusion becoming more critical at higher frequency.

The antenna or applicator is a crucial element for microwave ablation device and has a significant impact on the ablation pattern and ablating power efficiency. The major requirements of ablation antennas include (i) small diameter for ease of insertion; (ii) good impedance matching for efficient power transmission; and (iii) localized spherical ablation pattern for accurate treatment. Ablation patterns are often characterized in ex vivo animal tissue, with the size and shape of ablation zone defined by tissue discoloration at elevated temperatures after certain ablation time [112]. Semirigid coaxial cables have been widely used as feeding transmission lines between power generator and applicator, and most microwave ablation antennas are readily integrated by modifying the geometry of the end of cable. Some representative coaxial antennas are illustrated in A.9. The monopole antenna is formed by

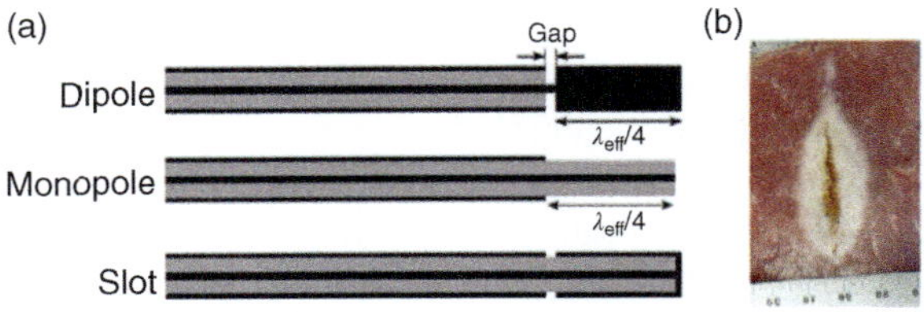

Figure A.9 (a) Examples of coaxial antennas commonly used for interstitial thermal ablation: dipole, monopole, and slot (black: metal, gray: dielectric). (b) Example of ablation pattern of dipole antenna [113]. (*Source*: Fallahi, H. and Prakash, P., 2018. © Begell House Inc.)

stripping off a section of the outer conductor at the end of the coaxial cable by length of $\lambda_{eff}/4$, where λ_{eff} represents the effective wavelength of the EM wave for the coaxial antenna consisting of an inner conductor wrapped with multiple dielectric layers and immersed into lossy dielectric medium [114]. Similarly, the coaxial dipole antenna is formed with a $\lambda_{eff}/4$ length of conductor separated from the cable, and the coaxial slot antenna is formed by shorting inner and outer conductors at the end of a coaxial dipole.

Based on these early antenna topologies, researches have been focusing on adding chokes and sleeves to suppress the backward current on the coaxial cable outer conductor [115]. In [116], a hemicylindrical reflecting structure was incorporated to achieve an asymmetrical and directional ablation pattern, which helped facilitate treatments in proximity to critical structures to prevent unintended tissue damage. Besides dipole and monopole topologies, helix and spiral antennas have also been integrated within flexible catheter-based devices for ablation purposes [117, 118], to achieve alternative radiation patterns. The antennas were typically constructed by stripping off part of the outer conductor and wrapping thin copper wire on the dielectric layer of the coaxial cable. The use of applicator array that consists of multiple ablation antennas has been investigated in [118, 119] to achieve a larger ablation volume, which helps to overcome the heat sink effect of local blood flow and reduce the chance of incomplete ablation.

A.3 Sensors for Wearable Medical Applications

A.3.1 Sensor Classification and Terminologies

In this section, the review and discussion focus on wearable sensing technologies that extract information from within the body, however, without implanting a sensor into the body. The sensing modalities based on motion capture or coupling between sensors through environment sensing are therefore not included.

There are several key analytical parameters that are critical in characterizing wearable sensors, including detection limit, sensitivity, dynamic range, selectivity, specificity, and stability [120]:

- Detection limit is defined as the lowest detectable measurement quantity, commonly related to the standard deviation of the noise level.
- Sensitivity is defined as the change in the sensor output signal per change in the input physical quantity.
- Dynamic range is the range of operation for a specific sensor, which spans the lowest measurable physical quantity to the highest measurable physical quantity.
- Selectivity is defined as the ability to distinguish between the target physical quantity and the coexisting interfering components.
- Specificity is defined as the accuracy against false positive results or the proportion of correct negative results.
- Stability is measured by the degree to which sensor performance and correct response remain constant over time. This is a major issue for chemical sensors that are continuously exposed to biochemicals and mechanical sensors that could degrade from strain or stress over time.

The interests in developing wearable sensing technologies first arouse in the 1960s, with the need of continuous health monitoring of astronauts during space missions [121]. Wireless electrocardiogram (EKG) heart rate monitors were then developed by the Finnish National Cross-Country Ski team in 1977 and quickly grew into commercial products in the early 1980s. About the same time, the first commercial pulse oximeter was announced by Biox (Colorado, USA) and was soon implemented as a standard modality of oxygen-level monitoring under general anesthesia.

The developments of chemical-based noninvasive sensing technologies took relatively longer than electrical sensing modalities, due to the presence of epidermis as strong chemical barrier. An impressive milestone is the development of GlucoWatch by Cygnus in 2002, providing noninvasive glucose sensing for diabetes patients [122]. Although it was not successful as a commercial product due to issues including frequently needed calibration and robustness with sweating, it remains one of the most important development for noninvasive diabetes monitoring. Today, diagnostic tools are available for nearly every analyte that a doctor would be interested to measure. Unfortunately, they are predominately not wearable and are mostly based on blood draw analysis.

Most of today's widely commercialized wearable sensing technologies are wrist-watch devices based on simple mechanical, electrical, or optical sensors that have been developed and smartly adapted for decades. Advanced fabrication technologies facilitate the innovations of miniaturized, conformal, and highly integrated wearable devices. However, the development of underlying sensing technologies that acquire data from human body is still facing fundamental challenges.

A.3.2 Mechanical Sensors

Wearable mechanical sensors transduce mechanical deformations into electrical signals for the applications including personalized health monitoring, human motion detection, human–machine interfaces, and soft robotics. A wearable strain sensor should be designed with certain requirements including high stretchability and flexibility, low hysteresis, high sensitivity, and large dynamic range. Many works on skin-mountable and wearable sensors have been proposed utilizing nanomaterials supported by mechanically flexible polymers, demonstrating superior stretchability, biocompatibility, and robustness [123]. Another type of skin-mountable electronics utilizes electrotextile, which is safe and easy to integrate into clothes [124]. The state-of-the-art flexible and stretchable strain sensors are mainly classified into resistive- and capacitive-type sensors [125], with the general mechanisms of each illustrated in A.10.

Mechanical strain sensors are responding or transducing with various mechanisms. Traditional strain responses are generated based on elongation (shrinkage) and piezoresistivity of bulk materials. Most of the commercially available piezoresistive and piezocapacitance wearable sensors are based on the mechanisms of dimension changes [126, 127]. Piezoresistivity effect denotes the change of resistivity due to applied mechanical strain. Semiconductor materials such as silicon and germanium exhibit resistance change of sensors

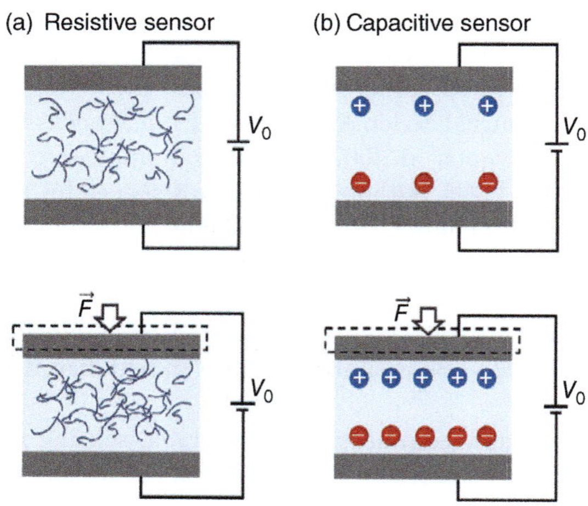

Figure A.10 Schematic illustrations for the different modalities of mechanical sensors: mechanisms of resistive (a) and capacitive (b) mechanical wearable strain sensors, before and after applying tensile strain [120]. (*Source*: Modified from Heikenfeld, J., Jajack, A., Rogers, J., et al., 2018.)

up to several orders of magnitudes, and therefore, achieve piezoresistive sensors with ultrahigh sensitivity. Nanomaterials such as individual carbon nanotubes (CNT) and zinc oxide nanowire (ZnONW) also show ultrahigh piezoresistivity [128].

In nanomaterial-based sensors, the effects of element disconnection are also utilized to generate strain responses. In nanomaterial-based thin-film conductors, the conductivity is determined by the overlapping connection within the network formed by nanoscale elements. Stretching of film causes loss of some electrical connection, and consequently, reduces the electrical conductivity. Stretchable and sensitive strain sensors were reported using thin films of nanowire (NW) networks [129] and graphene flakes [130]. The occurrence of microcracking of the nanomaterial has also been shown to contribute to strain responses. In [131], it has been reported that nanoscale crack in platinum (Pt) thin films becomes larger when experiencing strain, thereby increasing the electrical resistance of the material. However, a signal degradation at about 500 cycles was observed, bringing challenge on robustness and durability of the sensor [131].

The performance of wearable strain sensors is generally characterized by properties including stretchability, sensitivity or gauge factor (GF), linearity, hysteresis and recovery time, and durability. Stretchability depends on the property of the supporting elastic materials. Highly stretchable (300%) resistive-type sensors have been reported based on CNT-PDMS composite stretchable electrodes [132]. GF which represents the sensitivity denotes the slope of the relative change of the electrical signal over the applied strain. Ultrasensitive semiconductor-based strain sensors could exhibit GFs over 100 [133]. Silver nanowire (AgNW)-based elastic strain sensors reported GFs in the range of 2–14, while CNT composite-based sensors showed GFs of 1–2.5 [125]. In general, it has been found that a trade-off relationship between high GF and high stretchability is present in designing wearable strain sensors, those with ultrahigh sensitivity, typically small dynamic range and low stretchability, and vice versa. Hysteresis and recovery time are critical aspects of wearable sensors for continuous monitoring. Capacitive sensors in general exhibited better hysteresis performance and faster response and recovery than resistive strain sensors. As an example, AgNWs-based resistive strain sensors respond in around 200 ms and recover in seconds [134], while AgNWs-based capacitive sensors respond in 50 ms and recover in subseconds [135].

Wearable mechanical strain sensors hold great potential for several biomedical applications. The sensors with high sensitivity could detect skin strains induced by blood flow pulse, respiration, facial expression, tissue swelling, etc. Some of the representative biomedical applications are illustrated in Figure A.11. In [136], a resistive strain sensor was attached to the chest area for breath monitoring as well as the wrist for heartbeat monitoring. A capacitive sensor was applied on the knee for patellar reflex testing [135]. The use of CNT has also been implemented in conformal antennas that could bear mechanical loadings [137, 138].

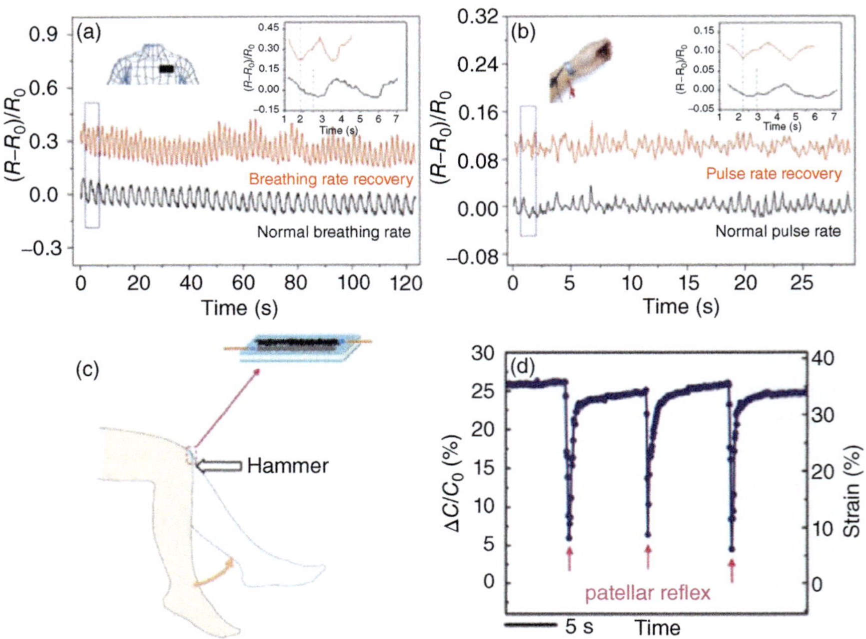

Figure A.11 Representative applications for wearable strain sensors. (a) Breath monitoring by attaching a wearable strain sensor in the chest; inset, location of attached strain sensor; (b) blood flow pulse monitoring by mounting a wearable sensor on the wrist [136]. (*Source*: Wang, Y., Wang, L,. Yang, T., et al., 2014. © John Wiley & Sons). (c and d) Patellar reflex monitoring by mounting a capacitive-type sensor on the knee for the strain measurement [135]. (*Source*: Yao, S. and Zhu, Y., 2014. © Royal Society of Chemistry.)

A.3.3 Electrical Sensors

Wearable electrical sensors interface with the skin and respond to the change in electrical resistance of the skin or change in accumulated charge at the skin interfaces. They transduce naturally occurring transients of ions in the human body into electrical signals. In order to drive the small signal from the skin into the sensor, the electrical contact between the skin and electrodes needs to be optimized.

The electrical interface between the skin and various types of electrodes can be modeled with circuit equivalence consisting of potential source, parallel and series resistors and capacitors, as illustrated in Figure A.12. A half-cell potential exists at the electrode–electrolyte interface, denoted by E_{hc}. The top layer of the skin, known as the epidermis, typically presents resistance and capacitance on the order of $10^5\ \Omega\,cm^2$ and $30\ nF\,cm^2$. The underlying layers of the dermis and hypodermis are more conductive than the epidermis with a negligible capacitance and, therefore, are modeled by a series resistance [139].

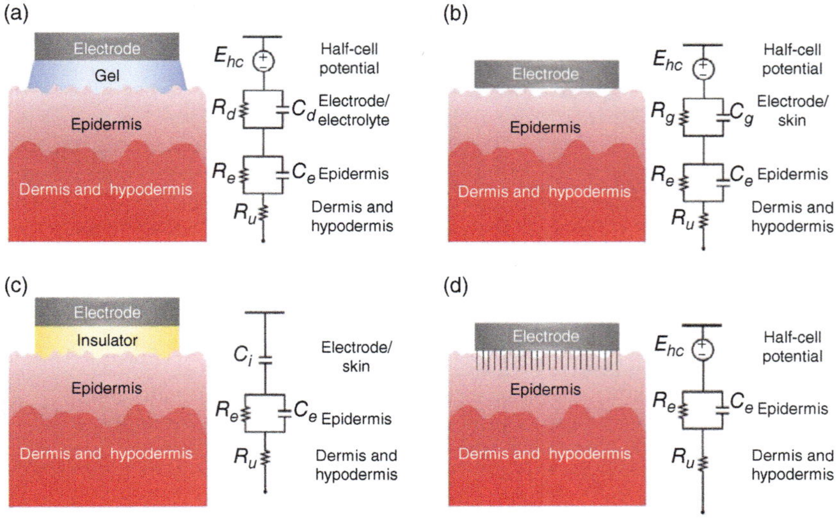

Figure A.12 Schematics and circuit models of electrode–skin interfaces for different types of wet and dry electrodes. (a) Gel electrodes, (b) dry contact electrodes, (c) dry capacitive electrode, and (d) dry penetrating electrode [139]. (*Source*: Yao, S. and Zhu, Y., 2016. © Springer Nature. © American Association for the Advancement of Science).

Wet electrodes interface with the skin with an electrolyte gel pad to minimize the contact impedance of the skin by introducing hydration and forming conformal contacts with the skin textures. Disposable Ag/AgCl wet electrodes are representative examples of wet-type electrodes. The major limitations of wet electrodes lie in the degradation over time due to gel dehydration as well as occurrence of dermal irritation and allergic reactions [140].

Dry electrodes are therefore developed to overcome such limitations. The goal is to eliminate the gel layer, while maintaining the signal quality. Dry electrodes with direct contact to the skin are typically not conformal to the skin texture, resulting in a relatively poor electrical contact than wet electrodes [141], which typically improves after a few minutes of application due to skin humidity and sweat [142]. Contact dry electrodes are designed to minimize the air gaps between the electrodes and the skin as well as motion artifacts. The work in [143, 144] presented some of the most successful designs of electronics integrated into ultrathin, low-modulus, lightweight, and stretchable "skin-like" membranes. The commonly adopted layout geometries of such designs including periodic serpentine or fractal with enhanced stretchability are illustrated in Figure A.13.

Another approach for dry electrodes is to insert an insulating layer without direct contact with the skin. The interface can be modeled by a series connection of the capacitor Ci with a parallel resistance and capacitance

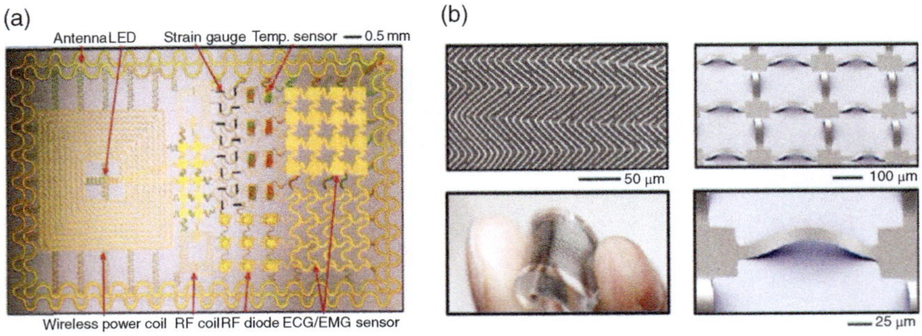

Figure A.13 (a) A soft electronics platform with multifunctional sensing and matched physical properties to the skin [143]. (*Source*: Kim, D.-H., Lu, N., Ma, R., et al., 2011. © American Association for the Advancement of Science). (b) Examples of stretchable electronic designs with wavy shape and meshed geometries [144]. (*Source*: Rogers, J. A., Someya, T., and Huang, Y., 2010 © American Association for the Advancement of Science.)

representing the epidermis. Such capacitive dry electrodes are electrically safe, easy to integrate into clothes, and therefore preferred in many long-term recording applications [145]. The capacitive electrodes generally tend to be more susceptible to motion artifacts compared to those with direct contact, which is commonly addressed by implementing proper shielding and buffering [146]. Wearable electrical interfaces enable real-time monitoring of a broad range of physiological biosignals, including electrocardiogram (ECG or EKG), electroencephalogram (EEG), galvanic skin response (GSR), and electrical impedance tomography (EIT) [120]. State-of-the-art technologies of soft and stretchable electronic platforms integrate sensors, microfluidics, circuits, and wireless modules, allowing for multifunctional and user-friendly wearable sensing systems for medical diagnostics and personal health care.

A.3.4 Optical Sensors

Optical sensing offers noninvasive and contactless approaches for acquiring essential information from the human body. Optical-based sensors generally rely on detecting interactions between the human body and the incident optical power. A light source introduces optical wave onto the skin, and by detecting the backscattered power from a photodetector, physiological information is revealed [147].

Transmission, absorption, and scattering properties of the skin layers determine the optical interface between the sensors and the skin. The optical properties of the skin layers have been well characterized in [148]. It was found that the epidermis layer mainly absorbs the ultraviolet (UV) radiation and partially absorbs visible spectrum, while the dermis layer which is highly vascularized dominates absorption of visible light. The stratum corneum, the outermost layer of the epidermis, mainly results in nonspecular reflection due to surface roughness. The total scattering is also dominated by the Mie and Rayleigh scattering from the dermis layer [147], since its thickness (about 4 mm) is much larger than that of the epidermis (about 100 μm).

Optical sensing is widely adopted for diagnostic purposes. One important example is the extraction of heart rate from blood flow detection utilizing the variations in optical properties of hemoglobin in its oxygenated and deoxygenated states, known as pulse oximetry [149, 150]. It measures human pulse rate and blood oxygen saturation with an optical sensor that consists of two LEDs with different peak frequencies of emission and a single photodiode. The LEDs are placed on one side of a finger, and the light transmitted through the tissue is captured by the photodiode placed on the opposite side of the finger. Applying the same mechanism in the computation of heart rate variability has been widely used as photoplethysmography (PPG) [151] in monitoring cardiovascular system. Measuring oxygenation and perfusion states of tissue and organs through near-infrared light spectroscopy also provides information of tissue health condition [152, 153]. Another approach of optical measurements is based on the scattering and fluorescence properties, which can be well correlated to tissue health in diagnosis of malignant or premalignant tissue [154, 155].

Conventional hardware for optical measurements such as PPG is typically large and bulky, bringing challenges in power consumption and miniaturization for developing wearable optical sensing devices. The advances in soft and biointegrated electronics facilitate the development of optical sensing devices that are human body friendly with "skin-like" properties and geometries [156]. Wireless power transferring and near-field communication (NFC) technology eliminate the need for batteries and enable ultrathin and highly miniaturized designs. The developments in organic semiconductors and electroluminescent materials also enable all-organic optical sensing platforms composed solely of organic optoelectronics, providing a highly biocompatible interface. One representative work is the demonstration of organic pulse oximetry [157, 158]. Accurate measurements are reported in these sensing platforms integrated with organic light-emitting diodes (OLEDs) and photodiodes (OPDs), enabling low-cost, disposable, and biocompatible optical sensing modalities (Figure A.14).

A.3.5 Chemical Sensors

Chemical sensing provides specific detection of chemical biomaker, revealing critical and comprehensive information regarding patient's health. Direct chemical detection has been extensively used in clinical blood and urine tests but still presents big challenges in noninvasive wearable sensors. The skin layers which provide defense and barrier for dehydration also block the

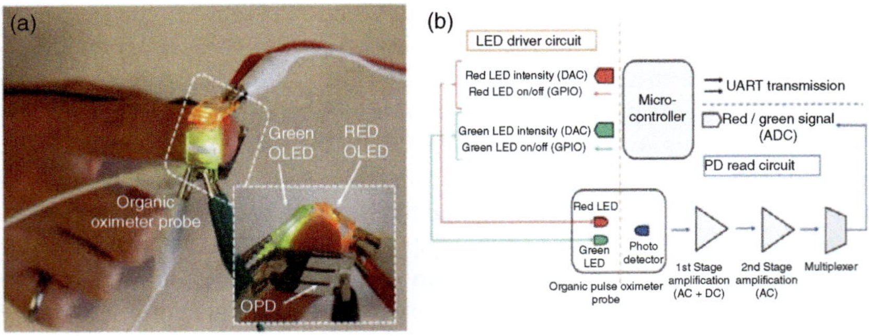

Figure A.14 (a) All-organic pulse oximetry placed on finger with red and green OLEDs transmitting light, which is collected with an OPD placed below the finger. (b) Hardware block diagram for the system setup with data reading and processing [157]. (*Source*: Lochner, C. M., Khan, Y., Pierre, A., et al., 2014. © Springer Nature.)

transport of chemicals. The vast majority of chemical analytes are accessible and measurable only through penetration of the skin layers. Wearable and noninvasive chemical sensing is mainly through measurements of biofluids secreted by the body (e.g. saliva, sweat, and tears). These biofluids are typically diluted in large molecules and proteins and are available only in very small sample volume, bringing additional challenges for developing reliable chemical sensing modalities [159]. The on-skin measurements are also subject to biochemical contaminations, further limiting the accuracy of evaluation of target analytes. An estimated density of microorganisms (including bacteria, viruses, and fungi) on human skin is on the order of billions per square centimeter [160]. The bacteria on the skin consume analytes such as glucose and proteins and alter the original concentration before the measurement is taken, causing occurrence of measurement errors.

A.3.5.1 Electrochemical Sensing Mechanisms

Electrochemical sensors form an important class of chemical sensors, which is based on measuring electrical quantities through sensing electrodes and relating it to the concentration of target analytes. It is commonly believed that electrochemical sensing holds great potential in highly integrated, label-free biosensing. Electrochemical sensing typically requires the use of two or more electrode elements, providing references to eliminate the effects of offset and device drift over time.

One class of well-demonstrated electrochemical sensors are the potentiometric devices. The measurement is based on ion-selective electrodes (ISEs), transducing an electrical potential response associated with the concentration of selective target ionic analyte. The generated potential is recorded as a voltage difference between the working electrode and the reference electrode [161, 162]. Another type of electrochemical sensor is known as amperometric sensors, which measure the electrical current signal formed by electron transfer across the electrode/electrolyte with an externally applied voltage potential across the working and reference electrodes. The majority of amperometric sensing devices rely on immobilization of specific enzyme to the target analyte. As an example, glucose sensing is achieved by the interaction of immobilized glucose oxidase enzyme on sensors [163]. Aptamer-based electrochemical sensing is another approach that has been widely investigated. They provide continuous detection with high sensitivity and selectivity. It requires immobilization of aptamer that selectively binds and releases the analyte in the biofluid, generating real-time electrical response [164].

A.3.5.2 Electrochemical Sensing: State of the Art

Significant progress in the field of wearable electrochemical sensing has been achieved in the past decade. The usage of sweat, saliva, and tears has been successfully demonstrated for noninvasive real-time electrochemical monitoring of various metabolites. Development of stress-enduring inks for screen printing of stretchable electrochemical sensors enables long-term mechanical robustness for continuous monitoring [165]. A noninvasive lactate sensor was reported in [166], with real-time perspiration monitoring during physical exercise using a flexible "tattoo-like" enzyme electrode. Glucose [167] and alcohol [168] tattoo biosensors were then demonstrated, which combine iontophoretic extraction with amperometric electrochemical sensing. The integration of sweat stimulation and extraction has been demonstrated for improving the sensing quality during continuous sweat analysis [169, 170]. The sensing and chemical stimulating blocks are integrated side by side to avoid cross-contamination. In [171], the authors demonstrated a sweat sensor platform that combines sweat collection and sodium content analysis with potentiometric sensors in a single device (SWEATCH). An integrated multianalyte sensing wristband with potentiometric/amperometric sensor wristband was demonstrated in [172, 173]. Simultaneous and multiplexed screening and detection of sweat metabolites (glucose and lactate), electrolytes (sodium and potassium ions), and skin temperature are achieved. It also merged silicon-based circuits for signal processing with elastic sensor array, achieving a fully integrated sensing system with advanced functionalities (Figure A.15).

Besides sweat analysis, noninvasive monitoring of glucose in tears has also been successfully demonstrated. The contact lens developed in [174] performs real-time glucose sensing with miniaturized amperometric sensor, wireless chip, and ring antenna. In [175], an integrated wireless platform for amperometric sensing in saliva was demonstrated, offering real-time uric acid sensing with high sensitivity and selectivity.

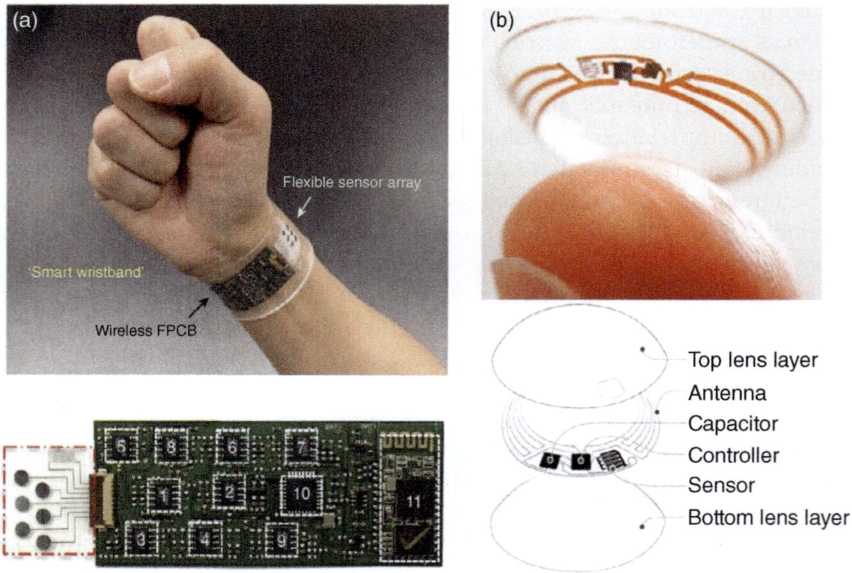

Figure A.15 (a) A multianalyte sensing wristband for real-time sweat analysis [172]. (*Source*: Gao, W., Emaminejad, S., Nyein, H. Y. Y., et al., 2016. © Springer Nature.) (b) The contact lens sensor for glucose concentration monitoring in tears [174]. (*Source*: Farandos, N. M., Yetisen, A. K., Monteiro, M. J., et al., 2015. © John Wiley & Sons.)

References

1 Gruber, B., Froeling, M., Leiner, T., and Klomp, D.W. (2018). RF coils: a practical guide for nonphysicists. *Journal of Magnetic Resonance Imaging* 48 (3): 590–604.

2 Hayes, C.E., Edelstein, W.A., Schenck, J.F. et al. (1985). An efficient, highly homogeneous radiofrequency coil for whole-body NMR imaging at 1.5 T. *Journal of Magnetic Resonance (1969)* 63 (3): 622–628.

3 Ginsberg, D. and Melchner, M.J. (1970). Optimum geometry of saddle shaped coils for generating a uniform magnetic field. *Review of Scientific Instruments* 41 (1): 122–123.

4 Bendall, M.R. and Gordon, R.E. (1983). Depth and refocusing pulses designed for multi-pulse NMR with surface coils. *Journal of Magnetic Resonance (1969)* 53 (3): 365–385.

5 Reykowski, A. (1996). Theory and Design of Synthesis Array Coils for Magnetic Resonance Imaging. Ph.D. thesis, Texas A&M University.

6 Bolinger, L., Prammer, M.G., and Leigh, J.S. Jr., (1989). A multiple-frequency coil with a highly uniform B1 field. *Journal of Magnetic Resonance (1969)* 81 (1): 162–166.

7 Smith, M., Zhai, X., Kurpad, K. et al. (2011). Excite and receive solenoid radiofrequency coil for MRI-guided breast interventions. *Magnetic Resonance in Medicine* 65 (6): 1799–1804.
8 Wright, A.C., Lemdiasov, R., Connick, T.J. et al. (2011). Helmholtz-pair transmit coil with integrated receive array for high-resolution MRI of trabecular bone in the distal tibia at 7 T. *Journal of Magnetic Resonance* 210 (1): 113–122.
9 Wald, L.L. and Adalsteinsson, E. (2009). Parallel transmit technology for high field MRI. *Magnetom Flash* 40 (1): 2009.
10 Kumar, A., Edelstein, W.A., and Bottomley, P.A. (2009). Noise figure limits for circular loop MR coils. *Magnetic Resonance in Medicine: An Official Journal of the International Society for Magnetic Resonance in Medicine* 61 (5): 1201–1209.
11 Wright, S.M. and Wald, L.L. (1997). Theory and application of array coils in MR spectroscopy. *NMR in Biomedicine: An International Journal Devoted to the Development and Application of Magnetic Resonance In Vivo* 10 (8): 394–410.
12 Pruessmann, K.P., Weiger, M., Scheidegger, M.B., and Boesiger, P. (1999). Sense: sensitivity encoding for fast MRI. *Magnetic Resonance in Medicine* 42 (5): 952–962.
13 Wiesinger, F., Boesiger, P., and Pruessmann, K.P. (2004). Electrodynamics and ultimate SNR in parallel MR imaging. *Magnetic Resonance in Medicine: An Official Journal of the International Society for Magnetic Resonance in Medicine* 52 (2): 376–390.
14 Keil, B. and Wald, L.L. (2013). Massively parallel MRI detector arrays. *Journal of Magnetic Resonance* 229: 75–89.
15 Roemer, P.B., Edelstein, W.A., Hayes, C.E. et al. (1990). The NMR phased array. *Magnetic Resonance in Medicine* 16 (2): 192–225.
16 Jevtic, J. (2001). Ladder networks for capacitive decoupling in phased-array coils. Proceedings of the 9th Annual Meeting of ISMRM, Glasgow, Scotland, vol. 17.
17 Lee, R.F., Giaquinto, R.O., and Hardy, C.J. (2002). Coupling and decoupling theory and its application to the MRI phased array. *Magnetic Resonance in Medicine: An Official Journal of the International Society for Magnetic Resonance in Medicine* 48 (1): 203–213.
18 Hurshkainen, A.A., Derzhavskaya, T.A., Glybovski, S.B. et al. (2016). Element decoupling of 7 T dipole body arrays by EBG metasurface structures: experimental verification. *Journal of Magnetic Resonance* 269: 87–96.
19 Slobozhanyuk, A.P., Poddubny, A.N., Raaijmakers, A.J. et al. (2016). Enhancement of magnetic resonance imaging with metasurfaces. *Advanced Materials* 28 (9): 1832–1838.
20 Corea, J.R., Flynn, A.M., Lech ˆ ene, B. et al. (2016). Screen-printed flexible MRI receive coils. *Nature Communications* 7: 10839.

21 Malko, J.A., McClees, E.C., Braun, I.F. et al. (1986). A flexible mercury-filled surface coil for MR imaging. *American Journal of Neuroradiology* 7 (2): 246–247.

22 Zhang, D. and Rahmat-Samii, Y. (2019). A novel flexible electro-textile 3T MRI RF coil array for carotid artery imaging: design, characterization and prototyping. *IEEE Transactions on Antennas and Propagation* 67 (8): 5115–5125.

23 Nordmeyer-Massner, J., De Zanche, N., and Pruessmann, K. (2012). Stretchable coil arrays: application to knee imaging under varying flexion angles. *Magnetic Resonance in Medicine* 67 (3): 872–879.

24 Venook, R.D., Hargreaves, B.A., Gold, G.E. et al. (2005). Automatic tuning of flexible interventional RF receiver coils. *Magnetic Resonance in Medicine: An Official Journal of the International Society for Magnetic Resonance in Medicine* 54 (4): 983–993.

25 Hassan, A.M. and El-Shenawee, M. (2011). Review of electromagnetic techniques for breast cancer detection. *IEEE Reviews in Biomedical Engineering* 4: 103–118.

26 Chandra, R., Zhou, H., Balasingham, I., and Narayanan, R.M. (2015). On the opportunities and challenges in microwave medical sensing and imaging. *IEEE Transactions on Biomedical Engineering* 62 (7): 1667–1682.

27 Afsari, A., Abbosh, A.M., and Rahmat-Samii, Y. (2018). Modified born iterative method in medical electromagnetic tomography using magnetic field fluctuation contrast source operator. *IEEE Transactions on Microwave Theory and Techniques* 67 (1): 454–463.

28 Afsari, A., Abbosh, A.M., and Rahmat-Samii, Y. (2018). A rapid medical microwave tomography based on partial differential equations. *IEEE Transactions on Antennas and Propagation* 66 (10): 5521–5535.

29 Pisa, S., Pittella, E., and Piuzzi, E. (2016). A survey of radar systems for medical applications. *IEEE Aerospace and Electronic Systems Magazine* 31 (11): 64–81.

30 Zakrzewski, M., Raittinen, H., and Vanhala, J. (2011). Comparison of center estimation algorithms for heart and respiration monitoring with microwave doppler radar. *IEEE Sensors Journal* 12 (3): 627–634.

31 Semenov, S.Y. and Corfield, D.R. (2008). Microwave tomography for brain imaging: feasibility assessment for stroke detection. *International Journal of Antennas and Propagation* 2008: 1–8.

32 Nikolova, N.K. (2011). Microwave imaging for breast cancer. *IEEE Microwave Magazine* 12 (7): 78–94.

33 O'Loughlin, D., O'Halloran, M., Moloney, B.M. et al. (2018). Microwave breast imaging: clinical advances and remaining challenges. *IEEE Transactions on Biomedical Engineering* 65 (11): 2580–2590.

34 Salvador, S.M., Fear, E.C., Okoniewski, M., and Matyas, J.R. (2010). Exploring joint tissues with microwave imaging. *IEEE Transactions on Microwave Theory and Techniques* 58 (8): 2307–2313.
35 Mahmud, M., Islam, M.T., Misran, N. et al. (2018). Ultra-wideband (UWB) antenna sensor-based microwave breast imaging: a review. *Sensors* 18 (9): 2951.
36 Ojaroudi, M., Ghobadi, C., and Nourinia, J. (2009). Small square monopole antenna with inverted T-shaped notch in the ground plane for UWB application. *IEEE Antennas and Wireless Propagation Letters* 8: 728–731.
37 Jafari, H.M., Deen, M.J., Hranilovic, S., and Nikolova, N.K. (2007). A study of ultrawideband antennas for near-field imaging. *IEEE Transactions on Antennas and Propagation* 55 (4): 1184–1188.
38 Nilavalan, R., Craddock, I., Preece, A. et al. (2007). Wideband microstrip patch antenna design for breast cancer tumor detection. *IET Microwaves, Antennas & Propagation* 1 (2): 277–281.
39 Hagness, S.C., Taflove, A., and Bridges, J.E. (1999). Three-dimensional FDTD analysis of a pulsed microwave confocal system for breast cancer detection: design of an antenna-array element. *IEEE Transactions on Antennas and Propagation* 47 (5): 783–791.
40 Bourqui, J., Okoniewski, M., and Fear, E.C. (2010). Balanced antipodal Vivaldi antenna with dielectric director for near-field microwave imaging. *IEEE Transactions on Antennas and Propagation* 58 (7): 2318–2326.
41 Amineh, R.K., Ravan, M., Trehan, A., and Nikolova, N.K. (2010). Near-field microwave imaging based on aperture raster scanning with TEM horn antennas. *IEEE Transactions on Antennas and Propagation* 59 (3): 928–940.
42 Li, X., Hagness, S.C., Choi, M.K., and van der Weide, D.W. (2003). Numerical and experimental investigation of an ultrawideband ridged pyramidal horn antenna with curved launching plane for pulse radiation. *IEEE Antennas and Wireless Propagation Letters* 2: 259–262.
43 Porter, E., Bahrami, H., Santorelli, A. et al. (2016). A wearable microwave antenna array for time-domain breast tumor screening. *IEEE Transactions on Medical Imaging* 35 (6): 1501–1509.
44 Gilmore, C., Mojabi, P., Zakaria, A. et al. (2009). A wideband microwave tomography system with a novel frequency selection procedure. *IEEE Transactions on Biomedical Engineering* 57 (4): 894–904.
45 Saenz, E., Guven, K., Ozbay, E. et al. (2010). Decoupling of multifrequency dipole antenna arrays for microwave imaging applications. *International Journal of Antennas and Propagation* 2010: 1–8.
46 Saenz, E., Ederra, I., Gonzalo, R. et al. (2009). Coupling reduction between dipole antenna elements by using a planar meta-surface. *IEEE Transactions on Antennas and Propagation* 57 (2): 383–394.

47 ITU. *International Telecommunications Union-Radiocommunications (ITU-R), Radio Regulations, SA1346*. Geneva, Switzerland: ITU.

48 F. C. Commission et al. (1999). Medical implant communications service (MICS) federal register. *Rules Regulations* 64 (240): 69 926–69 934.

49 IEEE Standards Coordinating Committee. (2006). IEEE standard for safety levels with respect to human exposure to radio frequency electromagnetic fields, 3 kHz to 300 GHz. IEEE Std C95.1-2005 (Revision of IEEE Std C95.1-1991), April 2006, 1–238.

50 Khan, M.W.A., Sydänheimo, L., Ukkonen, L., and Björninen, T. (2017). Inductively powered pressure sensing system integrating a far-field data transmitter for monitoring of intracranial pressure. *IEEE Sensors Journal* 17 (7): 2191–2197.

51 Moradi, E., Sydänheimo, L., Bova, G.S., and Ukkonen, L. (2017). Measurement of wireless power transfer to deep-tissue RFID-based implants using wireless repeater node. *IEEE Antennas and Wireless Propagation Letters* 16: 2171–2174.

52 Song, L. and Rahmat-Samii, Y. (2017). An end-to-end implanted brain–machine interface antenna system performance characterizations and development. *IEEE Transactions on Antennas and Propagation* 65 (7): 3399–3408.

53 Moncion, C., Balachandar, L., Bojja-Venkatakrishnan, S. et al. (2019). Fully-passive wireless implant for neuropotential acquisition: an in vivo validation. *IEEE Journal of Electromagnetics, RF and Microwaves in Medicine and Biology* 3 (3): 199–205.

54 Mark, M. (2011). Powering mm-size Wireless Implants for Brain-Machine Interfaces. Ph.D. dissertation, UC Berkeley.

55 Chen, Y. (2013). Reflective impulse radios: principles and design. Ph.D. dissertation, UC Berkeley.

56 Poon, A.S.Y., O'Driscoll, S., and Meng, T.H. (2010). Optimal frequency for wireless power transmission into dispersive tissue. *IEEE Transactions on Antennas and Propagation* 58 (5): 1739–1750.

57 Leelatien, P., Ito, K., Saito, K. et al. (2018). Channel characteristics and wireless telemetry performance of transplanted organ monitoring system using ultrawideband communication. *IEEE Journal of Electromagnetics, RF and Microwaves in Medicine and Biology* 2 (2): 94–101.

58 Rahmat-Samii, Y. and Kim, J. (2005). Implanted antennas in medical wireless communications. *Synthesis Lectures on Antennas* 1 (1): 1–82.

59 Azad, U., Jing, H.C., and Wang, Y.E. (2012). Link budget and capacity performance of inductively coupled resonant loops. *IEEE Transactions on Antennas and Propagation* 60 (5): 2453–2461.

60 Pichorim, S.F. and Abatti, P.J. (2004). Design of coils for millimeter-and submillimeter-sized biotelemetry. *IEEE Transactions on Biomedical Engineering* 51 (8): 1487–1489.

61 Best, S.R. (2009). A low Q electrically small magnetic (TE mode) dipole. *IEEE Antennas and Wireless Propagation Letters* 8: 572–575.
62 Khan, M.W.A., Rizwan, M., Sydänheimo, L. et al. (2017). Characterization of 3-D loop antenna to overcome the impact of small lateral misalignment in wirelessly powered intracranial pressure monitoring system. *IEEE Transactions on Antennas and Propagation* 65 (12): 7405–7410.
63 Qing, X., Goh, C.K., and Chen, Z.N. (2010). A broadband uhf near-field RFID antenna. *IEEE Transactions on Antennas and Propagation* 58 (12): 3829–3838.
64 Yakovlev, A., Jang, J.H., and Pivonka, D. (2016). An 11 μw sub-pJ/bit reconfigurable transceiver for mm-sized wireless implants. *IEEE Transactions on Biomedical Circuits and Systems* 10 (1): 175–185.
65 Biederman, W., Yeager, D.J., Narevsky, N. et al. (2013). A fully-integrated, miniaturized (0.125 mm2) 10.5 μw wireless neural sensor. *IEEE Journal of Solid-State Circuits* 48 (4): 960–970.
66 Mirbozorgi, S.A., Yeon, P., and Ghovanloo, M. (2017). Robust wireless power transmission to mm-sized free-floating distributed implants. *IEEE Transactions on Biomedical Circuits and Systems* 11 (3): 692–702.
67 Topsakal, E. (2014). Wireless medical telemetry: Current status and future directions. 2014 USNC-URSI Radio Science Meeting (Joint with AP-S Symposium). IEEE, 244–244.
68 Liu, C., Guo, Y.-X., and Xiao, S. (2016). A review of implantable antennas for wireless biomedical devices. *Forum for Electromagnetic Research Methods and Application Technologies (FERMAT)* 14 (3): 1–11.
69 Kiourti, A. and Nikita, K.S. (2012). Miniature scalp-implantable antennas for telemetry in the MICS and ISM bands: design, safety considerations and link budget analysis. *IEEE Transactions on Antennas and Propagation* 60 (8): 3568–3575.
70 Chien, T.-F., Cheng, C.-M., Yang, H.-C. et al. (2010). Development of non-superstrate implantable low-profile CPW-fed ceramic antennas. *IEEE Antennas and Wireless Propagation Letters* 9: 599–602.
71 Liu, C., Guo, Y.-X., and Xiao, S. (2012). Compact dual-band antenna for implantable devices. *IEEE Antennas and Wireless Propagation Letters* 11: 1508–1511.
72 Karacolak, T., Hood, A.Z., and Topsakal, E. (2008). Design of a dual-band implantable antenna and development of skin mimicking gels for continuous glucose monitoring. *IEEE Transactions on Microwave Theory and Techniques* 56 (4): 1001–1008.
73 Asili, M., Green, R., Seran, S., and Topsakal, E. (2012). A small implantable antenna for med radio and ISM bands. *IEEE Antennas and Wireless Propagation Letters* 11: 1683–1685.

74 Lee, C.-M., Yo, T.-C., Luo, C.-H. et al. (2007). Compact broadband stacked implantable antenna for biotelemetry with medical devices. *Electronics Letters* 43 (12): 660–662.

75 Quevedo-Teruel, O., Kehn, M.N.M., and Rajo-Iglesias, E. (2011). Dual-band patch antennas based on short-circuited split ring resonators. *IEEE Transactions on Antennas and Propagation* 59 (8): 2758–2765.

76 See, T.S., Qing, X., Liu, W., and Chen, Z.N. (2015). A wideband ultra-thin differential loop-fed patch antenna for head implants. *IEEE Transactions on Antennas and Propagation* 63 (7): 3244–3248.

77 Kim, J. and Rahmat-Samii, Y. (2004). Implanted antennas inside a human body: simulations, designs, and characterizations. *IEEE Transactions on Microwave Theory and Techniques* 52 (8): 1934–1943.

78 Bocan, K.N. and Sejdíc, E. (2016). Adaptive transcutaneous power transfer to implantable devices: a state of the art review. *Sensors* 16 (3): 393.

79 Kim, S., Ho, J.S., Chen, L.Y., and Poon, A.S. (2012). Wireless power transfer to a cardiac implant. *Applied Physics Letters* 101 (7): 073701.

80 Amin Karami, M. and Inman, D.J. (2012). Powering pacemakers from heartbeat vibrations using linear and nonlinear energy harvesters. *Applied Physics Letters* 100 (4): 042901.

81 Das, R. and Yoo, H. (2015). Biotelemetry and wireless powering for leadless pacemaker systems. *IEEE Microwave and Wireless Components Letters* 25 (4): 262–264.

82 Chow, E.Y., Ouyang, Y., Beier, B. et al. (2009). Evaluation of cardiovascular stents as antennas for implantable wireless applications. *IEEE Transactions on Microwave Theory and Techniques* 57 (10): 2523–2532.

83 Sun, Y., Greet, B., Burkland, D., et al. (2017). Wirelessly powered implantable pacemaker with on-chip antenna. 2017 IEEE MTT-S International Microwave Symposium (IMS), June 2017, 1242–1244.

84 Iddan, G., Meron, G., Glukhovsky, A., and Swain, P. (2000). Wireless capsule endoscopy. *Nature* 405 (6785): 417.

85 Munoz, F., Alici, G., and Li, W. (2014). A review of drug delivery systems for capsule endoscopy. *Advanced Drug Delivery Reviews* 71: 77–85.

86 Bertram, J.M., Yang, D., Converse, M.C. et al. (2006). A review of coaxial-based interstitial antennas for hepatic microwave ablation. *Critical Reviews in Biomedical Engineering* 34 (3): 187–213.

87 Khan, A.N., Ermakov, A., Sukhorukov, G., and Hao, Y. (2019). Radio frequency controlled wireless drug delivery devices. *Applied Physics Reviews* 6 (4): 041301.

88 Hao, Y., Khan, A.N., Giddens, H., and Sukhorukov, G. (2019). Characterization of microchamber arrays for targeted drug delivery. 2019 IEEE International Symposium on Antennas and Propagation and USNC-URSI Radio Science Meeting. IEEE, 2019, 1–2.

89 Than, T.D., Alici, G., Zhou, H., and Li, W. (2012). A review of localization systems for robotic endoscopic capsules. *IEEE Transactions on Biomedical Engineering* 59 (9): 2387–2399.

90 Yuce, M.R. and Dissanayake, T. (2012). Easy-to-swallow wireless telemetry. *IEEE Microwave Magazine* 13 (6): 90–101.

91 Ciuti, G., Caliò, R., Camboni, D. et al. (2016). Frontiers of robotic endoscopic capsules: a review. *Journal of Micro-Bio Robotics* 11 (1–4): 1–18.

92 Izdebski, P.M., Rajagopalan, H., and Rahmat-Samii, Y. (2009). Conformal ingestible capsule antenna: a novel chandelier meandered design. *IEEE Transactions on Antennas and Propagation* 57 (4): 900–909.

93 Rajagopalan, H. and Rahmat-Samii, Y. (2016). Novel antenna designs and characterization methodologies for medical diagnostics and sensing. In: *Electromagnetics of Body Area Networks: Antennas, Propagation, and RF Systems* (eds. D.H. Werner and Z.H. Jiang). Artech House.

94 Rajagopalan, P.I.H. and Rahmat-Samii, Y. (2011). Antennas in medicine: ingestible capsule antennas. In: *Frontiers in Antennas, Next Generation Design and Engineering* (ed. F.B. Gross). McGraw-Hill.

95 Thotahewa, K.M., Redoutè, J.-M., and Yuce, M.R. (2015). Propagation, power absorption, and temperature analysis of UWB wireless capsule endoscopy devices operating in the human body. *IEEE Transactions on Microwave Theory and Techniques* 63 (11): 3823–3833.

96 Garcia-Pardo, C., Andreu, C., Fornes-Leal, A. et al. (2018). Ultrawideband technology for medical in-body sensor networks: an overview of the human body as a propagation medium, phantoms, and approaches for propagation analysis. *IEEE Antennas and Propagation Magazine* 60 (3): 19–33.

97 Liu, C., Guo, Y.-X., and Xiao, S. (2014). Circularly polarized helical antenna for ISM-band ingestible capsule endoscope systems. *IEEE Transactions on Antennas and Propagation* 62 (12): 6027–6039.

98 Kwak, S., Chang, K., and Yoon, Y.J. (2006). Small spiral antenna for wideband capsule endoscope system. *Electronics Letters* 42 (23): 1328–1329.

99 Yun, S., Kim, K., and Nam, S. (2010). Outer-wall loop antenna for ultrawideband capsule endoscope system. *IEEE Antennas and Wireless Propagation Letters* 9: 1135–1138.

100 Yu, H., Irby, G., Peterson, D. et al. (2007). Printed capsule antenna for medication compliance monitoring. *Electronics Letters* 43 (22): 1179–1181.

101 Cheng, X., Wu, J., Blank, R. et al. (2012). An omnidirectional wrappable compact patch antenna for wireless endoscope applications. *IEEE Antennas and Wireless Propagation Letters* 11: 1667–1670.

102 Rajagopalan, H. and Rahmat-Samii, Y. (2012). Wireless medical telemetry characterization for ingestible capsule antenna designs. *IEEE Antennas and Wireless Propagation Letters* 11: 1679–1682.

103 Li, R., Guo, Y.-X., and Du, G. (2018). A conformal circularly polarized antenna for wireless capsule endoscope systems. *IEEE Transactions on Antennas and Propagation* 66 (4): 2119–2124.

104 Das, R. and Yoo, H. (2017). A wideband circularly polarized conformal endoscopic antenna system for high-speed data transfer. *IEEE Transactions on Antennas and Propagation* 65 (6): 2816–2826.

105 Li, Y., Guo, Y.-X., and Xiao, S. (2017). Orientation insensitive antenna with polarization diversity for wireless capsule endoscope system. *IEEE Transactions on Antennas and Propagation* 65 (7): 3738–3743.

106 Bao, Z. (2018). Comparative study of dual-polarized and circularly-polarized antennas at 2.45 GHz for ingestible capsules. *IEEE Transactions on Antennas and Propagation* 67 (3): 1488–1500.

107 Na, K., Jang, H., Ma, H., and Bien, F. (2014). Tracking optimal efficiency of magnetic resonance wireless power transfer system for biomedical capsule endoscopy. *IEEE Transactions on Microwave Theory and Techniques* 63 (1): 295–304.

108 Machnoor, M., Rodríguez, E.S.G., Kosta, P. et al. (2018). Analysis and design of a 3-coil wireless power transmission system for biomedical applications. *IEEE Transactions on Antennas and Propagation* 67 (8): 5012–5024.

109 Sawicki, J.F., Shea, J.D., Behdad, N., and Hagness, S.C. (2017). The impact of frequency on the performance of microwave ablation. *International Journal of Hyperthermia* 33 (1): 61–68.

110 Sawicki, J.F., Luyen, H., Mohtashami, Y. et al. (2018). The performance of higher frequency microwave ablation in the presence of perfusion. *IEEE Transactions on Biomedical Engineering* 66 (1): 257–262.

111 Asili, M., Colebeck, E., Green, R., and Topsakal, E. (2013). The effect of temperature on antenna return loss for microwave ablation antennas. 2013 US National Committee of URSI National Radio Science Meeting (USNC-URSI NRSM). IEEE, 1–1.

112 Mohtashami, Y., Luyen, H., Sawicki, J.F. et al. (2018). Tools for attacking tumors: performance comparison of triaxial, choke dipole, and balun-free base-fed monopole antennas for microwave ablation. *IEEE Antennas and Propagation Magazine* 60 (6): 52–57.

113 Fallahi, H. and Prakash, P. (2018). Antenna designs for microwave tissue ablation. *Critical Reviews in Biomedical Engineering* 46 (6): 495–521.

114 King, R.W., Trembly, B., and Strohbehn, J. (1983). The electromagnetic field of an insulated antenna in a conducting or dielectric medium. *IEEE Transactions on Microwave Theory and Techniques* 31 (7): 574–583.

115 Yang, D., Bertram, J.M., Converse, M.C. et al. (2006). A floating sleeve antenna yields localized hepatic microwave ablation. *IEEE transactions on biomedical engineering* 53 (3): 533–537.

116 McWilliams, B.T., Schnell, E.E., Curto, S. et al. (2015). A directional interstitial antenna for microwave tissue ablation: Theoretical and experimental investigation. *IEEE Transactions on Biomedical Engineering* 62 (9): 2144–2150.

117 Gu, Z., Rappaport, C.M., Wang, P.J., and VanderBrink, B.A. (1999). A 2 14-turn spiral antenna for catheter cardiac ablation. *IEEE Transactions on Biomedical Engineering* 46 (12): 1480–1482.

118 Sherar, M.D., Gladman, A.S., Davidson, S.R. et al. (2001). Helical antenna arrays for interstitial microwave thermal therapy for prostate cancer: tissue phantom testing and simulations for treatment. *Physics in Medicine & Biology* 46 (7): 1905.

119 Ryan, T.P. (1991). Comparison of six microwave antennas for hyperthermia treatment of cancer: SAR results for single antennas and arrays. *International Journal of Radiation Oncology Biology Physics* 21 (2): 403–413.

120 Heikenfeld, J., Jajack, A., Rogers, J. et al. (2018). Wearable sensors: modalities, challenges, and prospects. *Lab on a Chip* 18 (2): 217–248.

121 "Inventing the Apollo spaceflight biomedical sensors," https://airandspace.si.edu/stories/editorial/inventing-apollo-spaceflight-biomedical-sensors (accessed 2 July 2020).

122 Cunningham, D.D. and Stenken, J.A. (2009). *In Vivo Glucose Sensing*, vol. 174. John Wiley & Sons.

123 Pang, C., Lee, C., and Suh, K.-Y. (2013). Recent advances in flexible sensors for wearable and implantable devices. *Journal of Applied Polymer Science* 130 (3): 1429–1441.

124 Ukkonen, L. and Rahmat-Samii, Y. (2016). Embroidered textile antennas for body-centric wireless identification and sensing devices. In: *Handbook of Antenna Technologies* (ed. Z.N. Chen). Springer Science and Business Media.

125 Amjadi, M., Kyung, K.-U., Park, I., and Sitti, M. (2016). Stretchable, skin-mountable, and wearable strain sensors and their potential applications: a review. *Advanced Functional Materials* 26 (11): 1678–1698.

126 Cohen, D.J., Mitra, D., Peterson, K., and Maharbiz, M.M. (2012). A highly elastic, capacitive strain gauge based on percolating nanotube networks. *Nano Letters* 12 (4): 1821–1825.

127 Cai, L., Song, L., Luan, P. et al. (2013). Super-stretchable, transparent carbon nanotube-based capacitive strain sensors for human motion detection. *Scientific Reports* 3: 3048.

128 Zhao, J., He, C., Yang, R. et al. (2012). Ultra-sensitive strain sensors based on piezoresistive nanographene films. *Applied Physics Letters* 101 (6): 063112.

129 Xu, F. and Zhu, Y. (2012). Highly conductive and stretchable silver nanowire conductors. *Advanced Materials* 24 (37): 5117–5122.

130 Jing, Z., Guang-Yu, Z., and Dong-Xia, S. (2013). Review of graphene-based strain sensors. *Chinese Physics B* 22 (5): 057701.

131 Kang, D., Pikhitsa, P.V., Choi, Y.W. et al. (2014). Ultrasensitive mechanical crack-based sensor inspired by the spider sensory system. *Nature* 516 (7530): 222.

132 Yamada, T., Hayamizu, Y., Yamamoto, Y. et al. (2011). A stretchable carbon nanotube strain sensor for human-motion detection. *Nature Nanotechnology* 6 (5): 296.

133 Hempel, M., Nezich, D., Kong, J., and Hofmann, M. (2012). A novel class of strain gauges based on layered percolative films of 2D materials. *Nano Letters* 12 (11): 5714–5718.

134 Amjadi, M., Pichitpajongkit, A., Lee, S. et al. (2014). Highly stretchable and sensitive strain sensor based on silver nanowire–elastomer nanocomposite. *ACS Nano* 8 (5): 5154–5163.

135 Yao, S. and Zhu, Y. (2014). Wearable multifunctional sensors using printed stretchable conductors made of silver nanowires. *Nanoscale* 6 (4): 2345–2352.

136 Wang, Y., Wang, L., Yang, T. et al. (2014). Wearable and highly sensitive graphene strain sensors for human motion monitoring. *Advanced Functional Materials* 24 (29): 4666–4670.

137 Zhou, Y., Bayram, Y., Du, F. et al. (2010). Polymer-carbon nanotube sheets for conformal load bearing antennas. *IEEE Transactions on Antennas and Propagation* 58 (7): 2169–2175.

138 Zhong, J., Kiourti, A., Sebastian, T. et al. (2016). Conformal load-bearing spiral antenna on conductive textile threads. *IEEE Antennas and Wireless Propagation Letters* 16: 230–233.

139 Yao, S. and Zhu, Y. (2016). Nanomaterial-enabled dry electrodes for electrophysiological sensing: a review. *JOM* 68 (4): 1145–1155.

140 Connolly, M. and Buckley, D. (2004). Contact dermatitis from propylene glycol in ECG electrodes, complicated by medicament allergy. *Contact Dermatitis* 50 (1): 42–42.

141 Yeo, W.-H., Kim, Y.-S., Lee, J. et al. (2013). Multifunctional epidermal electronics printed directly onto the skin. *Advanced Materials* 25 (20): 2773–2778.

142 Yokus, M.A. and Jur, J.S. (2015). Fabric-based wearable dry electrodes for body surface biopotential recording. *IEEE Transactions on Biomedical Engineering* 63 (2): 423–430.

143 Kim, D.-H., Lu, N., Ma, R. et al. (2011). Epidermal electronics. *Science* 333 (6044): 838–843.

144 Rogers, J.A., Someya, T., and Huang, Y. (2010). Materials and mechanics for stretchable electronics. *Science* 327 (5973): 1603–1607.

145 Lim, Y.G., Kim, K.K., and Park, K.S. (2007). ECG recording on a bed during sleep without direct skin-contact. *IEEE Transactions on Biomedical Engineering* 54 (4): 718–725.

146 Jeong, J.-W., Kim, M.K., Cheng, H. et al. (2014). Capacitive epidermal electronics for electrically safe, long-term electrophysiological measurements. *Advanced Healthcare Materials* 3 (5): 642–648.

147 Tuchin, V. (2007). *Tissue Optics: Light Scattering Methods and Instruments for Medical Diagnosis.* Bellingham: SPIE Press.

148 Anderson, R.R. and Parrish, J.A. (1981). The optics of human skin. *Journal of Investigative Dermatology* 77 (1): 13–19.

149 Tremper, K.K. (1989). Pulse oximetry. *Chest* 95 (4): 713–715.

150 Yelderman, M. and New, J.W. (1983). Evaluation of pulse oximetry. *Anesthesiology* 59 (4): 349–352.

151 Allen, J. (2007). Photoplethysmography and its application in clinical physiological measurement. *Physiological Measurement* 28 (3): R1.

152 Thorniley, M.S., Sinclair, J., Barnett, N. et al. (1998). The use of near-infrared spectroscopy for assessing flap viability during reconstructive surgery. *British Journal of Plastic Surgery* 51 (3): 218–226.

153 Boushel, R., Langberg, H., Olesen, J. et al. (2001). Monitoring tissue oxygen availability with near infrared spectroscopy (NIRS) in health and disease. *Scandinavian Journal of Medicine &Science in Sports* 11 (4): 213–222.

154 Bigio, I.J. and Mourant, J.R. (1997). Ultraviolet and visible spectroscopies for tissue diagnostics: fluorescence spectroscopy and elastic-scattering spectroscopy. *Physics in Medicine & Biology* 42 (5): 803.

155 Alfano, R., Tata, D., Cordero, J. et al. (1984). Laser induced fluorescence spectroscopy from native cancerous and normal tissue. *IEEE Journal of Quantum Electronics* 20 (12): 1507–1511.

156 Kim, J., Gutruf, P., Chiarelli, A.M. et al. (2017). Miniaturized battery-free wireless systems for wearable pulse oximetry. *Advanced Functional Materials* 27 (1): 1604373.

157 Lochner, C.M., Khan, Y., Pierre, A., and Arias, A.C. (2014). All-organic optoelectronic sensor for pulse oximetry. *Nature Communications* 5: 5745.

158 Yokota, T., Zalar, P., Kaltenbrunner, M. et al. (2016). Ultra-flexible organic photonic skin. *Science Advances* 2 (4): e1501856.

159 Heikenfeld, J. (2016). Non-invasive analyte access and sensing through eccrine sweat: challenges and outlook circa 2016. *Electroanalysis* 28 (6): 1242–1249.

160 Grice, E.A. and Segre, J.A. (2011). The skin microbiome. *Nature Reviews Microbiology* 9 (4): 244.

161 Bandodkar, A.J., Molinnus, D., Mirza, O. et al. (2014). Epidermal tattoo potentiometric sodium sensors with wireless signal transduction for continuous non-invasive sweat monitoring. *Biosensors and Bioelectronics* 54: 603–609.
162 Cuartero, M., Parrilla, M., and Crespo, G.A. (2019). Wearable potentiometric sensors for medical applications. *Sensors* 19 (2): 363.
163 Windmiller, J.R. and Wang, J. (2013). Wearable electrochemical sensors and biosensors: a review. *Electroanalysis* 25 (1): 29–46.
164 Arroyo-Curras, N., Somerson, J., Vieira, P.A. et al. (2017). Real-time measurement of small molecules directly in awake, ambulatory animals. *Proceedings of the National Academy of Sciences* 114 (4): 645–650.
165 Bandodkar, A.J., Jeerapan, I., You, J.-M. et al. (2015). Highly stretchable fully-printed CNT-based electrochemical sensors and biofuel cells: combining intrinsic and design-induced stretchability. *Nano Letters* 16 (1): 721–727.
166 Jia, W., Bandodkar, A.J., Valdés-Ramírez, G. et al. (2013). Electrochemical tattoo biosensors for real-time noninvasive lactate monitoring in human perspiration. *Analytical Chemistry* 85 (14): 6553–6560.
167 Bandodkar, A.J., Jia, W., Yardımcı, C. et al. (2014). Tattoo-based noninvasive glucose monitoring: a proof-of-concept study. *Analytical Chemistry* 87 (1): 394–398.
168 Kim, J., Jeerapan, I., Imani, S. et al. (2016). Noninvasive alcohol monitoring using a wearable tattoo-based iontophoretic-biosensing system. *ACS Sensors* 1 (8): 1011–1019.
169 Sonner, Z., Wilder, E., Gaillard, T. et al. (2017). Integrated sudomotor axon reflex sweat stimulation for continuous sweat analyte analysis with individuals at rest. *Lab on a Chip* 17 (15): 2550–2560.
170 Emaminejad, S., Gao, W., Wu, E. et al. (2017). Autonomous sweat extraction and analysis applied to cystic fibrosis and glucose monitoring using a fully integrated wearable platform. *Proceedings of the National Academy of Sciences* 114 (18): 4625–4630.
171 Glennon, T., O'Quigley, C., McCaul, M. et al. (2016). 'SWEATCH': a wearable platform for harvesting and analyzing sweat sodium content. *Electroanalysis* 28 (6): 1283–1289.
172 Gao, W., Emaminejad, S., Nyein, H.Y.Y. et al. (2016). Fully integrated wearable sensor arrays for multiplexed in situ perspiration analysis. *Nature* 529 (7587): 509.
173 Nyein, H.Y.Y., Gao, W., Shahpar, Z. et al. (2016). A wearable electrochemical platform for noninvasive simultaneous monitoring of Ca^{2+} and pH. *ACS Nano* 10 (7): 7216–7224.

174 Farandos, N.M., Yetisen, A.K., Monteiro, M.J. et al. (2015). Contact lens sensors in ocular diagnostics. *Advanced Healthcare Materials* 4 (6): 792–810.

175 Kim, J., Imani, S., de Araujo, W.R. et al. (2015). Wearable salivary uric acid mouthguard biosensor with integrated wireless electronics. *Biosensors and Bioelectronics* 74: 1061–1068.

Index

Antenna and Sensor Technologies in Modern Medical Applications,
First Edition. Edited by Yahya Rahmat-Samii and Erdem Topsakal.

D

K

L

O

P

U

V

W

X

Z

Printed and bound by CPI Group (UK) Ltd, Croydon, CR0 4YY
17/09/2026
14964320-0003